FELINE INTERNAL MEDICINE SECRETS

Michael R. Lappin, DVM, PhD, DACVIM
Professor, Department of Clinical Sciences
College of Veterinary Medicine and Biomedical Sciences
Colorado State University
Fort Collins, Colorado

HANLEY & BELFUS, INC./Philadelphia

Publisher: HANLEY & BELFUS, INC.
                  Medical Publishers
                  210 South 13th Street
                  Philadelphia, PA 19107
                  (215) 546-7293; 800-962-1892
                  FAX (215) 790-9330
                  Web site: http://www.hanleyandbelfus.com

Note to the reader: Although the information in this book has been carefully reviewed for correctness of dosage and indications, neither the authors nor the editor nor the publisher can accept any legal responsibility for any errors or omissions that may be made. Neither the publisher nor the editor makes any warranty, expressed or implied, with respect to the material contained herein. Before prescribing any drug, the reader must review the manufacturer's current product information (package inserts) for accepted indications, absolute dosage recommendations, and other information pertinent to the safe and effective use of the product described.

Library of Congress Cataloging-in-Publication Data

Feline Internal Medicine Secrets / edited by Michael R. Lappin.
        p. ; cm. — (Secrets Series®)
     ISBN 1-56053-461-3 (alk. paper)
        1. Cats—Diseases—Examinations, questions, etc.   I. Lappin, Michael R. 1956–
     II. Series.

     SF985.F42 2001
     636.8'0896'0076—dc21

                                                              2001016579

FELINE INTERNAL MEDICINE SECRETS   ISBN 1-56053-461-3

Last digit is the print number: 9   8   7   6   5   4   3   2   1

DEDICATION

To those cat owners, friends, veterinary students, graduate students, interns, residents, technicians, and research associates who have accompanied me through my adult life with cats. Dr. Craig Greene at the University of Georgia first gave me the idea to study *Toxoplasma gondii*, which ultimately led to the strengthening of my bond with cats. In my office at Colorado State University resides a composite of photographs of my first 10 research cats that was presented to me by Pat Shroeder. Pat and Amanda Marks helped me care for these fine animals during that first project and ultimately helped me adopt them to private homes. Donald Dawe, Anne Prestwood, Cynthia Powell, Christie Cooper, Derek Burney, Chris McReynolds, Cindy Stubbs, Julia Veir, Lisa McReynolds, Sherrill O'Neil, Matthew Chavkin, Anthony Basher, Melissa Brewer, Kristy Dowers, Don Westfall, David Maggs, and Jennifer Ansbaugh are just a few of those who have directly or indirectly influenced me in the writing of this book.

To my parents, Barbara and Rex Lappin, and my partner in life, Catriona MacPhail, for tolerating my excessive work habits and supporting this endeavor.

To the multitude of people who have adopted our cats and have given them the lives they deserve—I cannot thank you enough.

MRL

CONTENTS

CONTRIBUTORS

Robin W. Allison, D.V.M.
Research Associate, Department of Pathology, Colorado State University College of Veterinary Medicine and Biomedical Sciences, Fort Collins, Colorado

Tammy E. Anderson, D.V.M.
Assistant Professor of Medicine, Department of Small Animal Clinical Sciences, University of Tennessee College of Veterinary Medicine, Knoxville, Tennessee

Dina A. Andrews, D.V.M., Ph.D., DACVP
Assistant Professor of Clinical Pathology, Department of Veterinary Pathobiology, Purdue University School of Veterinary Medicine; Clinical Pathologist, Purdue University Veterinary Teaching Hospital, West Lafayette, Indiana

Paul R. Avery, V.M.D.
Instructor, Department of Pathology, Colorado State University College of Veterinary Medicine and Biomedical Sciences, Fort Collins, Colorado

Joseph W. Bartges, B.S., D.V.M., Ph.D., DACVIM, DACVN
Associate Professor of Medicine and Nutrition, Staff Internist and Nutritionist, Department of Small Animal Clinical Sciences, University of Tennessee College of Veterinary Medicine, Knoxville, Tennessee

Jeff D. Bay, D.V.M.
Staff Veterinarian, Department of Internal Medicine, Rowley Memorial Animal Hospital, Springfield, Massachusetts

Ellen N. Behrend, V.M.D., M.S., Ph.D.
Assistant Professor, Department of Clinical Sciences, Auburn University College of Veterinary Medicine, Auburn, Alabama

Michelle L. Berry, D.V.M.
Department of Veterinary Clinical Sciences, Oklahoma State University College of Veterinary Medicine, Stillwater, Oklahoma

Laurie J. Blanco, D.V.M.
Department of Small Animal Clinical Sciences, University of Tennessee College of Veterinary Medicine, Knoxville, Tennessee

Cynthia L. Bowlin, D.V.M., DABVP (Feline)
Cats Only Veterinary Clinic, Columbus, Ohio

Hazel C. Carney, M.S., D.V.M., DABVP
Animal Emergency Clinic and Referral Center, Boise, Idaho; Four Rivers Feline Special Treatment Center, Ontario, Oregon

John M. Cheney, D.V.M., M.S.
Associate Professor, Department of Pathology, Veterinary Diagnostic Laboratory, Colorado State University College of Veterinary Medicine and Biomedical Sciences; Veterinary Teaching Hospital, Fort Collins, Colorado

Elizabeth J. Colleran, D.V.M., M.S.
Owner, Chico Hospital for Cats, Chico, California

Heather E. Connally, D.V.M., M.S.
Wheat Ridge Animal Hospital, Wheat Ridge, Colorado

Rick L. Cowell, D.V.M., M.S., DACVP
Professor, Department of Veterinary Pathobiology; Director, Clinical Pathology Laboratory, Oklahoma State University College of Veterinary Medicine, Stillwater, Oklahoma

Karen E. Dorsey, D.V.M.
Department of Veterinary Pathobiology, Oklahoma State University College of Veterinary Medicine, Stillwater, Oklahoma

Kristy L. Dowers, D.V.M.
Department of Clinical Sciences, Colorado State University College of Veterinary Medicine and Biomedical Sciences, Fort Collins, Colorado

Stephen J. Dullard, D.V.M., DABVP
Chief of Staff, Ancare Veterinary Clinic, Mendota, Illinois

Timothy M. Fan, D.V.M., DACVIM
Visiting Assistant Professor, Department of Small Animal Medicine, University of Illinois College of Veterinary Medicine, Urbana, Illinois

Julie R. Fischer, D.V.M., DACVIM
Staff Internist, South Bay Veterinary Specialists, San Jose, California

Deb Greco, D.V.M.
Department of Pathology, Veterinary Diagnostic Laboratory, Colorado State University College of Veterinary Medicine and Biomedical Sciences; Veterinary Teaching Hospital, Fort Collins, Colorado

Rebecka S. Hess, D.V.M., DACVIM
Senior Lecturer, Department of Clinical Studies, University of Pennsylvania School of Veterinary Medicine; Veterinary Hospital of the University of Pennsylvania, Philadelphia, Pennsylvania

Armando R. Irizarry-Rovira, D.V.M., DACVP
Department of Veterinary Pathobiology, Purdue University School of Veterinary Medicine, West Lafayette, Indiana

C. Bisque Jackson, V.M.D.
Department of Emergency and Critical Care, University of Pennsylvania School of Veterinary Medicine; Veterinary Hospital of the University of Pennsylvania, Philadelphia, Pennsylvania

Jordan Q. Jaeger, D.V.M.
Clinical Instructor, Department of Veterinary Clinical Sciences, Ohio State University College of Veterinary Medicine, Columbus, Ohio

Chad Johannes, D.V.M.
Department of Veterinary Medicine and Surgery, University of Missouri-Columbia College of Veterinary Medicine, Columbia, Missouri

Alice J. Johns, D.V.M., DABVP (Feline)
The Cat Doctor, Indianapolis, Indiana

Lynelle Johnson, D.V.M., Ph.D.
Research Assistant Professor, Department of Veterinary Biomedical Sciences, University of Missouri-Columbia College of Veterinary Medicine, Columbia, Missouri

Tina S. Kalkstein, D.V.M., M.A., DACVIM
Staff Internist, SouthPaws Veterinary Referral Center, Springfield, Virginia

Elyse M. Kent, D.V.M., DABVP
Hospital Director and Founder, Westside Hospital for Cats, Los Angeles, California

India F. Lane, D.V.M., M.S., DACVIM
Assistant Professor of Internal Medicine, Department of Small Animal Clinical Sciences, University of Tennessee College of Veterinary Medicine; Internist, Veterinary Teaching Hospital, Knoxville, Tennessee

Michael R. Lappin, D.V.M., Ph.D., DACVIM
Professor, Department of Clinical Sciences, Colorado State University College of Veterinary Medicine and Biomedical Sciences, Fort Collins, Colorado

Nicole Leibman, D.V.M., M.S., DACVIM (Oncology)
Ultravet Diagnostics, Mineola, New York

Jill Lurye, D.V.M.
Department of Small Surgery and Medicine, Auburn University College of Veterinary Medicine, Auburn, Alabama

Catriona M. MacPhail, D.V.M.
Surgical Fellow, Department of Clinical Sciences, Colorado State University College of Veterinary Medicine and Biomedical Sciences, Fort Collins, Colorado

Dennis W. Macy, D.V.M.
Department of Clinical Sciences, Colorado State University College of Veterinary Medicine and Biomedical Sciences, Fort Collins, Colorado

Elisa M. Mazzaferro, M.S., D.V.M.
Department of Small Animal Clinical Sciences, Colorado State University College of Veterinary Medicine and Biomedical Sciences, Fort Collins, Colorado

Elizabeth A. McNiel, D.V.M., Ph.D., DACVIM (Oncology)
Research Associate, Department of Radiological Health Sciences, Colorado State University College of Veterinary Medicine and Biomedical Sciences, Fort Collins, Colorado

Margo L. Mehl, D.V.M.
University of California, Davis, School of Veterinary Medicine; University of California, Davis, Veterinary Medical Teaching Hospital, Davis, California

James H. Meinkoth, D.V.M., Ph.D., DACVP
Associate Professor, Department of Veterinary Pathobiology, Oklahoma State University College of Veterinary Medicine, Stillwater, Oklahoma

Lynda Melendez, D.V.M., M.S., DACVIM
Assistant Professor, Department of Small Animal Medicine, Oklahoma State University College of Veterinary Medicine, Stillwater, Oklahoma

Tammy L. Miller, D.V.M., M.S.
Department of Ophthalmology, North Carolina State University College of Veterinary Medicine, Raleigh, North Carolina

James K. Olson, D.V.M.
Cat Specialist, Castle Rock, Colorado

Christine S. Olver, D.V.M., Ph.D.
Department of Pathology, Colorado State University College of Veterinary Medicine and Biomedical Sciences, Fort Collins, Colorado

Davyd Pelsue, D.V.M.
Department of Clinical Sciences, Colorado State University College of Veterinary Medicine and Biomedical Sciences, Fort Collins, Colorado

Cynthia C. Powell, D.V.M., M.S.
Assistant Professor, Department of Clinical Sciences, Colorado State University College of Veterinary Medicine and Biomedical Sciences, Fort Collins, Colorado

Marcella D. Ridgway, V.M.D., M.S.
Assistant Professor, Department of Small Animal Medicine, University of Illinois College of Veterinary Medicine, Urbana, Illinois

Tammy P. Sadek, D.V.M., DABVP (Feline)
Director, Kentwood Cat Clinic, Kentwood, Michigan

Margie Scherk, D.V.M., DABVP (Feline)
Cats Only Veterinary Clinic, Vancouver, British Columbia, Canada

Kim A. Selting, D.V.M.
Department of Oncology, Colorado State University College of Veterinary Medicine and Biomedical Sciences, Fort Collins, Colorado

Stacy B. Smith, D.V.M.
Department of Clinical Pathology, Oklahoma State University College of Veterinary Medicine, Stillwater, Oklahoma

John E. Stein, D.V.M.
Department of Clinical Sciences, Colorado State University College of Veterinary Medicine and Biomedical Sciences, Fort Collins, Colorado

Sara Stephens, D.V.M., DABVP (Feline)
Alpine Veterinary Service, Missoula, Montana

Cynthia J. Stubbs, D.V.M., M.S., DACVIM
Department of Internal Medicine, Cobb Veterinary Clinic, Marietta, Georgia

Séverine Tasker, B.Sc., B.V.Sc., DSAM, MRCVS
Feline Centre, Department of Clinical Veterinary Science, University of Bristol, Bristol, United Kingdom

Glenda F. Taton-Allen, B.S., M.S.
Microbiologist, Veterinary Diagnostic Laboratory, Department of Pathology, Colorado State University College of Veterinary Medicine and Biomedical Sciences; Veterinary Teaching Hospital, Fort Collins, Colorado

Helen Tuzio, D.V.M., M.S.
Associate Dean of Administration, Ross University School of Veterinary Medicine, New York, New York; Veterinary Associate, Forest Hills Cat Hospital, Glendale, New York

Julia K. Veir, D.V.M.
Department of Clinical Sciences, Colorado State University College of Veterinary Medicine and Biomedical Sciences, Fort Collins, Colorado

Craig B. Webb, D.V.M., Ph.D.
Department of Clinical Sciences, Colorado State University College of Veterinary Medicine and Biomedical Sciences, Fort Collins, Colorado

Drew D. Weigner, D.V.M., DABVP (Feline)
President, Academy of Feline Medicine; The Cat Doctor, Inc., Atlanta, Georgia

Donald S. Westfall, D.V.M., M.S.
Department of Clinical Sciences, Colorado State University College of Veterinary Medicine and Biomedical Sciences, Fort Collins, Colorado

PREFACE

My experiences with the feline species began with Mittens and Sport and the other barn cats that resided near my childhood home in Tonganoxie, Kansas, and at Deer Creek Ranch in Edmond, Oklahoma. These experiences influenced me through my formative years. As I progressed through veterinary college and my postgraduate training program, I realized that this wonderful and unique species would direct my research studies for the remainder of my career. Through interactions with cats in research projects, in the clinic, and with my personal "herd," I have had many wonderful experiences. I am pleased to be able to interact with my colleagues and present to you this compilation of chapters on feline internal medicine. I have tried to incorporate the problem-based approach to internal medicine with the well-received and easy-to-use question-and-answer format used in the Secrets Series®. This book is unique among current feline textbooks in that a significant percentage of our authors are board certified in feline medicine and work in exclusively feline practices. These individuals spend the entirety of their professional time working with cats and their diseases in the clinical setting. This has led to a very practical and user-friendly textbook.

A special thanks is extended to William Lamsback and Cecelia Bayruns at Hanley & Belfus for helping bring this book to the veterinary profession.

Michael R. Lappin, D.V.M., Ph.D.

I. *Cardiopulmonary Disorders*

Section Editor: Lynelle Johnson, D.V.M.

1. SNEEZING AND NASAL DISCHARGE: INITIAL DIAGNOSTIC PLAN

Michael R. Lappin, D.V.M., Ph.D.

1. What is sneezing?

A superficial reflex that originates in the mucous membranes lining the nasal cavity. Sneezing is easily induced by chemical or mechanical stimuli. The sneeze results in forceful, high velocity expulsion of air through the airways that clears the respiratory passageways. Most diseases of the nasal passages can induce sneezing.

2. What are the major nasal discharges?

- Serous
- Mucoid
- Mucopurulent
- Hemorrhagic

Depending on the primary cause of disease, mixed types of discharges also can occur. Respiratory epithelium has serous, mucous, and mixed tubuloalveolar glands. Goblet cells also are distributed throughout the nasal cavity. Most diseases of the nasal cavity result in serous nasal discharge that can become mucoid or mucopurulent depending on chronicity and secondary bacterial overgrowth.

Differential Diagnoses for Sneezing and Nasal Discharge in Cats

Local diseases

Congenital; palate defects
Nasopharyngeal or sinus masses (neoplasia, granulomas, or nasopharyngeal polyps)
Allergic
Dental disease with oronasal fistula
Trauma
Otitis media (if nasopharyngeal polyps are present)
Foreign body
Dysphagia, vomiting, regurgitation (resulting in food aspirated into the nasopharynx)
Infectious diseases

Bacterial
Primary pathogens
Bordetella bronchiseptica
Chlamydia psittaci
Mycoplasma spp.
Secondary floral overgrowth

Fungal
Cryptococcus neoformans
Aspergillus spp.
Viral
Feline herpesvirus 1
Calicivirus

Coagulation abnormalities

Systemic arterial hypertension

Vasculitis

3. What are the differential diagnoses for serous nasal discharge?
Serous nasal discharge is characteristic of most acute diseases of the nasal cavity. If the serous nasal discharge is chronic, viral, parasitic, and allergic diseases are most common. However, parasitic disease of the nasal cavity is extremely rare in cats of the United States.

4. What are the differential diagnoses for mucoid nasal discharge?
Mucoid nasal discharge occurs most commonly with allergic diseases, neoplasia, and fungal diseases.

5. What are the differential diagnoses of mucopurulent nasal discharge?
Appearance of neutrophils in nasal discharges suggests bacterial involvement. The disease may be associated with the primary bacterial pathogens or overgrowth of normal bacterial flora secondary to any chronic nasal disease, including neoplasia, oronasal fistula, foreign body, inflammatory polyp, or viral disease. Mucopurulent discharge also occurs with fungal rhinitis.

6. What are the differential diagnoses for hemorrhagic nasal discharge?
Acute epistaxis that occurs without other detectable discharges is most common with trauma, acute foreign body impaction, hypertension, vasculitis, and coagulopathy. However, vasculitis causing a nasal discharge is rare in cats. Epistaxis that develops after a mucoid to mucopurulent discharge is most common with fungal disease, neoplasia, and oronasal fistula.

7. How do you organize the diagnostic work-up in cats with sneezing and nasal discharge?
The diagnostic work-up can be divided into three phases that progress from least invasive to most invasive.

8. What physical examination techniques do you emphasize in phase 1 of a diagnostic work-up for sneezing and nasal discharge?
A thorough physical examination is performed first. Otic examination should be performed to evaluate for bulging or discoloration of the tympanum; these changes commonly occur with nasopharyngeal polyps (see Chapter 5). Oral examination and palpation should be performed to assess for oronasal fistula of the canine teeth, tooth root infections that may extend into the sinuses, and for defects in the soft palate. Ophthalmic examination may provide evidence of anterior uveitis (herpesvirus 1) and chorioretinitis (*Cryptococcus neoformans*).

9. What diagnostic tests should be considered during phase 1 of a diagnostic work-up for sneezing and nasal discharge?
Cytology of nasal discharge should be performed on all cats with mucoid to mucopurulent nasal discharge to evaluate for the presence of *Cryptococcus neoformans*. Neutrophils and bacteria are commonly detected if mucopurulent disease is present but do not prove primary bacterial disease. Secondary infections result in the same discharge as primary infections. Bacterial culture and antimicrobial susceptibility testing on nasal discharge collected from the nasal planum are usually not performed because results are difficult to interpret. It is better to collect tissue for culture from deep within the nasal cavity while under general anesthesia in phase 2 of the diagnostic workup. Complete blood cell count, feline leukemia virus antigen test, and feline immunodeficiency virus antibody test are usually performed in cats with nasal discharge. Results of the complete blood cell count rarely give a definitive diagnosis, but the presence of eosinophilia may support the diagnosis of allergic rhinitis. Feline leukemia virus and feline immunodeficiency virus infections do not cause sneezing and nasal discharge primarily but may induce immunodeficiency that predisposes to other infections. If epistaxis without other nasal discharge is present, a platelet count, activated clotting time, and systemic arterial blood pressure should be performed to evaluate for coagulopathies or hypertension. Virus isolation, fluorescent antibody staining or polymerase chain reaction (PCR) can be used to help detect infections by specific upper respiratory pathogens like herpesvirus 1 or calicivirus (see Chapter 3).

10. Do you perform therapeutic trials during phase 1 of the diagnostic work-up?

Therapeutic trials often are performed in cats with acute or chronic sneezing and nasal discharge, particularly if the client cannot afford further diagnostic procedures to be performed in phase 2. Antibiotics, antivirals, immunostimulants, anti-inflammatory agents, topical decongestants, or topical glucocorticoids are used in certain situations (see subsequent chapters for specific recommendations).

11. What diagnostic procedures do you consider in phase 2 of a diagnostic work-up for sneezing and nasal discharge?

If a definitive diagnosis is not made during phase 1 and routine therapeutic trials fail, more invasive diagnostic testing is indicated. Phase 2 diagnostics usually consist of laryngeal function examination, pharyngeal examination, skull and dental radiographs, rhinoscopy, bacterial and fungal cultures, and biopsy for histology. Since biopsies are generally made in phase 2, a platelet count, activated clotting time, and systemic arterial blood pressure are performed prior to anesthesia. General anesthesia is induced by administering approximately one-third of an induction dose of a thiobarbiturate. The arytenoids are examined to make sure both are abducting normally. Oropharyngeal examination is performed to evaluate thoroughly for masses, foreign bodies, or palate defects. The nasopharynx is examined with a dental mirror or rhinoscope. If a definitive diagnosis is not apparent, nasal, sinus, and dental radiographs are made. Rhinoscopy of the anterior nasal cavity is then performed. If indicated, bacterial and fungal cultures are made using tissue biopsy collected from within the nasal cavity. The nasal cavity is flushed with sterile saline to evaluate for the presence of foreign material. Placing the nipple of a 60-ml syringe filled with sterile saline into the anterior nares and flushing rapidly will usually drive foreign material into the mouth where it can be removed. Biopsies are then made using a bone curette or small biopsy instrument. Finally, teeth are probed for evidence of oronasal fistula or periodontal pockets > 3 mm in depth.

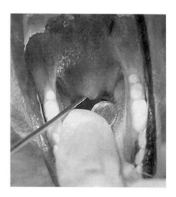

Dental mirror examination of the nasal pharynx.

12. What procedures are used in phase 3 of the work-up of sneezing and nasal discharge?

Rhinotomy is rarely indicated in cats but may be utilized in phase 3 evaluation of cats with sneezing and nasal discharge. For most cats with nasal cryptococcosis, medical therapy is successful, and debulking of a mass in the nasal cavity is usually not needed. There is also no added benefit to debulking nasal tumors prior to radiation therapy. Although removing turbinate tissue can increase airflow through the nasal cavities in cats with chronic rhinitis, bacterial osteomyelitis and some nasal discharge often remain.

BIBLIOGRAPHY

1. Hawkins EC: Chronic viral upper repiratory disease in cats: Differential diagnosis and management. Comp Cont Educ Pract Vet 10:1010–1013, 1988.
2. Lappin MR: Sneezing and nasal discharge. In, Lorenz MD, Cornelius LM (eds): Small Animal Medical Diagnosis, 2nd ed. Philadelphia, J.B. Lippincott, Philadelphia, 1993, pp 235–244.

2. BACTERIAL DISEASES

John E. Stein, D.V.M.

1. What clinical signs are most common in cats with bacterial upper respiratory disease?

Cats with sneezing and a mucopurulent nasal discharge most likely have a bacterial component to their disease, although it may be a primary or secondary condition. Some cats may have an ocular discharge as part of underlying disease or because the nasolacrimal duct has become obstructed. Coughing and retching occur in some cats when the nasal discharge is aspirated or swallowed or when pharyngitis is induced by the infectious agent. Epistaxis may be seen with invasive or chronic disease that disrupts the nasal mucosa, although this finding is rare with primary bacterial diseases alone. Noisy breathing is commonly noted, and open mouth breathing can be seen in cats with bilateral nasal obstruction due to discharge.

2. How common is primary vs. secondary bacterial rhinitis as a cause of clinical disease?

Bacterial rhinitis is rarely the primary cause of nasal disease in cats, but it is commonly noted as a secondary complication to other diseases affecting the nasal passageways and in cats with impaired immune systems. Secondary bacterial rhinitis can follow many diseases, including viral upper respiratory disorders, oronasal fistula, nasal foreign body, bony sequestrum, or nasal neoplasia.

3. What bacterial agents can be responsible for primary rhinitis in cats?

Bordetella bronchiseptica, Mycoplasma spp., and *Chlamydia psittaci.*

4. Describe the clinical manifestations of chlamydiosis.

C. psittaci is an intracellular bacterium that may account for 5–32% of feline respiratory tract diseases, depending on the study. In North America, however, the agent is associated most commonly with mild-to-severe conjunctivitis. In fact, primary infection with *C. psittaci* should be considered unlikely in cats with sneezing but no evidence of conjunctivitis. The most common clinical signs, therefore, are serous to mucopurulent ocular discharge, chemosis, blepharospasm, and eyelid swelling. Other clinical signs that may be noted include fever, submandibular lymphadenopathy, sneezing, nasal discharge, anorexia, and weight loss. Chlamydiosis is seen predominately in young cats, generally between 5 weeks and 9 months of age, and is more commonly diagnosed in the summer months.

5. What evidence suggests that *Mycoplasma* spp. are associated with rhinitis in cats?

Mycoplasma spp. have been cultured from the upper respiratory tract of both healthy and diseased cats. In one study, the organism was isolated from the nasopharynx of 35% of healthy cats. Because the organism is common in healthy cats, most species are probably opportunistic pathogens. *Mycoplasma felis* may cause conjunctivitis, mucopurulent nasal discharge, and sneezing in cats when it colonizes mucosal surfaces. *Mycoplasma* spp., however, are not found in the lower airways of healthy cats; thus the resident flora of the nasopharynx may represent a possible source of infection in cats that develop mycoplasmal pneumonia (see Chapter 12).

6. What evidence supports *Bordetella bronchiseptica* as a primary cause of rhinitis?

B. bronchiseptica is a common organism in cats and has been isolated from the oropharynx of both healthy and diseased cats. In one study, over 3% of cats without evidence of respiratory disease were found to have *B. bronchiseptica* on bacterial culture of oropharyngeal swabs. In addition, 24% of healthy cats were seropositive for *B. bronchiseptica*, indicating previous exposure to the organism. Its role as a potential primary pathogen has been confirmed by experimental induction of disease in specific pathogen-free kittens. Life-threatening pneumonia can develop, particularly if kittens are infected before 4– 6 weeks of age (see Chapter 12). Of importance, however, *B. bronchiseptica* appears much more likely to cause clinical disease in young kittens and group-housed cats, suggesting that concurrent disease, immune status, and stress factors such as overcrowding, poor hygiene, and recent weaning are also important in the pathogenesis of disease. Its role as a primary pathogen of adult household cats remains controversial.

7. What are the most common causes of secondary bacterial rhinitis?

A diverse population of gram-positive, gram-negative, aerobic, and anaerobic bacteria is found in the nasal passages of healthy cats, including *Streptococcus* spp., *Staphylococcus* spp., *Corynebacterium* spp., *Pasteurella multocida, Escherichia coli, Pseudomonas* spp., and *Enterobacter* spp. Anaerobic bacteria are commonly found under the mucus layer in the nose where oxygen tension is low. Any of these organisms or other normal inhabitants can overgrow and cause clinical signs of bacterial rhinitis in cats with concurrent local disease or compromised immune system. Overgrowth of normal nasal microflora can occur with viral, fungal, or (rarely) parasitic infections; trauma; foreign bodies such as plant material; aspiration of food into the nasopharynx following dysphagia, vomiting, or regurgitation; neoplasia; nasopharyngeal polyps; and extension of disease from the oral cavity, such as tooth root abscesses and oronasal fistulas (see Chapter 1). Specifically, cats with chronic viral respiratory tract infections may develop severe mucosal ulceration and turbinate destruction, resulting in chronic bacterial rhinitis/sinusitis. Patients with feline leukemia virus (FeLV) or feline immunodeficiency virus (FIV) infections may have impaired immune function and be particularly susceptible to secondary bacterial infections, although positive serologic tests for these agents do not prove the existence of immunodeficiency.

8. What is the initial diagnostic plan for cats with suspected bacterial rhinitis?

Because bacterial rhinitis is most commonly a secondary complication, cats with mucopurulent nasal discharge and sneezing should be evaluated carefully for an underlying primary disease (see Chapter 1). A thorough history and physical examination, with particular attention to otic, oral, and ophthalmic examinations to detect evidence of local or systemic disease, is paramount. Ideally, vaccine history and retroviral (FeLV/FIV) infection status should be known for every feline patient with chronic mucopurulent rhinitis. Cytology of nasal discharge is usually considered in the initial diagnostic plan to rule out infection with *Cryptococcus neoformans*. Whether more expensive and invasive tests are performed depends on history, physical examination, and initial diagnostic findings.

9. How does cytology potentially aid in the management of a cat with rhinitis?

Cytology of the nasal discharge confirms the presence of neutrophils and possibly bacteria, although it cannot differentiate primary from secondary infection or distinguish normal flora from pathogenic bacteria. *C. neoformans* may be detected in some cats (see Chapter 4).

10. Should I culture the nasal discharge?

Bacterial culture of the exudates from the nasal planum is not typically performed because of difficulty in interpreting the results. Since the nasal cavity has a rich normal flora, a mixed bacterial population is usually obtained from both healthy and diseased cats. If bacterial cultures are performed, samples are best obtained from deep tissue biopsies with the patient under general anesthesia and only after the presence of significant underlying disease has been ruled out (see Chapter 1). Isolation of a pure bacterial culture may be significant. *C. psittaci* is difficult to culture. Polymerase chain reaction is superior to culture for detection of the organism from conjunctival swabs but has not been evaluated for respiratory disease.

11. Are there radiographic abnormalities associated with bacterial rhinitis?

Few changes, if any, are seen on nasal radiographs, particularly if the disease course is acute. Rarely, turbinate destruction or bone lysis is caused by chronic bacterial disease alone. Either finding strongly suggests a more aggressive disease process, such as neoplasia or fungal infection.

12. How should I use systemic antibiotic therapy for management of bacterial rhinitis?

Acute, non–life-threatening cases of rhinitis may resolve spontaneously and often are managed with symptomatic care alone. Antibiotic therapy may prove unnecessary if an underlying disease is identified and treated effectively. In mild, relatively acute cases, a short course (7–10 days) of relatively broad-spectrum antibiotic may prove sufficient to alleviate clinical signs.

Treatment for **chronic bacterial rhinitis**, whether as a primary or secondary condition, generally involves long-term antibiotic therapy.

13. Which antibiotic agents are appropriate for bactrial rhinitis?

Drugs with anaerobic spectrum that penetrate bone and cartilage, such as amoxicillin or clindamycin, are effective in many cases. Clindamycin is a popular choice because of excellent gram-positive and anaerobic coverage, good tissue penetration, availability of a liquid preparation, and once-daily dosage. Although nausea, vomiting, and diarrhea occur in some cats, nausea may be lessened by storing the liquid in the refrigerator between administrations. Metronidazole is effective in some cats because of excellent anaerobic coverage as well as a potential anti-inflammatory effect due to T-lymphocytic modulation. However, an anti-inflammatory effect in nasal tissues has not been substantiated. Because metronidazole tablets are difficult to administer to cats, formulated suspensions may be indicated. If *B. bronchiseptica* or *Mycoplasma* spp. infection is suspected, doxycycline, chloramphenicol, a quinolone, or azithromycin should be administered. Many *B. bronchiseptica* isolates are susceptible to amoxicillin-clavulanate, but it is not an appropriate choice for *Mycoplasma* spp. Systemic doxycycline combined with topical tetracycline or chloramphenicol is the preferred treatment for suspected *C. psittaci* infections, although azithromycin is also effective. Administration of doxycycline tablets has been associated with esophageal strictures in cats (see Chapter 26). Thus, formulated suspensions should be used, or a small amount of water should be given orally after administration of tablets. Systemic tetracyclines may cause teeth enamel discoloration in kittens. Chronic bacterial rhinitis, usually associated with the feline viral rhinotracheitis, neoplasia, or fungal infections, may require long-term therapy (minimum of 4–6 weeks) in addition to addressing the underlying disease. In some cats with severe turbinate destruction, pulse therapy with antibiotics may be needed to control clinical signs of disease.

Drugs Commonly Used for Treatment of Bacterial Rhinitis in Cats

DRUG	DOSE REGIMEN	COMMENTS
Amoxicillin	11–22 mg/kg PO every 12 hr	Gram-positive, anaerobes
Amoxicillin-clavulanate	11–22 mg PO every 12 hr	Gram-positive, anaerobes, select gram-negative, *B. bronchiseptica*
Azithromycin	5–10 mg/kg PO every 24 hr for 3 days, then every 72 hr	*B. bronchiseptica, Mycoplasma* spp., *C. psittaci*, gram-negative, anaerobes
Cephalexin	22–50 mg/kg PO every 8–12 hr	Gram-positive, anaerobes
Chloramphenicol	25-50 mg/cat PO every 12 hr	*B. bronchiseptica, Mycoplasma* spp., *C. psittaci,* anaerobes, gram-positive
Clindamycin	11–24 mg/kg PO every 24 hr	Gram-positive, anaerobes; good tissue penetration
Doxycycline	5–10 mg/kg PO every 12–24 hr	*B. bronchiseptica, Mycoplasma* spp., *C. psittaci;* possibly anti-inflammatory
Enrofloxacin	5 mg/kg PO every 12–24 hr	Gram-negative, select gram-positive, B. bronchiseptica, Mycoplasma spp., but poor anaerobic coverage
Metronidazole	7.5–10 mg/kg PO every 8–12 hr	Anaerobes; possibly anti-inflammatory

PO = orally.

14. What adjunct treatments are used in addition to systemic antibiotics?

The nares should be kept clean and free of significant discharge. Humidification therapy to improve mucociliary apparatus function may be beneficial and can be achieved by humidifying the area where the cat sleeps, by bringing the cat into the bathroom while running hot water through the shower, or by nebulization. Some cats may tolerate nasal instillation of saline, which is mucolytic. Topical treatment with antibiotic nose drops or with nebulization of antibiotics may be beneficial for some cases, particularly with infection by *B. bronchiseptica* and *Mycoplasma* spp., which are thought to dwell on the surface (see Chapter 12). Nasal decongestants are generally not indicated if mucopurulent discharge is present. If a poor appetite is identified, feeding warm, soft food may increase the aroma and encourage cats to eat (see Chapter 62).

15. What is the prognosis for cats with bacterial rhinitis?

The overall prognosis for primary bacterial upper respiratory tract infections is excellent, with the possible exception of *C. psittaci* infections, which can be difficult to eliminate and may recur in times of stress. The prognosis for secondary bacterial infections of the upper respiratory tract depends on the successful identification and management of the underlying cause. Idiopathic chronic rhinitis generally is characterized by frequent recurrence of clinical signs with variable responsiveness to therapy.

16. Can bacterial rhinitis be prevented in cats?

Bacterial rhinitis in cats is generally a secondary complication; therefore, prevention centers on minimizing conditions that predispose the upper airways to invasion by bacteria. Careful husbandry practices, including adequate hygiene, appropriate weaning, good nutrition, and avoiding overcrowding, are critical to lessen exposure to infectious agents.

17. What is the role of vaccination?

Bolstering immunity through vaccinations against respiratory pathogens is also important. In particular, immunization against feline viral rhinotracheitis (FHV-1) and calicivirus (FCV) is crucial; these vaccines should be considered core vaccines, along with panleukopenia (FPV) and rabies virus, as recommended in the 1998 vaccine guidelines from the American Association of Feline Practitioners and the Academy of Feline Medicine (see Chapters 3 and 81).

Vaccines against the potential primary disease pathogens, *C. psittaci* and *B. bronchiseptica*, are available. Neither vaccine prevents infection or eliminates shedding. Additionally in most pet cats the diseases are relatively rare, non–life-threatening, and effectively treated with inexpensive antibiotics. Thus, it appears unnecessary to vaccinate all cats against these organisms. Use of *C. psittaci* and *B. bronchiseptica* vaccines probably are of most benefit in catteries and humane shelters with persistent respiratory problems (see Chapter 81).

BIBLIOGRAPHY

1. American Association of Feline Practitioners, Academy of Feline Medicine: 1998 Report of the American Association of Feline Practitioners and Academy of Feline Medicine Advisory Panel on Feline Vaccines. J Am Vet Med Assoc 212:227–241, 1998.
2. Boothe DM: Principles of drug selection for respiratory infections in cats. Comp Cont Educ Pract Vet 19:5–15, 1997.
3. Gaskell R, Dawson S: Feline respiratory disease. In Greene CE (ed): Infectious Diseases of the Dog and Cat, 2nd ed. Philadelphia, W.B. Saunders, 1998, pp 97–106.
4. Greene CE: Respiratory infections. In Greene CE (ed): Infectious Diseases of the Dog and Cat, 2nd ed. Philadelphia, W.B. Saunders, 1998, pp 582–594.
5. Hawkins EC: Disorders of the nasal cavity. In Nelson RW, Couto CG (eds): Small Animal Internal Medicine, 2nd ed. St. Louis, Mosby, 1998, pp 225–237.
6. Hoskins JD, Williams J, Roy AF, Peters JC, McDonough P: Isolation and characterization of *Bordetella bronchiseptica* from cats in southern Louisiana. Vet Immunol Immunopathol 65:173–176, 1998.
7. Randolph JF, Moise NS, Scarlett JM, et al: Prevalence of mycoplasmal and ureaplasmal recovery from tracheobronchial lavages and of mycoplasmal recovery from pharyngeal swab specimens in cats with or without pulmonary disease. Am J Vet Res 54:897–900, 1993.

8. Speakman AJ, Dawson S, Binns SH, et al: *Bordetella bronchiseptica* infection in the cat. J Small Anim Pract 40:252–256, 1999.
9. Sykes JE: Comparison of polymerase chain reaction and culture for the detection of feline *Chlamydia psittaci* in untreated and doxycycline-treated experimentally infected cats. J Vet Intern Med 13:146–152, 1999.
10. Sykes JE: Prevalence of feline *Chlamydia psittaci* and feline herpesvirus 1 in cats with upper respiratory tract disease. J Vet Intern Med 13:153–162, 1999.
11. Welsh RD: *Bordetella bronchiseptica* infections in cats. J Am Anim Hosp Assoc 32:153–158, 2000.

3. VIRAL DISEASES

Michael R. Lappin, D.V.M., Ph.D.

1. What are the common viral causes of feline upper respiratory disease?

Feline herpesvirus 1 (FHV-1), a double-stranded DNA virus and calicivirus (FCV), a single-stranded RNA virus, are thought to be most common. FHV-1 strains vary little and have similar pathogenicity, whereas FCV strains are variable. Coinfection with different FCV strains can occur with variation in clinical signs. Feline leukemia virus (FeLV) and feline immunodeficiency virus (FIV) do not directly cause respiratory disease. However, immunodeficient cats may be predisposed to chronic clinical disease due to FHV-1 or FCV.

2. How prevalent is FHV-1 infection?

In studies in the United States and Australia, the prevalence of FHV-1 infections in cats with and without upper respiratory tract disease or conjunctivitis was 13.7% and 21.2%, respectively. Prevalence varies by detection technique and study but was 31% by polymerase chain reaction (PCR) in one study of healthy cats.

3. How are the respiratory viruses transmitted?

Susceptible cats contract both FHV-1 and FCV infections after common exposure to infected animals in a crowded environment. Transmission can be by direct contact, fomites, or aerosalization. FCV survives outside the host for up to 1 week if it remains moist, whereas FHV-1 survives outside the host for up to 18 hours if it remains moist. Both viruses cause a carrier state in recovered cats despite vaccination status.

4. How does FHV-1 cause disease?

Epithelial infection causes local necrosis and neutrophilic inflammation. The upper respiratory tissues, conjunctiva, and cornea are affected most commonly. Local bacterial flora may cause secondary infection. Viremia is rare, but replication occurs in lower airways of some cats, particularly kittens, and may result in pneumonia.

After a 2–6-day incubation period, acute disease generally lasts for 1–3 weeks. Approximately 80% of recovered cats are thought to develop a latent infection that is maintained in the trigeminal ganglion. Repeat shedding is thought to occur in 50% and may be stress-induced (e.g., glucocorticoid administration, other infections). After a stressful event, shedding begins in approximately 1 week and lasts approximately 2 weeks. Clinical signs recur in some infected cats.

5. How does FCV cause disease?

The virus replicates primarily in oral and respiratory tissues. Ability to induce disease varies by strain. A form fatal to some adult cats was recently described. As with FHV-1, inflammation can result from viral replication or secondary bacterial overgrowth. Pneumonia in kittens is more likely to result from FCV than FHV-1 infection. Latent infection occurs, and the virus can be shed continually even without clinical signs of disease. After a 2–5-day incubation period, acute disease generally lasts for 2–3 weeks.

6. What are the clinical signs of viral upper respiratory tract disease?
- Both FHV-1 and FCV infections initially result in varying degrees of sneezing and serous nasal discharge that can progress to mucopurulent nasal discharge.
- Varying degrees of fever and inappetance occur with acute infection with both viruses.
- Chronic recurrent rhinitis and sinusitis can occur in some cats and is probably most common with FHV-1 infection.
- Conjuctivitis occurs with both viruses but is thought to be more prevalent with FHV1 infection.
- If keratitis with dendritic ulcer or corneal sequestrum is present, FHV-1 infection is most likely.
- Anterior uveitis may be related to FHV-1 infection with or without keratitis.
- Cough or dyspnea may occur in some infected kittens but is most common with FCV infection.
- Vesicles or erosions on the lips and tongue are most common with acute FCV infection but may occur with reactivated disease.
- Chronic lymphocytic plasmacytic stomatitis is possibly related to chronic FCV infection.
- Stiffness and lameness of short duration result from polyarthritis due to acute FCV infection or modified live vaccination in some kittens.

7. How is infection with FCV or FHV-1 diagnosed?
1. **Organism demonstration techniques**
   - Both viruses can be grown in appropriate culture (virus isolation).
   - Direct fluorescent antibody staining of conjunctival smears has been used to document the presence of FHV-1 infected cells.
   - PCR can be used to amplify DNA of the organisms and is the most sensitive technique for documenting presence of FHV-1.
   - Because both FHV-1 and FCV can be detected in healthy as well as sick cats, the value of these tests for proving disease is low. For example, in one study of cats with conjunctivitis, more healthy control cats were FHV-1–positive on PCR than cats with conjunctivitis.
2. **Detection of serum antibodies**
   - Serum neutralization and enzyme-linked immunosorbent assay (ELISA) have been used to detect antibodies against FHV-1 or FCV.
   - Most cats have been exposed to or vaccinated with FCV or FHV-1 antigens and so are seropositive.
   - Antibodies persist for years after exposure or vaccination.
   - Increasing FCV or FHV-1 antibody titers can be demonstrated for a short time after acute exposure, but titers usually do not rise on secondary exposure or with activation of chronic infection.
   - Because so many healthy cats are antibody-positive, the diagnostic utility of serology testing is minimal except for predicting whether vaccination is needed (see Chapter 81).
3. **Testing of aqueous humor**
   - In aqueous humor of cats suspected to have idiopathic anterior uveitis, local production of FHV-1 antibodies was documented frequently.
   - FHV-1 DNA was detected frequently in aqueous humor of cats with uveitis but infrequently in normal FHV-1–infected cats. These results suggest that FHV-1 infects the intraocular tissues of cats and may be associated with anterior uveitis in some cats.

8. How are viral upper respiratory tract infections treated?
Manifestations of acute disease resolve in most adult cats without specific treatment. Fever or mucopurulent nasal discharge suggests secondary bacterial infections, and antibiotic therapy

may be indicated. Antibiotics with an anaerobic and *Pasteurella* spp. spectrum often are used, including amoxicillin, amoxicillin-clavulanate, first-generation cephalosporins, and clindamycin (see Chapter 2). Ocular FHV-1 infections are managed systemically and topically. Symptomatic and supportive care is also important. Examples include:

- Airway humidification
- Nebulization or topical instillation of saline
- Topical antibiotic administration
- Appetite stimulants

9. Describe the role of interferon alpha.

Daily administration of interferon alpha (25 units orally) lessened clinical scores in acutely ill cats experimentally inoculated with FHV-1. Although controlled studies are lacking, some authorities believe that administration of interferon alpha at 30 U/day orally lessens clinical signs of disease in some cats with chronic FHV-1 infection. Information is not available for FCV infection.

Interferon alpha at 10,000–20,000 U/kg/day subcutaneously is thought to have antiviral effects and is indicated for treatment of acute FHV-1 or FCV infections, particularily if viral pneumonitis is suspected. Again, controlled studies are lacking.

10. What other treatments have been investigated?

- Lysine administered orally at 250 mg every 12 hours lessened viral shedding rates in cats experimentally inoculated with FHV-1. Although controlled studies are lacking, some believe that this dose of L-lysine helps to lessen chronic or recurrent clinical signs induced by FHV-1.
- Intranasal vaccines may lessen clinical signs of chronic FHV-1 infection in some cats. Controlled studies are lacking.
- Administration of acyclovir may be beneficial for the treatment of FHV-1 infections, but hematologic side effects may occur.

11. With what other disorder is FCV associated? How is it treated?

It is proposed that FCV is associated with chronic lymphocytic-plasmacytic stomatitis in cats. No therapeutic protocol has been shown to be 100% effective. Controlled studies are lacking, but the following approaches are recommended:

- Diseased teeth should be removed or repaired, and a biopsy should be procured to rule out neoplasia.
- Glucocorticoids help to control inflammation in some cats but are not curative.
- Antibiotics (metronidazole, clindamycin) with anaerobic bacterial spectrums aid in controlling secondary infections.
- Oral administraton of bovine lactoferrin has lessened disease in some cats.
- Immunostimulants (e.g., immunoreglan) and cytokines (e.g., interferon alpha) have been anecdoctally successful in some cats.
- Carbon dioxide laser ablation of diseased tissues has been beneficial in some cases.

12. How are viral upper respiratory tract infections prevented?

- The best way to avoid FCV and FHV-1 infections is to avoid infected cats. However, because of the presence of chronic, subclinical carriers, this strategy is almost impossible.
- Topical or parenteral vaccines lessen disease in exposed cats but do not provide sterilizing immunity (see Chapter 81).
- Intranasal vaccines are indicated in kittens in crowded environments because of the rapid development of secretory IgA but may cause mild clinical signs.
- Booster vaccines currently are recommended every 3 years after 1 year of age.
- Stress should be avoided in multiple-cat households.
- Hospital biosecurity should be maintained (see Chapter 80).

13. Do feline upper respiratory viruses infect humans?

To date, neither FHV-1 or FCV is considered a risk to human health.

BIBLIOGRAPHY

1. Burgesser KM, Hotaling S, Schiebel A, et al: Comparison of PCR, virus isolation, and indirect fluorescent antibody staining in the detection of naturally occurring feline herpesvirus infections. J Vet Diagn Invest 11:122–126, 1999.
2. Gaskell R, Dawson S: Feline respiratory disease. In Greene CE (ed): Infectious Diseases of the Dog and Cat, 2nd ed. Philadelphia, W.B. Saunders, 1998, pp 97–106.
3. Maggs DJ, Lappin MR, Nasisse MP: Detection of feline herpesvirus-specific antibodies and DNA in aqueous humor from cats with or without uveitis. Am J Vet Res 60:8 932–936, 1999.
4. Maggs DJ, Lappin MR, Reif JS, et al: Evaluation of serologic and viral detection methods for diagnosing feline herpesvirus-1 infection in cats with acute respiratory tract or chronic ocular disease. J Am Vet Med Assoc 214:4 502–507, 1999.
5. Maggs DJ, Nasisse MP: Effects of oral L-lysine supplementation on the ocular shedding rate of feline herpesvirus (FHV-1) in cats. Proceedings of the 28th Annual Meeting of the American College of Veterinary Ophthalmology, Santa Fe, NM, November, 1997, p 101.
6. Nassisse MP, Halenda RM, Luo H: Efficacy of low dose, oral, natural human interferon alpha (nHuIRN") in acute feline herpesvirus-1 infection. A preliminary dose determination trial. Proceedings of the 27th Annual Meeting of the American College of Veterinary Ophthalmology, Newport, RI, November 1996, p 79.
7. Pedersen NC, Elliott JB, Glasgow A, et al: An isolated epizootic of hemorrhagic-like fever in cats caused by a novel and highly virulent strain of feline calicivirus. Vet Microbiol 73:281–300, 2000.
8. Poulet H, Brunet S, Soulier M, et al: Comparison between acute oral/respiratory and chronic stomatitis/gingivitis isolates of feline calicivirus: Pathogenicity, antigenic profile and cross-neutralisation studies. Arch Virol 145:243–261, 2000.
9. Sato R, Inanami O, Tanaka Y, et al: Oral administration of bovine lactoferrin for treatment of intractable stomatitis in feline immunodeficiency virus (FIV)-positive and FIV-negative cats. Am J Vet Res 57:1443–1446, 1996.
10. Sykes JE, Anderson GA, Studdert VP, et al: Prevalence of feline *Chlamydia psittaci* and feline herpesvirus 1 in cats with upper respiratory tract disease. J Vet Intern Med 13:153–162, 1999.
11. White SD, Rosychuk RAW, Janik TA, et al: Plasma cell stomatitis-pharyngitis in cats: 40 cases (1973–1991). J Am Anim Hosp Assoc 200:1377–1380, 1992.

4. FUNGAL INFECTIONS

Stephen J. Dullard, D.V.M.

1. What are the primary upper respiratory fungal pathogens in cats?

Cryptococcus neoformans is the primary fungal pathogen that colonizes the nasal cavity of cats; systemic dissemination occurs in some cats. Rarely, *Aspergillus* spp. or *Penicillium* spp. infect the nasal passages of cats. Other fungal pathogens, such as *Blastomyces dermatitidis*, *Histoplasma capsulatum*, and *Coccidiomyces immitis*, initially colonize the lungs and then disseminate to various sites.

2. What causes cryptococcosis?

C. neoformans is a 3.5–7.0 micron, yeastlike organism with a thick polysaccharide capsule that may approach 30 microns in diameter. The organism reproduces by narrow-base budding. There are two varieties, *C. neoformans* var. *neoformans* and *C. neoformans* var. *gatti*. *C. neoformans* var. *gatti* occurs in tropical and subtropical climates such as Australia and is associated with eucalyptus trees. *C. neoformans* var. *neoformans* is found worldwide and has been associated principally with bird excrement and decaying plant matter. In the United States, southern California has the most cases. Cats of all ages may be affected, with no breed or sex predilection. The initial route of transmission is most likely through inhalation, which most commonly leads to nasal disease. Infection of skin, subcutaneous tissues, eyes, lymph nodes, and central nervous system (CNS) probably results from hematogenous or lymphatic dissemination from the nose. CNS infection also may result from direct invasion across the cribiform plate from the nasal cavity.

3. What factors predispose to cryptococcosis?

Approximately 50% of human cryptococcal infections occur in immunosuppressed patients. In most feline cases, an underlying cause of immune suppression cannot be found, but disseminated disease is more common in FIV-infected cats. Cats should be evaluated serologically for feline leukemia virus antigen and antibodies against feline immunodeficiency virus, although studies have not confirmed an increased prevalence of these viral infections in cats with cryptococcosis. Other predisposing causes may include glucocorticoid administration, neoplasia, or other diseases that compromise the immune system.

4. What are the presenting signs of feline cryptococcosis?

Clinical signs are variable and depend on lesion location. Infection of the nasal cavity resulting in sneezing, nasal obstruction, or nasal discharge occurs in 56–83% of cases. The nasal discharge may be serous, mucopurulent, or hemorrhagic, unilateral or bilateral. Stertorous breathing may result. Granulomatous lesions often arise within the nasal cavity, on the nasal planum, or over the facial bones. In one study, 33% of cases had single or multiple cutaneous or subcutaneous nodules of variable fluctuance. Nodules may ulcerate and exude a serous discharge that forms a crust. Regional lymphadenopathy often develops. Occasionally, ocular manifestations such as granulomatous chorioretinitis, retinal detachment, optic neuritis, lens luxation, or anterior uveitis occur. Ocular and CNS signs occur concurrently in some cats. In approximately 25% of cases of feline cryptococcosis, CNS disease results from diffuse or focal meningoencephalitis. Granulomatous masses may develop within the brain or spinal cord, resulting in signs of depression, ataxia, circling, seizures, blindness, and paresis. Signs of systemic disease, such as fever, weight loss, anorexia, and malaise, are uncommon but possible. Variability in presenting signs may relate to the thick polysaccharide capsule of the organism. The capsule inhibits plasma cell function, phagocytosis, and leukocyte migration, which enhances local infection and may account for the lack of systemic signs.

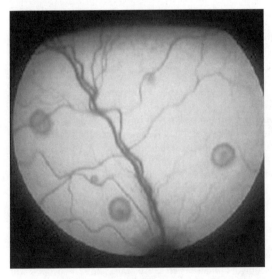

Chorioretinitis from *Cryptococcus neoformans* infection. (Courtesy of Dr. Cynthia Powell, Colorado State University.)

5. How do other nasal fungal diseases of cats manifest themselves?

Only a few cases of feline aspergillosis have been reported. The clinical findings are similar to those associated with cryptococcosis. Most cats have a chronic, unilateral nasal discharge that can be serous, purulent, or hemorrhagic. The disease may become bilateral and involve the sinuses or cribiform plate. Orbital cellulitis was reported in 1 case. Systemic mycoses such as blastomycosis, histoplasmosis, and coccidioidomycosis rarely are associated with nasal disease.

6. What are differential diagnoses for nasal fungal infections?

Other diseases to consider for cats with unilateral nasal discharge include nasal tumors, dental disease, oronasal fistula, nasopharyngeal polyps, and foreign bodies (see Chapter 1). Causes of bilateral nasal discharge include viral respiratory disease, nasal tumors (advanced disease), allergic rhinitis, cleft palate, and extranasal causes. Rarely, bacterial infections are the primary cause of disease; *Bordetella bronchiseptica, Mycoplasma* spp., and *Chlamydia psittaci* are most likely (see Chapter 2). Most bacterial infections result from damage caused by a primary disease process.

7. Which diagnostic tests should be performed initially to establish a diagnosis of nasal fungal disease?

Nonregenerative anemia and monocytosis are the most common hematologic abnormalities; biochemical panels are usually normal. Definitive diagnosis of nasal cryptococcosis can be made by demonstrating the organism cytologically. Microscopic examination of stained thin smears of nasal exudates or fine-needle aspiration of granulomas, cutaneous lesions, and lymph nodes often yields organisms. Cryptococcal organisms can be identified with routine hematologic stains, but new methylene blue, Gram stain and periodic acid-Schiff (PAS) provide better contrast. The capsule does not absorb staining and appears as a large, clear halo around the organism. The smaller and narrow-base budding helps to differentiate *C. neoformans* cytologically from *B. dermatitidis,* which tends to be larger (5–20 μm) and reproduces by broad-base budding.

Branching, septate fungal hyphae seen on 10% KOH wet mounts or thin smears of nasal discharge stained with new methylene blue or with routine hematologic stains suggest nasal aspergillosis. However, because the organism has been reported as a normal contaminant of the nasal cavity in dogs, presence of only a few hyphae should not be used to make a definitive diagnosis.

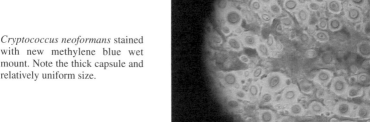

Cryptococcus neoformans stained with new methylene blue wet mount. Note the thick capsule and relatively uniform size.

8. How can serology aid in the diagnosis of fungal rhinitis?

Cryptococcal antigen can be detected in serum, aqueous humor, or cerebrospinal fluid in most cats with cryptococcosis via the latex cryptococcal antigen test (LCAT) or enzyme-linked immunosorbent assay (ELISA). Measurement of antibody is not useful. LCAT detects antigen from the polysaccharide capsule produced by the organism. Positive titers appear within 3 weeks of infection and strongly support the diagnosis. False-negative results can occur with acute disease, low-grade chronic infections, nondisseminated disease, and drug-induced remission without complete clearance. The incidence of false-positive and false-negative titers in cats is unknown. False-positive results have been reported in humans with *Klebsiella* infection or positive rheumatoid factor. Because the organism usually is demonstrated, serum antigen testing for *C. neoformans* is rarely needed to confirm the diagnosis. However, most authorities recommend measurement of titers for monitoring treatment (see question 14). Measurement of antibodies against *Aspergillus* spp. by agar gel immunodiffusion confirms exposure but not active disease. The percentage of cats with nasal aspergillosis that are seropositive is unknown.

9. What is the further diagnostic plan for cases of suspected fungal rhinitis for which a diagnosis is not made cytologically?

Definitive diagnosis of the cause of chronic nasal disease is made with the combination of radiology (computed tomography, if available), rhinoscopy, periodontal probing, histopathologic evaluation of nasal tissue, and, potentially, bacterial and fungal culture (see Chapter 1).

10. What radiographic abnormalities are seen with fungal rhinitis?

Radiographic abnormalities seen with cryptococcal infections are usually nondestructive with increased soft tissue/fluid opacity in the nasal cavities or sinuses. Occasionally, bony lysis in the nasal cavity and overlying tissues of the maxilla is seen. Thoracic radiographs are often normal but may reveal diffuse to miliary interstitial lung patterns with hilar lymphadenopathy. Radiographs in feline nasal aspergillosis may reveal turbinate bone loss, punctate bone lysis, and increased fluid opacity in the nasal cavity and sinuses due to secretions or direct fungal involvement.

11. What endoscopic abnormalities are associated with fungal rhinitis?

Typically, cryptococcal infection results in space-occupying granulomas with variable amounts of nasal discharge. These masses and the surrounding discharges should be sampled and examined cytologically because *C. neoformans* usually is found in high numbers in aspirates or biopsies. Infection by *Aspergillus* spp. often results in white, black, or yellow-green fungal plaques located within the turbinates. Granulation tissue or increased turbinate space resulting from destructive rhinitis may be seen. Necrotic debris and mucus may fill the turbinates and obscure visualization initially.

12. When is fungal culture useful in the diagnosis of fungal rhinitis?

In establishing a definitive diagnosis, fungal culture should be performed on any infected material, such as swabs from nasal or cutaneous exudates, aspirates of lesions, cerebrospinal fluid, or biopsy specimens. *C. neoformans* and *Aspergillus* spp. can be cultured from the nasal cavity of healthy cats; thus, a disease association cannot be based on positive cultures alone. Materials for culture should be placed in a media suitable for supporting the growth of fungi during transport to the laboratory.

13. How is cryptococcosis treated?

Several drugs have been used in the treatment of cryptococcosis—most frequently, ketoconazole, itraconazole, fluconazole, 5-flucytosine, and amphotericin B alone or in combination. Because ketoconazole commonly causes anorexia, vomiting, diarrhea, weight loss, and increased activity of liver enzymes, it is rarely used in cats. Oral fluconazole and itraconazole have been successfully used with minimal toxicity. Cats receiving 100 mg/day of itraconazole occasionally develop anorexia, depression, and increased alanine aminotransferase activity; these findings are rare at doses of 50 mg/day. Because of expense, most clinicians choose itraconazole. Fluconazole should be given to cats with CNS involvement because it is superior to itraconazole for penetrating the blood-brain barrier. Treatment with either agent should continue at least 1–2 months after resolution of clinical signs. Cats with immunosuppressive diseases may require longer-term therapy.

Antifungal Drugs Used in the Management of Feline Fungal Rhinitis

DRUG	DOSAGE
Amphotericin B	0.25 mg/kg, IV, 3 times/week*
	0.5-0.8 mg/kg SQ 2 times/week†
Amphotericin B (lipid or liposomal)	0.5 mg/kg IV as test dose, then 1.0 mg/kg IV 3–5 times/week‡
Fluconazole	50 mg PO every 12–24 hr

Table continued on following page

Antifungal Drugs Used in the Management of Feline Fungal Rhinitis (Continued)

DRUG	DOSAGE
Flucytosine	50 mg/kg PO every 8 hr
Ketoconazole	10 mg/kg PO SID
Itraconazole	5 mg/kg PO twice daily for 4 days; then 5 mg/kg PO SID

IV = intravenously, SQ = subcutaneously, PO = orally, SID = one time daily.
* In cats with normal renal function, dilute in 50–100 ml 5% dextrose and administer IV over 3–6 hours.
† Mixed in 0.45% saline and 2.5% dextrose. Total volume of 400 ml in cats and 500 ml in dogs. Subcutaneous route rarely leads to sloughing of tissues and is less toxic than IV route. To date, this regimen has been reported primarily for *C. neoformans*.
‡ Dilute the contents of a vial with 5% dextrose to a final concentration of 1.0 mg/ml, and shake for 30 seconds. Draw up needed volume, and filter through an 18-gauge monoject filter needle into 100 ml of 5% dextrose. Infuse IV over 15 minutes. (Abelcet, Liposome Co., Princeton, NJ.)

14. How is antigen testing used to monitor treatment of cryptococcosis?

Antigen titers can be used to monitor effectiveness of therapy because titers parallel severity of disease. Effective therapy and a good prognosis are indicated by a decline in antigen titer. Serum cryptococcal antigen titers are monitored every 1–2 months to evaluate treatment. Preferrably cats should be treated until serum antigen negative, however, many cats have had resolution of clinical disease but maintained serum titers. This may be suggestive of persistent infection, lack of susceptibility to a given antifungal agent, or a false positive titer. If this occurs, switching to a different treatment drug is indicated. If low titers are seen for several months, treatment can be discontinued. Titers can be monitored and treatment reinstituted if titers increase or clinical signs reoccur.

15. What should I do if my feline patient fails to respond to itraconazole or fluconazole?

Failure to respond to triazole therapy may be due to a number of reasons. For example, cure may be more difficult in immunosuppressed cats or cats with central nervous system (CNS) or ocular infections. Resistance to one triazole (itraconazole or fluconazole) does not confer resistance to the other, and a trial of an alternate drug in this class may be attempted.

In cats with poorly responsive CNS cryptococcosis, flucytosine can be administered concurrently with a triazole or amphotericin B. Flucytosine may cause vomiting, diarrhea, hepatotoxicity, cutaneous eruptions, and bone marrow suppression.

Amphotericin B also can be used to treat resistant cases, including those with CNS involvement. Regular amphotericin B administered intravenously is rarely used in cats because of renal toxicity. Use of liposomal or lipid encapsulated amphotericin B appears to be less toxic because of its renal epithelial cell-sparing effect. For clients unable to afford liposomal or lipid encapsulated amphotericin B, a subcutaneous protocol has proved to be safe and effective (see table in question 13).

16. What is the prognosis for cryptococcosis?

Most cats with nasal cryptococcosis can be cured or controlled. The prognosis is more guarded for those with ocular or CNS involvement.

17. Are cats with nasal cryptococcosis or aspergillosis a public health risk?

Infection by these organisms is acquired from the environment. There is minimal to no risk of acquiring infection from contact with affected cats (see Chapter 89).

BIBLIOGRAPHY

1. Flatland B, et al: Clinical and serologic evaluation of cats with cryptococcosis. J AmVet Med Assoc 209:1110–1113, 1996.
2. Jacobs GJ, et al: Cryptococcal infection in cats: Factors influencing treatment outcome, and results of sequential serum antigen titers in 35 cats. J Vet Intern Med 11:1–4, 1997.

3. Lappin M: Polysystemic mycotic diseases. In Nelson RW, Couto CG (eds): Small Animal Internal Medicine, 2nd ed. St. Louis, Mosby, 1998, pp 1302–1312.
4. Legendre AM, Toal RL: Diagnosis and treatment of fungal diseases of the respiratory system. In Bonagura JD (ed): Kirk's Current Veterinary Therapy XIII. Philadelphia, W.B. Saunders, 2000, pp 815–819.
5. Malik R, et al: Asymptomatic carriage of *Cryptococcus neoformans* in the nasal cavity of dogs and cats. J Med Vet Mycol 35:27–31, 1997.
6. Malik R, et al: Combination chemotherapy of canine and feline cryptococcus using subcutaneously administered amphotericin B. Aust Vet J 73:124–128, 1996.
7. Malik R, et al: Cryptococcosis in cats: Clinical and mycological assessment of 29 cases and evaluation of treatment using orally administered fluconazole. J Vet Med Mycol 30:133–144, 1992.
8. Malik R, et al: Nasopharyngeal cryptococcosis. Aust Vet J 75:483–488, 1997.
9. Medleau L, et al: Evaluation of ketoconazole and itraconazole for treatment of disseminated cryptococcosis in cats. Am J Vet Res 51:1454–1458, 1990.
10. Medleau L: Feline cryptococcus. In Kirk RW (ed): Current Veterinary Therapy X. Philadelphia, W.B. Saunders, 1989, pp 1109–1111.
11. Medleau L, et al: Itraconazole for the treatment of cryptococcosis in cats. J Vet Intern Med 9:39–42, 1995.
12. Rogers KS: Cytology of nasopharyngeal diseases. In August JR (ed): Consultations In Feline Internal Medicine, vol. 2. Philadelphia, W.B. Saunders, 1994, pp 279–286.
13. Wolf AM, Troy GC: Deep mycotic diseases. In Ettinger SJ, Feldman EC (eds): Textbook of Veterinary Internal Medicine, 4th ed. Philadelphia, W.B. Saunders, 1995, pp. 439-463.

5. NASOPHARYNGEAL POLYPS

Julia K. Veir, D.V.M.

1. What are nasopharyngeal polyps?
Benign, pedunculated masses typically arising from the middle ear. They are composed of a core of loosely arranged fibrovascular tissue covered by an epithelial layer that varies from stratified squamous to ciliated columnar epithelium. The core has scattered plasma cells, lymphocytes, and, occasionally, neutrophils. Sometimes there are small numbers of mucous secreting cells just beneath the surface, which is commonly ulcerated.

2. Why do nasopharyngeal polyps form?
No one really knows. The most popular theory currently is that they are secondary to an inflammatory stimulus, possibly associated with upper respiratory tract infections. In early case series, most cats were very young, leading to the hypothesis that they were remnants of the branchial arches.

3. What clinical signs are commonly associated with nasopharyngeal polyps?
Clinical signs depend on the physical location. The overwhelming number of cases are unilateral, although bilateral disease has been reported in the literature. Most polyps arise from the eustachian tube, protrude through the tympanic membrane into the middle ear, and extend into the nasopharynx or grow in both directions. Polyps in the middle ear and external ear lead to otitis interna, media, and externa. Signs range from mild otic discharge to constant head shaking with or without signs of vestibular disease (circling, head tilt), as well as Horner's syndrome or facial nerve paralysis. Polyps that grow into the naso- and oropharynx are associated with respiratory signs (stertorous breathing, wheezing, chronic nasal discharge, and sneezing) and oropharyngeal signs (dysphagia, gagging, and retching).

4. What is the typical signalment of cats with a nasopharyngeal polyp?
Cats with nasopharyngeal polyps are typically young. The reported median age of onset varies between 3 and 5 years. However, polyps have been reported in cats as old as 14 years. Gender and breed predilections have not been reported.

5. How do I diagnose nasopharyngeal polyps?

Because polyps can grow into the middle ear, otic examination may reveal a bulge or discoloration of the tympanic membrane. Polyps protruding through the tympanic membrane can be visualized by otic examination. Nasopharyngeal polyps sometimes can be palpated through the soft palate. Polyps in the nasopharyngeal or oropharyngeal regions sometimes can be seen on oral examination under anesthesia. Retraction of the soft palate rostrally with a spay hook helps to visualize polyps confined to the nasopharynx, and direct visualization is usually possible with caudal rhinoscopy using a flexible endoscope. Lateral skull radiographs can reveal a mass lesion in the nasopharyngeal region. Radiographs of the bullae usually are obtained to detect middle ear involvement and to assist in decisions about surgical treatment. Radiographs demonstrate a soft tissue opacity in the middle ear canal or bulla, and the bulla is often thickened. Computed tomography also can be used to delineate the tissues involved.

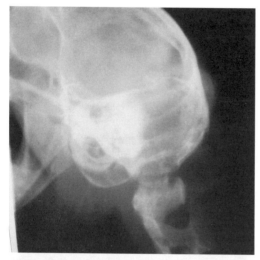

Plain radiographs of the bulla of a cat with a nasopharyngeal polyp. Note the thickened bulla wall.

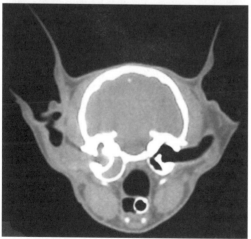

Computed tomography scan showing a nasopharyngeal polyp in the middle ear and external ear canal.

6. How are nasopharyngeal polyps treated?

Physical removal of the polyp is the only proven method of treatment. External ear canal and nasopharyngeal polyps can be removed successfully by the traction-avulsion technique that requires little expertise or special equipment. Removal is performed under general anesthesia. For polyps in the nasopharynx, the mass is visualized via retraction of the soft palate with a spay hook. Alternately, stay sutures can be placed in the soft palate to aid in manipulation. The soft palate usually does not need to be surgically incised unless the polyp is very large.

Polyps in the external ear canal can be visualized with an otoscope. The mass is grasped as close to the base of the stalk as possible, using an endoscopic cup biopsy instrument, alligator forceps, towel forcep, or hemostat, and pulled out with steady, firm traction. If bulla involvement is detected radiographically, surgical removal is performed via a ventral bulla osteotomy (VBO). The bulla is approached via the lateral aspect of the skull, the mass is removed, and the epithelial lining is curetted.

7. What is the recurrence rate after treatment with the traction-avulsion technique?

Polyps removed by simple traction-avulsion recur in about 40% of affected cats. Because recurrence with traction-avulsion is more common in cats with evidence of bulla involvement at the time of diagnosis, the author currently recommends VBO as the initial treatment in such cats. However, VBO requires an increased level of technical skill and a longer anesthetic period, has an increased chance of postoperative complications, and can be much more expensive for the owner. Risks and benefits of each option should be discussed with the owner.

8. What complications are associated with removal of nasopharyngeal polyps?

In some cats, polyps are quite large at diagnosis and occlude the oropharynx. If the polyp is in the oropharynx, endotracheal intubation can be difficult. Difficulty in gaining control of the airway during anesthetic induction can be life-threatening, and the need for an emergency tracheostomy should be anticipated. Little blood loss should be associated with removal of a nasopharyngeal polyp. Postoperatively, ipsilateral Horner's syndrome is not uncommon. It is usually transient, especially with the simple traction-avulsion technique, but may be permanent with VBO. Facial nerve paralysis and head tilt are also common postoperative complications that are usually transient but may be permanent.

9. What postoperative care is recommended after polyp removal?

If facial nerve paralysis is present after polyp removal, lubrication for the affected eye is mandatory until the problem resolves. Peri- and postoperative antibiotics for otitis media should be continued until results of culture and sensitivity testing of the removed tissue are available and for at least 21 days if the culture is positive.

10. What is the overall prognosis for cats with nasopharyngeal polyps?

Overall, the prognosis for surgical removal of a polyp is excellent, and a dramatic improvement in clinical signs is evident almost immediately after removal. Owners should be aware that some cats develop a polyp on the other side.

BIBLIOGRAPHY

1. Allen HS, Broussard J, Noone KE: Nasopharyngeal diseases in cats: A retrospective study of 3 cases (1991–1998). J Am Anim Hosp Assoc 35:457–461, 1999.
2. Bedford PG: Origin of the nasopharyngeal polyp in the cat. Vet Record 110:541–542, 1982.
3. Kapatkin AS, Matthiesen DT, Noone KE, et al: Results of surgery and long-term follow-up in 31 cats with nasopharyngeal polyps. J Am Anim Hosp Assoc 26:387–392, 1990.
4. Little CJ: Nasopharyngeal polyps. In August JR (ed): Consultations in Feline Internal Medicine, vol. 3. Philadelphia, W.B. Saunders, 1997, pp 310–316.
5. Parker NR, Binnington AG: Nasopharyngeal polyps in cats: Three case reports and a review of the literature. J Am Anim Hosp Assoc 21:473–478, 1985.
6. Pope ER: Feline inflammatory polyps. Semin Vet Med Surg (Small Anim) 10:87–93, 1995.

6. CONFORMATIONAL DISEASES

Lynelle Johnson, D.V.M., Ph.D.

1. What types of conformational diseases of the respiratory tract are seen in cats?
Conformational disorders of the respiratory tract may be structural or functional, congenital or acquired, and can be encountered at different levels of the respiratory tract.

2. Define the most common examples of conformational disease in the upper respiratory tract.
Stenotic nares is a congenital conformational abnormality of the upper respiratory tract.

Elongated, cleft, or deformed soft palate is usually a congenital lesion, but deformation may result from trauma.

Nasopharyngeal stenosis can be congenital but more often is due to chronic rhinitis. It has been proposed that chronic inflammation from rhinitis stimulates production of a web of scar tissue across the caudal opening of the nasal cavity.

Pharyngeal mucocoele is a rare cause of upper respiratory obstruction and respiratory distress due to a structural lesion.

Laryngeal paralysis is a functional conformational disease, in which a normally mobile structure has been rendered immobile and dysfunctional by peripheral or central damage to the recurrent laryngeal nerve. Damage may occur with trauma to the neck, iatrogenic injury to the recurrent laryngeal nerve (during thyroidectomy or other neck surgeries), or compression, infiltration, or interruption of the caudal laryngeal nerve anywhere in its course from the vagus trunk. In some cats, laryngeal paralysis may be a congenital condition.

3. Define the most common conformational lesions in the lower respiratory tract.
Bronchial dysgenesis is a rare conformational abnormality caused by malformation of the bronchial tree. Progressive signs of respiratory difficulty may be apparent, or the cat may be relatively asymptomatic, depending on the extent of involvement of lower airways.

Bronchiectasis, an irreversible dilatation of the airways, is more common in males than in females and results from long-standing inflammatory diseases of the lower airways. It does not appear to be primarily responsible for clinical signs, but it may worsen the clinical course of disease.

Cats with a **bronchoesophageal fistula** may have a history of recurrent pneumonia or present acutely with aspiration pneumonia. If the fistula is acquired secondary to a foreign body in the esophagus, a long history of dysphagia, gagging, or excessive salivation may be present.

4. Describe the typical signalment of cats affected by conformational diseases.
Brachycephalic cats may be predisposed to conformational abnormalities in the upper respiratory tract because of the breed preference for shortening of facial features. A true brachycephalic syndrome has not been reported, but it is wise to be aware that signs can occur in Persian and Himalayan cats. Cats with congenital lesions usually are presented at a young age, but the possibility of a congenital lesion should not be ruled out solely on the basis of age. Owners may fail to notice that the cat has a respiratory problem until later in life because of inexperience with pet ownership. Alternatively, owners may acquire an adult cat with a previously undiagnosed lesion, or a mild problem that was recognized at an early age may suddenly worsen because of concurrent disease.

5. Describe the typical history of cats with conformational diseases.
Cats with upper airway lesions such as stenotic nares or elongated, deformed, or cleft soft palate usually are presented for signs of abnormal, difficult, or noisy breathing. In mildly affected cats, signs may be apparent only with exercise. In contrast, bilateral laryngeal paralysis generally causes marked signs of respiratory distress at rest, and owners often note a voice change, dysphagia, coughing, or anorexia. The cause of laryngeal paralysis is inapparent in most cats, but questions

should be raised about a recent history of neck surgery, difficult intubation, or trauma to the neck. Acquired nasopharyngeal stenosis is more often found in older cats with a history of chronic rhinitis. Historically, such cats have longstanding, recurrent upper respiratory signs, such as sneezing and nasal discharge, that are gradually replaced by signs related to nasal obstruction.

6. What are common presenting complaints in cats with conformational diseases?

Presenting complaints depend on the site within the respiratory tract that is affected. Open-mouth breathing is a nonlocalizing sign because it can occur with respiratory distress at any level of the pulmonary system and can be seen in cats that are stressed. However, cats that are unable to breathe with the mouth held closed generally have disease of both nasal passages or the nasopharynx.

7. What complaints suggest conformational disease of the upper respiratory tract?

Diseases of the upper respiratory tract usually lead to loud and abnormal breathing sounds such as stertor and stridor. Stertor resembles a snoring noise and is heard when passage of air through the nose or pharynx is obstructed, as may occur with stenotic nares or an elongated soft palate. With an elongated soft palate, intermittent airway obstruction or stertor may be observed by the owner. Stridor classically is associated with laryngeal paralysis. Cats with laryngeal disease often present with a history of a voice change and inspiratory dyspnea.

8. What complaints suggest conformational disease of the lower respiratory tract?

Bronchial dysgenesis may lead to progressive signs of tachypnea and respiratory distress associated with obstruction of the airways. Cats with bronchoesophageal fistula may present with recurrent pneumonia associated with the presence of gastrointestinal organisms on airway culture. Clinical signs can include lethargy, depression, anorexia, and a respiratory pattern consistent with pneumonia. Eating or drinking may exacerbate clinical signs.

9. What physical examination abnormalities are seen in cats with stenotic nares?

Stenotic nares can be difficult to identify because the opening to the rostral portion of the nasal cavity is naturally small in cats. Significant breed variations in appearance also make it impossible to construct guidelines for the diagnosis. Young kittens should be examined carefully at each veterinary visit to assess the alar opening, particularly in brachycephalic breeds such as Himalayan and Persian. Normally, the opening to the nasal cavity increases slightly as the cat grows, and the kitten should have no difficulty with nasal respiration. Stenotic, slit-like openings to the nasal cavity cause difficulty in inspiration and may be associated with noisy respirations and increased effort on inspiration.

10. What physical examination abnormalities suggest obstruction of both nasal passages or obstruction of the caudal nasopharynx?

Cats with obstruction of both nasal passages (due to a mass lesion or bilateral nasopharyngeal polyps) or obstruction of the caudal nasopharynx (due to a mass or stenosis) can present with open-mouth breathing (see Chapter 5). Open-mouth breathing may be associated with respiratory distress, or the cat may simply hold its mouth slightly open at all times. In the latter case, it can be difficult to tell that the cat fails to breathe through the nose until it is forced to do so by closing the mouth. Nasal airflow should be assessed by holding a cooled microscope slide in front of the nose and watching for condensation or by holding a wisp of cotton in front of each naris and looking for subtle movement of the cotton. Airflow should be assessed as present or absent bilaterally or as decreased or absent unilaterally.

11. Describe the physical examination findings associated with palatal abnormalities.

Cats with palatal abnormalities may present with nasal discharge from passage of oral contents into the nasal cavity. After drinking, the cat can be observed for nasal discharge or sneezing. A deformed or cleft soft palate can be visible on physical examination but often requires sedation for complete evaluation. Stertor that varies in character as the soft palate obstructs respiration may be the most obvious physical examination finding in cats with an elongated soft palate. Stertor can be difficult to distinguish from stridor. Stridor is usually a more continuous sound and has less of a musical quality. Stridor and inspiratory dyspnea are suggestive of laryngeal paralysis. The cat with stridor should be closely examined for signs of neck injury.

12. Describe the physical examination findings of conformational lesions in the lower respiratory tract.

Cats with bronchiectasis or bronchial dysgenesis usually present with expiratory effort because both diseases are associated with obstructed airways. Cats with pneumonia secondary to a bronchoesophageal fistula typically have an increased respiratory rate, mild tracheal sensitivity, and crackles on auscultation. Fever may or may not be present.

13. What differential diagnoses should be considered in cats with conformational respiratory diseases?

Upper respiratory signs may be due to infectious or inflammatory diseases of the nasal cavity or mass lesions (abscess, granuloma, parasites, neoplasia) in the nose, pharynx, larynx, or trachea. **Lower respiratory signs** may indicate bacterial or aspiration pneumonia, asthma, pleural effusion, or congestive heart failure; however, auscultation and percussion findings usually help to rule out causes other than pneumonia.

14. How are stenotic nares and cleft palate diagnosed?

Stenotic nares and cleft palate can be diagnosed on visual inspection. Because the finding of an elongated soft palate is subjective and requires surgical correction, a full oral and laryngeal examination should be performed under anesthesia for accurate diagnosis.

15. Describe the diagnosis of nasopharyngeal stenosis.

Diagnosis of nasopharyngeal stenosis is relatively easy if a flexible endoscope can be retroflexed into the caudal nasopharynx to allow visualization of the caudal opening of the nares. Generally, this opening should be 5–6 mm across, and the nasal turbinates are seen on each side of the nasal cavity. In cats with nasopharyngeal stenosis, the opening to the nasal cavity is reduced by a fibrous web of tissue, and the caudal aspect of the turbinates cannot be visualized. The narrowed region can be present at any location within the nasopharynx. If an endoscope is not available, a spay hook should be used to retract the soft palate rostrally while a dental mirror is used to examine the nasopharynx (see Chapter 1). The patency of the ventral nasal meatus also can be assessed by attempting to pass a tom-cat catheter through the nasal cavity into the pharynx, similar to the way that a nasogastric tube is passed. Care should be taken to ensure that the catheter goes ventrally rather than into the dorsal meatus, which terminates in the ethmoid turbinates and brain. If an obstruction is met at the appropriate level within the ventral meatus, nasopharyngeal stenosis should be considered.

16. How is laryngeal paralysis diagnosed?

Laryngeal examination is generally quite straightforward in cats because of their marked laryngeal sensitivity. A light plane of anesthesia is induced (by giving $1/4$–$1/2$ the calculated dose of thiobarbiturate), and the arytenoid cartilages should be seen to abduct with inspiratory motions. Paresis or paralysis may be unilateral or bilateral. Thoracic and cervical radiographs are often abnormal in cats with laryngeal paralysis and are indicative of obstructive airway disease. Abnormalities included caudal displacement of the larynx, lung hyperinflation, and aerophagia.

17. How are conformational diseases of the lower respiratory tract diagnosed?

Evidence of bronchial dysgenesis and bronchiectasis may be visible radiographically, but definitive diagnosis requires histologic studies. A high index of suspicion is required for clinical diagnosis. It can be difficult to obtain a definitive diagnosis of pneumonia caused by a bronchoesophageal fistula. Radiographic changes may be similar to those expected in aspiration pneumonia, particularly if the fistula occurs in the dependent lung field or the middle lung lobes, which are common sites of aspiration. An atypical location for aspiration pneumonia, along with suggestive clinical findings, should encourage suspicion for a bronchoesophageal fistula. The presence of megaesophagus or an esophageal diverticulum in the region of a pulmonary infiltrate also should be considered suspect.

18. What other tests may be required in cats with conformational respiratory diseases?

To achieve a definitive diagnosis of bronchoesophageal fistula, an esophagram may be required. Fluoroscopy can reveal dynamic reflux of contrast material from the esophagus into the airways, or static radiography may be used to define a connection between the gastrointestinal and respiratory tracts.

19. Describe the management of stenotic nares and conformational diseases of the palate.

Stenotic nares can be opened by wedge resection of part of the alar fold. A deformed soft palate may require reconstructive surgery or use of an implant to close the defect. An elongated soft palate is trimmed to an appropriate length; complete apposition of mucosal edges should be ensured to avoid dehiscence. Trimming the palate too short should be avoided because it can lead to dysphagia.

20. How is nasopharyngeal stenosis managed?

Management of nasopharyngeal stenosis is problematic because the tough, fibrous band of tissue is difficult to break down and often reforms after surgery. Methods used to remove the obstruction include balloon dilation of the stricture, laser removal of excessive scar tissue, use of a stent to increase the diameter of the opening, conventional surgery to open the lesion, and surgical resection of the affected region with placement of a mucosal advancement flap to cover the defect. Variable results are encountered, and a tracheostomy may be required to allow adequate respiration.

21. Describe the management of laryngeal paralysis.

Treatment of laryngeal paralysis can involve lateralization of the arytenoid (as in dogs) or occasionally tracheostomy. Thus far, reasonable quality of life has been reported in cats treated with surgery.

22. How are bronchoesophageal fistulas and bronchiectasis managed?

A bronchoesophageal fistula requires surgical resection. Similarly, if bronchiectasis of a single lung lobe is believed to be contributing to clinical signs, lung lobectomy should be considered.

23. What is the expected treatment response in cats with conformational respiratory diseases?

In cats with stenotic nares and cleft or elongated soft palate, surgery is usually curative. Generally, cats with laryngeal paralysis respond well to treatment, although occasionally tracheostomy is required. Cats with nasopharyngeal stenosis are more problematic because excessive fibrous tissue can reform after the stricture is opened. Little clinical information is available about these cases, but control of inflammation and infection in the area is essential. Antibiotics effective against primary and secondary pathogens should be used. Doxycycline or enrofloxacin may be used to control *Bordetella bronchiseptica* and *Mycoplasma* spp. infections; these drugs are also effective against some of the normal upper respiratory flora. Coverage against anaerobes also should be considered, and long-term therapy is recommended in cats with chronic rhinitis (see Chapter 2). Anti-inflammatory dosages of corticosteroids may help to control excessive deposition of scar tissue, although the risk for poor wound healing at other surgical sites must be considered. Cats with bronchiectasis or bronchial dysgenesis require management of obstructive airway disease.

BIBLIOGRAPHY

1. Basher AWP, Hogan PF, Hanna PE, et al: Surgical treatment of a congenital bronchoesophageal fistula in a dog. J Am Vet Med Assoc 199:479–482, 1991.
2. Griffon DJ, Tasker S: Use of a mucosal advancement flap for the treatment of nasopharyngeal stenosis in a cat. J Small Anim Pract 41:71–73, 2000.
3. Larue MJ, Garlick DS, Lamb CR, et al: Bronchial dysgenesis and lobar emphysema in an adult cat. J Am Vet Med Assoc 197:886–888, 1990.
4. Mitten RW: Acquired nasopharyngeal stenosis in cats. In Bonagura JD, Kirk RW (eds): Current Veterinary Therapy XI. Philadelphia, W.B. Saunders, 1992, pp 801–803.
5. Norris CR, Samii VF: Clinical, radiographic, and pathologic features of bronchiectasis in cats: 12 cases (1987–1999). J Am Vet Med Assoc 216:530–534, 2000.
6. Novo RE, Kramek B: Surgical repair nasopharyngeal stenosis of in a cat using a stent. J Am Anim Hosp Assoc 35:152–156, 1999.
7. Schachter S, Norris CR: Laryngeal paralysis in cats: 16 cases (1990–1999). J Am Vet Med Assoc 216:1100–1103, 2000.

7. NASAL TUMORS

Stephen J. Dullard, D.V.M.

1. How common are nasal tumors in cats?

They represent approximately 1% of all tumors and 75% of all respiratory tumors in cats. Of primary nasal tumors, 80% are malignant; local invasion of surrounding tissue is the main biologic feature. Distal metastases are rarely found at the time of diagnosis (< 10%) but may occur late in the disease. The most common sites of metastases are regional lymph nodes, lung, and brain. Paraneoplastic syndromes are rarely associated with nasal neoplasia. Benign nasal tumors are quite rare, but inflammatory polyps (which have the gross appearance of a tumor) are common in cats (see Chapter 5). Males have twice the risk of females for developing a nasal tumor.

2. What are the most common types of feline nasal tumors?

Tumors of epithelial origin are more common than tumors of mesenchymal origin. Squamous cell carcinoma (SCC) is the most common type, followed by adenocarcinoma and lymphoma. Lymphoma of the nasal cavity can be solitary or part of a multicentric neoplastic disease. The most common types of mesenchymal tumors are osteosarcoma, fibrosarcoma, and chondrosarcoma.

3. What are the clinical signs of a nasal tumor?

Nasal tumors usually occur in older patients, but younger cats can be affected. SCC usually develops on the planum of the nose. Prolonged exposure to ultraviolet light results in preneoplastic changes to the nonpigmented planum, such as ulceration, crusting, swelling, and erythema. Tumor formation results in slow, progressive local invasion of the nasal cavity with destruction of underlying soft tissues and bone. In one study of 90 cats with nasal planum SCC, 73% had some white skin or hair. White-haired cats have a 13.4 times greater risk of developing SCC than cats of other colors.

Other tumors and advanced SCC often elicit a nasal discharge (unilateral or bilateral), sneezing, epistaxis, stertor, pain on examination of the nose or mouth, deformation of the facial bones or hard palate, and regional lymphadenopathy. Weight loss and anorexia may be evident. Rarely, the patient may present with neurologic disease (seizures, abnormal mentation) or ocular abnormalities (exophthalmos), which result from direct invasion of the cranial vault or orbit.

4. What nasal discharge is associated with tumors?

The nasal discharge can be serous, mucoid, mucopurulent, or hemorrhagic. One or both nostrils may be involved. Bilateral disease is suggestive of more extensive involvement, and often one side has more discharge than the other. History should note if the condition initially was unilateral and progressed. This observation may help to direct further examination to one side vs. the other.

5. How can nasal airflow be assessed?
Assessment of nasal airflow is easily accomplished by placing a cold microscope slide in front of the nasal planum and observing for symmetrical condensation on the slide.

6. What are the differential diagnoses for nasal tumors?
The main differential diagnoses for unilateral nasal discharge are nasal fungal infections, dental disease, oronasal fistula, nasopharyngeal polyps, and foreign bodies (see Chapter 1). Causes of bilateral nasal discharge include viral respiratory disease, fungal infections, allergic rhinitis, cleft palate, and extranasal diseases. Differentials for early SCC include pemphigus, mycoses, plastic dish syndrome, solar dermatitis, eosinophilic granuloma complex, and other rare skin diseases.

7. What diagnostic tests should be performed?
All patients should have a complete blood count, serum chemistry profile, and urinalysis to detect systemic disease. Definitive diagnosis is based on identifying abnormal tissue on the nasal surface or within the nasal cavity on physical examination, radiographs, rhinoscopy, fine-needle aspiration, or computed tomogram (CT). Once the abnormal tissue is identified, it must undergo biopsy and histologic examination. If lymphadenopathy is present, needle aspiration with a cytologic examination or biopsy of the lymph node is warranted. If lymphoma is suspected, the cat should be tested for feline leukemia and feline immunodeficiency virus. Cytologic examination of bone marrow and abdominal radiographs or ultrasound should be performed to determine the stage of the disease (see Chapter 68).

8. What is the best radiographic view for evaluating nasal disease?
Open-mouth ventral dorsal radiographic views are essential in evaluating patients with nasal disease. The open-mouth procedure requires anesthesia but allows radiographic evaluation of the entire nasal cavity without interference of the mandible as well as separate visualization of both nasal cavities. The use of ultraspeed nonscreen dental occlusal film sheets (2.25" × 3") works well in cats and allows detailed evaluation of the turbinates. The patient is placed in dorsal recumbency with the head parallel to the table. The x-ray tube is angled 10–15° from its normal position with the beam centered on the hard palate of the opened mouth. The head should be as centered and as parallel to the table as possible.

A lateral open-mouth view may be helpful in identifying a nasopharyngeal mass lying dorsal to the soft palate. Because such masses often originate in the middle ear, the bullae should be examined as well (see Chapter 5). Obtaining radiographs of the maxillary arcade of teeth using a bisecting angle technique allows evaluation of tooth roots to rule out sinusitis as a cause for nasal discharge. Thoracic radiographs should be taken to detect metastatic pulmonary disease.

9. What radiographic lesions are seen with nasal tumors?
Radiographs may show evidence of turbinate, vomer bone, or facial bone lysis. Deviation or lysis of the nasal septum may occur. Soft tissue mass lesions may be present along with increased fluid opacity of the nasal cavity resulting from increased nasal secretions. However, these findings are not diagnostic for nasal neoplasia because chronic rhinitis can result in similar radiographic changes.

10. What lesions are seen on rhinoscopy?
Rhinoscopy should be performed anteriorly through the naris and posteriorly over the soft palate, using a flexible endoscope or a dental mirror and light source. It is important to rule out masses in the nasopharyngeal region. On rostral rhinoscopy, the nasal cavity should be evaluated for increased or decreased air space. Neoplastic masses grow between the turbinates and decrease nasal air space. Frequently, nasal neoplasms elicit marked inflammation of the nasal mucosa with secondary bacterial or fungal infections. The nasal cavity may be filled with large

amounts of nasal discharge that must be flushed and suctioned to provide adequate visualization. Any mass lesions must be biopsied.

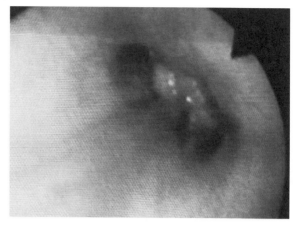

Chondrosarcoma occluding right and left posterior choanal openings.

11. How should a suspected mass be biopsied?

Suspicious areas should be biopsied with either an alligator cup biopsy forcep, Tru-cut biopsy needle (Travenol Laboratories, Inc., Deerfield, IL), or a sharpened plastic tube fashioned from the protective sleeve of an intravenous catheter or spinal needle. The sharpened tip of the plastic tube is forced into the suspected mass and rotated; a negative pressure is applied with a 12-ml syringe; and then the plastic tube is withdrawn. The biopsy instrument should never pass caudal to the medial canthus of the eye to avoid penetration of the cribiform plate and brain.

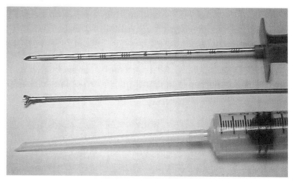

Different types of biopsy instruments: Tru-cut biopsy device, endoscopic biopsy forcep, and tissue core biopsy device made from a polypropylene catheter and a 12-ml syringe.

12. What should you do if lesions are not identified but neoplasia is still suspected?

Some cases of neoplasia are not diagnosed on initial examination. Diagnostic tests may need to be repeated in 1–3 months when a definitive diagnosis is not made but signs of nasal disease persist. Because viral respiratory disease is a common differential diagnosis in cats, client education about follow-up examinations and disease differentials is important. Observation of type, location, and change in nasal discharge volume should be attempted. CT may be recommended because it detects soft tissue changes that may not be evident on radiographs or endoscopy.

13. Can a diagnosis be made cytologically?

Care should be taken in diagnosing nasal neoplasia based on cytology. Chronic inflammation and metaplastic changes within the nasal cavity may cause alterations in cytology that mimic neoplasia. Some tumors can have similar cytologic characteristics, leading to incorrect classification and improper treatment. All nasal tumors should have histologic confirmation.

14. When should CT or magnetic resonance imaging be used?

Whenever possible, because they are more sensitive in detecting and determining the extent of abnormal tissue within the nasal cavity and paranasal sinuses than conventional radiography. In recent years, they have become increasingly available.

15. Once diagnosed, how are intranasal tumors treated?

Because most nasal tumors are malignant, the recommended treatment is usually radiation therapy with or without surgical debulking. Surgery alone does not prolong survival time; in fact, it may shorten survival times.

Chemotherapy can be used for tumors that do not respond to radiation or when radiation therapy is not a viable option. Carboplatin and various multiagent chemotherapy protocols for carcinomas can be tried. Cisplatin (which is toxic to cats) has resulted in palliation of clinical signs in some dogs for up to 12 months. Piroxicam, given orally at 0.3 mg/kg every 48 hours, has been used for treatment of epithelial tumors of the nasal cavity when the owner cannot afford other modalities. Liver, clotting and renal functions should be evaluated periodically because piroxicam is a potent nonsteroidal anti-inflammatory agent.

Lymphoma can be treated with various chemotherapy protocols or radiation (see Chapter 68). Local radiation avoids the systemic adverse effects of chemotherapy, but chemotherapy is recommended to minimize the development of systemic lymphoma. Cats with localized intranasal lymphoma had disease-free intervals that lasted more than 500 days.

16. How does radiation therapy affect survival in cats with nasal tumors?

Few studies have been performed in cats with intranasal tumors, but in dogs receiving localized radiation median survival times improved substantially from 8 to 36 months. Dogs receiving no therapy usually live < 6 months. In one study of cats receiving 48 Gy of telecobalt or orthovoltage radiation, survival times ranged from 1–36 months. The 1-year survival rate was 44.3%, and the 2-year survival rate was 16.6%. In another study, cats receiving orthovoltage radiation after rhinotomy had mean and median survival times of 27.9 and 20.8 months, respectively. Survival rates were 66% at 1 year, 44% at 2 years, and 33% at 3 years.

17. How should SCC of the nasal planum be treated?

SCC of the planum, if detected early, can be treated by surgical removal of the planum, localized radiation, photodynamic therapy, or carboplatin/cisplatin intralesional injection. If surgical resection is contemplated, advanced imaging techniques are recommended to assess extent of disease.

18. How is surgical resection done?

Surgical resection involves the removal of the planum, the underlying cartilage, and a portion of the turbinates. Surgical margins should be submitted for histopathology to ensure tumor-free borders. This procedure is well accepted by cats and owners as a treatment modality. In one series of 9 feline cases treated with aggressive resection of the planum, the median postoperative tumor-free period was 16 months with a range of 1–27 months.

19. How successful is localized radiation for treatment of SCC?

In cats with localized SCC of the nasal planum (1–2 cm diameter), 1-year control rates of 85% have been reported with localized radiation. Survival times for deeply invasive SCC tumors have improved with higher dose and modified dose-fractionation schemes. After irradiation, 1- and 5-year progression-free survival rates were 60.1 and 10.3%, respectively.

20. What is photodynamic therapy?

Photodynamic therapy is a new modality for cutaneous tumors. It involves the use of laser light to activate a dye that absorbs light and produces oxygen radicals that destroy surrounding tissue. The dyes themselves are nontoxic and have the advantage of localizing in abnormally proliferating tissues in preference to normal tissue. Cure rates in a group of 60 cats with SCC were reported at 60–90%. This modality is used for superficial tumors.

21. How is chemotherapy used for SCC?

Carboplatin or cisplatin given intralesionally has caused remission of small tumors. Cisplatin (10 mg in 1 ml of saline) may be mixed with 2 ml of sterilized sesame oil and injected intralesionally. Of cats treated with this regimen, 83% had > 50% reduction in tumor volume; complete resolution was reported in 64% of cats after 6 treatments with a similar protocol using cisplatin and a collagen-matrix vehicle. Because of the depot nature of the treatments and slow release of cisplatin, the systemic toxicity typically seen with cisplatin was not noted. Carboplatin has been used in a similar manner, resulting in a complete remission rate of 73% and a 1-year control rate of 55%. Carboplatin is safer to use in cats and can also be given as a systemic treatment.

22. What is the overall prognosis for nasal tumors?

The prognosis for cats with untreated malignant nasal tumors is poor. Survival is usually a few months. Persistent dyspnea, epistaxis, anorexia, weight loss, and neurologic signs are often reasons for euthanasia.

Radiation treatment is well tolerated, improves survival, provides palliation of clinical signs, and improves the quality of life in many cats. Reported adverse reactions to radiation therapy include radiation-induced dermatitis, cataract formation, and nasocutaneous fistula.

SCC of the planum can be cured if aggressive treatment is instituted before deep invasion of the nose. Early skin changes (crusting or hyperemic plaques) should be investigated immediately to obtain a diagnosis. A "wait-and-see" approach is not appropriate.

Prognosis for lymphoma is difficult to provide for individual cats (see Chapter 68). Important prognostic factors include stage of disease, anatomic site, response to therapy, and retroviral status.

BIBLIOGRAPHY

1. Beck ER: Shedding light on feline cancers: Photodynamic therapy on the brink of the 21st century. Proceedings of the 1997 Fall meeting of the American Association of Feline Practitioners, Atlanta, pp 219–220.
2. Carothers M, Couto CG: Respiratory Neoplasia. In Kirk RW, (ed), Current Veterinary Therapy X. Philadelphia, W.B. Saunders, 1989, pp 399–405.
3. Elmslie RE, Ogilvie GK, Gillette EL, et al: Radiotherapy with and without chemotherapy for the control of localized lymphoma in cats: 10 cases (1983–1989). Vet Rad 32:277–280, 1991.
4. Evans SM, Hendrick M: Radiotherapy of feline nasal tumors: A retrospective study of nine cases. Vet Radiol 30:128–132, 1989.
5. Hahn KA, Anderson TE: Tumors of the respiratory tract. In Bonagura JD (ed): Kirk's Current Veterinary Therapy XIII. Philadelphia, W.B. Saunders, 2000, pp 500–505.
6. Hawkins EC: Disorders of the nasal cavity. In Nelson RW, Couto CG (eds): Small Animal Internal Medicine, 2nd ed. St. Louis, Mosby, 1998, pp 231–232.
7. Ogilvie, GK, Moore AG: Tumors of the respiratory tract. In Managing the Veterinary Cancer Patient. Trenton, NJ, Veterinary Learning Systems, 1995, pp 314–326.
8. Ogilvie, GK, Moore AG: Tumors of the skin and surrounding structures. In Managing the Veterinary Cancer Patient. Trenton, NJ, Veterinary Learning Systems, 1995, pp 479–482.
9. Orenburg EK, Luck EE, Brown DM, et al: Implant delivery system: Intralesional delivery of chemotherapeutic agents for treatment of spontaneous skin tumors in veterinary patients. Clin Dermatol 9:561–568, 1992.
10. Peaston AE, Leach MW, Higgins RJ: Photodynamic therapy for nasal and aural squamous cell carcinoma in cats. J Am Vet Assoc 202:1261–1265, 1993.
11. Ruslander D, Kaser-Hotz B, Sardines JC: Cutaneous squamous cell carcinoma in cats. Comp Cont Educ Pract Vet 19:1119–1129, 1997.
12. Theon AP: Indications and applications of radiation therapy. In Bonagura JD (ed): Kirk's Current Veterinary Therapy XII. Philadelphia, W.B. Saunders, 1995, pp 467–474.
13. Theon AP, Madewell BR, Shearn VI: Prognostic factors associated with radiotherapy of squamous cell carcinoma of the nasal plane in cats. J Am Vet Med Assoc 206:991–996, 1995.
14. Theon AP, Peaston AE, Madewell BR, et al: Irradiation of nonlymphoproliferative neoplasms of the nasal cavity and parasinuses in 16 cats. J Am Vet Assoc 204:78–83, 1994.
15. Theon AP, VanVechten MK, Madewell BR: Intratumoral administration of carboplatin for treatment of squamous cell carcinomas of the nasal plane in cats. Am J Vet Res 57:205–210, 1996.
16. Withrow SJ, Straw RC: Resection of the nasal planum in nine cats and five dogs. J Am Anim Hosp Assoc 26:219–222, 1990.

8. COUGH AND DYSPNEA: INITIAL DIAGNOSTIC PLAN

Michael R. Lappin, D.V.M., Ph.D.

1. What is a cough?

The forceful expulsion of air from the lungs. Coughing is a normal physiologic response to airway irritation. Irritant receptors from the oropharynx throughout the airway epithelium can stimulate the afferent pathway, resulting in cough. Receptor density is greatest in the larynx and major lobar airways. Foreign body contact with the airway epithelium stimulates mechanoreceptors. Exogenous chemicals (e.g., smoke) and endogenous chemicals (e.g., histamine) stimulate chemoreceptors. It is possible that all causes of cough induce bronchospasm, which then acts as the primary stimulus to the cough receptors.

2. What are the physiologic components of a cough?

The vagus and glossopharyngeal nerves carry afferent impulses to the cough center in the dorsolateral region of the medulla. The efferent impulses resulting in cough are carried by the vagal nerves, phrenic nerves, recurrent laryngeal nerves, and some spinal motor nerves. Cough is divided into three phases: respiratory, compressive phase, and expiratory. Once a cough is induced, the animal inspires deeply (respiratory phase). The compressive phase begins with closure of the glottis and contraction of the expiratory musculature. The expiratory phase occurs as the glottis suddenly opens, leading to a sudden flow of air from the lungs through the airways.

3. What are the differential diagnoses for cough?

Differential diagnoses for cough in cats can be categorized into upper airway, lower airway, and cardiovascular causes. Dirofilariasis is the exclusive cardiovascular cause of cough in cats. Cardiac failure leads to dyspnea, not cough, in cats. Diseases resulting in coughing are relatively rare in cats compared with dogs.

Differential Diagnoses for Cough in Cats

Upper respiratory tract disease
Congenital disorders	Irritants
Masses	Foreign body
Allergic	Gastrointestinal disease with nasal aspiration
Anatomic	Infectious diseases (see table in question 7)
Trauma	

Lower respiratory tract disease
Congenital disorders	Dysphagia, vomiting, or regurgitation resulting in aspiration
Masses (neoplastic or granulomatous)	
Allergic	Pulmonary thromboembolic disease (dyspnea more common than cough)
Anatomic	
Irritants	Noncardiogenic pulmonary edema (dyspnea more common than cough)
Foreign body	
Infectious diseases (see table in question 8)	

4. Define dyspnea and orthopnea.

Dyspnea is a state of difficult, labored, or painful breathing. It can occur intermittently or continuously or may be more pronounced after exertion. **Orthopnea** is a state of difficult breathing in a recumbent position.

5. Define tachypnea, polypnea, and hyperpnea.

Tachypnea, polypnea, and hyperpnea describe conditions resulting in increased respiratory rates. **Tachypnea** generally refers to rapid shallow respirations; **polypnea** and **hyperpnea** refer to rapid deep respirations. Tachypnea, hyperpnea, and polypnea do not denote difficult breathing and may be due to physiologic changes.

6. What are the differential diagnoses for dyspnea?

Dyspnea is a pathologic event; conditions resulting in dyspnea can be divided into nasal/sinus diseases, pharyngeal diseases, airway diseases, pulmonary parenchymal diseases, pleural diseases, diseases of the muscles of respiration, diseases affecting erythrocyte oxygen carrying capability, central nervous system diseases, and pain. Several conditions including acidosis, fever, glucocorticoid excess, and psychological anxiety, can cause tachypnea, polypnea, or hyperpnea and are commonly confused with dyspnea.

Differential Diagnoses for Dyspnea in Cats

Cardiac disease	Diaphragmatic diseases
Airway diseases	Hernia
Pulmonary parenchymal diseases	Muscular weakness
Pleural diseases	Neurologic (paralysis)
Pneumothorax	Impingement
Hemorrhage pleural effusions	Organomegaly (especially hepatomegaly)
Transudative pleural effusions	Peritoneal effusions
Modified transudate pleural effusions	Obesity
Pyothorax	Masses
Chylothorax	Erythrocyte diseases
Feline infectious peritonitis	Anemia
Neoplasia	Methemoglobinemia
Peritoneopericardial hernia	Central nervous system diseases

7. What infectious diseases may cause cough and dyspnea in cats?

Infectious Causes of Cough and Dyspnea in Cats

INFECTIOUS AGENT	SYNDROME
Bacterial	
Mycoplasma spp.	URI, pneumonia (??)
Bordetella bronchiseptica	URI, pneumonia (??)
Yersinia pestis	Pneumonia
Chlamydia psittaci	URI
Aerobes and anaerobes	Pyothorax, secondary pneumonia
Viral	
Feline calicivirus	URI, pneumonia in kittens
Feline herpesvirus 1	URI, pneumonia in kittens
Feline leukemia virus	Mediastinal lymphoma, secondary URI or pneumonia
Feline immunodeficiency virus	Mediastinal lymphoma, secondary URI or pneumonia
Feline infectious peritonitis virus	Pleural or peritoneal effusion; granulomatous pneumonia
Fungal (rare in cats)	
Blastomyces dermatitidis	Pneumonia
Cryptococcus neoformans	URI, rarely pneumonia
Histoplasma capsulatum	Pneumonia
Coccidioides immitis	Pneumonia
Aspergillus spp.	URI

Table continued on following page

Infectious Causes of Cough and Dyspnea in Cats (Continued)

INFECTIOUS AGENT	SYNDROME
Parasitic	
Migratory	
Toxocara cati	Small airway disease, pneumonia
Strongyloides stercoralis	Small airway disease, pneumonia
Primary	
Aelurostrongylus abstrusus	Small airway disease, pneumonia
Paragonimus kellicotti	Small airway disease, pneumonia, pneumothorax
Capillaria aerophila	Small airway disease, pneumonia
Polysystemic	
Dirofilaria immitis	Small airway disease, pulmonary embolism
Toxoplasma gondii	Pneumonia

URI = upper respiratory infection.

8. Can the signalment help in ranking the differential diagnoses?

The age, breed, and gender of a cat with cough or dyspnea lends valuable information for localization of lesions and identification of primary differentials. Kittens are more likely than cats to present with congenital abnormalities resulting in cough or dyspnea. Young, nonvaccinated kittens commonly develop respiratory tract infections. Older cats commonly develop neoplasia, cardiac failure, and chronic bronchitis. Cough due to migratory parasitism is more likely in kittens. Feline leukemia virus (FeLV) and feline immunodeficiency virus (FIV) infection can lead to immunosuppression and predispose to infectious causes of respiratory disease. Clinical FeLV and feline infectious peritonitis virus (FIPV) infections are common in young cats; clinical FIV infection is common in older cats. Pulmonic toxoplasmosis is more common in neonatal cats than in older cats. Older cats with cough are likely to have chronic bronchitis and are more refractory to treatment than young cats. Male cats may be more likely to hunt and thus, in the Southwestern states, may become infected with *Yersinia pestis*.

9. How can the history help to rank differentials for cough and dyspnea?

- Severe, acute coughing occurs commonly with exposure to airway irritants, aspiration, foreign body inhalation, and acute infectious diseases.
- Coughing in cats with serous oculonasal discharge and pruritic skin disease that occurs seasonally may suggest allergic lung disease.
- Mucopurulent oculonasal discharge with or without oral erosions suggests feline rhinotracheitis, especially if the cat has been kenneled or a cattery problem is identified.
- Mild cough in cats with low-grade conjunctivitis may be consistent with chlamydiosis.
- Gagging and dysphagia are reported commonly in cats with pharyngeal or laryngeal causes of cough, especially cats with nasopharyngeal polyps.
- Fungal diseases, heartworm disease, and many parasitic diseases depend on travel to endemic areas for exposure.
- Respiratory parasites are more common in outdoor cats than indoor cats.
- Unvaccinated cats, particularly those in contact with other cats, are likely to have infectious causes of cough.
- Dirofilariasis commonly presents with a history of gagging or vomiting as well as cough.
- Slowly progressive cough is common with neoplasia.
- Hemoptysis is most common with dirofilariasis, pulmonary contusions, and neoplasia.
- Cough after eating may indicate diseases inducing dysphagia.

10. What historical evidence suggests respiratory tract abnormalities associated with diseases of other body systems?

Evidence of other clinical abnormalities, such as vomiting (aspiration pneumonia), polyuria/polydipsia (uremic pneumonitis), or weakness (diaphragmatic abnormalities).

11. How should clinical problems be characterized?

Owners should be asked to identify the predominant clinical signs of respiratory disease, including sneezing, nasal discharge, gagging, dysphagia, stridor (wheezing), stertor (snoring or snorting), cough, terminal retch, dyspnea, and tachypnea. They should be questioned to determine whether a perceived cough is truly vomiting, regurgitation, or gagging. Each clinical problem should be characterized for duration, frequency, time of occurrence, and progression. Nasal discharges should be characterized as continuous or intermittent, unilateral or bilateral, whether they occur with sneezing, and whether they are serous, mucoid, mucopurulent, or hemorrhagic.

12. What physical examination findings are most helpful?

A complete physical examination should be performed on all cats with respiratory tract disease, including the following:

- Emaciation commonly occurs with chronic respiratory tract diseases, including dirofilariasis, neoplasia, cardiac failure, and fungal pneumonia.
- Mucous membrane color (cyanotic or pale) and capillary refill time.
- Occasionally cats with gastrointestinal tract disease predisposing to aspiration have abdominal palpation abnormalities or evidence of megaesophagus on evaluation of the cervical region.
- Neurologic abnormalities occur with several causes of respiratory tract disease, including FIPV infection, toxoplasmosis, and systemic mycoses.
- Ocular abnormalities can be seen with infectious diseases (FIPV infection, toxoplasmosis, respiratory viruses, and systemic mycoses) as well as with coagulopathies, hypertension, and diseases inducing vasculitis.
- Abnormalities associated with cardiac dysfunction, including cardiac murmur or gallop rhythm, arrythmias, jugular pulse, jugular distention, tachycardia, weak arterial pulses, muffled heart or lung sounds, pulmonary crackles or wheezes, abdominal fluid wave, and hepatosplenomegaly.
- Lymph nodes should be palpated carefully; lymphadenopathy occurs commonly with lymphosarcoma and systemic mycoses.
- Cats with dyspnea due to uremic pneumonitis commonly have either large kidneys (acute nephrosis) or small kidneys (chronic renal failure) on abdominal palpation.
- The cat should be carefully assessed for evidence of pain; discomfort can lead to dyspnea or tachypnea.
- The nares should be examined for discharge and size. Airflow through the nares can be estimated by holding a cool microscope slide over the nares and observing the area of vapor condensation.
- The oral cavity should be evaluated carefully for evidence of masses, dental disease, phlegm, tonsillar changes, or foreign bodies.
- The skull should be palpated for evidence of trauma or asymmetry (tumor or fungal disease).
- The trachea and larynx should be gently palpated to assess for tracheal cough or masses.

13. How should respiratory patterns be assessed?

Respiratory rate should be assessed at rest and after minimal exercise. The respiratory rate should be 10–30 breaths/minute and should be effortless with minimal abdominal component. An abdominal press or increased expiratory time is characteristic of obstructive airway disease or asthma. If the respiratory rate or character is abnormal, attempt to characterize whether the primary abnormality is dyspnea, tachypnea, or orthopnea. An abnormal respiratory pattern should be characterized as **obstructive** (slow and deep) or **restrictive** (rapid and shallow). Respiration should be evaluated carefully for the presence of stertor or stridor. Stertor occurs most commonly with diseases of the nasal cavity, sinuses, and pharynx. Stridor occurs with laryngeal and tracheal diseases. Inspiratory stridor is most common with laryngeal paralysis and extrathoracic tracheal collapse. Inspiratory and expiratory stridor occur most commonly with fixed lesions of the larynx and trachea.

14. Discuss the proper technique for thoracic auscultation.

The thorax should be palpated gently for rib fractures, evidence of discomfort, compressibility (which can be decreased in cats with mediastinal disease), and evidence of cardiac thrill and or a decreased apex beat. Thoracic auscultation is best performed in a quiet room on a cat that is not panting or trembling. The respiratory tract should be ausculted prior to cardiac auscultation, and the trachea should be auscultated to differentiate lower respiratory tract wheezes or crackles from referred sounds from the trachea.

15. What are the relevant findings of respiratory tract auscultation?

Normal breath sounds vary based on the respiratory pattern, site of auscultation, and thickness of the thoracic wall. Normal breath sounds are designated as bronchial, vesicular, and bronchovesicular. Bronchial sounds are heard predominantly in the perihilar area and trachea; they are relatively loud and easy to detect. Bronchial sounds are slightly louder on expiration and the expiratory phase is slightly longer than the inspiratory phase. Vesicular sounds develop in the lobar and segmental bronchi and can be heard distal to the perihilar area. These sounds are described as similar to the rustling sound made by wind blowing through trees and are more prominent on inspiration than expiration. Bronchovesicular sounds are generated in the terminal airways and alveoli and are very soft or difficult to hear. These sounds are heard at the periphery of the thoracic cavity. Crackles, wheezes, or absence of breath sounds are abnormal. Crackles (rales) sound like crumpling cellophane and can be inspiratory, expiratory, or continuous. Crackles are most commonly induced by fluid in the alveoli or inflammatory diseases of the small airways. End-inspiratory crackles are consistent with fluid in the alveoli. Right-side and dependent lung lobe crackles are consistent with aspiration pneumonia. Wheezes (rhonchi) are continuous musical sounds heard best on expiration. Wheezes are most commonly heard with diseases of the airways. Cats with asthma often breathe with their neck extended and may appear to have a "barrel chest."

16. What findings of thoracic auscultation suggest cardiac disease?

In dyspneic cats, crackles may suggest hypertrophic cardiomyopathy. If crackles are due to cardiac disease, cardiac murmurs and elevated heart rate are usually present concurrently, and affected cats rarely cough.

17. What do muffled or absent breath sounds suggest?

They occur most commonly with diaphragmatic hernia, pleural effusions, pneumothorax, obesity, consolidated lung lobes, and collapsed lung lobes.

18. What is the differential diagnosis for wet vs. dry cough?

With the exclusion of bacterial bronchopneumonia, cats rarely develop moist or productive coughs. Dry cough occurs commonly with pharyngeal diseases, laryngeal diseases, tracheal diseases, and low-grade inflammation induced by allergic and parasitic etiologies.

19. Can a tracheal cough help to localize the lesion?

The presence of pharyngeal, laryngeal, or tracheal inflammation does not correlate only with upper airway disease; lower airway inflammation results in passage of inflammation cells up the mucociliary apparatus to the mouth, leading to secondary inflammation of the upper respiratory tract. This possibility precludes the use of a tracheal cough to localize the lesion; tracheal cough can occur just as readily with bacterial pneumonia as with a tracheal foreign body.

20. What is the initial diagnostic plan for most coughing cats?

After assessment of the signalment, history, and physical examination, diagnostic tests are commonly performed to identify the primary cause of the cough or dypsnea. Primary causes of cough in cats include asthma, heartworm disease, bacterial bronchitis, and respiratory parasitism. The initial diagnostic plan for coughing cats in a nonendemic area for dirofilariasis generally consists of a complete blood count (CBC), fecal examination, and thoracic radiographs.

In endemic areas for dirofilariasis, *Aelurostrongylus abstrusus*, or *Paragonimus kellicotti*, heartworm serology, Baermann assessment of feces, and fecal sedimentation, respectively, are performed as well. Further diagnostic testing depends on the results of these procedures.

21. What is the initial diagnostic plan for most dyspneic cats?
    The initial diagnostic plan for evaluation of dyspnea is based on the severity of clinical disease at presentation combined with signalment, physical examination, and history findings. Most cases ultimately require thoracic radiographs. Thoracocentesis may be necessary. Arterial blood gas assessment is indicated in some stable, dyspneic cats with pulmonary parenchymal diseases.

22. Which should be performed first—thoracic radiographs or thoracocentesis?
    This is one of the most important clinical decisions made by veterinary practitioners. Although relatively safe, thoracocentesis is not indicated for most causes of dyspnea. However, thoracocentesis is diagnostic as well as therapeutic for dyspnea due to pleural effusion or pneumothorax (see Chapters 13–15). The veterinary clinician should evaluate the signalment, history, and physical examination findings carefully; if evidence consistent with pneumothorax or pleural effusion is present, thoracocentesis should be performed as the initial diagnostic procedure. If dyspneic cats exhibit a restrictive breathing pattern and diminished breath sounds, thoracocentesis should be performed as soon as possible. If the clinician chooses to perform thoracic radiographs as the initial diagnostic procedure, oxygen should be delivered by facemask and a single dorsoventral radiograph should be made for evaluation of pneumothorax or pleural effusion.

23. How should cats be stabilized before performing diagnostic procedures?
    All cats with dyspnea should be stabilized before performing diagnostic procedures. The minimal stress associated with venipuncture, thoracocentesis, or thoracic radiographs is enough to induce cardiopulmonary arrest in many cats with severe compromise. Delivery of oxygen by facemask or, preferably, oxygen cage for 15–20 minutes often stabilizes dyspneic animals adequately to allow performance of minimal diagnostic tests.

24. How can the CBC aid in the diagnosis of cough or dyspnea in cats?
    Most cats with upper airway inflammation have normal leukograms. An inflammatory leukogram with or without a left shift is most common with bacterial pneumonia and pyothorax. However, the lack of an inflammatory leukogram does not rule out bacterial colonization of the lower airways. All cats with bacterial inflammation of the lower respiratory tract should be evaluated for the presence of an underlying etiology especially FeLV and FIV. Lymphopenia is commonly induced by FeLV and FIV and may be present in immunosuppressed cats. Monocytosis is also a component of a stress leukogram and so can be hard to interpret. Persistent monocytosis is consistent with chronic inflammation and occurs with many chronic respiratory diseases. Monocytosis is commonly identified in cats with dirofilariasis. Eosinophilia and basophilia most commonly occur with asthma, dirofilariasis and respiratory parasites. However, eosinophilia and basophilia also occur commonly with allergic and parasitic diseases of the skin and gastrointestinal tract. Cats with respiratory disease and eosinophilia or basophilia should be evaluated with heartworm serology; thoracic radiographs; transtracheal wash for cytology, culture, and sensitivity testing; fecal flotation and sedimentation (in areas endemic for *Paragonimus* spp.); and Baermann examination of feces.

25. When should you perform a serum biochemical panel or urinalysis in cats with cough or dyspnea?
    Occasionally cats with uremic pneumonitis present with cough; azotemia is noted on the biochemical panel. The serum biochemical panel should be used to screen all older cats with bacterial lower respiratory disease. Hyperglobulinemia occurs with some diseases of the respiratory tract, particularly, dirofilariasis, chronic bronchitis, neoplasia, and toxoplasmosis. All cats with cough and hyperglobulinemia should be evaluated for dirofilariasis. Total carbon dioxide is an indirect

measurement of serum bicarbonate and can be used to estimate acid-base status. Hypoalbuminemia can result in a transudative pleural effusion; the biochemical panel can be used to screen for potential abnormalities. Urinalysis should be performed in any cat for which a serum biochemical panel is justified. Proteinuria occurs most commonly with dirofilariasis, fungal diseases, retroviruses, FIPV, and neoplasia. However, any chronic antigenic stimulation in the respiratory tract may result in the production of circulating immune complexes, deposition at the glomerular basement membrane, and induction of proteinuria.

26. What are the major thoracic radiographic abnormalities in alveolar lung disease?

Alveolar lung disease is characterized by air bronchograms that develop as the alveolar sacs fill with fluid and outline air-filled airways. Air bronchograms occur most commonly with cardiogenic pulmonary edema, neurogenic pulmonary edema, bacterial bronchopneumonia, eosinophilic inflammation, and hemorrhage. Air bronchograms are seen occasionally with atelectatic lungs and granulomatous diseases. In general, a transtracheal wash should be performed in cats with cough and air bronchograms without physical or radiographic evidence of cardiac disease. Toxoplasmosis is a cause of alveolar lung disease in neonatal cats.

27. Discuss the significance of bronchial patterns.

Bronchial patterns develop as the peribronchiolar tissues become inflamed. Inflammation of the peribronchiolar tissues results in "doughnuts," or air-filled circles surrounded by soft-tissue density. Bronchial patterns develop most commonly with inflammation of the airways. Irritant gases, allergic disease, viral disease, and some bacterial diseases commonly lead to a bronchial pattern. Most cats with asthma have a marked bronchial pattern.

28. Discuss the significance of interstitial patterns.

The pulmonary interstitium is the supporting network of the lungs. The pulmonary blood supply courses through the interstitial space. Interstitial patterns can be divided into the following categories:

Diffuse interstitial patterns appear as an increased soft tissue density in the interstitium and may occur in older cats as a result of normal aging. Interstitial disease develops in the first stages of cardiogenic pulmonary edema. Mycoplasmal pneumonia can cause a diffuse interstitial pattern. Any cause of vasculitis or coagulopathy can present with a diffuse interstitial pattern.

Miliary interstitial patterns are characterized by 1–5-mm masses and occur most commonly with fungal disease and metastatic neoplasia.

Nodular interstitial patterns are characterized by 0.5–1-cm masses and are most common with fungal disease, metastatic neoplasia, and primary pulmonary neoplasia.

Tumorous interstitial patterns are characterized by masses > 1 cm and are most common with primary pulmonary neoplasia.

29. How do you assess for vascular patterns?

In the **dorsoventral or ventrodorsal radiograph**, the artery is located laterally, followed medially by the bronchus and vein. Pulmonary venous hypertension occurs most commonly with hypertrophic cardiomyopathy. Pulmonary arterial hypertension occurs most commonly with dirofilariasis. In the **lateral thoracic radiograph**, the cranial lobar artery is most dorsal, followed ventrally by the bronchus and vein.

30. What pleural diseases may result in restrictive breathing patterns?

Usually restrictive breathing patterns are associated with pneumothorax, pleural effusions, mass lesions, or diaphagmatic abnormalities.

31. When should an airway washing be performed?

Airway washings should be performed after assessment of the thoracic radiographs and is indicated for all coughing cats with interstitial, bronchial, or alveolar lung patterns that are not suspected to be due to cardiogenic disease or coagulopathy. The goal of transtracheal washing (TTW) is to collect fluids from the lower airways for cytology, culture, and sensitivity testing.

32. How should airway secretions be collected?

Bronchoscopy with bronchoalveolar lavage is the most sensitive technique but requires general anesthesia and a bronchoscope. Because cats commonly develop subcutaneous emphysema and pneumomediastinum after TTW, it is preferable to use a transoral approach. Materials needed include a sterile catheter or feeding tube (6 or 7 French), 2% lidocaine, sterile saline, sterile swab, transport media (Portacul, Bectin-Dickinson Microbiology Systems, Franklin Lakes, NJ), syringes, needles, and microscope slides.

33. How is transoral TTW performed?

1. Intravenous administration of 10–30 mg of ketamine (100 mg/ml) and an equal volume of diazepam (5 mg/ml) generally provides enough sedation to intubate the animal successfully but not to ablate the cough response.

2. After administration of ketamine and diazepam, place 1 drop of 2% lidocaine on each arytenoid.

3. Place the cat in sternal recumbency, and intubate with a sterile 3.5 tracheal tube, taking care to avoid contact with the oral cavity.

4. The carina is located approximately at the point where the elbow crosses the midthoracic region. Measure from this point up the trachea to estimate how far to insert the TTW catheter.

5. After intubation and placement of the sterile catheter, instill 2–3 ml sterile saline. As you are injecting, encourage the cat to cough by tracheal manipulation or thoracic compression.

6. After injection of saline, immediately aspirate with the sterile collection syringe. Recovered saline should contain respiratory secretions that are easily visualized as flocculent material.

7. The tracheal washing can be repeated up to 3–4 times until an adequate sample is obtained; 0.5–1.0 ml provides sufficient fluid for most analyses.

8. The washing can be performed in right or left lateral recumbency; if a unilateral lesion is present, place the diseased side down.

9. After collection of respiratory secretions, place a sterile swab into the fluid; then place the swab into the Portacul for aerobic culture, mycoplasmal culture, and antibiotic susceptibility testing.

10. The remainder of the respiratory secretions can be used for cytologic evaluation. Direct smears and cytospins are generally performed. Examine for infectious agents, including intracellular bacteria, white blood cells, and neoplastic cells.

11. Administer 100% oxygen through the tracheal tube while in sternal recumbency until ready to be extubated.

34. What are the most common abnormalities noted on cytology of airway washings in cats?

The presence of eosinophils is consistent with asthma, parasitism, and granulomatous disease. Neutrophils and macrophages are commonly increased with bacterial disease, and intracellular bacteria may be present, indicating bacterial infection. Bacteria can be found in airway washings from healthy cats because they are commonly present at the carina. The presence of a positive bacterial culture with no evidence of neutrophils on cytologic examination is difficult to interpret. Parasitic larvae are commonly identified by TTW. Neoplastic cells are sometimes retrieved, and pulmonary involvement of lymphoma can be documented. Fungal elements can be found in some cases.

35. When is transthoracic aspiration biopsy indicated?

Primary indications for transthoracic aspiration biopsy are interstitial (including masses) or alveolar diseases that were not diagnosed by cytology of transoral washings. This technique is more dangerous than TTW because of the increased risk for development of pneumothorax or hemothorax, particularly in cats with severe cough or dyspnea.

36. What materials are required for transthoracic aspiration biopsy?

Twenty-two–gauge spinal needles, 2% lidocaine, clipper blades, surgical preparation solutions, sterile saline, culturette, transport media, syringes, needles, and microscope slides.

37. How is transthoracic aspiration biopsy performed?

1. Use the thoracic radiographs or ultrasound to identify the area to be aspirated.

2. Entry through the seventh, eighth, or ninth intercostal space is preferred to avoid great vessels, large airways, and the liver.

3. Choose a spinal needle of appropriate length.

4. Clip a 3 × 3-cm area over the entry site, and perform a surgical preparation.

5. Administer 0.25–0.5 ml of 2% lidocaine subcutaneously over the entry site.

6. Position the spinal needle so that the entry avoids the periosteum (pain) and caudal area of the ribs (vessels).

7. Pass the needle on a single plane to the depth calculated for the aspiration.

8. Remove the stylet, place a sterile syringe, and aspirate. It is generally safe to advance the needle inward on a single plane, but do not move laterally.

9. Remove the needle from the animal.

10. Place a small amount of the aspirated material on a sterile swab and place in a Portacul; make thin smears with remainder of the aspirate.

11. Request aerobic, anaerobic, and mycoplasmal culture as well as antibiotic susceptibility testing from the Portacul and routine cytologic assessment of the thin smears.

12. If a poor yield is obtained, the aspirate can be repeated with injection of 0.5 ml of sterile saline before aspiration to mobilize respiratory cells and secretions.

38. When is transthoracic biopsy indicated?

Transthoracic biopsies are reserved for cases with nodular to tumorous interstitial lung disease for which airway washing and transthoracic aspiration fails to give a diagnosis. A primary indication is to differentiate granulomatous disease from neoplasia. Sedation or anesthesia is required. Biopsies are generally obtained by passing a small biopsy forceps (Biopty, CR Bard, Covington, GA) through the intercostal space into the mass. Primary disadvantages include hemothorax and pneumothorax. The procedure is performed as described for transthoracic aspiration. Ultrasound, fluoroscopy, or thoracoscopy should be used to help guide the biopsy instrument, if available. For solitary masses, surgical excision is often recommended for diagnosis and potential cure.

39. When should ultrasound be used in the work-up of coughing or dyspneic cats?

Echocardiography is a valuable aid for the diagnosis of cardiac diseases such as cardiomyopathy or pericardial effusion that may result in dyspnea. *Dirofilaria immitis* can be seen in the main pulmonary artery of many infected cats by ultrasound (see Chapter 10). Ultrasound can be used to identify diaphragmatic hernia or diaphragmatic-pericardial hernia. Transthoracic biopsy can be guided by ultrasound. Ultrasonic evaluation of the mediastinum can be used to document mass lesions.

BIBLIOGRAPHY

1. Hawkins EC: Clinical manifestations of lower respiratory tract disorders. In Nelson RW, Couto GC (eds): Small Animal Internal Medicine, 2nd ed. St. Louis, Mosby, 1998, pp 249–253.
2. Hawkins EC: Diagnostic tests for the lower respiratory tract. In Nelson RW, Couto GC (eds): Small Animal Internal Medicine, 2nd ed. St. Louis, Mosby, 1998, pp 254–284.

9. SMALL AIRWAY DISEASE

Elisa M. Mazzaferro, M.S., D.V.M.

1. What is feline asthma?

Feline asthma is a syndrome characterized by acute bronchoconstriction leading to cough and/or respiratory distress. Clinical signs may require immediate therapy or may resolve without treatment. The exact cause of asthma in cats has not been determined.

2. How does feline asthma differ from chronic bronchitis?

Chronic bronchitis is a condition in which other causes of cough, such as pneumonia, heartworm infestation, bronchopulmonary neoplasia, and lungworm infection, have been ruled out. Cats with chronic bronchitis typically cough on a daily basis for at least 2 months of the year. The cough associated with chronic bronchitis is usually refractory to bronchodilator therapy. **Asthma** is a disorder characterized by acute bronchoconstriction that causes signs ranging from intermittent coughing to life-threatening respiratory distress. The cat with asthma commonly has asymptomatic periods between episodes of respiratory signs. Usually the signs associated with asthma in the cat are exquisitely responsive to bronchodilator therapy.

3. What unique features of the feline pulmonary system predispose to asthma?

The feline pulmonary system is unique in that airway smooth muscle can be found distally as far as the alveolar duct. In addition, the ratio of airway smooth muscle to bronchial wall thickness is greater in cats than in other examined species. Feline bronchioles are abundant in goblet cells, and inflammatory stimulation results in mucus accumulation. Cilia extend to just beyond the level of mucus-producing structures.

4. Are certain breeds of cats predisposed to developing asthma?

Feline asthma has been documented in cats of all breeds and ages. The Siamese cat, however, may have an increased incidence of bronchial disease compared with the general cat population, suggesting a genetic predisposition.

5. What predisposing factors may contribute to development of chronic lower airway disease in cats?

- Congenital abnormalities in structure and function of airway cilia
- Parasitic infestation of the tracheobronchial tree
- Mycoplasmal infection
- Viral or bacterial infection
- Exposure to noxious substances or inhaled irritants
- Immune-mediated or allergic phenomena
- Airway hyperreactivity

6. What are the most common presenting complaints in cats with asthma?

Mild-to-moderate cough, wheezing, open-mouthed breathing, exercise intolerance or lethargy, or acute respiratory distress.

7. What is the pathogenesis of clinical signs in cats with asthma or bronchial disease?

Inflammation probably plays a key role in feline small airway disease. Mast cell degranulation and eosinophil–lymphocyte interactions result in the release of mediators and cationic proteins that affect the epithelium and smooth muscle. The respiratory epithelium responds to irritating or inflammatory stimuli by hypertrophy, metaplastic change, and erosion or ulceration. The underlying smooth muscle layer also becomes hyperplastic, and in some cats airway hyperreactivity is present. Such changes cause a reduction in the size of the airway lumen, and small changes in airway diameter cause tremendous increases in airway resistance. Increased airway resistance and inflammatory airway disease lead to clinical signs.

8. What are the mediators of bronchoconstriction in cats?

Studies in experimentally induced feline airway disease suggest that serotonin release from mast cells causes smooth muscle contraction in vitro. This response may result in bronchoconstriction and respiratory distress in cats with asthma. Stimulation of histamine receptors commonly causes bronchoconstriction in dogs and humans; however, cats have different histamine receptors within the airways. Activation of histamine receptors in cats may have no effect, cause bronchoconstriction, or result in bronchodilation. The role of leukotrienes in airway constriction in cats is unclear.

9. What physical examination findings are associated with asthma in cats?

Physical examination in cats with acute respiratory distress can be dangerous because handling can easily exacerbate dyspnea. Physical examination findings range from a normal respiratory pattern at rest to severe expiratory dyspnea. Tachypnea, adventitious lung sounds, increased tracheal sensitivity, and crackles or wheezes on auscultation are often present. Marked expiratory difficulty with an expiratory push may be apparent in severe cases. Some cats may develop a barrel-shaped appearance to the thorax or show decreased thoracic compressibility.

10. What are the most appropriate emergency treatments for cats with asthma?

Emergency therapy for cats presenting with respiratory distress includes administration of oxygen and use of minimal restraint or manipulation. Small changes in airway diameter with bronchodilating agents can cause rapid and marked improvement in the clinical signs of dyspnea associated with a feline asthmatic crisis. In addition to oxygen, bronchodilator therapy with subcutaneous terbutaline (0.01 mg/kg) or intramuscular aminophylline (4 mg/kg) can be used. Nebulization of terbutaline (0.01 mg/kg in deionized water) in a small oxygen cage also may be beneficial. If respiratory distress persists after 5–10 minutes of observation, rapidly acting glucocorticoids are administered to decrease airway inflammation. When the patient's respiratory pattern is more stable, diagnostic tests such as bloodwork and radiographs can be performed.

Emergency and Long-term Therapy for Feline Asthma

DRUG	DOSE	EMERGENCY OR LONG-TERM	MECHANISM
Antibiotics			
Chloramphenicol	12.5–20mg/kg PO every 12 hr	Long-term (2–4 wk)	Antibiotic
Doxycycline	5 mg/kg PO every 12–24 hr	Long-term (2–4 wk)	Antibiotic and anti-inflammatory
Enrofloxacin	5 mg/kg PO every 24 hr	Long-term (2–4 wk)	Antibiotic
Bronchodilators			
Aminophylline	4 mg/kg IM	Emergency	Phosphodiesterase inhibitor; increased or decreased histamine release, decreased release of slow-acting subtance of anaphylaxis, pulmonary smooth muscle relaxation
	5 mg/kg PO every 8–12 hr	Long-term	
Terbutaline	0.01 mg/kg SC	Emergency	Beta agonist, smooth muscle relaxation
	0.625 mg PO every 12 hr	Long-term	
Theophylline	50–100 mg/cat PO every 24 hr	Long-term	As for aminophylline
Epinephrine	20 mg/kg SC, IV, IM, or IT	Emergency	Beta agonist, smooth muscle relaxation

Table continued on following page

Emergency and Long-term Therapy for Feline Asthma (Continued)

DRUG	DOSE	EMERGENCY OR LONG-TERM	MECHANISM
Glucocorticoids			
Dexamethasone SP	1–2 mg/kg SC, IV, IM	Emergency	Anti-inflammatory, decreases eosinophil chemotaxis and adherence, decreases cytokine production
Dexamethasone	0.25 mg/kg PO every 8–24 hr; then taper to every 48 hr for 1–2 mo	Long-term	As for dexamethasone SP
Prednisolone	1 mg/kg PO every 12 hr for 10–14 days; then taper to 2.5 mg/kg every 48 hr	Long-term	As for dexamethasone SP
Prednisone sodium succinate	50–100 mg/cat IV 0.1–0.625 mg/kg PO every 12 hr	Emergency Long-term	As for dexamethasone SP
Triamcinolone	0.11 mg/kg PO every 12–24 hr, then taper; *or* 0.11 mg/kg SQ and repeat in 7–14 days if necessary	Long-term	As for dexamethasone SP
Others			
Cyclosporine-A	10 mg/kg PO every 12 hr	Long-term	Decreases activtated T-lymphocyte function
Cyproheptadine	2 mg/cat PO every 12 hr	Long-term	Serotonin antagonist, decreases smooth muscle contraction, may cause bronchodilation
Zafirkulase	5 mg PO every 12 hr	Long-term	Leukotriene D4 and E4 antagonist

PO = orally, IM = intramuscularly, SC = subcutaneously, IT = intratracheally, IV = intravenously.

11. What diagnostic tests should be performed in cats with asthma?
- Complete blood cell count
- Serum biochemistry profile
- Thoracic radiographs
- Occult heartworm test in endemic areas
- Fecal flotation and Baerman examination for parasite ova and larvae (see Chapter 11)
- Airway sampling for cytology and culture (see Chapter 8)

12. What are the radiographic signs of feline asthma?
- Bronchial markings with "doughnuts" and "tram lines" (see figure on following page)
- Hyperlucent lung areas
- Flattening and caudal displacement of the diaphragm
- Air trapping and hyperinflation
- Right middle lung lobe atelectasis with mediastinal shift to the right

13. Define bronchiectasis.
Bronchiectasis is the irreversible dilation of bronchi due to destruction of the airway wall from inflammation. Occasionally, these airway changes may be visible on radiographs. Bronchiectasis may be secondary to chronic bronchitis in cats.

14. What changes may be observed in airway fluid from cats with asthma?
Cats with airway disease have increased numbers of inflammatory cells in airway fluid, and the number of cells in bronchial fluid appears to correlate with the severity of clinical disease.

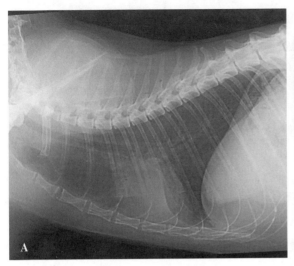

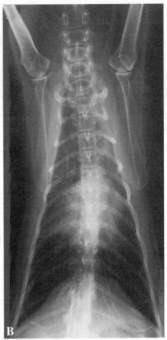

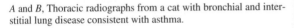

A and *B*, Thoracic radiographs from a cat with bronchial and interstitial lung disease consistent with asthma.

Eosinophils may predominate in some patients with asthma or bronchitis, but a large number of eosinophils (up to 25% of cells) may be present in airways of normal cats. Therefore, the presence of eosinophils supports a diagnosis of asthma or bronchitis but does not necessarily prove that the disease is present. In many studies, nondegenerate neutrophils were the predominant cell type found in airway cytology from cats with a clinical diagnosis of bronchial disease or asthma.

15. Are infectious agents involved in feline small airway disease?

Flavobacterium, Bordetella bronchiseptica, Streptococcus spp., *Acinetobacter* spp., *Enterobacter* spp., and lesser numbers of *Pseudomonas* spp., and *Klebsiella* spp. have been isolated from bronchial cultures of healthy cats. Bacteria also have been isolated from 25–42% of cats with bronchial disease, making it difficult to interpret positive bacterial culture results. *Mycoplasma* spp. have been cultured from the airways of approximately 25% of cats diagnosed with feline asthma but have not been cultured from the airways of healthy cats. Therefore, positive mycoplasmal cultures from airway fluid may indicate involvement of *Mycoplasma* spp. in clinical disease. Some cats with bronchopulmonary disease have clinical signs suggestive of upper respiratory tract infection, but the role of viruses in feline airway disease is unknown. Viral culture is often unrewarding.

16. How can infection with *Mycoplasma* spp. contribute to clinical signs in cats with small airway disease?

Experimental investigations in some species indicate that *Mycoplasma* spp. can degrade a neutral endopeptidase enzyme that breaks down substance P. Accumulation of substance P in the airways can cause smooth muscle constriction and edema. Thus, in some cats, doxycycline treatment can be beneficial both for its antimycoplasmal effects and for decreasing inflammation.

17. What are the differential diagnoses in cats with acute respiratory distress (see Chapter 8)?

• Lower airway disease
• Congestive heart failure/pulmonary edema

- Pleural space disease (pleural effusion, pneumothorax, mediastinal masses)
- Pain
- Fear
- Pneumonia
- Anemia
- Methemoglobinemia (e.g., secondary to acetaminophen toxicity)
- Trauma (flail chest, pneumothorax, hemothorax, diaphragmatic hernia)
- Smoke inhalation
- Carbon monoxide intoxication

18. What is the mainstay of long-term therapy for cats with asthma or bronchial disease?

Long-term therapy (see table in question 10) is directed at suppressing inflammation with sustained administration of glucocorticoids. Most commonly, prednisolone is administered at 1 mg/kg orally every 12 hours for 10–14 days. The dose then is tapered gradually to 2.5 mg/kg orally every 48 hours. The primary benefit of glucocorticoid therapy is inhibition of phospholipase A_2, that is necessary for metabolism of arachidonic acid to prostaglandins, leukotrienes and platelet-activating factor. Glucocorticoids also can minimize airway inflammation by decreasing eosinophil chemotaxis and epithelial adherence. Some cats that fail to respond to prednisolone respond to dexamethasone or triamcinolone.

19. When is bronchodilator therapy useful?

In cats with reversible airway constriction, bronchodilator therapy may be added. Terbutaline (0.625 mg orally every 12 hr) and extended-action theophylline (Theodur, Key Schering-Plough Corporation, Kenilwirth, NJ; Slo-bid gyrocaps, Rhone Poulenc Rorer, King of Prussia, PA) administered orally at 50–100 mg once daily in the evening are used most frequently. In addition, there are anecdotal reports of some cats tolerating nebulization with terbutaline or aminophylline diluted in deionized water as a nightly treatment.

20. What other options are available?

In cats that are intolerant of glucocorticoids or have an inadequate response to glucocorticoids and bronchodilators, a trial of the antiserotonin drug **cyproheptadine** (2 mg orally every 12 hr) is recommended. In addition, adjunctive use of serotonin antagonist drugs with glucocorticoids may be useful for long-term therapy. **Cyclosporine-A** decreases activated T-lymphocyte function and, in experimentally induced feline airway disease, histologic alterations that may be responsible for signs of chronic airway disease. Therapy may prove beneficial in selected cases of severe feline bronchial disease. Trough cyclosporine levels should be 500–1000 ng/ml. **Anti-interleukin-5 antibody** treatment has been effective in alleviating clinical signs of bronchoconstriction in cats with experimentally induced asthma. **Fish oil** supplementation, with high omega-3 fatty acid concentrations, can decrease the amount of arachidonic acid available for leukotriene release and may be beneficial in long-term therapy. Finally, there are anecdotal reports of success with the antileukotriene **zafirlukast** (Accolate, Merck & Co., West Point, PA) for treating cats with lower airway disease.

21. What effects do beta₂ agonists have on airways?

- Inhibition of cholinergic neurotransmission
- Stabilization of mast cell membranes with inhibition of mast cell mediator release
- Decreased vascular permeability
- Increased mucociliary clearance

22. Are antibiotics beneficial in the treatment of feline asthma?

If a bacterium is grown in pure culture or if *Mycoplasma* spp. are isolated, antibiotic therapy should be instituted for a minimum of 3 weeks. Routine use of antibiotics in feline asthma, however, is controversial. Various bacterial species have been cultured from airways of healthy cats, and tracheobronchial cultures are often negative in cats with airway disease. Most cultured bacteria probably represent colonization secondary to chronic airway inflammation rather than primary infections. The exception is *Mycoplasma* spp., which may be a primary pathogen, causing structural damage to the airway epithelium. The use of doxycycline, enrofloxacin, or chloramphenicol is indicated when *Mycoplasma* spp. are cultured (see table in question 10).

23. Why is N-acetylcysteine contraindicated in the treatment of acute feline bronchoconstriction?

N-acetylcysteine (Mucomyst, Apothecon, Inc., Princeton, NJ) is a mucolytic agent that breaks disulfide bonds in proteins present in airway secretions, thereby decreasing the viscocity of airway mucus. However, aerosol therapy with N-acetylcysteine can promote bronchoconstriction by irritating the airway epithelium.

24. What other drugs are contraindicated in the treatment of feline asthma?

Beta-adrenergic blocking drugs, such as propranolol, are contraindicated because decreasing adrenergic tone may aggrevate bronchoconstriction and worsen respiratory difficulty. Sedatives that suppress respiration can exacerbate hypoventilation and hypoxemia. Atropine, as a single injection, may temporarily relieve bronchospasm, but long-term use is contraindicated because it increases viscocity of airway mucus. Similarly, inappropriate diuretic therapy can dry respiratory secretions and decrease mucociliary clearance. Because histamine may be beneficial in cats with asthma by causing bronchodilation, the use of antihistamines may be contraindicated or not useful in cats with airway disease.

25. What is the long-term prognosis for cats with asthma?

Most cats with asthma experience additional acute episodes. Clients should be instructed that immediate veterinary attention is necessary as soon as clinical signs develop. In addition, avoidance of noxious gases, particulate matter (such as aerosol sprays or carpet powders), and smoke can avoid or delay recurrence. Bronchiectasis may be a long-term sequela of feline lower airway disease. With time, respiratory function can become severely compromised to such an extent that humane euthanasia is warranted.

BIBLIOGRAPHY

1. Bauer T: Pulmonary hypersensitivity disorders. In Kirk RW (ed): Current Veterinary Therapy X. Philadelphia, W.B. Saunders, 1989, pp 369–376.
2. Corcoran BM, Foster DJ, Fuentes VL: Feline asthma syndrome: A retrospective study of the clinical presentation in 29 cats. J Small Anim Pract 36:481–488, 1995.
3. Dye TL, Teague HD, Poundstone ML: Lung lobe torsion in a cat with chronic feline asthma. J Am Anim Hosp Assoc 34:493–495, 1998.
4. Moise NS, Wiedenkeller D, Yeager AE, et al: Clinical, radiographic, and bronchial cytologic features of cats with bronchial disease: 65 cases (1980–1986). J Am Vet Med Assoc 194:1467–1473, 1989.
5. Moses BL, Spaulding GL: Chronic bronchial disease of the cat. Vet Clin North Am Small Anim Pract 15:929–948, 1985.
6. Padrid P: Chronic lower airway disease in the dogs and cat. Probl Vet Med 4:320–344, 1992.
7. Padrid P: New strategies to treat feline asthma. Vet Forum Oct:46–50, 1996.
8. Padrid P: CVT Update: Feline Asthma. In Kirk RW (ed): Current Veterinary Therapy XIII. Philadelphia, W.B. Saunders, 2000, pp 805–810.
9. Padrid, PA, Mitchell RW, Ndukwu IM, et al: Cyproheptadine-induced attenuation of type I immediate hypersensitivity reactions of airway smooth muscle from immune-sensitized cats. Am J Vet Res 56:109, 1995.
10. Wingfield WE: Allergic airway disease (asthma) in cats. In Wingfield WE (ed): Veterinary Emergency Medicine Secrets, 2nd ed. Philadelphia, Hanley & Belfus, 2000, pp 170–173.

10. DIROFILARIASIS

Jeff D. Bay, D.V.M.

1. What causes dirofilariasis?

Dirofilaria immitis, a nematode parasite transmitted by mosquitoes, is the causative agent in both dogs and cats.

2. How does dirofilariasis differ in cats and dogs?
- Cats are more resistant hosts than dogs and are less easily infected.
- Cats usually are infected with fewer worms (usually 6 or less and commonly 1 or 2) because of a more aggressive immunologic response.
- The heartworm life span in cats is only about 2–3 years compared with 5–7 years in dogs.
- Caval syndrome (dirofilarial hemoglobinuria) is rare in cats because of the low worm burden.
- Cats more often exhibit signs associated with aberrant migration of heartworms.

3. What is the prevalence of *D. immitis* infection in cats?

Feline heartworm disease (FHD) has been found practically everywhere in the world that it is seen in dogs, but its incidence is generally lower. A recent survey analyzed the prevalence of positive heartworm antibody tests in subclinically infected cats from endemic and nonendemic areas of the United States. This survey suggests regional differences in prevalence, with rates ranging from 4–33%. Of the cats that were antibody-positive, 3% were also positive for heartworm antigen. However, correlation of antibody and antigen detection test results have varied among studies.

4. Which cats are susceptible to *D. immitis* infection?

Cats may be infected at any age. In some natural and experimental infections, male cats were infected more frequently and more heavily. Indoor cats may be at lower risk for encountering infected mosquitoes, but approximately one-third of cats with FHD live totally indoors.

5. Describe the life cycle of *D. immitis* in cats.

Cats are infected by *D. immitis* when an infected mosquito injects stage L_3 larvae during feeding. The larvae develop through an L_4 stage to adult worms (L_5), which usually arrive in the pulmonary arteries at approximately 5–6 months after infection. An antibody response is mounted against migrating larvae, and positive titers may be detected 3 months after infection. If at least one adult male and one adult female worm are present, microfilaria (L_1 larvae) can be found between 6 and 8 months after infection, but it appears that occult infections are common in cats because their immunologic response rids the body of microfilaria. Thus, it is unlikely that cats serve as a source of L_1 larvae to infect mosquitoes. For undetermined reasons, aberrant migration of heartworm occurs more commonly in cats than in dogs.

6. Are microfilaria prevalent in cats with FHD?

Cats with FHD are rarely microfilaria-positive. The period in which infected cats demonstrate microfilaremia is small (approximately 1 month, between 195 and 228 days after infection). In addition, feline heartworm infection is typified by a low worm burden or infection with immature worms, thus limiting the number of microfilaria produced. However, heartworm is the only filarial disease in cats. Therefore, if microfilaria are detected, the diagnosis is confirmed.

7. What are the clinical signs of FHD?

The most common clinical signs involve the respiratory tract; cough, dyspnea, and tachypnea are common. Vomiting is also common, either alone or in combination with respiratory signs in some cats. Central nervous system signs (e.g., blindness, seizures), probably due to aberrant worm migration, can be appreciated in rare cases. Sudden death may occur without prior signs apparent to the owner. A small percentage of infected cats exhibit no clinical signs, apparently because the infection is cleared before worm maturation or the cat outlives the worm's life span with inapparent infection.

8. How is FHD diagnosed?

Diagnosing FHD can be difficult. In many cases, the tentative diagnosis is based on a variety of suggestive findings rather than a single definitive test. Detection of *D. immitis* microfilaria in blood confirms the diagnosis of FHD (high specificity) but has poor sensitivity. When concentration methods such as the modified Knott or filter tests are used, a larger volume of blood (3 ml) should be used than the amount recommended for dogs (1 ml).

9. What routine laboratory abnormalities may be seen in FHD?

Peripheral eosinophilia and basophilia should increase suspicion of *D. immitis* infection, but these findings are not specific because they can be caused by any internal or external parasitic disease or hypersensitivity reaction. Polyclonal gammopathy and proteinuria also occur in some cats but are not specific for FHD.

10. Discuss the role of serologic tests in the diagnosis of FHD.

Positive test results for serum host antibody (i.e., feline heartworm antibody titers) against *D. immitis* antigens generally become positive 90 days after infection. These titers are highly sensitive but not specific for FHD because antibodies can develop against larvae that never become adult heartworms. In addition, antibodies may persist in cats that were exposed to *D. immitis* but are not currently infected. Serologic tests detecting female heartworm antigen (i.e., occult heartworm tests) are nearly 100% specific, but their sensitivity is lower because of parasite immaturity at the time of the test or because too few female worms infected the cat. When FHD is suspected, antibody serology can be used as a screening test; a positive antigen test confirms infection. However, antibody tests can be negative in cats with FHD. For example, in one study of 25 antigen-positive cats, only 4 or 5 cats were positive for antibody when tested with two different commercially available kits. In addition, a negative antigen test result does not rule out active disease. Thus, serum tests should not be used alone to make the diagnosis of FHD.

11. What signs of FHD may be seen on thoracic radiographs?

Thoracic radiographs of cats with FHD commonly show enlarged caudal lobar arteries, with the artery > 1.6 times the width of the ninth rib. This finding is generally evident 6–7 months after infection. A diffuse bronchointerstitial pattern may be seen, but radiographic abnormalities can be transient. Radiographic changes in the cardiac silhouette are rarely seen in cats infected with FHD. Uncommon findings include pleural effusion and lung lobe collapse. Thoracic radiographs are also valuable for assessing the severity of disease and monitoring its progression or regression over time. (See figure on following page.)

12. Is echocardiography helpful in diagnosing FHD?

Sometimes. Echocardiography is a highly specific test if heartworms are seen in the right heart. *D. immitis* typically appear as multiple, parallel, double-linear, hyperechoic objects in the right ventricle or main pulmonary artery segment. However, because the organism commonly resides in the pulmonary arteries, it may not be visualized by echocardiography.

13. Discuss the role of airway washing procedures in the diagnosis of FHD.

Because other diffuse pulmonary diseases (e.g., asthma, lungworm infection, neoplasia) are typically on the differential list in a cat with FHD, transtracheal washes or bronchoalveolar lavages are commonly performed. Airway wash cytology may reveal a preponderance of eosinophils 4–7 months after infection with *D. immitis*; however, airway eosinophilia is not specific for heartworm infection. In addition, the absence of eosinophils does not preclude heartworm infection.

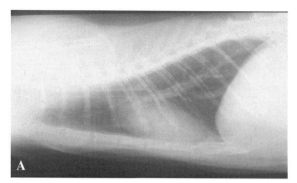

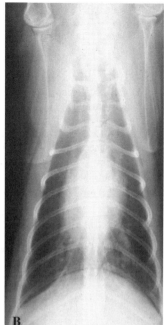

Thoracic radiographs consistent with dirofilariasis in cats. Note the enlarged pulmonary arteries in the VD view *(B)*. (Courtesy of Dr. Jan Bright, Colorado State University.)

14. Can FHD be diagnosed at necropsy?
Unfortunately, some cats with FHD are diagnosed via necropsy, especially those that die suddenly. Look for intact or fragmented worms in the heart, pulmonary arteries, systemic veins, and central nervous system (if neurologic symptoms were present). However, some cats that die from sequelae of FHD may have cleared the infection; in such cases, worms are absent.

15. How is FHD treated?
Supportive care for secondary respiratory tract inflammation is most important; use of adulticide treatment is controversial. Acutely ill cats should be stabilized with appropriate supportive care such as supplemental oxygen, parenteral fluids, bronchodilators, and glucocorticoids. Glucocorticoids decrease reaction to the worms in the pulmonary arteries and thus reduce clinical signs. They can be used over the long term in cats with mild-to-moderate symptoms while waiting for adult worms to die (up to 2–3 years). This approach usually decreases pulmonary arteritis caused by the chronic presence of worms, but acute thromboembolic complications caused by death of worms are still possible. Supportive treatment protocols are similar to those for asthma and chronic bronchitis (see Chapter 9).

16. Should adulticide treatment be considered?
Thiacetarsamide was found to be effective in cats with FHD, but its use does not increase survival rates over the use of glucocorticoids alone, and death has resulted from its administration in some cats. Thiacetarsamide usually is reserved for stable cats that continue to manifest clinical signs despite glucocorticoid treatment. The dose is 2.2 mg/kg intravenously twice daily for 2 days. Cage confinement and close observation are recommended for 3–4 weeks because pulmonary thromboembolic complications can be expected in about one-third of treated cats. Aspirin should not be used in cats with FHD.
The safety and efficacy of **melarsamine** have not been firmly established in cats; therefore, its use cannot be recommended. One study found that a single intramuscular dose of 2.5 mg/kg reduced worm burdens by only 30%.

17. When should surgical removal of adult worms be considered?

In cats with caval syndrome, surgical removal may be considered if adult worms are visualized echocardiographically in the right side of the heart. However, success rates are largely undetermined because of limited information.

18. What preventive measures can be used against heartworms in cats?

Monthly ivermectin at an oral dose of 24 µg/kg is highly effective in preventing heartworm infection in cats. Milbemycin is effective at the canine preventive dose (0.5–0.99 mg/kg/month orally) but has not been labeled for use in cats. Selamectin, a monthly topical heartworm preventive labeled for cats, is an alternative for cats that refuse oral preventive medications. Because even indoor cats are at risk in endemic areas, preventive drugs should be considered for them as well as for cats who live predominantly outdoors. Depending on the product, heartworm preventives have the added benefit of aiding in the control of other helminth parasites.

BIBLIOGRAPHY

 1. Atkins C: The diagnosis of feline heartworm infection. J Am Anim Hosp Assoc 35:185–187, 1999.
 2. Atkins CE, Atwell RB, Dillon R, et al: American Heartworm Society Guidelines for the diagnosis, treatment, and prevention of heartworm (*Dirofilaria immitis*) infection in cats. Comp Cont Educ Pract Vet 19:422–429, 1997.
 3. Atkins CE, DeFrancesco TC, Coats JR, et al: Heartworm infection in cats: 50 cases (1985–1997). J Am Vet Med Assoc 217:355–358, 2000.
 4. Atkins CE, DeFrancesco TC, Miller MW, et al: Prevalence of heartworm infection in cats with signs of cardiorespiratory abnormalities. J Am Vet Med Assoc 212:517–520, 1998.
 5. Dillon R: Clinical significance of feline heartworm disease. Vet Clin North Am Small Anim Pract 28:1547–1565, 1998.
 6. Dillon AR, Brawner WR, Robertson-Plouch CK, et al: Feline heartworm disease: Correlations of clinical signs, serology, and other diagnostics: Results of a multicenter study. Vet Therapeut 1:176–182, 2000.
 7. Goodwin JK: The serologic diagnosis of heartworm infection in dogs and cats. Clin Tech Small Anim Pract 13:83–87, 1998.
 8. Kalkstein TS, Kaiser L, Kaneene JB: Prevalence of heartworm infection in healthy cats in the lower peninsula of Michigan. J Am Vet Med Assoc 217:857–861, 2000.
 9. McCall JW, Dzimianski MT, McTier TL, et al: Biology of experimental heartworm infection in cats. In Soll MD, Knight DH (eds): Proceedings of the American Heartworm Symposium 1992. Batavia, IL, American Heartworm Society, 1992, pp 71–79.
10. Miller MW, Atkins CE, Stemme K, et al: Prevalence of exposure to *Dirofilaria immitis* in cats in multiple areas of the United States. Vet Therapeut 1:169–175, 2000.
11. Robertson-Plouch CK, Dillon AR, Brawner WR, et al: Prevalence of feline heartworm infections among cats with respiratory and gastrointestinal signs: Results of a multicenter study. Vet Therapeutics 1:88–95, 2000.
12. Selcer BA, Newell SM, Mansour AE, et al: Radiographic and 2-D echocardiographic findings in eighteen cats experimentally exposed to *D. immitis* via mosquito bites. Vet Radiol Ultrasound 37:37–44, 1996.
13. Snyder PS, Levy JK, Salute ME, et al: Performance of serologic tests used to detect heartworm infection in cats. J Am Vet Med Assoc 216:693–700, 2000.
14. Venco L, Calzolari D, Mazzocchi D, et al: The use of echocardiography as a diagnostic tool for detection of feline heartworm (*Dirofilaria immitis*) infections. Feline Pract 26:6–9, 1998.

11. RESPIRATORY PARASITES

Elizabeth J. Colleran, D.V.M., M.S.

1. What are the most common primary lung parasites?

Paragonimus kellicotti is a trematode in the family Troglotrematids, all of which are lung parasites. This lung fluke causes pulmonary disease in the states surrounding the Great Lakes and in the Midwestern and Southern United States. *P. westermani* is more common on the West Coast.

Aelurostrongylus abstrusus is a nematode in the family Angiostrongylidae. This small lungworm is distributed throughout the United States and is considered the most common respiratory parasite.

Capillaria aerophila is a small worm in the superfamily Trichuroidea that contains several common parasites of domestic animals including *C. trichuris*, the whipworm found in dogs and rarely in cats. *Capillaria* spp. may cause mild cough in cats, but infection is usually subclinical.

2. What are the most common migratory respiratory parasites?

Toxocara cati and *Strongyloides stercoralis* migrate through the lungs of cats after primary infection (see Chapter 19). Tissue migration leads to eosinophilic inflammation and cough in some cats. Infection and visceral larva migrans resulting in cough may be more common in kittens.

3. What are the common polysystemic respiratory parasites?

Toxoplasma gondii and *Dirofilaria immitis* (see Chapter 10).

4. How are cats infected by *Paragonimus* spp.?

Paragonimus spp. eggs from a host are passed in feces about 6 weeks after infection. If the eggs reach water, the miracidia stage develops and hatches in about 2 weeks. These organisms enter the snail *Pomatiopsis lapidaria*. Several stages of development take place until the organism becomes a cercaria. The cercariae leave the snail and encyst in crayfish as metacercariae. Cats that hunt near water containing crayfish may ingest the encysted cercariae with the crayfish or consume paratenic hosts that have recently eaten crayfish. The flukes "excyst" from the intestines, migrate through the diaphragm, and encyst in lung parenchyma. The adults and eggs that become trapped in alveoli and airways result in lung pathology.

5. What are the clinical signs of *Paragonimus* spp. infection?

The primary sign of *Paragonimus* spp. infection is chronic cough. Clinical signs are associated with the inflammatory reaction to the parasite, secondary bacterial infection, or cyst rupture. Lung sounds are often normal, but crackles and wheezes can be auscultated when inflammatory disease is present and may be confused with feline bronchitis. Acute respiratory distress occurs when encysted organisms rupture, causing pneumothorax.

6. How is *Paragonimus* spp. infection diagnosed?

Thoracic radiographic abnormalities include well-defined cystic lesions approximately 1 cm in diameter and pneumothorax may be present if a cyst ruptures. A nodular, interstitial pattern may result from diffuse inflammation. Definitive diagnosis is made by identification of eggs either in tracheal washings or feces after fecal sedimentation. Fecal sedimentation can be done by an outside laboratory or by the following procedure:

1. Mix 5 gm of feces in 200 ml of water in a beaker.
2. Pour the mixture through a tea strainer, and discard the material in the strainer.
3. After 10 minutes, decant approximately 70% of the supernatant, and refill the beaker with fresh water.
4. Repeat step 3 3–5 times until the supernatant is clear.

5. Pour off 90% of the supernatant, and pour the sediment into a petri dish.

6. Examine the sediment under a dissecting microscope (20–30 ×) or scanning objective (4 ×) of the microscope (total magnification = 40 ×) for large, single-operculated eggs.

7. Which cats are most at risk for *A. abstrusus* infection?

The life cycle of *A. abstrusus* requires a mollusk (slug or snail) as an intermediate host and a small mammal or bird as a transport host. Thus, cats that hunt in areas with sufficient moisture for slugs and snails to thrive are at risk.

8. What are the clinical signs of *A. abstrusus* infection?

Clinical signs are related to parasite burden. Larvae in feces are an incidental finding in some subclinically infected cats. Clinical signs range from mild cough to respiratory distress and even death. Crackles and wheezes may be auscultated, mimicking feline bronchitis. Occasionally, secondary bacterial pneumonia can complicate the diagnosis.

9. Describe the radiographic appearance of *A. abstrusus* infection.

On thoracic radiographs, poorly defined nodular densities are observed, particularly in caudal lung fields. These densities are deposits of egg "nests" in the lung parenchyma. Bronchial and diffuse interstitial patterns are also common.

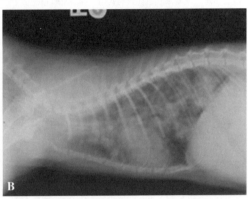

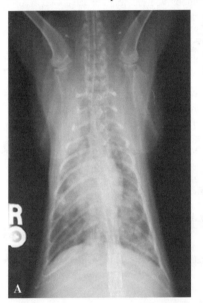

A and *B*, Thoracic radiographs from a cat with *Aelurostrongylus abstrusus* infection.

10. How is *A. abstrusus* infection diagnosed?

Diagnosis is made by identifying the parasite in feces or airway washings. Eggs hatch into first-stage larvae while in the lungs. The larvae are then coughed up and swallowed and appear in the cat's feces 5–6 weeks after infection. First-stage larvae can be recovered in tracheal wash samples or by Baermann examination of feces. This test requires a Baermann apparatus, which consists of a ring stand and ring holder and a glass funnel covered by a wire net or cheesecloth with a piece of rubber tubing on the end. Approximately 3–5 gm of fresh feces are placed on the cheesecloth or wire mesh immediately above the water filled funnel. Over several hours, larvae migrate out of the feces into the fluid and sink to the bottom of a funnel for collection and identification.

Zinc sulfate fecal flotation also can be diagnostic (see Chapter 19). The author has found this technique useful for the diagnosis of *A. abstrusus* larvae in clinically ill cats. The larvae are distinguished from other parasitic infections by the spines on their tails.

Cytologic evaluation of airway washings often demonstrate eosinophilic inflammation suggestive of parasitism, but larvae may or may not be identified.

11. What is the life-cycle of *C. aerophila*? How is infection diagnosed?

The life cycle of *C. aerophila* is unclear but probably involves an earthworm host or ingestion of eggs from the soil. *C. aerophila* infects the trachea and large bronchi of cats. Eggs are coughed up, swallowed, and passed in the feces. Occasionally, clinical signs of cough or wheeze are present, but most infected cats are subclinical. Diagnosis is made by identification of eggs in tracheal wash fluid or in feces after fecal flotation (see Chapter 19). The eggs of *C. aerophila* are morphologically similar to the double-operculated egg of *Trichuris vulpis* but are slightly smaller.

12. How are the primary lung parasites treated?

If clinical signs of disease worsen during treatment, prednisolone at 2 mg/kg orally every 12 hour may be needed to lessen eosinophilic inflammation.

13. What are the clinical signs of the migratory parasites?

Toxocara cati and *S. stercoralis* infections of cats may be subclinical. Alternately, gastrointestinal signs may occur, including vomiting and diarrhea. Infected kittens may be unthrifty. Mild cough can occur in some kittens and adult cats.

14. How are the migratory parasites diagnosed and treated?

Fecal flotation reveals the ova of *T. cati*, and the Baermann technique can be used to demonstrate larvae of *S. stercoralis*. Although drugs such as pyrantel pamoate and fenbendazole (see Chapter 19) can clear the intestinal tract, it is unknown whether migrating tissue stages can be treated successfully.

15. Does *Toxoplasma gondii* infection cause respiratory disease?

Cats are the definitive host for *Toxoplasma gondii*, and virtually all other warm-blooded animals are intermediate hosts (see Chapters 19 and 84). After primary infection of the host, *T. gondii* replicates in most body tissues, including the lungs. In most immunocompetent hosts, primary infection results in minimal-to-no clinical signs. Thus, *T. gondii* is rarely diagnosed clinically as a cause of respiratory disease in cats. In some infected cats, particularly young cats with acute disease, coughing, dyspnea, and polypnea occur. Toxoplasmic pneumonia is most common in transplacentally or neonatally infected kittens. Proliferative interstitial pneumonia was the most consistent finding in a study of neonatally induced toxoplasmosis. Of 100 cats with histologically confirmed, fatal toxoplasmosis, 26 had pulmonary lesions. Organisms were found in 76.7% of 86 lungs examined. Other clinical signs may include pyrexia (104–106°F, 40.0–41.1,C), anorexia, anterior uveitis, posterior uveitis, and abdominal discomfort.

16. How is toxoplasmosis diagnosed?

Antemortem diagnosis may be difficult. Thoracic radiographs reveal a patchy, diffuse infiltrative pattern resembling bacterial or viral pneumonia. Hematologic findings are nonspecific. Oocysts are small, intermittently shed, and easily overlooked in fecal preparations. Bronchoalveolar lavage may or may not contain tachyzoites. Definitive diagnosis is made by a combination of the following:
- Serologic evidence of infection (IgG indicates exposure and IgM active disease)
- Clinical signs of toxoplasmosis
- Response to treatment
- Identification of organism histologically associated with inflammation

17. How is toxoplasmosis treated?

Because of the minimal number of cases of pulmonic toxoplasmosis, optimal treatment is undetermined. Clindamycin HCl (Antirobe, Pharmacia and Upjohn Co., Kalamazoo, MI) at 12.5 mg/kg/day orally every 12 hours for a minimum of 4 weeks has been used most frequently for syndromes other than respiratory disease. Loose stool and emesis have been reported as potential side effects in cats. Potentiated sulfas and azithromycin are effective alternative choices. In general, pulmonic toxoplasmosis suggests overwhelming tissue replication and carries a guarded-to-poor prognosis.

BIBLIOGRAPHY

1. Bowman DD, Lynn CR, Georgi JR: Parasitology for Veterinarians, Philadelphia, W.B. Saunders, 1999.
2. Dubey JP, Carpenter JL: Histologically confirmed clinical toxoplasmosis in cats: 100 cases (1952–1990). J Am Vet Med Assoc 203:1556–1566, 1993.
3. Dubey JP, Lappin MR: Toxoplasmosis and neosporosis. In Greene CE (ed): Infectious Diseases of the Dog and Cat. Philadelphia, W.B. Saunders, Philadelphia, 2nd ed. 1998, pp 493–503.
4. Dubey, JP, Mattix, ME, Lipscomb TP: Lesions of neonatally induced toxoplasmosis in cats. Vet Pathol 33:290–295, 1996.
5. Hawkins EC: Pulmonary parenchymal diseases. In Ettinger SJ, Feldman EC (eds): Textbook of Veterinary Internal Medicine. Philadelphia, W.B. Saunders, 2000, pp 1068–1071.
6. Hawkins EC, Davidson MG, Meuten DJ, et al: Cytologic identification of *Toxoplasma gondii* in bronchoalveolar lavage fluid of experimentally infected cats. J Am Vet Med Assoc 210:648–650, 1997.
7. King L, Drake D, Scott F, et al: Roundtable: Feline respiratory diseases, Pt 2. Feline Pract 26:6–10, 1998.
8. Knowlen JR: The coughing cat. In August JR (ed): Consultations in Feline Internal Medicine. Philadelphia, W.B. Saunders, 1991, pp 180–181.
9. Lappin MR, Greene, CE, Winston S, et al: Clinical feline toxoplasmosis: Serologic diagnosis and therapeutic management of 15 cases. J Vet Intern Med 3:139–143, 1989.

12. PNEUMONIA

John E. Stein, D.V.M.

1. What is pneumonia?

Pneumonia refers to inflammation of the lung. It is generally due to infectious causes such as bacteria, viruses, fungi, or parasites, but it also may result from a noninfectious cause such as aspiration of material into the lower airways. The chemical inflammation induced by aspiration often results in secondary bacterial pneumonia.

2. What historical findings suggest pneumonia in cats?

Pneumonia in cats may develop from a wide variety of causes. A thorough history provides valuable clues to the underlying cause. Cats, and in particular kittens, that have recently been housed in stressful, multicat environments such as shelters are at increased risk of developing bacterial pneumonia. In sick cats with a history of vomiting or a recent procedure requiring general anesthesia, aspiration pneumonia should be considered. Hunting cats are at increased risk of developing parasitic pneumonia and, during summer months in endemic areas, can encounter pneumonic plague caused by *Yersinia pestis* (see Chapter 86). Although serologic tests by themselves do not prove immunodeficiency, the retroviral status of all sick cats should be known because coinfection with feline leukemia virus (FeLV) and/or feline immunodeficiency virus (FIV) may predispose to infectious pneumonia.

3. What clinical signs of illness does pneumonia generally cause in cats?

The most common clinical signs are cough, which may be moist and productive, and dyspnea. Some cats demonstrate vague, nonspecific signs, including anorexia, lethargy, dehydration, and weight loss. Some cats also have a nasal discharge and/or ocular abnormalities, depending on the underlying cause of pneumonia. Aspiration pneumonia occurs most frequently in cats that have a history of vomiting, regurgitation, or recent anesthetic event.

4. What physical examination findings suggest pneumonia?

Fever, tachypnea or dyspnea, and weight loss are common physical examination findings in cats with pneumonia. In addition, thoracic auscultation may demonstrate the presence of increased bronchovesicular or adventitial sounds, such as "crackles," that indicate fluid-filled alveoli. The presence of submandibular lymphadenopathy in a hunting cat during summer months in plague endemic regions should be cause for immediate quarantine until *Y. pestis* has been ruled out (see Chapter 86). Generalized peripheral lymphadenopathy may be noted in cats with pulmonary mycoses. A fundic examination may reveal evidence of uveitis or chorioretinitis with systemic infectious agents such as *Toxoplasma gondii* or fungal agents, both of which can cause pneumonia in cats.

5. Which bacterial agents have been associated with pneumonia in cats?

Bacteria can enter and colonize the lower airways of cats via either the inhalation/aspiration or hematogenous routes, and many possible agents can be involved. As with bacterial infection of the upper respiratory tract, the resident population of bacteria in the oropharynx and trachea can overgrow under certain circumstances and descend into the distal airways. Careful evaluation for an underlying condition that may predispose the patient to bacterial pneumonia is always indicated. Many bacteria, whether present as a primary or secondary infection, possess virulence factors that further disrupt the normal mucociliary apparatus, interfere with local immunity, and/or damage respiratory epithelium. Among the more common bacterial agents found in feline bacterial pneumonia are *Pasteurella multocida*, *Moraxella* spp., *Klebsiella pneumoniae*, *Proteus* spp., *Pseudomonas aeruginosa*, *Mycoplasma* spp., and *Bordetella bronchiseptica*, in addition to the ubiquitous *Staphylococcus* spp., *Streptococcus* spp., and *Escherichia coli*. These infections may represent overgrowth of resident microflora, opportunistic invaders, or possibly primary pathogens arriving either via the airway or hematogenously.

6. Which organisms may cause primary bacterial pneumonia in cats?

Although, in general, secondary bacterial pneumonia is more common in cats, the following organisms are known to cause primary disease:

1. *B. bronchiseptica* has been shown to be a potential primary pathogen but appears to cause severe pneumonia only in kittens less than 4–6 weeks of age, particularly those housed in overcrowded, unsanitary conditions. Overall, *B. bronchiseptica* is commonly detected in healthy cats and appears to be an unlikely cause of primary bacterial pneumonia in adult, household cats.

2. *Mycoplasma* spp. are not normally found in the lower airways of healthy cats and undoubtedly may be opportunistic invaders; however, their role as primary bacterial pathogens remains somewhat controversial.

3. In the southwest portion of the United States, from late spring to early fall, pneumonic plague caused by *Y. pestis* is an important and zoonotic differential for primary bacterial pneumonia in outdoor cats that hunt (see Chapter 86).

7. Discuss the role of canine distemper virus and *Chlamydia psittaci* in lower respiratory tract disease.

The role of canine distemper virus and *C. psittaci* in lower respiratory tract disease was evaluated in a retrospective study (1987–1996) of 245 cases of feline pneumonia or conjunctivitis/rhinitis. Patients were evaluated histologically and by immunohistochemical staining for both organisms. Neither organism could be demonstrated in the lungs of household cats, suggesting that they are not involved with feline lower respiratory disease.

8. What other infectious agents may cause pneumonia in cats?

Viral, fungal, and parasitic pneumonia occur in some cats. Secondary bacterial infection may result from colonization of the damaged airways after the primary infection.

9. What are the most common causes of viral pneumonia in cats?

Viral pneumonia has been noted with calicivirus and, less commonly, feline herpesvirus 1 (feline viral rhinotracheitis), almost exclusively in kittens (see Chapter 3). Feline infectious peritonitis has been reported to result in pyogranulamatous pneumonia with patchy interstitial to alveolar densities noted radiographically (see Chapter 38). Although not responsible for primary viral pneumonia, both FeLV and FIV may result in decreased immune function in cats and increased incidence of pneumonia due to infectious agents.

10. What causes mycotic pneumonia in cats?

Mycotic pneumonia is relatively rare in cats compared with dogs. The most common feline fungal infection, *Cryptococcus neoformans*, typically results in rhinitis with possible ocular or central nervous system manifestations rather than pneumonia (see Chapter 4). Cats with evidence of pneumonia and concurrent rhinitis should be examined carefully for evidence of cutaneous lesions, central nervous system signs, and ocular abnormalities, such as exudative retinal detachment, granulomatous chorioretinitis, or anterior uveitis associated with cryptococcal infection. *Blastomyces dermatitidis, Histoplasma capsulatum,* and *Coccidiodes immitis* are possible, though less common, causes of pneumonia in cats. Because these organisms often establish systemic infections, cats with fungal pneumonia may demonstrate abnormalities in multiple body systems, including the eye, central nervous system, bones, lymph nodes, intestinal tract, kidneys, and skin. *Blastomyces* spp. are found most commonly in soil in the regions of the Mississippi, Missouri, and Ohio River valleys and may cause anterior uveitis, optic neuritis, and/or retinal hemorrhage as well as dyspnea and potentially draining skin lesions in cats with systemic disease. *Histoplasma* spp. are also found most commonly in the central United States and may cause pneumonia as well as lymphadenopathy, hepatosplenomegaly, and, occasionally, ocular, central nervous system, skin, bony, or gastrointestinal lesions. *Coccidioides* spp. are found in the southwestern United States and are more likely to cause skin lesions than pneumonia in cats; on occasion they also cause bony or ocular lesions.

11. Can respiratory parasites be involved with lung disease in cats?

Multiple parasites are associated with respiratory tract disease in cats. Some, like *Toxoplasma gondii*, are polysystemic parasites that may cause pneumonia as well as ocular, central nervous system, and other multisystemic signs (see Chapter 11). The two most common migratory parasites are *Toxocara cati* and *Strongyloides stercoralis* (see Chapter 11). The three most common primary lung parasites are the lungworms, *Aleurostrongylus abstrusus* and *Capillaria aerophila*, and the lung fluke, *Paragonimus kellicotti* (see Chapter 11). *Dirofilaria immitis* can cause severe lower respiratory disease, but pneumonia is uncommon (see Chapter 10).

12. What causes sterile pneumonia?

Aspiration of gastric secretions results initially in chemical inflammation that is sterile. However, because of the rich normal flora of the mouth, pharynx, and proximal trachea, bacteria are usually aspirated as well. Chemical inflammation usually allows secondary bacterial colonization. Aspiration pneumonia should be suspected in cats with a history of vomiting, regurgitation, or recent anesthetic event that develop acute signs of respiratory distress. Examples of underlying conditions reported in cats include regurgitation and megaesophagus secondary to congenital or acquired esophageal strictures. Esophagitis with stricture formation has been seen after esophageal reflux under general anesthesia and also in some cats given oral doxycycline tablets (see Chapter 26).

13. How is pneumonia generally diagnosed in cats?

Evaluation of cats with evidence of respiratory disease must be tempered with caution. A patient that appears stable when initially examined may decompensate rapidly under stress. Supplemental oxygen therapy is indicated before and during examination of dyspneic cats with suspected pneumonia. In addition, in areas of the country where *Y. pestis* is endemic, it is vitally important to minimize exposure to personnel and to take proper precautions until this disease has been ruled out. In general, a presumptive diagnosis of pneumonia is based on assessment of the signalment, history, and physical examination, along with results of a complete blood count (CBC), thoracic radiographs, serum FeLV antigen test, serum FIV antibody test, and fecal examination techniques, including flotation, sedimentation, or Baermann test, depending on geographic location and travel history (see Chapter 8). A definitive diagnosis of pneumonia requires cytologic evaluation and culture of fluid obtained via transoral airway washings or bronchoalveolar lavage, although these procedures may not be advisable in unstable, critically ill patients (see Chapter 8).

14. What are the characteristic abnormalities of the CBC?

With bacterial or fungal pneumonia, CBC may demonstrate an inflammatory leukogram with or without a left shift; however some patients have a normal leukogram. In septic cats, neutropenia with a degenerative left shift may be seen. Eosinophilia may be noted in some cats with parasitic pneumonia. Normocytic, normochromic, nonregenerative anemia may be noted in response to chronic inflammation with fungal pneumonia. Total protein can be increased in some cats with systemic mycoses due to hyperglobulinemia. A macrocytic, normochromic, nonregenerative anemia may be seen in patients with bone marrow suppression due to concurrent FeLV infection. Anemia, neutropenia, and lymphopenia are relatively common abnormalities in patients with FIV.

15. What are the characteristic thoracic radiographic findings of pneumonia?

Thoracic radiographic findings vary with the cause of pneumonia. In acute aspiration pneumonia, radiographs may be normal. Patients with bacterial pneumonia typically show evidence of an alveolar pattern characterized by air bronchograms, often distributed in the cranial ventral lung region. Mycotic pneumonia usually causes a miliary-to-nodular interstitial pattern throughout the lungs. Viral or mycoplasmal pneumonia often causes a diffuse interstitial pattern, particularly early in the course of disease.

16. Should airway washing be performed?

In stable patients, cytologic evaluation and culture of airway fluids are indicated to aid diagnosis and determination of appropriate treatment (see Chapter 8). Washings can be obtained by either bronchoscopy and bronchoalveolar lavage or transoral wash. Rarely, a transthoracic aspirate may be required when other diagnostic techniques have been attempted without success. Transthoracic aspiration is most beneficial in cats with interstitial pneumonia (see Chapter 8).

17. How can arterial blood gas analysis be used in the care of pneumonia cases?

Arterial blood gas measurements help to determine the severity of pulmonary parenchymal disease and to monitor response to therapy. Although arterial blood sampling may be difficult in cats, particularly those in respiratory distress, the changes are more sensitive than those noted on radiographs.

18. What is the alveolar-arterial gradient? How is it calculated and interpreted?

The alveolar-arterial (A-a) gradient on room air (21% oxygen) is calculated to determine relative oxygenation with the following formula:

$$\text{A-a gradient} = \text{Calculated alveolar oxygen} - \text{measured PaO}_2$$
$$= [(\text{Barometric pressure} - 47)(0.21) - \text{PaCO}_2/0.8] - \text{PaO}_2$$

where PaO_2 = partial pressure of oxygen in arterial blood and $PaCO_2$ = partial pressure of carbon dioxide in arterial blood. A normal A-a gradient in a well-oxygenated patient is 0–10. An A-a gradient of 10–20 is suspicious for impaired oxygenation ability. An A-a gradient of 20–30 indicates oxygenation impairment, and a gradient > 30 indicates severe disease.

19. What formula is used for patients receiving supplemental oxygen therapy?

When the patient is receiving supplemental oxygen therapy, the following formula for the oxygenation ratio must be used instead:

$$\text{Oxygenation ratio} = PaO_2/FIO_2$$

where FIO_2 = concentration of inspired oxygen. FiO_2 may be presumed to be 40% (0.40) in patients receiving oxygen supplementation via a face mask and 100% (1.0) in patients receiving oxygen from an anesthetic machine or ventilator via an endotracheal tube. A patient with an oxygenation ratio > 200 mmHg is considered to have normal oxygenation ability.

20. How do I treat bacterial pneumonia?

The mainstay of treatment for bacterial pneumonia remains adequate systemic hydration and antibiotic therapy. Ideally, therapy should be guided by results of bacterial culture and antibiotic sensitivity testing. However, while you are awaiting results, particularly in patients not stable enough to undergo respiratory tract fluid collection procedures, empiric antibiotic therapy is usually necessary. In cats suspected to have severe pneumonia or bacteremia, parenteral administration of four-quadrant antibiotics is indicated. The combination of a quinolone plus a penicillin or first-generation cephalosporin provides excellent coverage, but this regimen should be reserved for life-threatening or resistant infections. The maximal recommended daily dosage of enrofloxacin in cats has recently been reduced because of reports of sudden blindness in some cats. If toxoplasmic pneumonia is suspected, clindamycin or azithromycin should be considered in lieu of penicillin or cephalosporin. After initial therapy, cats without evidence of bacteremia may be maintained on penicillin, first-generation cephalosporin, or clindamycin alone (see table in Chapter 2 for doses and spectrums).

21. What additional therapy is important?

Additional therapy for all patients with pneumonia should include replacement of fluid deficits and maintenance of adequate hydration to ensure adequate function of the mucociliary apparatus. For the same reason, diuretics and drugs that interfere with the normal cough response, such as direct antitussives, should be avoided. Finally, supplemental oxygen therapy may provide some relief to cats in respiratory distress with poor oxygenation due to significant pulmonary parenchymal disease.

22. Should other adjunct treatments be considered for bacterial pneumonia?

Nebulization and coupage (repeated gentle chest percussion) may facilitate clearance of mucus and exudates but may not be well tolerated in cats (nebulization is tolerated in a cage or box, but coupage may not be). Nebulization for 10 minutes 3 times/day may be performed using 3–5 ml of sterile saline, which acts as a mucolytic agent and enhances hydration, alone or in combination with an aminoglycoside such as gentamycin (25 mg). Drugs such as theophylline may be of benefit as mild, indirect antitussives and aid in mucociliary apparatus clearance.

23. How is fungal pneumonia diagnosed?

Mycotic pneumonia is suspected based on clinical signs, history, and radiographic findings. Organism identification by culture, cytology, or histopathology gives a definitive diagnosis. Serology is of variable usefulness in diagnosing mycotic infections and monitoring response to therapy, depending on the fungal organism involved. Serology is particularly useful in cases of *C. neoformans* because antigen can be detected and may be used to evaluate response to therapy (see Chapter 4). Serum, cerebrospinal fluid, and aqueous humor can be tested effectively for cryptococcal antigen. Serology for the other systemic fungal organisms is based on antibody titers, and a positive result indicates exposure to the organism rather than a definitive diagnosis. Serologic test results for most cats with blastomycosis or coccidiomycosis are positive. Serologic test results for cats with histoplasmosis are extremely variable.

24. How is fungal pneumonia treated?

In general, mycotic pneumonia is a difficult disease to treat, requiring long-term therapy with expensive, systemic antifungal drugs. Treatment should continue for at least 2 months after resolution of clinical signs. Although itraconazole has been effective in cats with *C. neoformans* infection, fluconazole has superior penetration into the central nervous system and should be used in cats with central nervous system or ocular involvement (see Chapter 4). Ketoconazole has serious side effects in cats and is not recommended. Although these drugs are effective in treating chronic disease, a fungicidal drug such as amphotericin B is indicated in cats with life-threatening systemic infections. Liposome-encapsulated microsomal amphotericin B is expensive but potentially safer because it is less nephrotoxic. For *C. neoformans*, monitoring of serum antigen titers can be beneficial. Ideally, a two-fold decrease in serum titer per month should be detected in a resolving case, although at least 10% of cats may remain seropositive despite effective treatment and resolution of clinical signs.

25. What is the prognosis for pneumonia?

The prognosis for pneumonia depends greatly on the underlying disease process. With secondary pneumonia, resolution depends on accurately identifying and treating the primary condition. In general, bacterial pneumonia responds well to aggressive antibiotic therapy, as discussed above. Viral and aspiration pneumonia may resolve with symptomatic care and antibiotics to treat secondary bacterial infections. Fungal pneumonia may resolve with appropriate therapy, particularly in the case of *C. neoformans*. Parasitic pneumonia usually responds well to antiparasitic therapy, with the exception of severe *Toxoplasma gondii*-induced pneumonitis, which warrants a more guarded prognosis.

BIBLIOGRAPHY

1. Bart M, Guscetti F, Zurbriggen A, et al: Feline infectious pneumonia: A short literature review and a retrospective immunohistological study on the involvement of *Chlamydia* spp. and distemper virus. Vet J 159:3220–3230, 2000.
2. Boothe DM: Principles of drug selection for respiratory infections in cats. Comp Cont Educ Pract Vet 19S:5–15, 1997.
3. Dye JA, McKiernan B, Rozanski EA, et al: Bronchopulmonary disease in the cat: Historical, physical, radiographic, clinicopathologic, and pulmonary functional evaluation of 24 affected and 15 healthy cats. J Vet Intern Med 10:385–400, 1996.
4. Greene CE: Respiratory infections. In Greene CE (ed): Infectious Diseases of the Dog and Cat, 2nd ed. Philadelphia, W.B. Saunders, 1998, pp 582–594.
5. Hawkins EC: Disorders of the pulmonary parenchyma. In Nelson RW, Couto CG (eds): Small Animal Internal Medicine, 2nd ed. St. Louis, Mosby, 1998, pp 297–312.
6. Hoskins JD, Williams J, Roy AF, et al: Isolation and characterization of *Bordetella bronchiseptica* from cats in southern Louisiana. Vet Immunol Immunopathol 65:173–176, 1998.
7. Legendre AM, Toal RL: Diagnosis and treatment of fungal diseases of the respiratory system. In Greene CE (ed): Infectious Diseases of the Dog and Cat, 2nd ed. Philadelphia, W.B. Saunders, 1998, pp 815–819.
8. Randolph JF, Moise NS, Scarlett JM, et al: Prevalence of mycoplasmal and ureaplasmal recovery from tracheobronchial lavages and of mycoplasmal recovery from pharyngeal swab specimens in cats with or without pulmonary disease. Am J Vet Res 54:897–900, 1993.
9. Speakman AJ, Dawson S, Binns SH, et al: *Bordetella bronchiseptica* infection in the cat. J Small Anim Pract 40:252–256, 1999.
10. Wingfield WE: Acid-base disorders. In Wingfield WE (ed): Veterinary Emergency Medicine Secrets. Philadelphia, Hanley & Belfus, 1997, pp 288–293.
11. Welsh RD: *Bordetella bronchiseptica* infections in cats. J Am Anim Hosp Assoc 32:153–158, 2000.

13. PYOTHORAX

Elizabeth J. Colleran, D.V.M., M.S.

1. Define pyothorax.

An accumulation of purulent material in the pleural space.

2. What causes pyothorax?

Bacterial infection generally is involved with pyothorax. In cats, the inciting cause for pyothorax often remains unknown. Infection may result from direct extension due to bite or puncture wounds, migrating foreign bodies, pneumonia, pulmonary or thoracic trauma, or neoplasia. Alternately, infection may result from hematogenous spread from other infection sites such as an abscess or gingivitis. Immunocompromised cats may be at higher risk for pleural infection.

3. Which cats are more likely to be affected?

Young cats that roam freely outdoors are at risk for bite wounds and foreign bodies. Older cats are at increased risk for neoplasia and immunosuppressive disorders. In all cases, other underlying causes should be investigated.

4. What are the signs of pyothorax?

Dyspnea, exercise intolerance, and cyanosis are common presenting complaints with diseases of the pleural space (see Chapter 8). Cats also may present with nonspecific signs of anorexia, lethargy, and depression.

5. What are the common physical examination findings in pyothorax?

The cat may or may not be febrile, but usually an altered breathing pattern is noted because pleural effusion results in restrictive breathing (rapid and shallow breaths). Auscultation reveals muffled heart sounds, with decreased respiratory noises ventrally. Thoracic compressibility may be decreased.

6. What is the role of thoracic radiographs in the diagnosis of pyothorax??

Thoracic radiographs reveal pleural effusion, increased fluid density ventrally that obscures the cardiac shadow, lung lobes are retracted from the thoracic cage, and rounded lung borders outlining individual lung lobes. Rarely, a foreign body may be identified with radiographs or ultrasound.

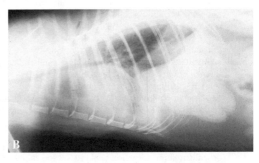

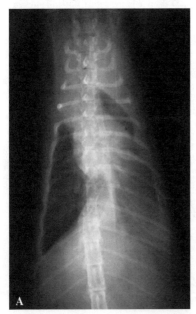

A and *B*, Thoracic radiographs from a cat with pyothorax taken before chest tube placement.

7. Explain the role of thoracocentesis in the diagnosis of pyothorax.

In cats with marked respiratory distress, thoracocentesis may be required for stabilization before chest radiographs are obtained. Thoracocentesis is both diagnostic and therapeutic.

8. How is thoracocentesis performed?

A small area on the ventral portion of the chest at the seventh-to-eighth intercostal space is clipped and surgically prepared. Thoracocentesis is performed with a syringe connected to a three-way stopcock, extension set, and needle or catheter. The needle or catheter is inserted behind the caudal border of the rib to avoid intercostal vessels and nerves. The needle should be directed ventrally, with the needle and syringe nearly parallel to the chest wall to minimize lung laceration. This positioning becomes most important when the lung lobes reinflate as fluid is removed. The extension set and three-way stopcock should be placed in line and are closed off to the patient when the chest is entered. Once the needle is in place, connections are opened and fluid is aspirated. In some cases, fluid may be too thick to be removed via a 22-gauge needle or small catheter, necessitating a larger-bore catheter or placement of a chest tube. In some cats, the mediastinum is complete, and thoracocentesis on both sides of the thorax is required. Fluid samples should be analyzed cytologically and submitted for both aerobic and anaerobic culture and susceptibility testing. Fungal elements may be present but are uncommon.

9. Describe the fluid from a pyothorax.
The fluid is usually a highly cellular exudate, with bacteria visible cytologically in over 90% of cases. Protein concentrations are high, and the fluid varies in color from amber to red to white. It may be extremely malodorous, particularly in the presence of anaerobes such as *Bacteroides* spp. Nucleated cells in the fluid are usually degenerate neutrophils, macrophages, and mesothelial cells. If active phagocytic cells are present, they normally contain bacteria.

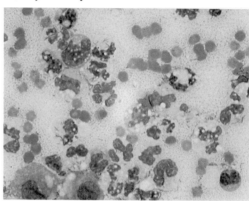

Cytology of a direct smear from a cat with pyothorax. Multiple degenerative and non-degenerative neutrophils are present.

10. Are additional diagnostic procedures needed?
Sepsis, moderate-to-severe dehydration, and electrolyte abnormalities may be present in addition to respiratory signs. Therefore, a complete blood count, chemistry profile, and urinalysis are generally performed when the cat is stable. Serum tests for feline leukemia virus (FeLV) antigens and feline immunodeficiency virus (FIV) antibodies are usually performed because most cats with pyothorax roam outdoors and immunosuppression may worsen the prognosis. Fluid may have obscured underlying causes, such as foreign bodies, lung abscesses, or intrapleural masses, that alter treatment decisions and prognosis for recovery. Thoracic ultrasound is helpful in the search for underlying diseases, for detecting the amount of fluid in the pleural cavity, and for assessing the efficacy of fluid removal.

11. What kind of supportive care is important initially?
Oxygen therapy is started immediately in dyspneic animals, although removal of thoracic fluid is more advantageous in improving gas exchange. Fluids are given intravenously when the cat is stable, and parenteral antibiotics effective against gram-positive, gram-negative, aerobic, and anaerobic organisms (four-quadrant approach) are administered after cultures have been submitted. A good four-quadrant antibiotic regimen is the combination of a fluoroquinolone combined with a first-generation cephalosporin, clindamycin, or ampicillin. Adjustments in antibiotic selection should be based on culture and susceptibility results. Many specimens yield multiple organisms.

12. What treatment course is most likely to be successful?
A chest tube should be placed after diagnosis because drainage and lavage are the mainstays of successful treatment. Bilateral chest tubes may be necessary. Vigorous monitoring of cytologic characteristics is important to assess resolution of disease. Radiographs or ultrasound also can be used to assess drainage and presence of fluid pockets. Long-term antibiotics are needed and are based on culture results. Antibiotic therapy should continue for at least 4–6 weeks.

13. What materials are needed for chest tube placement?

- 12-French Sovereign red rubber catheter or feeding tube (Sherwood Medical, St. Louis) or similar tube from Cook Veterinary Products (Bloomington, IN). In general, a stylet is not required. If the tube has a closed end, carefully cut it off at an angle, and remove any sharp edges. Multiple fenestrations can be made in the distal half, taking care not to weaken the tube. A catheter cap, three-way stopcock, or other closed-end tubing is used to close the tube.
- Sterile gloves
- 2 Mosquito or Kelly hemostats or other small hemostats with a fairly sharp point
- Scalpel and blade
- Nonabsorbable suture material
- Scissors
- Needle holders
- Thumb forceps
- Sterile antibiotic ointment
- Bandaging material
- Soft Elizabethan collar (optional but helpful)

14. How is a chest tube placed?

Because cats have more compliant chest walls and less muscle to penetrate, a simpler technique can be used than that required for dogs. In cats that present with respiratory distress, thoracocentesis should be performed first, and as much fluid is removed as is practical. The technique for tube placement described below applies to a normal-sized adult cat.

1. If one tube is planned, the side most affected should be selected. If the mediastinum is occluded by fibrin clots, chest tube placement is repeated on the second side.

2. Manual restraint should be kept to a minimum, particularly in cats with signs of respiratory distress. Mild sedation can be given intravenously to effect. If the cat is fractious or if struggling continues, general anesthesia is used with a cuffed endotracheal tube.

3. The skin of the lateral chest wall is clipped and aseptically prepared.

4. Local anesthetic can be infiltrated into the intercostal muscles in the dorsal third of the chest near the tenth rib space and in a second site lower on the thorax at the seventh or eighth rib space.

5. A small skin incision is made in the dorsal third of the chest by the tenth rib space. The skin is pulled cranially to the area of the seventh or eighth intercostal space.

6. The tube is tunneled subcutaneously to the region at the seventh or eighth intercostal space, where it will enter the thorax.

7. A hemostat is used to separate the intercostal muscles gently at the site of insertion.

8. Light, controlled pressure is exerted downward (perpendicular to the table) to penetrate the thoracic cavity. A low "pop" of air usually is heard as the tube enters the thorax.

9. The hemostat is released, and the tube is advanced gently into the thoracic cavity. About two-thirds of the tube should lie within the thoracic cavity on the ventral surface.

10. The tube is secured to the skin with nonabsorbable suture. A lightly placed pursestring suture begins the process.

11. Half of the length of the suture is pulled through the skin so that an even amount of suture is on either end of the pursestring.

12. A Chinese fingertrap pattern is used to secure the tube to the chest wall. This simple pattern is composed of the first throw of a surgeon's knot in the front.

13. The two ends are then passed around the tube, one in each direction, and another double throw is made.

14. Continue this pattern for 5–7 throws, and end with a complete surgeon's knot.

15. Cut off the long ends of the suture.

16. Use sterile antibiotic ointment at the thoracostomy site, and wrap the thorax with a light bandage. Cats often object to thoracic bandages, and minimal material is better tolerated.

17. A soft Elizabethan collar, such as the Recovery Collar (Trimline Manufacturing, Boca Raton, FL), is advised.

18. Radiographs are performed after the procedure to confirm proper placement of the tube.

15. What is the difference between continuous and intermittent suction for pleural lavage?

Continuous suction is considered ideal because it offers the advantage of maximal drainage. However, intermittent suction is simpler and easier to manage.

16. How do I perform pleural lavage?

1. To a 1-L bag of sterile isotonic solution (lactated Ringer's solution or 0.9% sodium chloride), add 1500 units of heparin/100 ml of fluid. Heparin may lessen further fibrin formation. The addition of antibiotics to the lavage fluid is no longer recommended by most authorities.

2. After the fluid is warmed to near body temperature, flush 10 ml/kg into each hemithorax and leave for 1 hour, if the cat will tolerate it. Some absorption of fluid occurs during this time.

3. Aspirate fluid from the pleural space. You should recover 50–60% of the original fluid volume. Greater recovery is an indication that a pocket of exudate has been aspirated; less may suggest some pocketing of fluid.

4. A single lavage should not be used as a measure of success or failure; the cumulative amount of fluid over several intervals indicates the efficacy of therapy. Ultrasound or radiographs will demonstrate how successful the lavage has been.

17. How often should lavage and suction be performed?

Initially, lavage and suction should be performed every 3–5 hours. As the fluid becomes clearer and the volume declines, the interval between lavage and suction treatments can be increased. Treatment should continue until the fluid is clear and no organisms are seen cytologically. Usually this goal is achieved within 4–5 days, although intervals of 3–6 and 5–10 days have been recommended.

18. Discuss the role of fibrinolytic agents in pleural lavage.

In human cases of pyothorax (empyema), fibrinolytic agents are often added to the lavage fluid to enhance breakdown of adhesions and improve fluid drainage. Streptokinase is used in patients who have not responded well to drainage and antibiotics. Some studies demonstrated shortening of the duration of treatment, improved drainage, and avoidance of surgical intervention. The dose of streptokinase varied from 50,000 U in children to 250,000 U in adults. This approach may be considered when "pockets" of fluid have localized with fibrin adhesions. However, streptokinase is quite expensive, and no studies have been done in cats.

19. How is nutrition managed after pleural lavage?

Nutrition is critical to resolution of pyothorax in cats. Once the cat is afebrile, a good appetite often returns. On the other hand, thoracic bandages, discomfort, and unfamiliar surroundings may cause inappetance or anorexia. Warming food, providing a variety of flavors, and covering the cat's cage for a certain period each day may be helpful (see Chapter 62). Privacy or quiet or a combination of the two seems to improve appetite. Otherwise, force-feeding or the use of esophagostomy tubes may be required. It is essential to feed the calculated amount of calories necessary to maintain a positive nutritional balance.

20. Discuss the role of analgesia after pleural lavage.

Analgesia may speed recovery. Human patients report that chest tubes are uncomfortable, and some cats seem restless. Therefore, use of a fentanyl patch (25µg/10 lb cat) or intermittent treatment with oxymorphone or buprenorphine should be considered. The fentanyl patch seems to offer the best combination of continuous pain relief and ease of administration. If the cat remains in pain after 3 days with a patch, a second patch may replace the first.

21. Summarize proper care of the thoracostomy site.
The thoracostomy site should be checked daily for leaks and cleaned and rewrapped with a sterile antibiotic ointment at the insertion site, if needed. Take care to avoid entry of bacteria or air into the thorax during bandage changes.

22. How are patients monitored to determine when the chest tube can be removed?
Fluid pockets are easily visualized with ultrasound. Volume of fluid at each aspiration and daily volumes of recovered fluid should be recorded. Declining fluid volume and changes in fluid character indicate successful therapy. Fluid evaluation should begin no later than the third day, if adequate fluid is recovered. Cellularity decreases, as does bacterial count. The absence of organisms indicates resolution of pyothorax. Fluid aspirated from the chest tube before lavage should decrease to ≥ 2 ml/kg/day before tube removal.

If fluid recovery appears to be inadequate, repeated radiographs help to assess chest tube(s) position and fluid drainage. Complications of chest tube placement include kinking, occlusion by fibrin clots, or migration from the ventral thorax. It is sometimes possible to reposition the chest tube. The site should be aseptically prepared, sutures removed, and the tube withdrawn and shifted ventrally. A second tube may be required. Surgical intervention may be indicated if fluid recovery remains poor. Regular assessment of electrolytes is useful throughout treatment. Even when electrolyte abnormalities are not found on presentation, aggressive IV fluid administration and pleural lavage may create imbalances that require correction.

23. When is surgical intervention recommended?
If no improvement in clinical signs, fluid recovery, or fluid character is seen after the first 3 days of therapy, surgical intervention is indicated. Thoracotomy is needed when extensive pleural adhesions prevent adequate drainage and lavage. Pyothorax in conjunction with lung abscessation, thoracic foreign bodies, and intrapleural masses generally requires surgery. Complications associated with chest tube placement also may require surgical intervention.

24. What is necessary after the chest tube is removed?
Long-term administration of oral antibiotics is indicated. After discharge, reevaluation should take place in 1 week and then 1 month later. Antibiotic intervals depend on the organisms isolated but are recommended for a minimum of 1 month. One week after discontinuation of antibiotics, another reevaluation should be scheduled. Relapse is uncommon if lavage has been successful and no underlying cause remains.

25. What are the potential complications of pyothorax?
Lung lobe perforation and pneumothorax can occur if the chest tubes are improperly placed. Other potential complications of pyothorax include fibrinous pleural adhesions, lung lobe entrapment, pneumonia, and overwhelming sepsis. However, the success rate of intermittent lavage, aggressive antibiotic therapy, careful monitoring, and supportive care exceeds 80% in some studies. In one study, cats with pyothorax had the best prognosis compared with other types of pleural effusion.

BIBLIOGRAPHY

1. Davies C, Forester SD: Pleural effusion in cats: 82 cases (1987–1995). J Small Anim Pract 37:217–224, 1996.
2. Dunning D, Orton EC: Pulmonary surgical techniques. In Bojrab MJ (ed): Current Techniques in Small Animal Surgery, 4th ed. Baltimore, Williams & Wilkins, 1998, pp 408–411.
3. Fendin J, Obel N: Catheter drainage of pleural fluid collections and pneumothorax. J Small Anim Pract 38:237–242, 1997.
4. Fooshee SK: Managing the cat with septic pleural effusion. Vet Med 83:907–913, 1988.
5. Fossum TW, Relford RL: Pleural effusion: Physical, biochemical and cytologic characteristics. In August JR (ed): Consultations in Feline Internal Medicine, 2n ed. Philadelphia, W.B. Saunders, 1994, pp 292–293.
6. Fossum T: Pleural and extrapleural diseases. In Ettinger SJ (ed): Textbook of Veterinary Internal Medicine, 5th. Philadelphia, WB Saunders, 2000, pp 1106–1107.
7. Fox SM: The best methods of wound drainage in pets. Vet Med 83:462–472, 1988.

8. Frey DJ, Klapa J, Kaiser D: Irrigation drainage and fibrinolyis for treatment of parapneumonial pleural empyema. Pneumologie 53:596–604, 1999.
9. King L, et al: Roundtable discussion: Feline respiratory disease. Feline Pract 26:16–17, 1998.
10. Jerges-Sanchez C, et al: Intrapleural fibrinolysis with streptokinase as an adjunctive treatment in hemothorax and empyema: A multicenter trial. Chest 109:1514–1519, 1996.
11. Rosen H, et al: Intrapleural streptokinase as adjunctive treatment for persistent empyema in pediatric patients. Chest 103:1190–1193, 1993.
12. Walker AL, Jang SS, Hirsh DC: Bacteria associated with pyothorax in dogs and cats: 98 cases. J Am Vet Med Assoc 216:359–363, 2000.

14. PNEUMOTHORAX

Elisa M. Mazzaferro, M.S., D.V.M.

1. What are the most common causes of pneumothorax in cats?

The most common cause of pneumothorax in cats is trauma, including being hit by a motor vehicle, bite wounds, penetrating injuries (e.g., bullets, arrows), and high-rise syndrome. Other documented causes of pneumothorax include barotrauma secondary to anesthetic equipment malfunction, tracheal rupture, and dirofilariasis. Spontaneous pneumothorax has been documented in dogs but not in cats.

2. What are the three categories of pneumothorax?

Simple pneumothorax usually is associated with nonpenetrating trauma that damages lung parenchyma, resulting in leakage of air into the pleural space.

Open pneumothorax results from a penetrating injury to the chest wall that allows communication between the pleural space and the atmosphere.

Tension pneumothorax occurs when a one-way valve develops in either an airway (bronchopleural fistula) or the chest wall (pleurocutaneous fistula). Negative intrapleural pressure during inspiration aspirates air into the pleural cavity, but air cannot leave during expiration because the one-way valve closes. Once intrapleural pressure exceeds atmospheric pressure, tension pneumothorax develops and rapidly leads to a fatal reduction in gas exchange and cardiac output.

3. What are the clinical signs of pneumothorax?

Cats with pneumothorax typically are presented with respiratory distress, tachypnea, open-mouth breathing, cyanosis or pale pink-to-gray mucous membranes, and a rapid, shallow restrictive respiratory pattern. Pneumothorax should be considered in any cat with known trauma. However, the clinical signs associated with pneumothorax are not pathognomonic and may be observed with other pleural space problems, including pleural effusion and diaphragmatic hernia. Auscultation of the thorax usually reveals muffled heart and lung sounds.

4. What is the most appropriate emergency treatment for pneumothorax?

Therapeutic and diagnostic thoracocentesis should be performed to relieve respiratory distress and stabilize the patient before radiographs are performed. Emergency treatment in patients displaying signs of pneumothorax or a restrictive respiratory pattern includes immediate oxygen supplementation in the form of flow-by oxygen. Analgesia and sedation may be required to alleviate stress of breathing, anxiety, and pain. Morphine (0.025 mg/kg subcutaneously) decreases work of respiration and anxiety in patients requiring thoracocentesis.

5. How is a therapeutic and diagnostic thoracocentesis performed?

1. Clip a 4-inch square section of fur from each side of the thorax.
2. Quickly prepare each area aseptically.

3. Insert a 1-inch, 20–22-gauge needle connected to an extension set, three-way stopcock, and 60-ml into the mid thorax between the seventh-to-tenth intercostal space, carefully avoiding the caudal border of the rib.

4. After inserting the needle into the pleural space, direct the needle parallel with the thoracic wall to avoid penetrating the lung parenchyma.

5. Aspirate air from the chest, and record the volume.

6. If negative pressure is encountered, redirect the needle in several spots, because pockets of air may persist and restrict breathing or cause lung collapse.

7. Once negative pressure is obtained, the entire procedure should be repeated on the other side of the thorax.

5. When are radiographs necessary in patients with pneumothorax?

Radiographs should be performed only after the patient's respiratory and cardiovascular system have been stabilized. Therapeutic thoracocentesis, oxygen therapy, and intravenous fluids for vascular support are often necessary before radiographs. After successful stabilization, radiographs can be performed to evaluate the patient for continued air accumulation, rib fractures, pulmonary contusions, and diaphragmatic hernia.

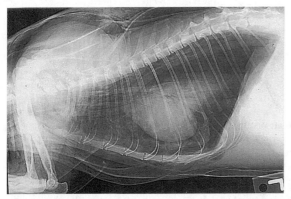

Severe posttraumatic pneumothorax in a cat. Note the subcutaneous emphysema.

6. What concurrent injuries are often observed in patients with pneumothorax secondary to trauma?

When pneumothorax is secondary to trauma, concurrent injuries may include pulmonary contusions, rib fractures or flail chest, myocardial contusions, and diaphragmatic hernia. Penetrating wounds into the thorax also may be associated with vessel laceration and hemothorax, myocardial contusion or hemorrhage, and presence of foreign bodies.

7. What treatment is appropriate for simple pneumothorax?

In most cases, the leak is self-limiting, requiring conservative management with thoracocentesis.

8. How is open pneumothorax managed?

If the wound causing the pneumothorax is small relative to the size of the glottis, adequate ventilation can be maintained. If the wound is large relative to the size of the glottis, severe hypoventilation results. Open pleural wounds should be covered immediately with sterile ointment and bandages. Insertion of a thoracic drain and aspiration of the pleural space can then be done to stabilize the patient.

9. Describe the appropriate management of tension pneumothorax.

Because respiratory impairment develops rapidly, therapeutic thoracocentesis must be performed immediately. Management then proceeds as for open pneumothorax.

10. Define flail chest.

A flail chest occurs when three or more contiguous ribs are fractured in two or more spaces, causing instability of the chest wall. The flail segment often moves paradoxically with respiration: inward during inspiration and outward during expiration. Hypoxemia results from hypoventilation and underlying pulmonary contusions. The pain associated with flail chest contributes significantly to inefficient gas exchange.

11. What is the most appropriate treatment of flail chest?

Treatment of flail chest is directed at alleviating the pain associated with rib fractures. Local anesthesia (bupivacaine at 0.10–0.25 ml/site, taking care not to exceed 2 mg/kg) should be infused at the caudal aspect of each affected rib proximally and distally. The ribs cranial and caudal to the flail segment also should be blocked. Typically, the treatment can be performed up to 3 times/day. However, caution must be taken if lidocaine is used for local anesthesia, because excessive doses have been associated with seizures and hemolytic anemia. In rare cases, external stabilization of the flail segment may be required.

12. What are the indications for placement of a chest tube in cats with pneumothorax?

A chest tube should be placed in cats that develop respiratory distress due to continued accumulation of air within the thorax and cats that require performance of thoracocentesis more than 2–4 times/day.

13. Is sedation appropriate for placement of a chest tube in cats with pneumothorax?

The chest tube should be placed in a way that minimizes stress. When sedation is needed, a 1 µg/kg intravenous bolus of fentanyl or 2–4 mg/kg of intravenous propofol, given to effect, can be used for sedation and chemical restraint. The skin should be aseptically prepared on the side of the thorax generating the air. Local anesthetic (0.75 mg/kg 2% lidocaine or maximum of 2 mg/kg bupivicaine) is then infused near the tenth intercostal space and at a second site where the chest tube will enter the mid-thorax (between the seventh and eighth intercostal space).

14. Describe the technique for placement of a chest tube after appropriate sedation.

1. Use an 8- or 10-French trocarized tube.
2. Make a stab incision with a scalpel blade at the tenth intercostal space, and tunnel the tube under the skin to the seventh or eighth intercostal space. An assistant can pull the skin cranioventrally to aid tunneling.
3. Compress the thorax over the sternum to increase intrathoracic pressure while placing the trocar through the body wall.
4. Once the trocar enters the pleural space, push the tube rapidly off the trocar in a cranioventral direction.
5. Use a large hemostat to clamp off the chest tube and prevent further leakage of air into the chest.
6. The tip of the chest tube should lie on the ventral floor of the thoracic cavity at approximately the third intercostal space, just cranial to the heart.
7. Connect a Christmas tree adapter with extension tubing, three-way stopcock, and 60-ml syringe to the chest tube, open the hemostat, and begin suctioning immediately.
8. Secure the chest tube to the skin with a horizontal mattress suture around the tube.
9. Use a pursestring suture to close the point of entry of the tube into the skin, and further secure the tube with a Chinese finger trap.
10. Cover the entrance point of the tube with betadine-soaked sponges, and bandage the thorax with layers of gauze. The tubing should be incorporated into the bandaging in a way that covers all connections in the system and discourages withdrawal of the tube with traction.
11. The chest tube can be suctioned intermittently as needed or connected to a continuous suction system.
12. If patient discomfort continues, 0.75 mg/kg bupivacaine can be flushed into the chest tube 3 times/day.

15. Describe an alternate method of chest tube placement if a trocarized tube is not available.

1. Use a sterile red rubber feeding tube and a sterile polypropylene urinary catheter.

2. Insert the urinary catheter into the feeding tube to provide rigid support while the feeding tube is placed into the chest.

3. Grasp only the distal end of the red rubber tube with large, curved hemostats.

4. Place the hemostat through the stab incision in the skin and tunnel it with the trocar. Using blunt force, insert the tips of the hemostat through the chest wall at the seventh intercostal space.

5. Pass the red rubber tube into the pleural cavity, and direct it cranially and ventrally to the third intercostal space.

6. Withdraw the urinary catheter, and clamp the red rubber tube with the hemostats.

7. After placement of a Christmas tree adapter, proceed as described for the trocar tube.

8. Take thoracic radiographs after insertion of the chest tube to ensure proper placement within the chest cavity.

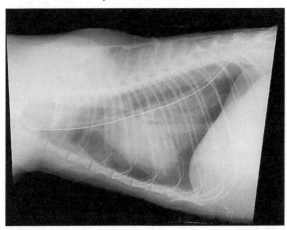

Correct chest tube placement in a cat with pneumothorax.

16. Are Heimlich valves appropriate for treating pneumothorax in cats?

Heimlich valves require sufficient respiratory excursions and generation of positive intrapleural pressure during expiration to force the free air past the one-way Heimlich valve. Because cats typically do not generate enough pressure during expiration to force air past the valve, Heimlich valves are contraindicated in feline patients with pneumothorax.

17. Is continuous suction usually required for treatment of pneumothorax in cats?

Most cats with pneumothorax have small volumes of air in the pleural space and can be handled by hand aspiration intermittently.

19. When should surgical intervention be considered in a cat with pneumothorax?

Conservative therapy is successful in the majority of cases with pneumothorax. When a chest tube is required to alleviate tension pneumothorax or persistent air accumulation, seal of the air leak is expected within 5 days. If air continues to leak, surgical intervention should be considered, since devitalized lung tissue, pleural blebs, or bullae may be limiting resolution of disease.

20. What is the pathogenesis of hypotension in patients with pneumothorax?

Accumulation of free air within the thorax impedes venous return to the heart, resulting in decreased cardiac output and hypotension. With trauma, hypotension is often complicated by acute hypovolemia secondary to hemorrhage.

BIBLIOGRAPHY

1. Berkwitt L, Berzon JL: Thoracic trauma: Newer concepts. Vet Clin North Am Small Anim Pract 15:1031–1038, 1985.
2. Brown DC, Holt D: Subcutaneous emphysema, pneumothorax, pneumomediastinum, and pneumoperi-cardium associated with positive-pressure ventilation in a cat. J Am Vet Med Assoc 206:997–999, 1995.
3. Caylor KB, Moore RW: What is your diagnosis? Severe cervical trachea and substantial subcutaneous emphysema in a cat. J Am Vet Med Assoc 205:561–562, 1994.
4. Evans AT: Anesthesia case of the month. Pneumothorax, pneumomediastinum and subcutaneous emphysema in a cat due to barotraumas after equipment failure during anesthesia. J Am Vet Med Assoc 212:30–32, 1998.
5. Frendin J, Obel N: Catheter drainage of pleural fluid collections and pneumothorax. J Small Anim Pract 38:237–242, 1997.
6. Godfrey DR: Bronchial rupture and fatal tension pneumothorax following routine venipuncture in a kitten. J Am Anim Hosp Assoc 33:260–263, 1997.
7. Hackner SG: Emergency management of traumatic pulmonary contusions. Comp Cont Educ Pract Vet 17:677–686, 1995.
8. Kagan KG: Thoracic trauma. Vet Clin North Am Small Anim Pract 10:641–653, 1980.
9. Kapatkin AS, Matthiesen DT: Feline high-rise syndrome. Comp Cont Educ Pract Vet 13:1389–1396, 1991.
10. Kolata RJ: Management of thoracic trauma. Vet Clin North Am Small Anim Pract 11:103–120, 1981.
11. Malik R, Gabor L, Hunt GB, et al: Benign cranial mediastinal lesions in three cats. Aust Vet J 75:183–187, 1997.
12. Manning MM, Brunson DB: Barotrauma in a cat. J Am Vet Med Assoc 205:62–64, 1994.
13. McKiernan BC, Adams WM, Huse DC: Thoracic bite wounds and associated internal injury in 11 dogs and 1 cat. J Am Vet Med Assoc 184:959–964, 1984.
14. Murtaugh RJ: Acute respiratory distress. Vet Clin North Am Small Anim Pract 24:1041–1055, 1994.
15. Smith JW, Scott-Moncrieff JC, Rivers BJ: Pneumothorax secondary to *Dirofilaria immitis* infection in two cats. J Am Vet Med Assoc 213:91–93, 1998.

15. CHYLOTHORAX

Elisa M. Mazzaferro, M.S., D.V.M., and Davyd Pelsue, D.V.M.

1. Define chylothorax.
Chylothorax is the accumulation of chylomicron-containing fluid within the thoracic cavity. This fluid typically has a white or pink milky appearance, although if the cat is anorectic or on a low-fat diet, the fluid may be less opaque.

2. What conditions have been associated with chylothorax in cats?
Conditions associated with chylothorax in cats include right heart failure, cranial mediastinal mass (lymphosarcoma, thymoma), thrombosis of the jugular vein(s), infection, dirofilariasis, traumatic diaphragmatic hernia, rupture of the thoracic duct, and lung lobe torsion. In many cases, however, the cause of chylothorax is unknown (idiopathic chylothorax).

Conditions Associated with Chylothorax

Right heart failure	Trauma	Postoperative disorders
Persistent atrial standstill	Diaphragmatic hernia	Pulmonary thromboembolism
Restrictive pericarditis	Lung lobe torsion	Thrombosis of cranial vena cava
Tetralogy of Fallot		Jugular catheter placement
Tricuspid dysplasia	**Neoplasia**	
Restrictive cardiomyopathy	Lymphoma	**Infection**
Hypertrophic cardiomyopathy	Thymoma	Feline infectious peritonitis
Dilative cardiomyopathy	Chemodectoma	Dirofilariasis
	Metastatic pulmonary	
	adenocarcinoma	**Idiopathic chylothorax**

3. What diagnostic tests should be performed in cats with chylothorax?

Complete blood cell count, serum biochemistry profile, urinalysis, and serum tests for feline leukemia virus antigens and feline immunodeficiency virus antibodies should be performed in all cats with chylothorax. Echocardiography and thoracic radiographs help to determine whether dilated, restrictive, or hypertrophic cardiomyopathy is present. In addition, thoracic radiographs (horizontal beam) and thoracic ultrasonography help to determine whether the anterior vena cava is occluded by an intrathoracic mass. Determination of total T4 concentrations can be used to rule out hyperthyroidism. In endemic areas, serum *Dirofilaria immitis* antigen and antibody tests should be performed. In cats with dilated cardiomyopathy, plasma taurine levels should be considered, because levels < 30 nmol/ml are suggestive of systemic taurine depletion as a cause for cardiac insufficiency. A fundic examination also should be performed because central retinal degeneration may occur with taurine deficiency.

4. Does idiopathic chylothorax result from rupture of the thoracic duct?

Numerous studies have documented chylothorax without leakage of the thoracic duct. Positive contrast lymphangiography often reveals lymphangiectasia of the cranial mediastinal lymphatic vessels in cats with chylothorax. Although rupture of the thoracic duct has been documented secondary to blunt trauma, the duct often quickly heals and does not result in chylous effusion.

5. What are the presenting complaints in cats with chylothorax?

The most common presenting complaints from owners include dyspnea (respiratory distress), tachypnea, cough, anorexia or inappetance, weight loss, dysphagia, regurgitation, lethargy or weakness, exercise intolerance, depression, salivation, cyanosis, and acute collapse.

6. What are the physical examination findings in cats with chylothorax?

Physical examination findings in cats with chylothorax (or other causes of pleural effusion) include tachypnea, muffled heart sounds, decreased or absent lung sounds below the effusion, increased bronchovesicular sounds over aerated lung fields, and a rapid shallow respiratory pattern consistent with restrictive pulmonary disease. Other signs, which depend on the underlying disease process, may include jugular venous distention (right heart failure, obstruction of the cranial vena cava), arrhythmias, gallop rhythm, murmurs, noncompliant thorax (due to fluid or an anterior mediastinal mass), dehydration, and cachexia due to chronic weight loss.

7. What are the radiographic findings of chylothorax?

Radiographic findings often include unilateral or bilateral pleural effusion with increased opacity throughout the thorax, elevation of the trachea (due to effusion or an anterior mediastinal mass), rounding or scalloping of the lung lobes, loss of the cardiac silhouette, widened interlobar fissures, and retraction of the lung lobes from the thoracic wall. However, these findings are not pathognomonic.

8. How do you perform thoracocentesis?

Thoracocentesis should be performed bilaterally in patients with a restrictive respiratory pattern, often before radiographs are performed. An ethylenediamine tetraacetic acid (EDTA) tube, red-top tube, sterile swab for culture, transport media for culture, microscope slides, and collection bowl should be readily accessible.

1. Clip a 4-inch area over the midthorax on both sides.
2. Prepare the area septically.
3. Use a 21-gauge butterfly catheter, 20–22-gauge fenestrated catheter, or 22-gauge needle for thoracocentesis.
4. An extension set with three-way stopcock and syringe is attached to the tubing of the butterfly catheter or should be available to connect to the catheter as soon as the stylet is removed.
5. Insert the needle or catheter between the seventh and ninth intercostal space in the ventral portion of the thorax, taking care to avoid the intercostal vessels at the caudal aspect of the rib.

6. Gently aspirate fluid from the thorax. The needle may need to be repositioned within the thorax.

7. Bilateral aspiration is recommended to maximize fluid removal.

9. What are the characteristics of chylous effusions?

Chylous effusions typically are opaque and white to pinkish-white; they have a protein content of 2.5–6.0 gm/dl. The protein content may be increased artifactually by the triglyceride concentration. Fibrin content is variable. The fluid is typically nonseptic. Sudan III stain allows visualization of fat droplets. Nucleated cell count varies, ranging from 500–20,000/μl, depending on the cause and chronicity of the chylous effusion. Early in the course of the disease, lymphocytes are typically the predominant cell type, accounting for more than 50% of total nucleated cells. Lymphocyte morphology should be evaluated closely for characteristics of malignancy (see Chapter 16). As the chylous effusion becomes more chronic, necessitating repeated thoracocentesis, nondegenerate neutrophils or macrophages may predominate. Chylous effusions characteristically have elevated triglyceride levels in comparison to serum concentrations. Therefore, an accurate diagnosis of chylous effusion is made by measuring pleural effusion triglyceride and cholesterol levels. A cholesterol:triglyceride ratio in pleural fluid < 1:1 is found in chylothorax.

Characteristics of Chylous Effusions

Color	Milky white, pinkish
Turbidity	Clear to opaque
Specific gravity	1.019–1.038
Cell count	500–20,000
Protein content	2.5–7.8 gm/dl
Fibrin	Variable
Triglyceride	Elevated (higher than serum levels)
Cholesterol	Normal
Cholesterol:triglyceride ratio	< 1
Bacteria	Absent

10. How do you distinguish between chylous effusion and pseudochylous effusion?

It is often difficult to distinguish chylous effusions from pseudochylous effusions visually or cytologically. Triglyceride concentrations are higher in chylous effusion than in serum, whereas pseudochylous effusions have higher cholesterol concentrations and lower triglyceride concentrations than serum.

11. What are the metabolic and pathologic consequences of chronic chylothorax?

Negative consequences of chronic chylothorax include fluid loss and subsequent dehydration, loss of fat-soluble vitamins, electrolyte imbalances (hyponatremia, hyperkalemia), hypoproteinemia, caloric depletion resulting in weight loss and cachexia, and infections secondary to a compromised immune system, lymphopenia, and repeated thoracocentesis. Chronic chylothorax in cats can result in life-threatening fibrosing pleuritis, a thickening of the pleura in response to chronic fluid exudation. Fibrosing pleuritis can occur even after successful management of chylothorax, resulting in restrictive pleural disease and severe respiratory difficulty.

12. What is the most appropriate form of medical management for chylothorax in cats?

Medical management of chylothorax involves repeat thoracic drainage when clinical signs of tachypnea or respiratory distress are noted. If an inciting cause of chylothorax is established, the primary disease should be treated. For example, diuretics, beta blockers, angiotensin-converting inhibitors, and calcium-channel blockers have been used to treat hypertrophic cardiomyopathy (see Chapter 17). Methimazole, surgical thyroidectomy, or radioactive iodine therapy can be used to treat hyperthyroidism (see Chapter 53). Surgery, radiation therapy, or chemotherapy can be used to treat neoplasia of the anterior mediastinum, depending on tissue type (see Chapter 16).

13. How can dietary management assist in the treatment of chylothorax in cats?

A low-fat diet has been used successfully. Commercial diets or homemade diets can be used. A commonly used homemade diet consists of 1 cup boiled rice, potato, oatmeal or pasta; 1 cup low-fat (2%) cottage cheese (or skinned chicken breast or water-packed tuna instead of cottage cheese), and ½ teaspoon calcium carbonate. Medium-chain triglycerides have been advocated, with the rationale that they do not enter the lymphatic system and, therefore, do not contribute to the development of chylothorax. However, medium-chain triglycerides have been documented in the thoracic duct of humans and dogs with chylothorax. Therefore, their efficacy is questionable.

14. What drugs may be helpful?

Diuretics are not routinely recommended for cats with chylothorax. There is no definitive proof that they decrease production of chylous fluid, and diuretic therapy may lead to dehydration. Benzopyrones, such as rutin, have been used with some success to decrease lymph production and increase lymph removal.

15. Describe the mechanism of action of rutin in the treatment of chylothorax.

Benzopyrone derivatives, such as the bioflavinoid rutin (250–500 mg/cat orally every 8 hr), have been used successfully with low-fat diets in the treatment of chylothorax—with or without surgical intervention. Bioflavinoids have several proposed mechanisms of action, including decreased leakage from blood vessels, increased protein removal from lymphatic vessels, increased phagocytosis via macrophage stimulation, and increased proteolysis and lymph removal from tissues.

16. Is administration of glucocorticoids beneficial?

Some authoritites have advocated the administration of glucocorticoids to cats with chronic, idiopathic chylothorax. The rationale is that glucocorticoids decrease inflammation due to pleuritis and may decrease chylous effusion production. However, no controlled studies document the efficacy of glucocorticoids for this syndrome.

17. Should pleurodesis be attempted?

Chemical pleurodesis achieved by instilling sterile talc or tetracyclines through previously placed chest tubes has not been documented to be effective for the treatment of idiopathic chylothorax. However, it does increase inflammation and discomfort for the cat.

18. Name several surgical options for treatment of chylothorax.

- Ligation of the thoracic duct and its tributaries
- Passive pleuroperitoneal shunting, which shunts chyle into the abdomen for absorption by a large surface area,
- Active pleuroperitoneal or pleurovenous shunting
- Pleurodesis

Surgery may be more difficult in cats because of their small size. Ligation of the thoracic duct successfully resolved chylothorax in approximately 53% of cats in which the procedure was performed.

19. How is thoracic duct ligation performed?

A thoracic duct lymphangiogram typically is performed before a left tenth intercostal thoracotomy. Alternatively, a transdiaphragmatic approach may be used. Injection of methylene blue into a mesenteric lymph vessel may improve visualization of the thoracic duct. Once identified, it is ligated with silk or hemoclips. The lymphangiogram helps to define the anatomy of the thoracic duct and demonstrate abnormalities, if present. A postoperative lymphangiogram may be performed to demonstrate complete occlusion of the duct.

20. When should I consider surgery for cats with chylothorax?

When clinical signs require thoracic drainage more often than once a week and medical management does not appear to be reducing chyle formation, surgical intervention should be considered. Cats that have developed significant protein or caloric malnutrition are poor surgical candidates; therefore, surgery should be considered before the animal becomes debilitated.

21. What is the prognosis for cats with chylothorax?

The prognosis for cats with chylothorax is guarded to poor, unless definitive treatment for an underlying disease is successful. Spontaneous remission has been reported, and medical therapy may benefit a certain percentage of cases. Use of rutin may improve management of cats with chylothorax. In a recent study, 3 of 4 cats treated with low-fat diets and rutin had long-term resolution of chylothorax. Surgery also can be considered for cats with chylothorax. Regardless of treatment, however, fibrosing pleuritis can decrease quality of life and increase mortality rates.

BIBLIOGRAPHY

1. Birchard SJ, Fossum TW: Chylothorax in the dog and cat. Vet Clin North Am Small Anim Pract 17:271–283, 1987.
2. Birchard SJ, Smeak DD, McLoughlin MA: Treatment of idiopathic chylothorax in dogs and cats. J Am Vet Med Assoc 212:652–657, 1998.
3. Davies C, Forrester SD: Pleural effusions in cats: 82 cases (1987–1995). J Small Anim Pract 37:217–224, 1996.
4. Fossum TW, Jacobs RM, Birchard SJ: Evaluation of cholesterol and triglyceride concentrations in differentiating chylous and nonchylous pleural effusions in dogs and cats. J Am Vet Med Assoc 188:49–51, 1986.
5. Fossum TW, Miller MW, Rogers KS, et al: Chylothorax associated with right-sided heart failure in five cats. J Am Vet Med Assoc 204:84–89, 1994.
6. Fossum TW, Forrester D, Swenson CL, et al: Chylothorax in cats: 37 cases (1969–1989). J Am Vet Med Assoc 198:671–678, 1991.
7. Harpster NK. Chylothorax. In Kirk RW (ed): Current Veterinary Therapy IX. Small Animal Practice. Philadelphia, W.B. Saunders, 1986, pp 393–399.
8. Hawkins EC, Fossum TW: Medical and surgical management of pleural effusion. In Kirk RW (ed): Current Veterinary Therapy XIII. Small Animal Practice. Philadelphia, W.B. Saunders, 2000, pp 819–825.
9. Kerpsack SJ, McLoughlin MA, Birchard SJ, et al: Evaluation of mesenteric lymphangiography and thoracic duct ligation in cats with chylothorax: 19 cases (1987–1992). J Am Vet Med Assoc 205:711–715, 1994.
10. Smeak DD, Kerpsack SJ: Management of feline chylothorax. In Kirk RW (ed): Current Veterinary Therapy XII. Small Animal Practice. Philadelphia, W.B. Saunders, 1995, pp 921–927.
11. Thompson MS, Cohn LA: Use of rutin for medical management of idiopathic chylothorax in four cats. J Am Vet Med Assoc 215:345–348, 1999.
12. Tyler RD, Cowell RL: Evaluation of pleural and peritoneal effusions. Vet Clin North Am Small Anim Pract 19:743–768, 1989.

16. LOWER RESPIRATORY TRACT NEOPLASIA

Nicole Leibman, D.V.M.

1. What are the most common tumors in the larynx and trachea of cats?

Neoplasia of the larynx and trachea are rare in cats. The most common histologic types of tumors in these areas are squamous cell carcinoma, adenocarcinoma, and lymphoma.

2. What are typical clinical signs in cats with laryngeal or tracheal neoplasia?

- Voice change
- Ptyalism
- Respiratory stridor
- Dysphagia
- Cyanosis
- Dyspnea
- Gagging
- Anorexia
- Hemoptysis
- Cough

Affected cats also may carry the neck in an extended position.

3. What diagnostic tests should be performed in cats with suspected laryngeal or tracheal neoplasia?

Radiography often reveals a distinct mass, although sometimes only narrowing of the airway lumen may be evident. Laryngoscopy, tracheoscopy, computed tomography, and magnetic resonance imaging may be required alone or in combination to determine the extent of disease. A disadvantage of these procedures is the need for general anesthesia in a potentially compromised patient. If obstruction of a large airway is suspected, it is wise to anticipate the need for a tracheotomy. Often anesthesia is reserved for a surgical procedure that is both therapeutic and diagnostic. Usually, laryngeal tumors can be visualized intraorally; therefore, they can easily be biopsied. Surgery or endoscopy is often necessary to gain biopsy samples from tracheal tumors.

Routine blood work generally is performed, depending on the cat's age. Thoracic radiographs should be performed to rule out metastatic disease and pneumonia. Regional lymph nodes should be aspirated and cytology examined, regardless of whether or not they are enlarged. If lymphoma is suspected, chest and abdominal radiographs, complete blood cell count, serum biochemical panel, urinalysis, serum tests for feline leukemia virus (FeLV) angitens and feline immunodeficiency virus (FIV) antibodies, and cytology of a bone marrow aspirate may be indicated.

4. What are the treatment options for cats with laryngeal or tracheal neoplasia?

Lymphoma is best treated with combination chemotherapy and/or radiation therapy. Benign tumors on a stalk can be removed via endoscopy. Resection and anastamosis can be used to remove small tracheal tumors that involve only 3–4 tracheal rings. Laryngeal or tracheal tumors with metastatic spread are not candidates for curative surgical procedures, although debulking surgery may prolong life and result in temporary improvement in clinical signs. Palliative surgical, chemotherapeutic, and radiation treatments also may be used, depending on tumor type.

5. What is the prognosis for cats with tumors of the trachea or larynx?

Because these tumors are so rare, there is little information about prognosis.

6. What is the most common primary lung tumor of cats?

Primary lung tumors are rare, but histologically the most common type is the bronchial or bronchial-alveolar adenocarcinoma. Tumors of mesenchymal origin are very uncommon. Conversely, the lung is a common site for metastatic disease.

7. Describe the typical signalment of a cat with a primary lung tumor.

Most cats are 10–12 years of age, and spayed females seem to be overrepresented. Domestic shorthairs also are overrepresented.

8. What clinical signs are common in cats with primary lung tumors?

Cats often present with dyspnea, coughing, lethargy, and anorexia. Nonrespiratory signs, including general lethargy, weight loss, and pyrexia, may be predominant in some cats. Lameness occurs in some cats because of metastatic disease or hypertrophic osteopathy.

9. What diagnostic tests should be performed to stage suspected pulmonary neoplasia?

Radiographic findings suggestive of a primary lung tumor include a single, circumscribed mass or marked lobar consolidation. A diffuse, mixed pattern composed of severe peribronchial infiltration, a reticulonodular pattern, and alveolar filling also can be found with pulmonary neoplasia.

The possibility of metastatic pulmonary neoplasia should be excluded by completing a complete blood cell count, serum biochemical panel, urinalysis, FeLV serum antigen test, FIV serum antibody test, abdominal radiographs and/or ultrasound, and potentially bone radiographs.

If pleural effusion is present, it is often necessary to remove the fluid to evaluate the lung parenchma appropriately on radiographs. Cytologic evaluation of the effusion should be performed to help differentiate heart failure, lymphoma, mesothelioma, feline infectious peritonitis, and thymoma.

Fine-needle aspiration (FNA) of pulmonary masses, with or without ultrasound guidance, can be a useful tool. Neoplastic seeding of the pleura has not been reported, and in one study FNA was diagnostic for primary lung tumors in 80% of cases. Cytology of primary carcinomas usually reveals round epithelial cells forming glands or arranged in rows. Other markers of malignancy include anisocytosis and anisokaryosis, basophilic cytoplasm, and a high nuclear-to-cytoplasma ratio. Biopsy may be necessary for definitive diagnosis in some cats. Biopsies can be obtained through surgical exploratory, thoracoscopy, or ultrasound-guided procedures.

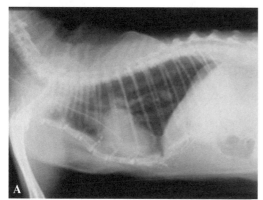

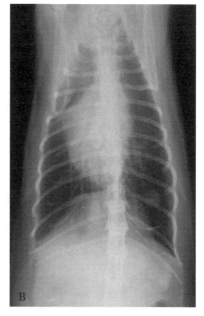

Primary pulmonary adenocarcinoma in the left caudal lung lobe of a middle-aged cat.

10. What is the most common anatomic site for primary lung tumor in cats?
The left caudal lung lobe is involved in most cases.

11. What are the differential diagnoses for solitary lung masses in cats?
Differential diagnoses include metastatic neoplasia, cyst, infarct, granuloma, localized hemorrhage, localized pneumonia, fungal disease, lung lobe torsion, and abscess.

12. What is the treatment of choice for cats with primary pulmonary neoplasia?
Surgery is the treatment of choice if less than 3 nodules are visible on radiographs and the cat does not demonstrate negative prognostic factors, such as lymph node metastases and distant metastatic disease.

13. What is the prognosis for cats treated with surgery for primary lung tumors?
In one study, cats with primary lung tumors treated with surgery alone had a median survival of 115 days. Cats with tracheobronchial lymph node enlargement treated with surgery had a median survival time of 73 days, whereas cats without tracheobronchial lymph node enlargement at the time of surgery had a median survival of 412 days. Cats with poorly differentiated tumors have a worse prognosis after surgery than cats with moderately differentiated tumors (median survival time of 75 days vs. 698 days).

14. What is the most common tumor of the mediastinum in cats?
Lymphoma in the most common mediastinal tumor and is thought to originate from mediastinal lymph nodes or thymic tissue. Differential diagnoses include thymoma, thymic cyst, ectopic

thyroid tumors, and chemoreceptor tumors. In general, mediastinal lymphoma affects younger cats, whereas thymic neoplasia develops in older cats.

15. What clinical signs and physical examination findings are typical in cats with mediastinal disease?

Cats often present with dyspnea, cough, and dysphagia. Because of mass effect or pleural effusion, most have a restrictive breathing pattern if dyspnea is present. Pleural effusion is secondary to tumor compression of lymphatics and decreased venous return to the heart, causing congestion and secondary transudation. Many cats with a mediastinal mass have a cranial thoracic cavity that cannot be compressed.

16. What diagnostic tests should be performed when mediastinal disease is suspected?

Radiography, thoracocentesis with cytologic evaluation of pleural fluid, and FNA of mass lesions are performed when possible. For staging suspected mediastinal lymphoma, a complete blood count, serum chemistry profile, urinalysis, abdominal ultrasound, FeLV serum antigen test, FIV serum antibody test, and cytology of a bone marrow aspiration should be performed. Of cats with mediastinal lymphoma, 80% are positive for FeLV. These diagnostic tests are also important to rule out other diseases.

17. How do effusions associated with lymphoma differ from those associated with thymoma?

Both tumors lead to effusions that usually are characterized as modified transudates. Effusions induced by thymoma contain primarily small, mature lymphocytes, epithelial cells, and sometimes mast cells. Effusions induced by lymphoma usually contain large lymphoblastic lymphocytes. However, small lymphocytes are the predominant cell in some cases.

18. What are the chemotherapeutic options for cats with mediastinal lymphoma?

Several chemotherapuetic options have been described in the literature. Historically, the cyclophosphamide, vincristine, and prednisone (COP) protocol has been the basis for treatment. In one study, 12 cats treated with a COP protocol attained a 92% complete remission rate, with a median remission duration of 6 months. In another study, cats with mediastinal lymphoma were treated with vincristine, cyclophosphamide, and methotrexate. Only 45% responded, with a median remission of 2 months. In cats with stage I and II lymphoma treated with combination chemotherapy consisting of L-asparaginase, vincristine, methotrexate, cyclophosphamide, and prednisone, the median survival was 7.6 months. Lastly, cats with lymphoma in several anatomic locations that were treated with induction chemotherapy with the COP protocol and maintained with 5 doses of doxorubicin enjoyed a median remission duration of 281 days. Overall, combination chemotherapy is recommended, although each patient should be evaluated individually. In some cases single agent therapy may be more appropriate.

19. Can radiation be effective for treatment of mediastinal lymphoma?

Cats with severe respiratory signs secondary to a mediastinal mass can respond favorably to radiation therapy. Because malignant lymphocytes are extremely radiation-sensitive, radiation therapy can cause a rapid reduction in tumor burden during life-threatening episodes. Chemotherapy should be administered with radiation treatment because lymphoma is considered a systemic disease.

20. What is the treatment of choice for cats with a thymoma?

Surgery is the treatment of choice. The median survival is 16 months for cats that survive the perioperative period. Encapsulated tumors seem to have a better prognosis.

21. Are paraneoplastic syndromes associated with thymomas and lymphomas in cats?

Paraneoplastic syndromes, such as myasthenia gravis, polymyositis, and hypercalcemia, are much more common in dogs. In one study, only 2 of 12 cats developed paraneoplastic syndromes, and both developed acquired myasthenia gravis. Paraneoplastic syndromes associated with lymphoma have been described in cats, although hypercalcemia associated with mediastinal lymphoma is rare.

BIBLIOGRAPHY

1. Barr IF, Gruffydd-Jones TJ, Brown PJ, et al: Primary lung tumors in the cat. J Small Anim Pract 28:1115–1125, 1987.
2. Bell FW: Neoplastic diseases of the thorax. Vet Clin North Am Small Anim Pract 17:387–409, 1987.
3. Carlisle CH, Biery DN, Thrall DE: Tracheal and laryngeal tumors in the dog and cat: Literature review and 13 additional patients. Vet Radiol 32:229–235, 1991.
4. Carpenter JL, Holzworth J: Thymoma in 11 cats. J Am Vet Med Assoc 181:248–251, 1982.
5. Cotter SM: Treatment of lymphoma and leukemia with cyclophosphamide, vincristine, and prednisone. II. Treatment of cats. J Am Anim Hosp Assoc 19:166–172, 1983.
6. Elmslie R, Ogilvie G, Gillette E, et al: Radiotherapy with and without chemotherapy for localized lymphoma in 10 cats. Vet Radiol 32:277–280, 1991.
7. Gores BR, Berg J, Carpenter JL: Surgical treatment of thymoma in cats:12 cases (1987–1992). J Am Vet Med Assoc 204:1782–1785, 1994.
8. Hahn KA, McEntee MF: Primary lung tumors in cats: 86 cases (1979–1994). J Am Vet Med Assoc 211:1257–1260, 1997.
9. Hahn KA, McEntee MF: Prognosis factors for survival in cats after removal of a primary lung tumor: 21 cases (1979–1994). Vet Surg 27:307–311, 1998.
10. Hahn KA, Anderson TE: Tumors of the respiratory tract. In Bonagura JD (ed): Kirk's Current Veterinary Therapy XIII. Philapelphia, WB Saunders, 2000, pp 500–505.
11. Jeglum KA, Whereat A, Young K: Chemotherapy of lymphoma in 75 cats. J Am Vet Med Assoc 190: 174–178, 1987.
12. Melhalf CJ, Mooney S: Primary pulmonary neoplasia in the dog and cat. Vet Clin North Am Small Anim Pract 14:1061–1075, 1985.
13. Miles KG: A review of primary lung tumors in the dog and cat. Vet Radiol 29:122–133, 1988.
14. Mooney SC, Hayes AA, MacEwen EG, et al: Treatment and prognostic factors in lymphoma in cats: 103 cases (1977–1981). J Am Vet Med Assoc 194:696–699, 1989.
15. Moore AS, Cotter SM, Frimberger AE, et al: A comparison of doxorubicin and COP for maintenance of remission in cats with lymphoma. J Vet Intern Med 10:372–375, 1996.
16. Saik JE, Toll SL, Diters RW, et al: Canine and feline laryngeal neoplasia: A 10 year survey. J Am Anim Hosp Assoc 22:359–365, 1986.

17. MYOCARDIAL DISEASES

C. Bisque Jackson, V.M.D.

1. Define cardiomyopathy.
Cardiomyopathies represent a heterogeneous class of diseases characterized by primary structural abnormalities and functional impairment of the heart muscle. **Idiopathic or primary cardiomyopathy** excludes conditions that result from valvular, pulmonary, vascular, pericardial, congenital, or systemic disease. **Secondary cardiomyopathy** refers to abnormalities of the heart muscle related to systemic disease. Examples include hypertrophic cardiomyopathy associated with hyperthyroidism or arterial hypertension.

2. What are the different types of cardiomyopathies?
The primary myocardial diseases in cats can be divided morphologically and functionally into hypertrophic, restrictive, and dilated cardiomyopathy.

3. What is hypertrophic cardiomyopathy?
Hypertrophic cardiomyopathy (HCM) is the most common feline myocardial disorder. It affects a broad range of ages, although young to middle-aged male cats seem to be affected most frequently. The hallmark characteristic of HCM is a hypertrophied, nondilated left ventricle in the absence of other cardiac, systemic, or metabolic diseases. Left atrial or biatrial enlargement (dilation) is common, and mild-to-moderate right ventricular hypertrophy is often present. The

functional abnormality associated with HCM is diastolic dysfunction due a reduction in both left ventricular chamber size and distensibility secondary to hypertrophy. Systolic function tends to be normal to increased. Left ventricular hypertrophy has many morphologic expressions and variable distributions; hypertrophy may be symmetric, affecting all wall segments proportionally, or asymmetric, affecting only segments of the interventricular septum, left ventricular free wall, and/or papillary muscles. Morphologic changes may include septal hypertrophy that leads to narrowing of the left ventricular outflow tract and dynamic outflow obstruction. Systolic anterior motion (SAM) of the mitral valve also can contribute to outflow obstruction. The typical histopathologic lesion in HCM is ventricular myofiber disorganization.

4. Which breeds are predisposed to HCM?
    Domestic shorthair, Maine coon, and Persian cats seem to be predisposed to HCM, and evidence for genetic transmission in these breeds is mounting. Recent studies suggest that HCM is a familial disorder with an autosomal dominant pattern of transmission. The mutation is thought to involve a defect in the cardiac β-myosin heavy chain gene (the gene that encodes the cardiac sarcomere protein).

5. Define restrictive cardiomyopathy.
    Recently attention has focused on a newly classified feline myocardial disease termed restrictive cardiomyopathy (RCM). Although RCM shares many structural and functional features with HCM, its unique feature is severe diastolic dysfunction with little-to-no ventricular hypertrophy. Significant left atrial or biatrial enlargement is another hallmark. Systolic function is usually well preserved or only slightly impaired. The disease is not well characterized but seems to result from impaired ventricular compliance and filling due to infiltration of the myocardium or endomyocardium by fibrous tissue or some other infiltrative process. The disease, however, is frequently classified as idiopathic. Histopathologically, extensive endocardial scar formation and myocardial fibrosis are present.

6. What is dilated cardiomyopathy?
    The hallmark characteristic of dilated cardiomyopathy (DCM) is dilation of all chambers of the heart and severe systolic dysfunction. In 1987, the association between taurine deficiency and DCM in cats was recognized. At that time, supplemental taurine was added to most commercial feline diets, and the number of cats affected with DCM markedly declined. Presently, DCM due to taurine deficiency is a rare disease in cats. The few cats affected tend to be on unsupplemented homemade diets or some other unconventional food. Idiopathic DCM is diagnosed more commonly in cats with systolic myocardial failure. Myocyte degeneration and necrosis are the common histopathologic findings.

7. Why is taurine important for cardiac function?
    Taurine is an essential amino acid for cats. Cats have a low concentration of cysteine-sulfinic acid decarboxylase, an enzyme required for taurine biosynthesis. As a result, their ability to synthesize taurine from cysteine and methionine is limited. Taurine is essential for normal structural and functional integrity of the heart and tapetum. Evaluation of the heart and retina should be performed on cats that are fed noncommercial diets.

8. What are the normal taurine values?
    Cats with myocardial failure have plasma taurine concentrations < 30 nmol/ml (normal = > 60 nmol/ml) or whole blood taurine concentrations < 100 nmol/mL (normal = > 200 nmol/ml). In addition, most of these cats were found to have concurrent retinal lesions, consisting of bilateral elliptical hyperreflective lesions in the area centralis in the early stages and diffuse retinal degeneration and blindness in the later stages.

9. Are myocardial changes reversible with taurine supplementation?
    Treatment with oral taurine supplementation probably improves clinical signs, restores myocardial function, and improves survival when taurine deficiency is responsible for DCM.

Echocardiographic improvements can be seen within 1 month of treatment, and some cats may be normal after 2–3 months of therapy. The recommended dose of taurine is 250–500 mg/cat/day. Cats with idiopathic DCM show little-to-no improvement on oral taurine supplementation.

10. What are the common clinical signs in cats with heart disease?

The broad range of clinical abnormalities depends on the severity of the underlying cardiac disease. Many cats are affected subclinically, and evidence of heart disease is detected during routine examination. Clinically affected cats tend to have a history of inactivity, depression, anorexia, and vomiting. Some cats may present for syncope secondary to bradyarrythmias or tachyarrhythmias, and others present with acute pelvic limb paralysis secondary to a distal aortic thrombus. Cats with distal aortic thrombus have absent femoral pulses and cool pelvic limbs and tend to experience significant pain. In addition, some cats display paresis of a front limb associated with embolization.

11. What are the common physical examination features in cats with heart disease?

Common physical examination findings include tachypnea, dyspnea, and crackles due to pulmonary congestion from left-sided heart failure. Decreased lung or heart sounds also may be present and suggest pleural and/or pericardial effusion. Ascites, hepatomegaly, and jugular venous distention may be present with right-sided heart failure. Because cats rarely present with exclusive right-sided heart failure, biventricular failure is likely if these findings are present. Heart rates can vary, but typically cats are tachycardic with heart rates > 200 beats/min. Systolic murmurs, abnormal heart sounds (gallop rhythms), arrhythmias, and possible pulse deficits are also frequently present. Other physical examination findings may include hypothermia, pale mucous membranes, and weak femoral pulses secondary to a low output state due to myocardial dysfunction.

12. What is the initial diagnostic plan for cats with myocardial disease?

After a thorough history and physical examination, the diagnostic work-up for cats with myocardial disease should include a complete blood count, biochemistry profile, urinalysis, total T4 concentration, thoracic radiographs, arterial blood pressure, electrocardiogram, and echocardiogram. The diagnostic work-up should not be initiated until the patient has stabilized completely.

13. What are the common laboratory findings in cats with heart disease?

Cats are often mildly azotemic as a result of decreased renal perfusion, decreased water consumption, and fluid sequestration. Mild elevations in liver enzyme activities may be seen from hypoxia due to decreased liver perfusion. A stress leukogram is usually present, along with hyperglycemia. If aortic thromboembolism is present, increased creatine phosphokinase (CPK), lactate dehydrogenase (LDH), and aspartate aminotransferase (AST) activities usually are detected.

14. How is hyperthyroidism associated with heart disease?

Hyperthroidism results in a high-output cardiac state with low peripheral vascular resistance. The high-output state causes an increase in myocardial metabolic rate (work load) and oxygen consumption. The resulting cardiac compensatory change is an increase in myocardial protein synthesis and subsequent hypertrophy. Circulating thyroid hormone also interacts with the sympathetic nervous system, causing an increase in the number of ß-receptors and in their sensitivity to catecholamines. This change also causes an increase in the metabolic rate of the myocardium. Reduced peripheral vascular resistance causes volume retention via renal mechanisms that conserve fluid (renin-angiotensin-aldosterone system). The cardiac compensatory changes seen with increased blood volume lead to chamber dilation.

15. When should hyperthyroidism be considered a possible diagnosis?

Hyperthyroidism should be considered in any cat over 6 years of age that exhibits clinical signs of hyperthyroidism (tachycardia, weight loss, polyuria, polydipsia, hyperactivity) and heart disease. Therefore, careful palpation of the cervical region to detect thyroid nodules is recommended for cats with historical or physical exam features consistent with cardiomyopathy.

Cardiomyopathy associated with hyperthyroidism tends to be reversible with appropriate treatment in an otherwise healthy heart.

16. What are the radiographic findings in cats with cardiomyopathies?

The purpose of thoracic radiographs is to evaluate heart size and shape, pulmonary parenchyma, and pulmonary vasculature. Left-sided heart enlargement or generalized cardiomegaly are the most common radiographic findings. Pulmonary parenchymal changes can include an interstitial and/or alveolar pattern that may be diffuse, patchy, or focal in distribution. Pulmonary venous distension may be present secondary to left-sided heart failure. Other findings may include pleural effusion, hepatomegaly, or ascites.

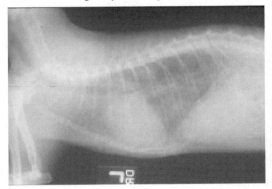
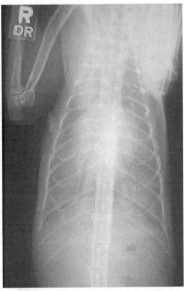

Thoracic radiographs of a cat with hypertrophic cardiomyopathy and heart failure. (Courtesy of Dr. Chris Orton, Colorado State University.)

17. Are cats with heart disease hypertensive?

Systemic arterial hypertension does not usually occur secondary to heart disease, but hypertension should be considered in the differential diagnoses for any cat with left ventricular hypertrophy. Myocardial changes usually result from rather than cause hypertension. Common causes for systemic hypertension in cats include renal disease, and hyperthyroidism (see Chapter 63). Other less common diseases include pheochromocytoma, primary aldosteronism due to an adrenal tumor or hyperplasia (Conn's syndrome), and hyperadrenocorticism. Primary (essential) hypertension is now a recognized disease in cats.

18. What electrocardiographic (EKG) findings are associated with cardiomyopathies?

The EKG of cats with cardiomyopathy is often unremarkable. When present, electrocardiographic abnormalities are highly variable and do not distinguish among the forms of cardiomyopathy. The purpose of the EKG is to determine heart rate and to evaluate for the presence and type of arrhythmias as well as left and/or right-sided heart enlargement. Typically, cats with heart disease are tachycardic. Some, however, may have normal rates, and others may be syncopal as a result of severe bradyarrhythmias.

Among the more common EKG abnormalities are supraventricular tachycardia, atrial premature contractions, first-degree atrioventricular block, left anterior fascicular block, left bundle-branch block, ventricular premature contraction, and ventricular tachycardias. Measurement of EKG complexes helps to determine whether left- and/or right-sided heart enlargement is present. Left atrial enlargement is present if the P-wave duration is > 0.04 sec; right atrial enlargement if the P-wave amplitude is > 0.2mV; and left ventricular enlargement if the QRS duration is

> 0.04 sec and the R wave amplitude is > 0.8mV. Low-voltage QRS complexes can be seen with severe pleural and pericardial effusion.

19. What echocardiographic findings are associated with cardiomyopathy?

The morphologic patterns encountered on echocardiography are complex and depend on the type and severity of underlying cardiomyopathy. In brief, HCM is characterized by thickening of the left ventricular free wall or septum at end-diastole; measured wall thickness is > 6 mm. Typically, cats with RCM demonstrate severe left atrial enlargement in the absence of severe left ventricular dilation or hypertrophy. Abnormal echogenicity of the left ventricular free wall may be present. DCM is typified by increased left ventricular end-systolic dimension (> 12 mm) with decreased fractional shortening (< 30%). Often, all four cardiac chambers are dilated.

20. What cardiovascular emergencies are commonly seen in cats?

The most common medical emergency is left-sided heart failure resulting in pulmonary edema and, less commonly, pleural effusion. Such cats usually present in severe respiratory distress with pulmonary crackles. Acute arterial thromboembolism resulting in pelvic limb paralysis is another frequently encountered emergency. Less common emergencies include biventricular failure resulting in pulmonary edema and systemic venous congestion (ascites, pericardial effusion) and syncope from brady- or tachyarrhythmias.

21. What other diseases can cause an acute onset of respiratory distress?

Cats that present with an acute onset of respiratory distress (tachypnea, dyspnea, open mouth breathing) usually have cardiac disease, lower airway disease (asthma), or pleural space disease (see Chapter 8). Thorough thoracic auscultation can determine accurately whether pleural space disease is present, requiring thoracocentesis. A history of cough and/or the presence of tracheal sensitivity indicates that airway disease is more likely, whereas a heart murmur or gallop rhythm is more typical in cats with cardiac disease. In compromised cats, oxygen should be administered, and treatment for both cardiac disease (diruretic) and asthma (glucocorticoids) may be required to stabilize the cat before diagnostic testing.

22. What are the initial goals of therapy for left-sided congestive heart failure?

Important initial therapy includes cage rest and supplemental oxygen therapy. It is imperative not to stress a cat in severe respiratory distress, because pulmonary edema can be rapidly and progressively life-threatening.

23. What drugs may be used to treat left-sided congestive heart failure?

Furosemide should be administered intravenously as soon as possible, although the intramuscular route is sufficient in a severely compromised cat. Furosemide, a loop diuretic, inhibits tubular reabsorption of sodium, chloride, and potassium in the ascending loop of Henle, thereby decreasing water reabsorption. Decreased water reabsorption reduces vascular volume and preload, thus decreasing left ventricular filling pressures and pulmonary edema. The dose of furosemide therapy ranges from 0.5–2.0 mg/kg every 1–12 hr. The goal of diuretic therapy is to resolve congestion within 24 hours so that the cat can breathe comfortably and oxygen therapy can be discontinued. At that time, maintenance doses of furosemide can be initiated. Recommended doses range from 1.1–2.2 mg/kg orally every 24–48 hr.

Nitroglycerine ointment (2%) also should be used in the treatment of acute, life-threatening pulmonary edema. Nitroglycerine is a potent, direct-acting vasodilator that increases venous capacitance, thus reducing preload. The recommended dose is ½ inch cutaneously to the pinna every 6–8 hours for the first 24–48 hours. Gloves are worn during application of nitroglycerine to prevent systemic absorption.

24. Describe the treatments for acute aortic thromboembolism.

Most cats with thromboembolism (TE) have accompanying signs of congestive heart failure; therefore, treatment for heart failure should be instituted as previously discussed. Judicious use of analgesics is appropriate for the first 24–48 hours because the ischemic insult is very painful. Butorphanol (0.05–0.2 mg/kg intravenously or intramuscularly every 8 hr) or morphine (0.05–0.1 mg/kg intramuscularly every 8 hr) provides good analgesia. Various medical treatments have been advocated for the treatment of TE, but most are empirical and no data support any single treatment. Current therapy is aimed at lysing the existing clot with thrombolytic agents or at preventing new thrombus formation or growth with anticoagulants. The current thrombolytic agents include tissue plasminogen activator (t-PA), streptokinase, and urokinase. Bleeding, severe reperfusion injury, and death are severe complications that can be associated with these drugs, and they should be used cautiously in cats. The anticoagulants used to impair clotting factor synthesis or enhance inactivation are warfarin and heparin, respectively. These drugs should be used with caution because they can result in severe bleeding complications without appropriate monitoring. Monitoring of bleeding times (one-stage prothrombin time or international normalized ratio for warfarin and activated partial thromboplastin time for heparin) is imperative if an anticoagulant is used. Aspirin often is used to retard thrombus formation or growth, because inhibition of thromboxane production theoretically should block platelet aggregation. The clinical effects of aspirin therapy are controversial, and most cats reembolize despite aspirin therapy.

25. What are the goals of maintenance therapy for HCM and RCM?
- To prevent congestion (diuretic therapy);
- To control heart rate and rhythm (beta blockers, calcium channel blockers)
- To block the neurohormonal mediators of heart failure, notably angiotensin, aldosterone, and epinephrine, and thus induce regression of the hypertrophy, (angiotensin-converting enzyme [ACE] inhibitors, spironolactone, beta blockers)
- To reduce the likelihood of TE with anticoagulants (heparin, warfarin, aspirin)

26. What is the recommended therapy for HCM and RCM?
There is no single treatment recommendation for heart disease. Therapy must be tailored to the particular type, severity, and duration of the cardiomyopathy. Frequent monitoring of patients is advocated. and drug therapy should be adjusted accordingly. Most cats affected with HCM or RCM are treated with furosemide, calcium channel blocker or a beta blocker, and an ACE inhibitor.

Drugs Used Frequently in the Management of Cardiac Disease in Cats

DRUG/CLASS	INITIAL DOSE
ACE inhibitors	
Enalopril	0.25–5.0 mg/kg PO every 12–24 hr
Benazepril	0.50 mg/kg PO every 24 hr
Beta blockers	
Atenolol	6.25–12.5 mg/cat PO every 12–24 hr
Metoprolol	2–15 mg/cat PO every 8 hr
Calcium channel blocker	
Diltiazem (Dilacor XR: extended release)	30 mg/cat PO every 12 hr
Digitalis	
Digoxin	Cats < 3.0 kg: 0.031 mg PO every 48–72 hr Cats 3.0–6.0 kg: 0.031 mg PO every 24 hr Cats > 6.0 kg: 0.031mg PO every 12–24 hr
Diruetic	
Furosemide	6.25 mg/cat PO every 24–48 hr–12.5 mg/cat PO every 8 hr
Anticoagulants	
Aspirin	25 mg/cat PO every 72 hr
Warfarin (Coumadin)	0.25–0.5 mg/cat PO every 24 hr
Heparin	100–200 U/kg IV once; then 100–300 U/kg SQ every 8 hr

Table continued on following page

Drugs Used Frequently in the Management of Cardiac Disease in Cats (Continued)

DRUG/CLASS	INITIAL DOSE
Others	
Nitroglycerine	½ inch cutaneously to the pinna every 6–8 hr for the first 24–48 hr
Taurine	250–500 mg/cat PO every 12 hr

ACE = angiotensin-converting enzyme, PO = orally, SQ = subcutaneously, IV = intravenously.

27. Why is the use of ACE inhibitors controversial in cats with HCM?

It has been well documented in dogs that activation of the renin-angiotensin-aldosterone system negatively affects the natural history of heart failure, primarily mediated by increased angiotensin II levels. Despite the many beneficial effects of ACE inhibitors for cardiac disease, their use in cats with HCM may be controversial. ACE inhibitors cause mild arteriolar dilation by inhibiting production of the vasoconstrictor angiotensin II. A decrease in afterload theoretically may result in an increased pressure gradient in cats with dynamic outflow obstruction and/or SAM of the mitral valve. In practice, however, ACE inhibitors are sometimes used in cats with HCM.

28. What are the treatment options and goals of maintenance therapy for DCM?

- To prevent congestion (diuretic therapy)
- To promote increased forward cardiac output and improve myocardial contractility (positive inotropy)

29. What is the recommended therapy for DCM?

Most cats affected with DCM are maintained on furosemide and digitalis. Furosemide therapy is the same as for HCM or RCM: 1.2–2.2 mg/kg orally every 24–48 hr. The inotropic effects of digoxin are mediated through inhibition of the sodium-potassium-adenosine triphosphatase-pump. By increasing the concentration of sodium in the cell, more calcium enters the cell via the sodium-calcium exchanger, ultimately producing a more forceful cardiac contraction. Therapy is based on a calculated dose of 0.005–0.01 mg/kg. The 0.125-mg tablet is more easily administered to most cats than the elixir form. The recommended doses are listed in question 26. Serum digoxin concentrations should be monitored as well as renal values because digoxin is eliminated by the kidneys. In addition, taurine is administered empirically (250–500 mg/cat orally every 12 hr).

BIBLIOGRAPHY

1. Abbott JA: Digoxin therapy. Proc Am Coll Vet Intern Med 18:131–133, 2000.
2. Bonagura JD: Feline restrictive cardiomyopathy. Proc Am Coll Vet Intern Med 13:205, 1995.
3. Bonagura JD, Fox PR: Restrictive cardiomyopathy. In Bonagura JD (ed): Kirk's Current Veterinary Therapy XII. Philadelphia, W.B. Saunders, 1995, pp 863–867.
4. Bright JM, Golden AL, Daniel GB: Feline hypertrophic cardiomyopathy: Variations on a theme. J Small Anim Pract 33:266–274, 1992.
5. Fox PR: Feline cardiomyopathies. In Fox PR, Sisson D, Moise NS (eds): Textbook of Canine and Feline Cardiology: Principles and Clinical Practice, 2nd ed. Philadelphia, W.B. Saunders, 1999, pp 621–678.
6. Hamlin RL: Feline heart disease. Proc Am Coll Vet Intern Med 18:114–115, 2000.
7. Harpster NK: Feline myocardial diseases. In Kirk RW (ed): Current Veterinary Therapy IX. Philadelphia, W.B. Saunders, 1986, pp 380–398.
8. Kienle RD: Feline unclassified and restrictive cardiomyopathy. In MD Kittleson, RD Kienle (eds): Small Animal Cardiovascular Medicine. St. Louis, Mosby, 1998, pp 363–369.
9. Kittleson MD: Hypertrophic cardiomyopathy. In MD Kittleson, RD Kienle (eds): Small Animal Cardiovascular Medicine. St. Louis, Mosby, 1998, pp 347–362.
10. Kittleson MD: Thromboembolic disease. In MD Kittleson, RD Kienle (eds): Small Animal Cardiovascular Medicine. St. Louis, Mosby, 1998, pp 540–551.
11. Medinger TL, Bruyette DS: Feline hypertrophic cardiomyopathy. Comp Cont Educ Pract Vet 14:479–490, 1992.
12. Pion PD, Kittleson MD, Rogers QR, et al: Myocardial failure in cats associated with low plasma taurine: A reversible cardiomyopathy. Science 237:764–768, 1987.

II. Gastrointestinal Problems

Section Editor: Lynda Melendez, D.V.M., M.S.

18. OVERVIEW AND DIAGNOSTIC PROCEDURES

Michael R. Lappin, D.V.M., Ph.D.

1. What differentiates vomiting from regurgitation?

Vomiting is the forceful ejection of stomach and proximal duodenal contents through the mouth. Vestibular, vagal, chemoreceptor trigger zone, or direct input to the emetic center can induce vomiting. **Regurgitation** is the passive expulsion of food or fluid from the oral cavity, pharyngeal cavity, or esophagus (see Chapter 26). Esophageal diseases are rare in cats compared with dogs.

2. How is diarrhea characterized?

Diarrhea is characterized by increased frequency of defecation, increased fluid content of the stool, or increased volume of stool. Markedly increased frequency of defecation, small-volume stools, tenesmus, urgency, hematochezia, and mucus are consistent with **large bowel diarrhea**. Slight increase in frequency of defecation, large volume, melena, steatorrhea, and polysystemic clinical signs are more consistent with **small bowel diarrhea**. **Mixed bowel diarrhea** is a combination of characteristics or clinical signs. The clinical differential diagnoses for vomiting and small bowel diarrheas are similar.

3. What are the major differential diagnoses for vomiting and small bowel diarrhea?

Causes can be grouped as either primary or secondary gastrointestinal (GI) tract diseases:

Differential Diagnoses for Vomiting and Small Bowel Diarrhea in Cats

	PREDOMINANT SIGN
Primary GI diseases	
Obstruction: masses, foreign body, intussusception	Vomiting or diarrhea
Dietary intolerance	Vomiting or diarrhea
Drugs or toxins	Vomiting or diarrhea
Inflammatory gastric and bowel diseases	Vomiting primarily, some diarrhea
Neoplasia	Vomiting or diarrhea
Infectious diseases	See table in question 4
Parasites	See table in question 4
Secondary GI diseases	
Renal disease	Vomiting primarily
Hepatic disease	Vomiting primarily, some diarrhea
Pancreatitis	Vomiting primarily
Hypoadrenocorticism (rare in cats)	Vomiting or diarrhea
Diabetes mellitus with ketoacidosis	Vomiting primarily
Peritonitis	Vomiting or diarrhea
Central nervous system/vestibular disease	Vomiting primariliy
Pancreatic exocrine insufficiency	Diarrhea primarily

4. What are the major differential diagnoses for large bowel diarrhea?

Most causes of large bowel diarrhea involve the GI tract primarily and include inflammatory disease, neoplasia, obstruction (ileocecocolic valve), spastic disorder (idiopathic), dietary intolerance, infection, and parasitism. Secondary GI diseases usually are not associated with large bowel or mixed bowel diarrhea. Inflammation of the cecum, large intestine, and rectum can result in vomiting; the mechanism is vagal afferent nerve transmission to the emetic center.

Infectious Disease Differential Diagnoses for Vomiting and Diarrhea in Cats*

Bacterial agents	**Helminths**
Salmonella spp. (S, M)	*Ancylostoma/Uncinaria* spp. (S, M, L)
Enterotoxigenic *Escherichia coli* (S, M)	*Strongyloides cati* (S, M, rare)
Clostridium perfringens (L, rare)	*Dirofilaria immitis* (V)
Helicobacter felis and *H. heilmannii* (V)	*Toxocara cati* (V)
Bacterial overgrowth (S)	*Ollulanus tricuspis* (V)
Bacterial peritonitis (S)	*Physaloptera* spp. (V)
Bacterial cholangiohepatitis (S)	**Flagellates**
Viral agents	*Giardia* spp. (S, M)
Feline coronaviruses (S)	*Trichomonas hominis* (L, rare)
Feline lymphoma (S, M, L)	**Amoeba**
Feline immunodeficiency virus (S)	*Entamoeba histolytica* (L, rare)
Feline panleukopenia (V only frequently, S)	**Coccidian**
Fungal	*Cystoisospora* spp. (M, L)
Histoplasma capsulatum (L)	*Cryptosporidium* spp. (S, M)
Saprophytic fungi (S, M, L)	*Toxoplasma gondii* (V, S, rare GI diseases)

S = small bowel diarrhea, M = mixed bowel diarrhea, L = large bowel diarrhea, V = vomiting.
* All diseases resulting in diarrhea also can cause vomiting.

5. Is a diagnostic work-up always indicated for cats with vomiting or diarrhea?

Vomiting or diarrhea due to drugs, toxins, and dietary intolerance can be excluded by history and diet change. Otherwise healthy cats with acute vomiting and normal physical examination findings often can be managed conservatively by withholding food for 24 hours, followed by introduction of bland food for several days.

6. What is the minimal diagnostic plan for cats with vomiting or diarrhea?

Fecal flotation and complete blood cell count (CBC) are indicated for most cats with vomiting. Although the CBC generally does not lead to a specific diagnosis, the presence of eosinophilia makes inflammatory bowel diseases and parasitism more likely. If diarrhea is present, wet mount examination for trophozoites, rectal cytology, and *Cryptosporidium* screen (fecal enzyme-linked immunosorbent assay [ELISA] or acid-fast stain of a thin fecal smear) also are indicated. Fecal fat assessment with Sudan IV stain with and without acetic acid helps to confirm malabsorption/maldigestion but is not specific for a single disease.

7. How do you screen for secondary GI tract diseases associated with vomiting and diarrhea?

A serum biochemical profile, urinalysis, feline leukemia virus (FeLV) antigen assay, and feline immunodeficiency virus (FIV) antibody assay generally are performed in cats with chronic vomiting and diarrhea (see Chapter 25). The author generally assesses serum total T4 concentration in all cats with vomiting or small bowel diarrhea that are older than 5 years. Although amylase and lipase are poor predictors of pancreatitis in cats, a trypsin-like immunoreactivity assay has now been validated (Texas A & M University, College Station, TX). It can be used to support the diagnosis of acute pancreatitis (increased) or exocrine pancreatic insufficiency (decreased) in cats (see Chapter 36). If a cat with suspected pancreatitis has abdominal effusion, measure lipase concentrations in the serum and effusion; if pancreatitis is present, effusion lipase is usually greater than serum lipase.

8. What are the indications for direct smears? What techniques are used?

Liquid feces or feces that contain large quantities of mucus should be microscopically examined immediately for the presence of protozoal trophozoites, including *Giardia* spp. (flagellate) and *Pentatrichomonas hominis* (flagellate). A direct saline smear can be made to facilitate observation of these motile organisms. The amount of feces required to cover the head of a match is mixed thoroughly with one drop of 0.9% sodium chloride (NaCl). After application of a coverslip, the smear is evaluated for motile organisms by examining it under $100 \times$ magnification.

9. How does rectal cytology aid in the diagnostic evaluation of cats with diarrhea?

A thin smear of feces should be made from all cats with diarrhea. Material should be collected by rectal swab, if possible, to increase chances of finding white blood cells. A cotton swab is gently introduced 3–4 cm through the anus into the terminal rectum, directed to the wall of the rectum, and gently rotated several times. Placing a drop of 0.9% NaCl on the cotton swab facilitates passage through the anus but does not adversely affect cell morphology. The cotton swab is rolled on a microscope slide gently multiple times to give areas with varying thickness; three slides are usually made. After air drying, one of the slides can be stained with Diff-Quick or Wright's-Giemsa stains. The slide should be examined for white blood cells and bacteria morphologically consistent with *Campylobacter jejuni* or *Clostridium perfringens*. *Histoplasma capsulatum* or *Prototheca* spp. may be observed in the cytoplasm of mononuclear cells. Methylene blue in acetate buffer (pH = 3.6) stains trophozoites of the enteric protozoans. Iodine stains and acid methyl green also are used for the demonstration of protozoans. Acid-fast or monoclonal antibody staining (Meridian Diagnostics, Cincinnati, OH) of a fecal smear should be performed in cats with diarrhea to aid in the diagnosis of cryptosporidiosis. *Cryptosporidium parvum* is the only enteric pathogen of approximately 4–6 μm in diameter that stains pink to red with acid-fast stain. Presence of neutrophils on rectal cytology may suggest inflammation induced by *Salmonella* spp., *C. jejuni,* or *C. perfringens*; fecal culture is indicated in such cases.

10. What fecal flotation solutions should be used for cats?

Ability to float parasite ova, oocysts, or cysts is based on the specific gravity of the solution; most ova, oocysts, and cysts are easily identified after zinc sulfate centrifugal flotation (see Chapter 19). This procedure is considered by many to be optimal for the demonstration of protozoan cysts, in particular *Giardia* spp.; it is a good choice for a routine flotation technique. Sugar centrifugation can be used for routine parasite evaluation and may be superior to many techniques for the demonstration of oocysts of *Toxoplasma gondii* and *C. parvum*. Giardial cysts are distorted by sugar centrifugation but can still be easily identified. Fecal sedimentation recovers most cysts and ova but also contains debris. This technique is superior to flotation procedures for the documentation of fluke eggs.

Zinc Sulfate Centrifugation Procedure

1. Place 1 gm of fecal material in a 15-ml conical centrifuge tube.

2. Add 8 drops of Lugol iodine, and mix well.

3. Add 7–8 ml of zinc sulfate (1.18 specific gravity),* and mix well.

4. Add zinc sulfate until there is a slight positive meniscus.

5. Cover the top of the tube with a coverslip.

6. Centrifuge at 1500–2000 rpm for 5 minutes.

7. Remove the coverslip, and place on a clean microscope slide for microscopic examination.

8. Examine the entire area under the coverslip for the presence of ova, oocysts, or larvae at $100 \times$ magnification.

---

* Add 330 gm of zinc sulfate to 670 ml of distilled water.

11. If a delay is expected before feces are evaluated, should a preservative be used?

Feces should be refrigerated, not frozen, until assayed. If a fecal sample is to be sent to a diagnostic laboratory for further analysis and will not be evaluated within 48 hours, it should be preserved. Polyvinyl alcohol, merthiolate-iodine-formalin, and 10% formalin can be used; 10% formalin is commonly used because of its routine availability. Add 1 part feces to 9 parts formalin, and mix well.

12. How can I increase the likelihood of diagnosing *Salmonella* or *Campylobacter* spp. infections?

Approximately 2–3 gm of fresh feces should be submitted to the laboratory immediately for optimal results; however, *Salmonella* and *Campylobacter* spp. are usually viable in refrigerated fecal specimens for 3–7 days. The laboratory should be notified of the suspected pathogen so appropriate culture media are used. Cary-Blair medium (Bectin-Dickinson Microbiology Systems, Sparkes, MD) is appropriate for transport.

13. Are any of the fecal antigen techniques beneficial in the evaluation of cats with gastrointestinal disease?

Parvovirus, *C. parvum*, and *Giardia* spp. antigen detection procedures are available for feces. In a limited number of feline samples assessed at Colorado State University, canine parvovirus assays detected feline parvovirus antigen and correlated well with results from electron microscopy. Sensitivity and specificity of *C. parvum* and *Giardia* antigen assays have not been determined when used with feces from cats. They should be interpreted in conjunction with results of fecal examination techniques.

14. How can viruses other than parvovirus be detected in feces?

Electron microscopy can be used to detect viral particles in feces of cats with GI signs of diseases. Approximately 1–3 gm of feces without fixative should be transported to the laboratory (Diagnostic Laboratory, Colorado State University, College of Veterinary Medicine and Biomedical Sciences, Fort Collins, CO) by overnight mail on cold packs. In some research laboratories, virus isolation can be performed. In addition, reverse transcriptase-polymerase chain reaction (RT-PCR) can be used to detect coronavirus particles in stool (see Chapter 21).

15. How can I assess cats for helicobacteriosis?

Gastric biopsies should be placed on urea slants to assess for urease, which is found in the cell wall of *Helicobacter* spp. but not in nonpathogenic spirochetes. A presumptive diagnosis of helicobacteriosis can be based on the identification of inflammatory cells and spirochetes in the gastric biopsies plus a positive urease test and exclusion of other causes of GI disease (see Chapter 20).

16. What imaging techniques are beneficial in evaluating primary GI tract diseases?

Imaging techniques such as radiographs, contrast radiographs, and ultrasound can aid in the diagnosis of diseases resulting in obstruction. Abdominal radiographs should be used to support palpation findings, particularly to help prove or deny obstructive disease. Contrast radiographs are beneficial to document obstructive disease and localize lesions. Ultrasound of the GI tract can be difficult to interpret; its value depends on the skill of the operator. However, ultrasound is quite valuable in the diagnosis of secondary GI tract diseases such as pancreatitis, renal diseases, and hepatic diseases.

17. When should endoscopy be considered in the work-up of a GI case?

The esophagus, stomach, proximal duodenum, rectum, colon, and distal ileum can be assessed endoscopically. The technique is most valuable to diagnose and retrieve foreign bodies and to obtain biopsies for evaluation of inflammatory and neoplastic diseases. Because endoscopic biopsies are small and lesions may be focal, at least 8–10 biopsies should be made from the stomach, duodenum, colon, and ileum, if possible. Full-thickness biopsies may be required to make a definitive diagnosis in some cats. There is no benefit to performing duodenal aspirates for quantitative bacterial cultures or giardial trophozoite evaluations in cats. The normal bacterial count range is broad in cats, and *Giardia* spp. are found in the distal small intestine.

BIBLIOGRAPHY

Lappin MR: Laboratory diagnosis of infectious diseases. In Nelson RW, Couto CG (eds): Small Animal Internal Medicine, 2nd ed. St. Louis, Mosby, 1998, pp 1240–1252.

19. GASTROINTESTINAL PARASITES

Glenda Taton-Allen, M.S., and John Cheney, D.V.M., M.S.

1. What internal parasites infect the gastrointestinal (GI) system?

Nematodes, cestodes, protozoans, and trematodes can be harbored in the GI tract of cats. Several of these organisms also infect humans; zoonotic aspects are discussed in depth in Chapter 84.

Morphologic Characteristics of Feline Gastrointestinal Parasites

ORGANISM	LIFE STAGE AND DESCRIPTION
Helminths	
Toxocara cati	Egg: 65–75μ
Toxascaris leonina	Egg: up to 80 μ
Ancylostoma cati	Egg: 55–65 μ × 34–45 μ
Ancylostoma braziliense	Egg: 55–76 μ × 35–45 μ
Uncinaria stenocephalia	Egg: 60–75 μ × 33–50 μ
Spirocerca lupi	Egg; 12 μ × 40 μ
Strongyloides stercoralis	Egg: 55μ × 30 μ; larvated
	Larvae: rhabditiform first-stage larva
Ollulanus tricuspis	Adult: 0.7–2.00 mm long
Physoloptera spp.	Adult: 3–6cm
	Egg: 30–33 μ × 45–55 μ; larvated
Trichuris spp.	Egg: 35–38 μ × 75–80 μ, bipolar plugs
Cestodes	
Dipylidium caninum	Proglottid; double pored
	Egg packet: 25–40 μ × 30–45 μ
Taenia spp.	Proglodttid; single pored
	Egg: 37 μ × 32 μ
Echinococcus multilocularis	Egg: 37 μ × 32 μ
Mesocestoides lineatus	Proglottid: central genital pore
	Egg: 22–25 μ × 25–30 μ
Flukes	
Alaria	Egg: 70 μ × 134 μ; operculated
Protozoans	
Coccidians	
Toxoplasma gondii	Oocyst: 10 μ × 12 μ
Isospora felis	Oocyst: 21–31 μ × 38–51 μ
Isospora rivolta	Oocyst: 20–26 μ × 23–29 μ
Sarcocystis spp.	Oocyst: 12–16 μ × 7–9 μ
Cryptosporidium spp.	Oocyst: 4–6 μ × 4–7 μ
Flagellates	
Giardia lamblia	Cyst: 7–10 μ × 8–12 μ
	Trophozoite: 10–12 μ × 15–18 μ
Pentatrichomonas hominis	Trophozoite: 4–6 μ × 7–14 μ

2. What are the most common GI helminthes?

The large roundworms (ascarids) *Toxocara cati* and *Toxascaris leonina* and the tapeworms *Taenia taeniaeformis* and *Dipylidium caninum* are very common in cats. *T. cati* is the most common parasite of kittens, and *T. taeniaeformis* and *D. caninum* are the most common parasites in adult cats.

3. How are cats infected with ascarids?

Adult *T. cati* live in the small intestine of cats, and eggs are passed with the feces into the environment. The eggs become infective in as little as 1 month, and when the infective eggs are ingested by another cat, the larvae migrate via the liver and lungs to the small intestine, where they mature. Rodents can serve as transport hosts, and larvae of the organism can be transmitted lactationally to kittens. The larval stage does not migrate through tissues when transmitted through milk but goes directly to the small intestine to mature. Prenatal infection does not occur with *T. cati*.

T. leonina eggs develop in the environment and become infective in as little as 1 week. Cats become infected after ingestion of the egg or infected transport hosts (primarily rodents). Transplacental and transmammary infection do not occur. Instead of migrating through tissues, the larvae burrow into the intestinal wall, undergo development, and then return to the lumen to mature into the adult stage. *T. cati* but not *T. leonina* can cause visceral larva migrans in people (see Chapter 84).

4. What are the clinical signs of ascarid infections?

Ascarid infections in adult cats are usually subclinical. In kittens and young cats, vomiting, small bowel diarrhea, and abdominal distention are common clinical findings. Kittens may be listless, fail to thrive, and have a poor hair coat.

5. What hookworms infect the GI tract of cats?

Ancylostoma braziliense, A. tubeforme, and *Uncinaria stenocephala* infect cats. Prevalence of hookworm infections varies by region of the United States. Both *Ancylostoma* spp. prefer warm, humid climates, whereas *U. stenocephala* survives well in colder climates. Hookworm infections in cats are more common in the southern and southeastern United States.

6. Describe the life cycle of feline hookworms.

The hookworm has a direct life cycle. Eggs passed in the feces larvate and hatch in the environment. If the environment is moist and warm, the larvae can hatch in a matter of hours; cats are infected by skin penetration or ingestion of infective larvae. There is no evidence that feline hookworms are transferred transplacentally or lactationally. Rodents can act as transport hosts.

7. What are the clinical manifestations of hookworm infection?

Hookworm infection is not nearly as devastating in cats as in dogs. Intestinal bleeding may occur, but it is usually minimal. Heavy infection must be present to manifest clinical signs such as poor hair coat, weight loss, and melena. Adult cats are infected more heavily than kittens because transplacental and lactational transmission do not occur. Infected people can develop cutaneous larva migrans (see Chapter 84).

8. What diagnostic techniques best recover hookworm, ascarid, and other nematode eggs?

The centrifugation fecal flotation technique is the best method to recover nematode eggs from fecal samples (see Chapter 18). The specific gravity of the salt solution used for flotation should be 1.18–1.25. Zinc sulfate at a specific gravity of 1.18 is a good solution because it is optimal for recovery of giardial cysts as well as most helminth eggs.

The prepatent period for *Toxocara* spp. is 6–8 weeks; eggs are not present in infected kittens younger than this age. Eggs of *T. cati* are large (65–75 µ) and dark brown with a thick, roughened outer (corticate) wall. Eggs of *T. leonina* are slightly larger than *T. cati* eggs (up to 80µ) and have a light golden brown color with a smooth outer wall and an undulating interior wall. Finding the unembryonated oval eggs in fresh feces establishes the diagnosis of hookworm infection. The eggs range from 55–95 µ in length, depending on the species of hookworm (see table in question 1).

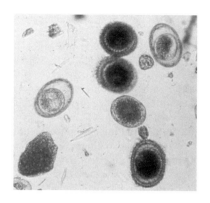

Comparison of *Toxocara* spp. eggs (dark brown eggs with corticated outer wall) with *Toxascaris* spp. eggs (lighter, more diffuse egg with smooth outer wall).

9. What stomach worms may infect cats?

Physaloptera spp. is the only common stomach worm of cats but can be found in the small intestine as well. This parasite requires insects, including crickets, various beetles, and cockroaches, as the intermediate host. Transport hosts are primarily mice. Cats become infected when they ingest the intermediate or transport host. Diagnosis can be difficult because the eggs do not float well in most salt solutions except in saturated magnesium sulfate (specific gravity = 1.30). Eggs are larvated and measure 30–33 μ × 45–55 μ. Immature or mature worms (1–6 cm) may be vomited, although these nematodes have small teeth and attach strongly to the gastric mucosa to suck blood. Endoscopy is a useful diagnostic tool since usually few eggs are found. Clinical abnormalities include vomiting and gastric ulcers.

Rare infections with two other parasites, *Ollulanus tricuspis* and *Gnathostoma spinigerum*, have been reported in the United States. The entire life cycle of *O. tricuspis* can take place within the stomach of the cat. It is an extremely small worm, only 0.7–1.0 mm long. Cats become infected from eating vomitus containing L3, L4, or adult nematodes, and the larvae can live in the vomitus up to 10 days, depending on environmental conditions. Microscopic examination of vomitus or gastric fluids is the primary way to diagnose *O. tricuspis* infection. *G. spinigerum* requires two intermediate hosts, first a crustacean and then a freshwater fish, amphibian, or reptile. The cat ingests the intermediate host. The parasites migrate throughout the body and cause severe ulceration and necrosis of the stomach wall, where the adults live. Diagnosis is difficult because few eggs are produced and usually are not present in feces. There is no treatment, and the infection is often fatal.

10. If adult worms are present in vomitus, how can *T. cati* be distinguished from *Physaloptera* spp.?

Adult *Physaloptera* spp. are similar to *Toxocara* and *Toxascaris* spp. except that they are shorter and usually coiled. The head of the ascarid has a small mouth opening surrounded by three lips. Physaloptera spp. are unique in that adults have two spines at the anterior end and a "collar" type structure around the head area.

11. What other nematodes are found on rare occasions in the feline GI tract?

Strongyloides stercoralis is an unusual parasite because it has both a parasitic life cycle and a free-living life cycle. This organism is generally a parasite of younger animals; the finding of larvated eggs (30 μ × 55 μ) or, more commonly, rhabditiform larvae in the feces is diagnostic. The entire life cycle can be completed in cats; diarrhea is the primary clinical sign. The organism can cause cutaneous larva migrans in people (see Chapter 84).

Spirocerca lupi adults generally live in the esophagus but can be harbored in the stomach. This organism uses coprophagic beetles as intermediate hosts as well as numerous paratenic hosts, including lizards, mice, and chickens. Infection is diagnosed by the finding of small, thick-walled larvated eggs in feces. The eggs measure 12 μ × 40 μ. Endoscopy is also a useful diagnostic tool to find esophageal granulomas and make a definitive diagnosis. Clinical signs of disease are rare in cats.

Trichuris campanula and *T. serrata* infections (whipworms) occur sporadically in cats in the United States. Adult worms live in the large intestine and cecum. The life cycle is direct; cats can become infected by ingestion of the eggs that have developed in the environment. Development of *Trichuris* spp. eggs takes from 10 days to 2 months. Infections normally do not cause severe disease in cats. Eggs are recovered using a fecal float and identified by the characteristic barrel shape and bipolar plugs; they range in size from 35–38 μ × 75–80 μ. Differentiation from the lungworm, *Capillaria aerophilia*, is necessary.

12. What are the principal anthelmintics used for treatment of nematodes infecting cats?
Several anthelmintics are used in cats to treat ascarids, hookworms, and other nematodes. Pyrantel pamoate, although not approved for use in cats, is extremely safe and efficacious in the treatment of ascarids and hookworms. It must be given in two doses about 2–3 weeks apart because the drug kills only parasites in the GI tract, not the tissue migratory stages. Fenbendazole, also extremely safe, is not approved for use in cats. It is effective for the treatment of ascarids, hookworms, whipworms, *S. stercoralis*, and other less common nematodes. The liquid formulation of fenbendazole is usually given for 3–5 days. Treatment must be repeated in 2–3 weeks for ascarids and hookworms. Treatment needs to be repeated at 4 weeks and 8 weeks for whipworms. Fenbendazole also has antigiardial activity (see question 30). The combination of praziquantel and pyrantel is approved for use in cats and is also effective for the treatment of tapeworms. Piperazine is approved for use in cats, but efficacy is variable and less than desirable. Selamectin is approved to treat *T. cati* and hookworms in cats. Ivermectin is effective for the control of hookworms.

Drugs Used for Control of Gastrointestinal Tract Parasites in Cats

GENERIC DRUG	COMMON FELINE DOSAGE
Alaria marcianae	
Praziquantel*	5 mg/kg/day PO for 2–3 days
Cestodes	
Epsiprantel*	2.75 mg/kg once PO
Fenbendazole (*Taenia* spp. only)	50 mg/kg/day PO for 3 days
Praziquantel*	23 mg/cat PO or 56.8 mg/ml SC or IM once
Cryptosporidium parvum	
Azithromycin	7–15 mg/kg every 12 hr PO for 5–7 days
Paromomycin	150 mg/kg every 12–24 hr PO for 5 days
Tylosin	10–15 mg/kg every 8–12 hr PO for 21 days
***Isospora* spp.**	
Trimethoprim-sulfonamide	15 mg/kg every 12 hr PO for 5 days
Sulfadimethoxine	50–60 mg/kg/day PO for 5–20 days
Furazolidone	8–20 mg/kg every 12–24 hr PO for 5 days
Amprolium	60–100 mg/day for 5 days
Paromomycin	165 mg/kg every 12 hr PO for 5 days
***Giardia* spp.**	
Metronidazole	10–25 mg/kg every 12 hr PO for 8 days
Fenbendazole	50 mg/kg every 24 hr PO for 3–7 days
Furazolidone	4 mg/kg every 12 hr PO for 7 days
Helminths	
Fenbendazole[†]	50 mg/kg/day for 3–5 days PO; repeat in 2–3 wk
Ivermectin[‡]	Label dose PO monthly
Pyrantel pamoate[#]	20 mg/kg once PO; repeat in 2–3 wk
Pyrantel plus praziquantel*[§]	72.6 mg pyrantel/18.2 mg praziquantel, 1 tablet PO
Piperazine*[∞]	110 mg/kg once PO; repeat in 2 wk
Selamectin*[£]	6 mg/kg topically once monthly

Table continued on following page

Drugs Used for Control of Gastrointestinal Tract Parasites in Cats (Continued)

GENERIC DRUG	COMMON FELINE DOSAGE
Pentatrichomonas hominis	
Metronidazole	10–25 mg/kg every 12 hr PO for 8 days
Paromomycin	150 mg/kg every 12–24 hr PO for 5 days
Toxoplasma gondii	
Azithromycin	7–15 mg/kg every 12hr PO for 5–7 day
Clindamycin hydrochloride	12.5 mg/kg every 12 hr PO, IM for 28 days
Clarithromycin	5–10 mg/kg PO every 12 hr for 7 days
Pyrimethamine	Rarely used because of toxicity
Trimethoprim-sulfonamide	15 mg/kg every 12 hr PO for 28 days

IM= intramuscular, IV = intravenous, SC = subcutaneous, PO = oral, NA = not applicable
* Drugs are approved for use in cats
† Effective against hookworms, roundworms, whipworms, and stomach worms.
‡ Heartgard for cats, Merck, Whitehouse Station, NJ; effective for hookworms.
# Effective against hookworms and roundworms.
§ Drontal Plus, Bayer Animal Health, Shawnee Mission, KS; effective against hookworms, roundworms, and tapeworms.
∞ Effective against hookworms and roundworms.
£ Revolution, Pfizer Animal Health, Exton, PA; effective against hookworms and roundworms.

13. How do cats become infected with tapeworms?

The most common tapeworms in cats are *T. taeniaeformis* and *D. caninum*. Adult tapeworms live in the small intestine, and both species require an intermediate host to complete their life cycles. Gravid proglottids containing many eggs are released from adult worms either singly or in chains attached to each other. These proglottids may rupture in the intestine, liberating the eggs, or, more commonly, intact proglottids may be expelled in or on the feces. The white proglottids may crawl out of the anus spontaneously and remain motile for a time. Occasionally, multiple proglottids still attached to one another are passed in vomitus. The intermediate host must ingest eggs from proglottids; then the larval stage develops. Rodents (mice) are the intermediate host for *T. taeniaeformis,* and dog and cat fleas are the intermediate hosts for *D. caninum*. Cats become infected with tapeworms by ingesting the intermediate host. The prepatent period is 4–6 weeks.

14. Do tapeworm infections cause clinical manifestations?

Usually no clinical signs are associated with tapeworm infections. Heavy infections occasionally cause anal pruritus, diarrhea, vomiting, or intestinal obstruction. People can be infected by *D. caninum* if they ingest infected fleas (see Chapter 84).

15. How are tapeworm infections diagnosed?

Tapeworm proglottid identification is probably the most common way to diagnose infections. Owners may observe the dried proglottids, which appear as "rice granules" on the perianal area. A squash mount, which causes release of eggs from the proglottid, facilitates identification. The proglottid is placed on a microscope slide with a drop of distilled water or saline. A large coverglass is pressed over the proglottid to force the eggs from the genital pore. *Taenia* eggs are mid-sized (30–35 µ × 35–40 µ) and expelled as single, thick-walled, round eggs with the hexacanth embryo visible inside. The wall has a striated or "sunburst" effect. Each proglottid has a genital pore on one side only. *Dipylidium* eggs are expelled in egg packets with 4–15 oncospheres per packet. Each proglottid has two genital pores, one on each side. Dried tapeworm proglottids can be hydrated in water first before a squash mount is performed. When fecal samples are submitted, it is important to look for tapeworm proglottids not only on the feces, but also on the walls of the container, because the proglottids may crawl off the feces. Eggs of *Taenia* spp. can be recovered with the zinc sulfate centrifugation concentration technique, but this technique is not as common as finding proglottids. *Dipylidium* egg packets range in size from 25–40 µ × 30–45 µ and are rarely recovered in a fecal float.

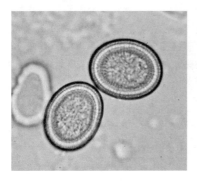

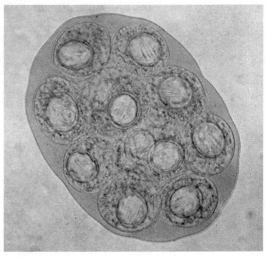

Above, Taenia-type eggs with thick, striated wall and hexacanth embryo. *Right, Dipylidium caninum* egg packet.

16. What other tapeworm infections occur in cats?

Taenia pisiformis and *T. hydatigena* are transmitted to cats by ingestion of rodents or rabbits. Clinical and diagnostic issues are the same as for *T. taeniaeformis*.

Cats can complete the lifecycle of *Echinococcus multilocularis*; infection usually is subclinical. *E. multilocularis* is acquired by eating infected rodents, which serve as intermediate hosts. Tiny proglottids and *Taenia*-type eggs (32 μ × 37 μ) are passed in the feces after a prepatent period of about 2 months. The eggs are infective to humans and, if ingested, can invade tissues to develop into hydatid cysts (see Chapter 84). *E. multilocularis* is most common in northern and central parts of North America.

Cats can be the definitive hosts of *Diphyllobothrium latum* and *Spirometra mansonoides.* Both agents require two intermediate hosts; the first intermediate host is a copepod, and the second a vertebrate. *D. latum* uses a freshwater fish for the second intermediate host, whereas S. *mansonoides* uses mammals, tadpoles, or water snakes. Eggs rather than gravid proglottids are passed in feces. Eggs of *D. latum* are heavy and do not float well in salt solutions except at higher specific gravity solutions (magnesium sulfate at 1.30 specific gravity). The eggs are operculated and are 45 μ × 70 μ. Spirometral eggs are smaller (30 μ × 60 μ) and operculated. Clinical manifestations include diarrhea and secondary anemia. Cats and dogs can serve as reservoir hosts for infections in humans. *D. latum* occurs in more temperate areas; humans can be a definitive host and become infected from eating raw fish. *S. mansonoides* occurs throughout North America, and humans can become infected from eating pork.

Mesocestoides lineatus occurs worldwide and requires two intermediate hosts. The first host includes beetles or orbatid mites; the second may be mammals, birds, or reptiles. This tapeworm is unusual in that cats can be the intermediate or definitive host, and the organism can multiply asexually in the peritoneal cavity to cause massive infections. The proglottids are about the size of sesame seeds. Identification is made by examining the proglottid to find the central genital pore. Eggs (22–25 μ × 25–30 μ) also may be recovered in a centrifugation fecal float.

17. How are tapeworm infections of cats treated?

Praziquantel and epsiprantel are the drugs of choice to treat most tapeworms. Both drugs are approved for use in cats. Efficacy against *Taenia* spp. and *D. caninum* tapeworms is 100% with either drug in a single treatment. Praziquantel but not epsiprantel has efficacy against *Echinococcus* spp. Because of public health concerns in areas where *E. mutilocularis* is endemic, cats allowed to hunt may be treated as often as monthly with praziquantel to control shedding of eggs into the environment.

18. What trematodes infect the GI tract of cats?

Alaria marcianae, Nanophyetus salmincola, and *Cryptocotyle lingua* rarely occur in the small intestine of cats in North America. These parasites require two intermediate hosts and may use transport hosts. A snail is the first intermediate host, and a fish is usually the second intermediate host. Cats become infected with trematodes by ingesting the second intermediate host or mice, frogs, and snakes, which serve as transport hosts. Intestinal fluke infections are usually subclinical in cats. Eggs are best recovered from the feces by use of sedimentation techniques. The eggs are dense and do not float well with fecal flotation salt solutions. Fluke eggs are large, ranging from 80–130 μ × 50–80 μ, depending on the species of fluke. In dogs, *N. salmincola* transmits *Neorickettsia helmintheca* (salmon poisoning), but the disease is not transmitted to cats.

19. How are GI trematode infections treated?

Praziquantel is the drug of choice to treat flukes. Usually the same dose is administered as for tapeworms, but it may need to be given daily for 2–3 days to be fully effective. Albendazole has shown some efficacy against flukes, but treatment requires 2–3 weeks. This drug is not approved for use in cats, and it is not as safe to administer to cats as praziquantel.

20. What are the most common protozoan GI parasites in cats?

Coccidians and flagellates commonly infect the GI tract of cats (see table in question 1). The coccidians, *Isospora felis* and *I. rivolta,* are the most common protozoans in kittens. *Toxoplasma gondii* and *Cryptosporidium parvum* are other coccidians of clinical importance. Infection with *Hammondia* spp., *Besnoitia* spp., and *Sarcocystis* spp. is usually subclinical in cats. The flagellates *Giardia lamblia* and *Pentatrichomonas hominis* infect cats and occasionally are associated with clinical illness. Infection of cats with *Entamoeba histolytica,* an amoeba, has rarely been reported.

21. What are the clinical findings of *Isospora* spp. infections in cats?

Infections in kittens may be subclinical or cause symptoms ranging from transient diarrhea to severe hemorrhagic diarrhea. Adult cats tend to be more resistant to clinical coccidiosis because immunity develops, although stressed or immunocompromised cats occasionally become clinically ill. Subclinically infected adult cats may shed oocysts sporadically, thus contributing to environmental contamination. Oocysts sporulate in the environment to become infective. Cats become infected directly by ingestion of sporulated oocysts or rodents harboring cyst stages. Enzootic infections are found frequently in catteries where animals are housed together or in close quarters. Diagnosis is made by demonstrating oocysts in feces after flotation. *I. felis* oocysts range in size from 27–31 μ × 38–51μ, and *I. rivolta* oocysts range from 20–26 μ × 23–29 μ. Because *I. felis* and *I. rivolta* can infect cats directly or indirectly, taxonomists have created a new genus name, *Cystoisospora. Isospora* consists of one-host species. Because tissue infections can occur in mice, rats, hamsters, rabbits, and sheep, Cystoisospora genus better describes these coccidian species. However, *Isospora* is still more commonly used.

22. Describe the other enteric coccidians of cats.

Cats serve as the definitive hosts for *Besnoitia besnoiti* and *Hammondia hammondi*; cattle and rodents are intermediate hosts, respectively. Because the oocysts are indistinguishable from those of *T. gondii,* animal inoculation is used for definitive diagnosis of *T. gondii* infection. *B. besnoiti* and *H. hammondi* are considered nonpathogenic in cats. However, because the oocysts are indistinguishable, *T. gondii* should always be suspected and precautionary measures taken.

Sarcocystis spp. also use two hosts; the cat can be a definitive host. Several *Sarcocystis* spp. use cattle, sheep, mice, and rabbits as intermediate hosts. Cats become infected by ingesting tissue cysts from the intermediate hosts. The sexual cycle occurs in cat intestinal cells, and fully sporulated oocysts are passed in the feces. Unlike other feline coccidians, *Sarcocystis* spp. are infective when passed and require no development in the environment. *Sarcocystis* spp. usually cause no illness in cats or other carnivores, but infection of herbivores can result in serious illness. The sporulated oocyst may be recovered from the feces by use of the centrifugation fecal flotation method. The oocysts resemble giardial cysts in shape, but *Sarcocystis* spp. oocysts are slightly larger (12–16 μ × 7–9 μ), and contain 4 sporozoites.

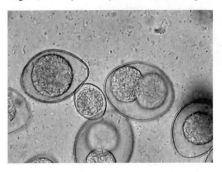

Isospora (Cystoisospora) felis unsporulated oocysts (larger oocysts; 1 sporoblast), *I. felis* sporulated oocysts (larger oocysts; 2 sporocysts), and *I. rivolta* oocysts (smaller oocyst; 1 sporoblast).

23. Does enteric coccidiosis require treatment?

If *Isospora* spp. oocysts are detected in cats with GI signs, treatment is usually administered. Sulfa drugs are generally effective (see table in question 12). Treatment of subclinically infected cats may lessen oocyst shedding and environmental contamination but does not clear infection because the treatment drugs are coccidiostats. *Hammondia* spp., *Sarcocystis* spp., and *Besnoitia* spp. infection do not require treatment.

24. Is *T. gondii* infection associated with GI disease?

Cats are the only known definitife hosts of *T. gondii* (see Chapter 84) and the only species known to shed oocysts. However, most cats are subclinically infected when shedding *T. gondii* oocysts. Because of rapid development of immunity, oocyst shedding occurs only for 7–14 days. If diarrhea occurs, it is of short duration (days) and involves the small bowel. The centrifugation fecal flotation method is the choice for recovery of oocysts (10 μ × 12 μ) from cat feces, but because the shedding period is so short, it is uncommon to find them in a routine sample. Clinical illness due to toxoplasmosis in cats is usually polysystemic. Uveitis (see Chapter 67) and fever (see Chapter 64) are common manifestations. Clindamycin hydrochloride administered orally at 10–12 mg/kg every 12hr is effective for polysystemic toxoplasmosis and may shorten the oocyst shedding period.

25. What are *Cryptosporidium* spp.?

Cryptosporidium spp. are the smallest of the coccidians found in cats. The organism infects a large number of animals, including humans. Transmission between other animal hosts and people occurs with some genotypes; thus the organism is an important zoonotic protozoan parasite (see Chapter 84). *Cryptosporidium* spp. are unusual in that they form autoinfective oocyts and can cause life-threatening infections in immune deficient animals and humans, especially those with acquired immunodeficiency syndrome.

Cryptosporidium spp. oocysts are sporulated when shed in the feces and thus are infective. The thick-walled oocysts may remain viable for several months in favorable environments. It takes extreme temperatures (> 65°C and< 0°C) to kill the oocysts. Desiccation and strong disinfectants also kill the oocysts, but disinfectants require extended contact to be effective. When the oocysts are ingested, sporozoites invade the microvillous border of the gastric glands (*C. muris*) or the lower half of the small intestine (*C. parvum*). Approximately 20% of oocysts have a thin wall that breaks open in the GI lumen. The released sporozoites reinvade host cells, which may account for chronic shedding of oocysts by some cats. Most clinical infections are probably due to *C. parvum*, but evidence of *C. felis* infection is increasing (see Chapter 84).

26. Does clinical cryptosporidiosis occur in cats?

In a study performed at Colorado State University, *Cryptosporidium* spp. oocysts or antigens were detected in 5.4% of the cats with diarrhea. However, oocysts also can be detected in feces of clinically normal cats. Lymphocytic plasmacytic duodenitis has been detected in some infected cats. Acute or chronic small bowel diarrhea is the primary clinical sign of cryptosporidiosis in cats.

Cryptosporidium spp. float in salt solutions, but they are difficult to differentiate from small yeast organisms. The oocysts are very small (4–7 μ × 4–6 μ). Staining of a thin fecal smear helps to identify the oocysts; modified acid-fast stain is commonly used. Immunofluorescent staining techniques are also useful diagnostic tools. Fecal antigen tests used for human cryptosporidiosis is under evaluation for use with cat feces.

Although no drug is consistently efficacious for treating cryptosporidiosis, tylosin and paromomycin apparently have been effective in some infected cats (see table in question 12). Chronic infection of immunocompetent cats has been documented.

27. Describe *Giardia* spp. infections.

Giardia spp. are probably among the most commonly diagnosed intestinal protozoan parasites in humans and animals. Their distribution is worldwide in tropical and temperate areas, and the organism does not appear to be host-specific. *Giardia* spp. can be harbored in virtually any animal. It is questionable how many species exist. At present three species are accepted: *G. duodenalis (G. lamblia)* in mammals, *Giardia muris* in mice, and *Giardia ranae* in frogs. Some feline isolates are identical genetically to human isolates. However, new genetic information suggests that a feline-specific species may exist (see Chapter 84).

Giardia spp. have a direct life cycle. Cats, other animals, and humans become infected by ingestion of cysts shed in the feces, and the cysts are infective when passed. Infection occurs by the fecal-oral route and occurs most commonly via contaminated drinking water and food. Excystment takes place in the duodenum, where two trophozoites are released. The trophozoites attach to the intestine by a sucking disc and multiply by binary fission. In cats, the jejunum and ileum are the primary areas of multiplication instead of the duodenum. Encystment occurs as the trophozoites pass through the GI tract. Trophozoites also may be passed in cases of severe diarrhea. The cyst stage is resistant in the environment, particularly to cold, and even chlorination may not be totally effective at killing cysts. Drying kills cysts more rapidly. Trophozoites do not survive long in the environment and are not the infective stage.

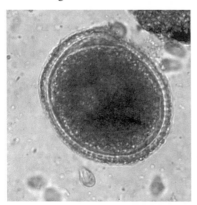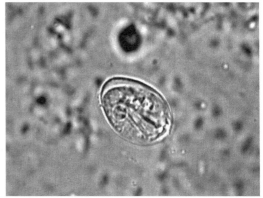

Left, Toxocara cati egg and *Giardia* spp. cyst. *Right, Giardia* spp. cyst

28. What are the clinical findings of giardiasis?

Giardial cysts are commonly excreted in cat feces. Some cats are subclinically infected, whereas others may be presented with acute, chronic, or episodic small bowel diarrhea. Intestinal malabsorption may contribute to persistent diarrhea that is mucoid, soft, and malodorous. Diagnosis is made by the zinc sulfate centrifugation concentration flotation technique, using Lugol's iodine to stain the cysts. Other salts and sugar distort giardial cysts rapidly, making them difficult to recognize. The cysts range in size from $8–12\ \mu \times 7–10\ \mu$. If diarrhea is present, a direct saline fecal smear should be examined to look for trophozoites, which range in size from $10–12\ \mu \times 15–18\ \mu$. In the vast majority of cases, however, diagnosis is made by finding the cysts in a fecal float. Unfortunately, giardial cysts are shed sporadically in the feces; thus, serial fecal samples over the course of 1 week may need to be collected to rule out giardiasis. The fecal antigen ELISA appears to be fairly accurate for diagnosis of giardiasis in cats.

29. How is giardiasis treated?

Commonly used drugs include metronidazole, fenbendazole, and albendazole (see table in question 12). Because albendazole has significant hematologic side-effects, it is not recommended. None of these drugs is approved for use in cats. Repeated treatments may be required. Addition of insoluble fiber may lessen trophozoite adherence to the microvillus. Vaccination is under evaluation as a therapy. In some chronically infected dogs, administration of 2 subcutaneous vaccines controlled diarrhea and lessened cyst shedding. It may be impossible to clear the infection in some cats.

30. How can giardiasis be prevented?

Giardial infection rates may be very high in catteries and difficult to control because the cysts are infective immediately when passed in the feces. Environmental disinfection helps control contamination. Dilute solutions of bleach or quaternary ammonium, heat, and drying kill the cysts. It is important to clean litter trays once or more daily to control reinfection. Environmental clean-up may be impossible because almost any animal may harbor *Giardia* spp. and thus contaminate water sources. In problem catteries, the combination of treatment of all cats, environmental disinfection, bathing to lessen cyst transmission, and vaccination may be helpful.

31. What are *Trichomonas* spp.?

Trichomonas spp. are flagellates occasionally seen in direct wet-mount fecal samples. They usually are considered to be commensal organisms but have been associated with diarrhea. It is questionable whether they are the primary cause of diarrhea or opportunistic organisms that multiply because of the changes in the intestinal environment due to diarrhea. Naturally occurring trichomonads have been reported in cats, but the organism associated with illness generally is *Pentatrichomonas hominis*, the same trichomonad that infects monkeys, dogs, rats, and humans. Thus it is unclear whether the cat is an accidental host. Large or mixed bowel diarrhea occurs in most clinically affected cats. The life cycle is direct, by contact or through contaminated food or water. Trichomonal trophozoites do not live long outside the host. Diagnosis is based on demonstration of the $7–14\ \mu \times 4–6\ \mu$ trophozoite with an anterior flagella, undulating membrane, and posterior flagellum on fecal wet mount. The organism also can be cultured.

32. Should trichomonal infection of cats be treated?

If *Trichomonas* spp. are detected in the stool of cats with mixed or large bowel diarrhea and there is no other explanation for the diarrhea, treatment is indicated. Many drugs, including metronidazole, fenbendazole, enrofloxacin, and paromomycin, have been used, but none has been shown to lead to cure. Paromomycin was associated with acute renal failure in 4 cats with bloody diarrhea and should be used with care. None of these drugs is approved for use in cats.

BIBLIOGRAPHY

1. Arrioja-Dechert A (ed): Compendium of Veterinary Products, 5th ed: Feline anthelmintics and parasiticides. Port Huron, North American Compendium, Ltd., 1999, p 339.
2. Bowman DD: Georgi's Parasitology for Veterinarians, 7th ed. Philadelphia, W.B. Saunders, 1999.
3. Courtney CH, Sundlof SF: Veterinary Antiparasitic Drugs. Gainesville, FL, University of Florida, 1999, pp 186–205.
4. Finley T: How to Prevent Transmission of Intestinal Roundworms from Pets to People. Atlanta, Centers for Disease Control and Prevention/Division of Parasitic Diseases, 1996, publication MSF22.
5. Foreyt WJ: Veterinary Parasitology Reference Manual, 4th ed. Philadelphia, W.B. Saunders, 1997.

6. Grieve RB (ed): Small Animal Practice. Veterinary Clinics of North America, vol. 17, no. 6. Philadelphia, W.B. Saunders, 1987.
7. Holzworth J: Diseases of the Cat: Medicine and Surgery. Philadelphia, W.B. Saunders, 1987.
8. Sherding RG (ed): The Cat: Diseases and Clinical Management, 2nd ed. New York, Churchhill Livingstone, 1994.
9. Urquhart GM, Armour J, Duncan JL, et al: Veterinary Parasitology, 2nd ed. Oxford, Blackwell Science, 1996.

20. BACTERIAL DISEASES

Margie Scherk, D.V.M.

1. What bacteria should be considered on a differential list for vomiting or diarrhea in cats?

- *Helicobacter* spp.
- *Salmonella* spp.
- *Campylobacter jejuni* and *C. coli*
- *Clostridium perfringens*
- *Escherichia coli*

2. Summarize the morphologic characteristics of each.

Morphologic Characteristics of Gastrointestinal Bacterial Pathogens

Campylobacter jejuni	Gram-negative; slender, curved or gull-shaped; motile rods (singles, pairs, chains of 3–5 spirals)
Clostridium perfringens	Gram-positive, spore-forming rods
Escherichia coli	Gram-negative, medium-sized, short rods
Helicobacter spp.	Gram-negative, spiral-shaped, highly motile spirochetes
Salmonella spp.	Gram-negative, non–spore-forming, motile rods

3. Do any of these bacteria pose a potential public health concern?

C. jejuni, C. coli, Helicobacter spp., *E. coli,* and *Salmonella* spp. have potential zoonotic implications, especially in immunocompromised people. Thus, a thorough diagnostic work-up is warranted in cats with vomiting or diarrhea that does not resolve with initial, symptomatic therapy (see Chapter 84).

4. What initial symptomatic therapy is recommended for suspected gastrointestinal bacterial infections?

Fluid and electrolyte support, withholding food for 24 hours followed by gradual introduction of a bland, enteric-type diet are non-specific, supportive measures for the cat who is not seriously ill with vomiting or diarrhea.

5. What antibiotic should be used empirically in cats with diarrhea?

Oral antibiotics should *not* be administered non-specifically for the treatment of diarrhea in cats.

6. What tests are usually performed initially on cats with diarrhea?

Because there are multiple infectious and parasitic causes of vomiting and diarrhea in cats, fecal flotation, fecal wet mount examination, and rectal cytology are usually performed (see Chapter 18 and 19). Romanowsky and Gram stains of thin fecal smears are simple techniques used to assess cats with suspected bacterial enteritis (see Chapter 18). With bacterial enteritis, neutrophils are common and morphologic forms consistent with *Campylobacter* spp. and *Clostridium perfringens* may be noted. If evidence suggests that a zoonotic pathogen may be involved, culture and antimicrobial sensitivity testing of feces should be recommended.

7. What are the clinical findings of *Helicobacter* spp. infection?

Since 1984, a pathogenic role has been recognized for some *Helicobacter* spp. in humans. In people, *H. pylori* causes most cases of peptic ulcer disease and type B gastritis; gastric carcinoma and B cell lymphoma occur secondarily in some cases. Cats are commonly infected by *H. felis, H. heilmannii, H. pametensis,* and, rarely, by *H. pylori.* The failure of one study to isolate *H. pylori* from stray cats indicates that in cats it may be an animal infection with a human pathogen.

Because *Helicobacter* spp. can be found in the stomach of healthy as well as ill cats, it is difficult to determine a disease association. The organisms may be commensal with opportunistic tendencies. The prevalence of *Helicobacter*-like organisms in gastric tissues ranges from 41–100% of healthy cats and 57–100% of vomiting cats. Transmission is probably by ingestion of food or water contaminated by vomitus, feces, and possibly saliva.

Chronic lymphocytic or lymphofollicular gastritis has been detected in some cats, suggesting that infection occasionally results in disease. Clinical signs in infected cats range from none to intermittent vomiting and weight loss due to chronic gastritis and gastroduodenal ulcers (rare). In the small number of cats with *H. pylori* infection, clinical signs were absent despite persistent colonization and presence of mucosal lesions.

8. How is a diagnosis of *Helicobacter* spp. gastritis made?

A presumptive diagnosis of *Helicobacter* spp. gastritis is based on exclusion of other causes of gastritis as well as the following tests:

- The characteristic endoscopic findings include multifocal mucosal punctate hemmorhages with rugal thickening.
- *Helicobacter* spp. produce urease. To screen for urease, mucosal biopsies are placed on a urea slant medium that contains urea and phenol red indicator. If urease is present, ammonia is liberated, raising the pH and turning the indicator red.
- Cytology of impression smears or mucosal brushings may reveal numerous motile spiral bacteria.
- Histopathology of gastric mucosal biopsies shows lymphocytic gastritis with prominent lymphoid follicles, fibrosis, erosions, and spiral bacteria in the gastric glands, surface mucus, and occasionally in the gastric parietal cells. Warthin-Starry silver staining increases visibility of the spiral bacteria in gastric biopsies.
- Culture, mouse inoculation, and polymerase chain reaction are used in research settings.

9. How is *Helicobacter* spp. infection treated?

In humans, combinations of antimicrobials and antacids have been used. Amoxicillin or doxycycline, combined with metronidazole and bismuth subsalicylate, was used most frequently initially. The combination of clarithromycin and other antacids, including famotidine or omeprazole), also is frequently prescribed. Because of the difficulty in medicating cats, the clarithromycin protocol may be more practical; both drugs can be given once daily. If a positive response occurs within 7–10 days, treatment should be continued for a minimum of 3 weeks. Reinfection and incomplete elimination occur.

Drugs Used in the Treatment of Bacterial Gastrointestinal Diseases

DRUG	DOSE	INDICATIONS
Amoxicillin	10–20 mg/kg PO every 8 hr	*Clostridium perfringens, Helicobacter* spp.
Ampicillin	10–20 mg/kg PO every 8hr	*C. perfringens*
Ampicillin	10–20 mg/kg IV or SC every 8 hr	Anaerobic or gram-positive sepsis (use with aminoglycosides or quinolones)
Bismuth sub-salicylate	17.5 mg bismuth/kg every 8 hr (Pepto-Bismol liquid: 17.5 mg/ml bismuth, 8.7 mg/ml salicylate)	*Helicobacter* spp.
Cephalothin	22–44 mg/kg IV or IM every 8 hr	Anaerobic or gram-positive sepsis (use with aminoglycosides or quinolones)

Table continued on following page

Drugs Used in the Treatment of Bacterial Gastrointestinal Diseases (Continued)

DRUG	DOSE	INDICATIONS
Chloramphenicol	10–15 mg/kg PO or SC every 12 hr	*Campylobacter* spp.
Clarithromycin*	7.5 mg/kg PO every 12–24 hr	*Helicobacter* spp.
Erythromycin	10 mg/kg PO every 8 hr	*Campylobacter* spp.
Enrofloxacin	5 mg/kg PO or SC every 12 hr	*Campylobacter* spp., gram-negative sepsis (including *Escherichia coli* and *Salmonella* spp.), *Clostridium difficile*
Famotidine	0.5–1.0 mg/kg PO every 24 hr	*Helicobacter* spp.
Gentamicin	2.2 mg/kg IV or SC every 8 hr	Gram-negative sepsis (including *E. coli* and *Salmonella* spp.)
Metronidazole	10–15 mg/kg PO every 12 hr	*C. perfringens, Helicobacter* spp.
Omeprazole	0.7–1.0 mg/kg PO every 24 hr	*Helicobacter* spp.
Tylosin	15 mg/kg PO every 12 hr	*C. perfringens*, bacterial overgrowth (?)

PO = orally, IV = intravenously, IM = intramuscularly, SC = subcutaneously
* Usually combined with either famotidine or omeprazole.

10. How common is salmonellosis in cats?
Salmonella spp. have been isolated from feces in up to 18% of healthy cats. The prevalence is thought to be even higher in cats with diarrhea. However, in a recent study of healthy cats and cats with diarrhea in Colorado, *Salmonella* spp. were identified in feces from 0.8% of client-owned cats and 1.3% of shelter cats with or without diarrhea.

11. How do cats become infected with *Salmonella* spp.?
The route of infection is almost always oral-fecal; airborne transmission is rare. Contact with contaminated food (especially raw meat or poorly processed diets), water, or fomites is the common mode of transmission. Poultry products are commonly contaminated. Moistened food left at room temperature may pose a risk to cats. Cats should not be fed undercooked meats. Ingestion of infected transport hosts, such as songbirds, may result in salmonellosis in cats; cats should not be allowed to hunt. Animal caregivers are most likely infected with nontyphoid *Salmonella* strains; these infections are generally self-limiting and do not pose an anthropomorphic risk.

12. How can salmonellosis in cats be prevented?
The organism is hardy and survives well in the environment in fecal-contaminated material, including hospital cages and litter trays, endoscopic equipment and sinks, food dishes, and grooming equipment. Cages and kennels should be cleaned and disinfected between each animal (see Chapter 80). Hand washing between each patient as well as after contact with feces is crucial. Bedding and clothing contaminated with fecal material should be washed, with bleach added to the laundry. Clinic resident cats and long-term boarders should not be housed with the hospital population because they may become infected and shed *Salmonella* spp. in the future.

13. What are the clinical findings of salmonellosis?
Bacteremia and endotoxemia are the most life-threatening form of infection. Acute episodes may occur as soon as 3–5 days after exposure, and patients may present with fever, anorexia, and lethargy with subsequent diarrhea, vomiting, and apparent abdominal discomfort. Diarrhea may be watery to mucoid with the presence of fresh blood. Localized infections, such as abscesses, cellulitis, osteomyelitis, pyothorax, pneumonia, or meningitis, occur in some cats. Poor reproductive performance (genital tract infection, abortions, stillbirths, fading kittens) is of concern in a breeding cattery.

14. What factors determine the clinical form of *Salmonella* spp. infection?
Salmonella spp. can cause subclinical infection. However, isolation of the organism from the gastrointestinal tract of diseased animals or normally sterile areas such as blood, urine,

cerebrospinal fluid, joint fluid, tracheal washings, or bone marrow is significant. Repeat shedding occurs in previously infected animals suffering from stress or other illness. The immune status of the host, the presence of concurrent disorders, and bacterial burden at presentation affect what form of disease will result.

15. Should salmonellosis be treated?

Parenteral administration of antibiotics should be reserved for treatment of endotoxemia, bacteremia, or other forms of systemic infection (see table in question 9). Oral administration of antibiotics not only reduces the host's intestinal resistance to salmonellosis by altering the balance of normal enteric flora but also has been shown to prolong the disease course in experimental animals. In addition, the organism may develop plasmid-mediated antibiotic resistance. Thus, the use of antibiotics is not recommended in uncomplicated gastroenteritis.

16. How is campylobacteriosis transmitted?

As with the other bacterial agents of diarrhea, fecal-oral, water-borne, or food borne routes of infection are the norm. Most human *Campylobacter* infections are due to ingestion of undercooked meat (especially chicken). Infected cats may be a source of infection for humans.

Privately owned animals are less likely to contract the disease than animals housed in kennels or catteries, stray animals, and animals in hospitals where nosocomial infections are prevalent. In a study from north central Colorado, 0% of cats from a shelter and 1.6% of client-owned cats with or without diarrhea were culture-positive.

17. What are the clinical findings of *Campylobacter* spp. infection?

In many cats, infection with *C. jejuni* or *C. coli* is subclinical. Diarrhea usually occurs in cats younger than 6 months and is usually watery with mucous or blood. Often the development of clinical signs is associated with coinfection with other enteric pathogens.

18. How is campylobacteriosis diagnosed?

Because the infection is localized to the colon, rectal cytology is helpful in establishing the diagnosis. Gram-negative, slender, gull wing-shaped organisms may be seen along with neutrophils. Confirmation is by fecal culture. It is unknown whether serum antibody titers reflect current infection.

19. How is diarrhea due to *Campylobacter* spp. treated?

Supportive care is administered as indicated. It is unknown whether antibiotics alter the course of infection. In severe cases, antibiotic therapy is indicated (erythromycin, second-generation cephalosporins, or enrofloxacin may be considered (see table in question 9). It is important to base treatment on antimicrobial susceptibility results and to treat for a complete course of 21 days; failure to do so may allow development of an antibiotic-induced carrier state.

20. What are the clinical findings of *Clostridium perfringens* gastrointestinal infections?

Clostridium perfringens is a normal intestinal flora; thus, not all culture-positive cats are diseased. Some types of *C. perfringens* produce enterotoxin that may induce disease. If diarrhea occurs, it is usually watery to mucohemmorhagic. Anal tissues may become inflamed, and occasionally colonic epithelium may slough. Diarrhea usually subsides after a few days. However, some authorities believe that the organism is associated with chronic intermittent diarrhea.

21. How is *C. perfringens*-associated diarrhea diagnosed?

Detection of > 5–10 safety-pin shaped spore-forming rods per high-power field, combined with the appropriate clinical findings, is suggestive. As previously discussed, culture of stool can document carriage of *C. perfringens* but does not prove a disease association. Enterotoxin can be detected in stool by reverse passive latex agglutination or enzyme-linked immunosorbent assay (ELISA); positive results were previously thought to have the best predictive value for disease.

However, positive results can occur in both healthy and diseased animals. In addition, false-negative enterotoxin results occur in cats with severely watery diarrhea and cats with chronic disease.

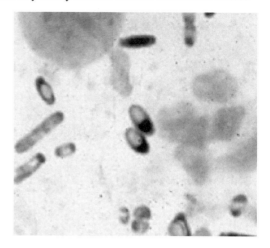

Spore-forming bacteria morphologically consistent with *Clostridium perfringens*.

22. Can diet prevent clostridial diarrhea?

Diets high in soluble fiber provide short-chained fatty acids through fiber fermentation. These acids acidify the colonic environment and alter microbial flora, which may help to reduce the proliferation of clostridial organisms.

23. Are oral antibiotics indicated in the treatment of suspected clostridial diarrhea?

In acute cases of suspected clostridial diarrhea, withholding food for 24 hours and then feeding small amounts of a high-fiber diet usually results in resolution of clinical signs within 2–3 days. Administration of oral antibiotics with presumed activity against *C. perfringens* (amoxicillin, tylosin, or metronidazole) may speed resolution of clinical signs. In addition, in some cats *C. perfringens* overgrowth may relate to coinfection with other pathogens. Thus, administration of tylosin (*Cryptosporidium* spp.) or metronidazole (*Giardia* spp.) may be effective for other reasons.

24. Is *Escherichia coli* infection associated with disease in cats?

E. coli is most commonly a normal enteric flora in cats. Some strains are true enteropathogens and cause inflammation resulting in severe watery diarrhea. Some enterotoxigenic strains also release toxins in the small intestine that inhibit resorption of sodium and chloride, resulting in water loss. Enteroinvasive forms actively invade the colonic cells and other cells, causing septicemia and endotoxemia.

25. How is *E. coli* transmitted?

Most cases of zoonotic *E. coli* infection result from ingestion of inadequately cooked ground beef or raw milk products; however, it is possible for people to become infected via fecal material of cats. *E. coli* is a hardy organism that survives in fecal material, dust, and water for long periods. The route of transmission is oral; fomites such as dishes, brushes, hospital equipment and instruments, respiratory equipment, floors, and even disinfectant solutions, may harbor the organism.

26. How is *E. coli* infection managed clinically?

Routine fecal culture cannot differentiate nonpathogenic *E. coli* from enteropathogenic strains; thus, *E. coli*-associated disease is usually not proven in small animal practice. Treatment is reserved for cats with systemic signs of infection. Supportive fluid treatment and parenteral antibiotic therapy is indicated in such cases. Because *E. coli* is a gram-negative organism, quinolones are appropriate empirical antimicrobial choices.

27. Do cats develop small intestinal bacterial overgrowth?

The range of quantitative bacterial counts from the duodenum of normal cats varies from 0 to > 10^8. Thus, in contrast to dogs, it is unclear whether small intestinal bacterial overgrowth occurs as a disease entity in cats.

BIBLIOGRAPHY

1. Deming MS, Tauxe RV, Blake PA, et al: *Campylobacter* enteritis at a university: Transmission from eating chickens and from cats. Am J Epidemiol 126:526–534, 1987.
2. El-Zaatari FAK, Woo JS, Badr A, et al: Failure to isolate *Helicobacter pylori* from stray cats indicated that *H. pylori* in cats may be an antroponosis—an animal infection with a human pathogen. J Med Microbiol 46:372–376, 1997.
3. Foley JE, Orgad U, Hirsh DC, et al: Outbreak of fatal salmonellosis in cats following use of a high-titer modified-live panleukopenia virus vaccine. J Am Vet Med Assoc 214:67–70, 1999.
4. Greene CE. Fox, JG: Enteric bacterial infections. In Greene CE (ed): Infectious Diseases of the Dog and Cat, 2nd ed. Philadelphia, W.B. Saunders, 1998, pp 226–248.
5. Hill S, Lappin MR, Cheney J, et al: Prevalence of enteric zoonotic agents in cats. J Am Vet Med Assoc 216:687–692, 2000.
6. Kruth SA: Gram-negative bacterial infections. In Greene CE (ed): Infectious Diseases of the Dog and Cat, 2nd ed. Philadelphia, W.B.Saunders, 1998, pp 217-226.
7. Marks SL, Melli A, Kass PH, et al: Evaluation of methods to diagnose *Clostridium perfringens*-associated diarrhea in dogs. J Am Vet Med Assoc 214:357–360, 1999.
8. Scott FW: *Salmonella* implicated as cause of songbird fever. Feline Health Top 3:5, 1988.
9. Simpson K, Neiger R, DeNovo R, et al: The relationship of *Helicobacter* spp. infection to gastric disease in dogs and cats. J Vet Intern Med 14:223–227, 2000.
10. Papasouliotis K, Sparkes AH, Werrett G, et al: Assessment of the bacterial flora of the proximal part of the small intestine in healthy cats, and the effect of sample collection method. Am J Vet Res 59:48–51 1998.
11. Zoran DL: Diet and drugs: The keys to managing feline colonic disease. Compend Cont Educ Pract Vet 21:731–748, 1999.

21. VIRAL DISEASES

Jordan Q. Jaeger, D.V.M.

1. What are the common viral causes of gastrointestinal (GI) disease?

Vomiting or diarrhea has been associated most frequently with feline panleukopenia virus (FPV), coronaviruses, feline leukemia virus (see Chapter 76), and feline immunodeficiency virus (see Chapter 77).

2. What causes feline panleukopenia?

Feline panleukopenia is caused by FPV, a small parvovirus. This single-stranded, DNA-type virus is related closely to canine parvovirus. Cats also can be infected by canine parvovirus and occasionally have clinical signs of disease. The name was derived from the clinical observation that many cats develop severe leukopenia, but this finding is not considered pathognomonic. The disease syndrome also has been called feline distemper. Clinical findings of FPV infection in cats are similar to those associated with canine parvovirus infection.

3. How is FPV transmitted and maintained in the environment?

FPV is shed in all body secretions; large quantities are present in the feces during active stages of infection. Cats continue to shed virus in feces and urine for a maximum of 6 weeks after infection. The virus is ubiquitous in the environment and can survive readily for more than 1 year. Susceptible animals are infected via fecal-oral transmission. Fomites are believed to play an important role in transmission because the virus can survive for prolonged periods on contaminated surfaces. Examples of fomites include clothing, shoes, hands, food dishes, and cages. Flies and other insects may serve as transport hosts during warmer periods of the year.

4. Which species are susceptible to FPV? What areas of the body does it infect?

All species of Felidae as well as raccoons, coatimundi, and mink are susceptible to the virus. Feline panleukopenia infects rapidly dividing cells; thus it has a predilection for the GI tract, lymphoid tissue, and bone marrow. In prenatal and early neonatal infections, the cerebrum, cerebellum, retina, and optic nerves are also commonly infected, resulting in clinical abnormalities.

5. Is FPV passed in utero?

The virus is passed from queen to fetus. Infection early in pregnancy results in fetal death and resorption with infertility, abortions, or birth of mummified fetuses. If infection occurs closer to term, the kittens are born alive with varying degrees of damage to the late developing neural tissue. Littermates may be affected to varying degrees.

6. What are the effects of FPV infection on the CNS and other developing neuronal tissue in late uterine and early prenatal infection?

About 70–80% of small neurons in the cerebellar cortex and granular cell layer of the cerebellum do not develop until after birth. FPV inhibits the normal cerebellar cortical development and migration of cells. The results are the gross pathologic finding of small or hypoplastic cerebellum and histologic findings of distorted cell layers and marked depletion of the granular cells and Purkinje's cells. Less commonly the spinal cord, optic nerve, and retina also may be affected.

7. What is the pathogenesis of FPV-associated GI tract disease?

After oral exposure, the virus induces a plasma viremia. GI disease develops as cells in the intestinal crypts are destroyed. leading to sloughing of the villi. Increased absorption of bacteria and bacterial toxins leads to systemic bacteremia or sepsis.

8. What is the typical signalment of cats with clinical feline panleukopenia?

The incidence is highest in cats under 1 year of age. There is no sex or breed predisposition. Often there is a seasonal increase in late summer to early fall, when the major annual crop of kittens is at the end of maternal antibody protection. The frequency of clinical disease is much lower than the actual number of cats infected with the virus. Most adult cats have subclinical infection. The finding of a high infection rate with low incidence of clinical disease in older cats is supported by a high prevalence of FPV antibody titers in the adult cat population; up to 75% of presumably unvaccinated feral cats are seropositive.

9. Describe the clinical presentation of kittens with prenatal or early postnatal FPV infection.

Kittens infected transplacentaly or shortly after birth often appear normal until they start to walk. At that time, varying degrees of ataxia, incoordination, intention tremors, broad-based stance, hypermetria, and falling are frequently observed. Affected kittens have normal mental status, which is typical of cerebellar hypoplasia. Some may have signs of forebrain involvement , such as seizures, behavioral abnormalities, or postural reaction deficits accompanied by a normal gate. The ataxia is nonprogressive.

10. Describe the clinical presentation in kittens with late postnatal FPV infection.

Generalized infection in young unvaccinated cats is the most common form of FPV disease. Severe disease may result in acute death. In less severe cases, fever (104–107°F), anorexia, and depression precede presentation by 3–4 days. At some time during the course of the disease, vomiting that is not associated with eating often develops. Diarrhea is a common but not consistent finding. The intestines may be painful and feel thickened during abdominal palpation. In complicated cases, bloody diarrhea, icterus, and severe dehydration may develop.

11. What laboratory abnormalities are associated with feline panleukopenia?

Specific laboratory abnormalities are found most often in the complete blood count. Severe panleukopenia is seen often but not in every case. In severe infections, the total white cell count varies between 50 and 3,000 cells/µl; in more moderate cases, between 3000 and 7000 cells/µl. Complete blood counts should be repeated because other diseases also may present with panleukopenia. The leukopenia associated with FPV resolves within a few days of recovery from illness. Thus, it can be differentiated from other causes of chronic leukopenia. If prolonged panleukopenia exists, other diseases, such as feline leukemia or septic salmonellosis, should be considered. The severity of the leukopenia often reflects the severity of clinical illness. A mild decrease in hematocrit and absolute reticulocyte count may be present in cats with viremia but should not result in marked anemia, unless severe GI bleeding occurs. The anemia remains mild because of the short course of the disease and the long life span of red blood cells. In cases of severe infection, thrombocytopenia may develop. Clotting abnormalities consistent with disseminated intravascular coagulation (DIC) also can be detected in severe infection.

Biochemical abnormalities are usually nonspecific. Azotemia due to dehydration is most often detected. Mild renal damage also may result from viral replication. In rare cases, mild elevations of liver enzyme activities may be detected. Hypoglycemia and hypokalemia result from sepsis and GI losses, respectively.

12. How is feline panleukopenia diagnosed?

A presumptive diagnosis is based on the presence of appropriate clinical findings in a susceptible host after exclusion of other diseases that produce acute GI signs or leukopenia. Peracute and acute cases must be differentiated from intoxication or foreign body ingestion; careful history taking is vital. Abdominal radiographs as well as fecal examination for parasites should be performed to rule out intestinal obstruction or extreme parasite burden. Clinical signs also may be compatible with acute toxoplasmosis. Toxoplasmosis often has accompanying respiratory signs, which may be helpful in differentiating between the two diseases. Negative feline leukemia virus status also should be confirmed.

Exposure to FPV can be confirmed by documenting increasing antibody titer on samples taken at the time of presentation and 2 weeks later. A fourfold rise in titer is supportive of acute infection. Presence of viral particles in feces on electron microscopy or viral antigens in feces by enzyme-linked immunosorbent assay (ELISA) also can confirm exposure to FPV. However, canine parvovirus ELISA has not been validated for use with feline feces, and neither electron microscopy nor ELISA can distinguish modified live vaccine strains from virulent strains.

13. How is FP treated?

Symptomatic and supportive care are the cornerstones of therapy. Fluid therapy, control of GI signs, antimicrobial therapy, potassium replacement, maintenance of euglycemia, and control of oncotic pressure are key components. Specific antiviral treatment is not available. The key is to support the patient until the immune response is able to overcome the infection.

14. What fluid therapy is suggested?

Fluid deficits and ongoing losses should be corrected parenterally. Use of a jugular catheter is preferred over other sites because the jugular catheter is usually not positional, can be used to obtain blood samples, is not likely to be contaminated with feces, is unlikely to develop phlebitis, and allows monitoring of central venous pressure. The fluid deficit (body wt [kg] × percent dehydrated × 1000 = ml) is replaced over 24 hours, along with estimates of ongoing losses and maintenance. Balanced isotonic fluid replacement is used with potassium supplementation. Electrolytes should be measured intermittently to aid in determining potassium needs; a minimum of 20 mEq/L should be used. Blood glucose should be monitored and supplemented as indicated. If clinical evidence of decreased oncotic pressure (peripheral or pulmonary edema) is present concurrently with hypoalbuminemia, plasma or colloids should be administered. Anemia due to severe GI blood loss may develop in addition to hypoproteinemia; therefore, blood transfusion may be needed.

Platelet count, fibrin degradation products (FDPs), and clotting times should be assessed in moribund or septic cats to evaluate for possible DIC.

15. How are GI signs of FP managed?

Eliminating oral intake of food and water decreases the amount of vomiting and slows replication of intestinal cells in the GI tract, which is needed for viral replication. Antiemetics may be used to control vomiting, if necessary. Anticholinergic medications should not be used because they produce ileus. First-line antiemetic therapy is metoclopramide, administered subcutaneously at 0.2–0.5 mg/kg every 6–8 hr. If vomiting persists, a continuous infusion of metoclopramide (1–2 mg/kg/day) is often helpful. Water can be reintroduced no sooner than 24 hours after cessation of vomiting. Initially, small amounts of water should be offered. If no vomiting occurs for 24 hours, small amounts of a bland food (specifically a commercial GI diet or rice with small amounts of baby food) may be introduced. If feedings are tolerated, the amount should be increased gradually. After the patient is consuming normal amounts, a slow transition over 4–6 days should be made to regular maintenance diet.

16. What antibiotics should be used if findings of bacteremia or sepsis exist?

Broad-spectrum antibiotics, such as ampicillin (22 mg/kg intravenously every 6–8 hr) or a first-generation cephalosporin (20–25 mg/kg intravenously every 6–8 hr) should be used to help prevent systemic bacterial infection. If sepsis is suspected, a fluoroquinolone (5–10 mg/kg intramuscularly or intravenously every 24 hr) or an aminoglycoside (3 mg/kg intravenously every 8hr) can be added to improve the gram-negative spectrum. Aminoglycosides should not be administered until the cat is well hydrated and potassium deficits have been corrected to lessen the chance of nephrotoxicity. Alternatively, a second-generation cephalosporin can be used. Antibiotic therapy also may decrease bacterial counts in the GI tract, which are known to increase mitotic rate of intestinal epithelia. In germ-free kittens, the clinical manifestations are not as severe.

17. Is passive immunotherapy of benefit in the treatment of FP?

In dogs, administration of lyophilized serum from hyperimmune dogs decreases morbidity associated with canine parvovirus infection. Although data from cats are not available, the same principle probably applies because the pathogenesis is similar to that in dogs. Administration of 1 ml/kg of plasma or serum from a well-vaccinated cat or survivor of feline panleukopenia may be administered intravenously, intraperitoneally, or subcutaneously.

18. How long do colostral antibodies and maternal virus-neutralizing (VN) antibodies persist in kittens?

Colostral antibodies have a half-life of 9.5 days. Thus, maternal VN antibodies may interfere with vaccination until 12–14 weeks of age.

19. When should kittens be vaccinated? With what type of vaccine?

Kittens presented for vaccination before 12 weeks of age should receive either inactivated or modified live vaccines every 3 weeks until they are 12 weeks of age. Kittens presented for vaccination after 12 weeks of age should receive two inactivated vaccines, 3 weeks apart, or 1 modified live vaccine. Boosters should be given at 1 year of age and then no more frequently than every 3 years. In one study, cats vaccinated with two inactivated vaccines had 100% protection when challenged with virulent FPV 7.5 years later. There is no benefit from use of intranasal products. Queens should be vaccinated before pregnancy; if vaccinated during gestation, they should receive only inactivated products because modified live vaccines may infect the fetal or neonatal cerebellum. Kittens born to naive queens may be vaccinated as soon as 4 weeks of age with inactivated products.

20. How is the virus inactivated once in the environment?

If FP is diagnosed in a household, a 1:32 dilution of household bleach should be used on all cages, bowls, litter pans, and floors. Plastic litter pans should be discarded because of the difficulty in disinfecting. New cats with past infection of FPV should not be introduced into the household without prior vaccination. Other susceptible cats in the household usually show initial signs (anorexia, lethargy, and vomiting) in 2–6 days. Passive immunity, as described in question 17, should be considered for exposed susceptible cats that need immediate protection.

21. What are feline coronaviruses? How are they transmitted?

The coronaviruses are ubiquitous RNA viruses transmitted by the fecal-oral route. Some isolates are limited to the intestinal tract, leading to subclinical infection in most (feline enteric coronavirus [FECV]). Other isolates have the ability to infect macrophages, disseminate through the body, and induce the clinical syndrome known as feline infectious peritonitis (see Chapter 38).

22. What are the clinical signs in cats infected with FECV?

When clinical signs occur, mild small bowel diarrhea is usually present. Occasionally, mucus and fresh blood also may be seen. Occasionally, vomiting, low-grade fever, anorexia, and lethargy may accompany the diarrhea. Clinical signs often resolve within 2–4 days. Although enteric coronaviruses are limited to the GI tract, spontaneous mutation to feline infectious peritonitis (FIP)-inducing strains can occur in the host.

23. How is a diagnosis of FECV infection made?

FECV infection is often a diagnosis of exclusion. It is important to rule out more common causes of mild diarrhea and vomiting, such as foreign body ingestion, parasite infestation, dietary intolerance, intestinal perforation, and other enteric viruses. Documentation of increasing coronavirus antibody titers suggests recent infection. FECV can be documented in feces with electron microscopy or virus isolation. Reverse transcriptase polymerase chain reaction also can be used to detect RNA of the organism in feces.

24. How is clinical FECV infection treated?

Treatment consists of supportive care (as in feline panleukopenia), but sepsis is less likely. Fluid therapy and gut rest are the most important components.

25. How is FECV infection prevented?

In crowded environments, most cats are seropositive for coronavirus antibodies. It is estimated that approximately 30% of seropositive cats are shedding coronaviruses in stool at any one time. The spread of the virus in catteries is highly efficient, and prevention of spread is essentially impossible. Stress should be avoided if possible, and care should be taken to lessen crowding of litter boxes. Vaccination with the intranasal coronavirus vaccine is not warranted because of the mild clinical signs seen in cats and associated low morbidity.

26. Can serology be used to differentiate FECV from FIP-inducing strains?

Currently no serologic test can differentiate antibodies against FECV from those against FIP-inducing strains (see Chapter 38).

BIBLIOGRAPHY

1. AAFP Vaccination Guidelines: 1998 Report of the American Association of Feline Practitioners and Academy of Feline Medicine Advisory Panel on Feline Vaccinations. J Am Vet Med Assoc 212:227–241, 1998.
2. Addie DD, Jarrett O: Feline coronavirus Infection. In Greene CE (ed): Infectious Diseases of the Dog and Cat. Philadelphia, W.B. Saunders, 1998, pp 58–59.
3. Barr MC, Olsen CW, Scott FW: Feline viral diseases. In Ettinger SJ, Feldman EC (eds): Textbook of Veterinary Internal Medicine, 4th ed., Philadelphia, W.B. Saunders, 1995, pp 409–439.
4. Birchard SJ, Sherding RG: Saunders Manual of Small Animal Practice, 2nd ed, Philadelphia, W.B. Saunders., 2000, pp 115–117.
5. Green CE: Feline panleukopenia. In Greene CE (ed): Infectious Diseases of the Dog and Cat, 2nd ed. Philadelphia, W.B. Saunders, 1998, pp 52–57.

6. Harbour DA: Feline enteric viral infections. Feline coronavirus infection. In Greene CE (ed):. Infectious Diseases of the Dog and Cat. Philadelphia: W.B. Saunders, 1998, pp 58–59.
7. Willard M: Disorders of the intestinal tract. In Nelson RW, Couto CG, King C: Manual of Small Animal Internal Medicine. St. Louis, Mosby, 1999, pp 433–467.
8. Scott FW, Geissinger CM: Long-term immunity in cats vaccinated with an inactivated trivalent vaccine [see comments]. Am J Vet Res 60:652–658, 1999 [published erratum appears in Am J Vet Res 60:763, 1999].
9. Sherding RG: The Cat: Diseases and Clinical Management, 2nd ed. New York, Churchill Livingstone, 1994, pp 357–365.

22. FUNGAL AND MISCELLANEOUS DISEASES

Chad Johannes, D.V.M.

1. What is the most common gastrointestinal (GI) fungal disease in cats?

Cats tend to be highly susceptible hosts for *Histoplasma capsulatum*. This systemic fungal infection results from inhalation or ingestion (less likely in cats) of infective conidia and subsequent hematogenous and lymphatic dissemination. The organism grows best under moist, humid conditions in nitrogen-rich soil (high in organic material such as bird and bat excrement). It is most prevalent in the central United States in regions of the Ohio, Missouri, and Mississippi Rivers as well as in Texas. Clinical histoplasmosis is most commonly seen in cats younger than 4 years of age, although cats of any age can be affected.

2. What signs are typically seen with GI histoplasmosis?

Although GI involvement with systemic histoplasmosis tends to be observed less commonly in cats than in dogs, it can produce chronic small or large bowel diarrhea. As all layers of the intestinal wall are disrupted by granulomatous inflammation, severe chronic malabsorption results in voluminous watery diarrhea. Protein-losing enteropathy is a potential sequela. If the large bowel is also affected, tenesmus, hematochezia, and fecal mucus can be seen. Physical examination often identifies diffusely thickened loops of bowel, along with palpably enlarged mesenteric lymph nodes. Additional systemic signs may include anorexia, rapidly progressive weight loss, fever, and lethargy. Intestinal histoplasmosis should be considered in any young cat with intractable large or small bowel diarrhea that has lived in or traveled through an endemic region.

3. How is GI histoplasmosis diagnosed?

Definitive diagnosis requires identification of *H. capsulatum* organisms (usually within macrophages) on cytology or biopsies. Although primary intestinal histoplasmosis has been reported, intestinal involvement most often results from systemic infection. Radiographs of the thoracic cavity may reveal a diffuse interstitial pattern, with infiltrates coalescing to produce a miliary or nodular interstitial appearance. Other signs of systemic involvement include peripheral lymph node enlargement, abdominal organomegaly, clinical icterus, and occasionally skin nodules or ulcerated lesions. Therefore, diagnosis is often aided by bone marrow, lung, lymph node, liver, splenic, or skin nodule aspirates. Ocular involvement is also possible, and physical examination should include a thorough evaluation of the fundus.

With intestinal involvement, *H. capsulatum* organisms may be seen on cytology from rectal mucosal scrapings and impression smears made from intestinal (endoscopic or surgical) or mesenteric lymph node biopsy samples. The yeasts are round to oval in shape with a distinct wall and are approximately 2–4 μm in diameter (about one-fourth to one-half the diameter of an erythrocyte). With Romanowsky type stains, the interior portion of the organism typically stains pale to medium blue to purple. In addition, organisms can be visualized on histopathology sections with appropriate fungal stains. Serologic tests for *H. capsulatum* antibodies are available, but their reliability is poor.

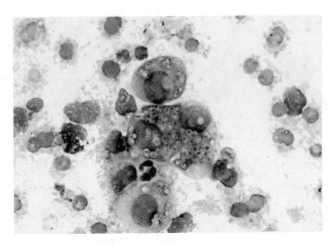

Macrophage containing numerous *Histoplasma capsulatum* yeasts. (Courtesy of Dr. Steven L. Stockham, Department of Veterinary Pathobiology, University of Missouri–Columbia.)

4. What laboratory values are commonly seen in disseminated histoplasmosis?

Normocytic, normochromic, nonregenerative anemia is the most common hematologic abnormality in cats with disseminated histoplasmosis. The anemia may result from chronic inflammatory disease, bone marrow infiltration by *H. capsulatum*, or intestinal blood loss. Leukocyte counts are quite variable, but neutrophilia and monocytosis are observed most frequently. Thrombocytopenia, resulting from increased platelet utilization or destruction, has been reported in as many as one-third of affected cats. With extensive bone marrow involvement, pancytopenia may be present. On occasion, *H. capsulatum* organisms may be visualized within monocytes or neutrophils on a blood smear.

Hypoalbuminemia, the most consistent serum biochemistry profile finding in cats with systemic histoplasmosis, may result from GI loss or liver dysfunction. Globulins may be elevated (chronic antigen stimulation), but this finding varies, depending on concurrent intestinal loss. Hypercalcemia has been reported in several cats and probably is due to systemic granulomatous disease. Elevations in serum alanine aminotransferase, alkaline phosphatase, and total bilirubin indicate possible hepatic involvement. Most affected cats that were tested for feline leukemia virus (FeLV) and feline immunodeficiency virus (FIV) have been negative.

5. What treatment options are available for intestinal histoplasmosis?

Itraconazole is the drug of choice for treatment of disseminated histoplasmosis. Treatment is initiated at 10 mg/kg orally every 24 hours, and if no signs of hepatotoxicity (elevated liver enzymes) develop, dosing can be increased to twice daily. An oral suspension (10 mg/ml) is available and is more consistently absorbed than the capsules. Combination therapy of itraconazole with liposome-encapsulated amphotericin B (0.25–0.5 mg/kg intravenously every 48 hr until a cumulative dose of 4–8 mg/kg is reached) may be necessary in severe or fulminating cases. Owners should be aware that treatment is needed for at least 4–6 months, sometimes as long as 12 months, depending on response to therapy. The prognosis for intestinal histoplasmosis is fair to good, depending on the severity of involvement. Relapse several months after discontinuing oral antifungal therapy is possible.

6. Is histoplasmosis a zoonotic disease?

Although concurrent common-source infections of animals and people have been reported, direct transmission of *H. capsulatum* between animals or from animals to humans has not been shown. Cats and humans in endemic regions are at risk of exposure from infected soil; prevention lies in minimizing this contact.

7. What other fungal organisms can cause diarrhea in cats?

Opportunistic fungal organisms that can cause enteritis and diarrhea in cats include *Aspergillus* spp., *Candida* spp., and *Mucor* spp. FPV, FIP, or FeLV infection, antibiotic therapy, or glucocorticoid therapy appear to be important predisposing factors that increase susceptibility to tissue invasion by these fungi. Both small and large bowel are often affected, causing a chronic mixed bowel diarrhea. Antemortem diagnosis of intestinal mycoses can be quite difficult and requires histopathologic identification of organisms in tissue sections. In some animals with renal involvement, fungal hyphae may be visualized on routine urine sediment examination.

Most reported cases have been identified on necropsy, providing limited information about treatment, drug dosages, and length of therapy. Ketoconazole (10 mg/kg orally every 12 hr), itraconazole (2.5–5 mg/kg orally every 12 hr), or liposomal amphotericin B (3–5 mg/kg intravenously every 48 hr until a cumulative dose of 12 mg/kg is reached) may be options for treating disseminated aspergillosis. Treatment with an oral imidazole may be needed for months to years, and long-term prognosis is generally grave. Nystatin (100,000 units/cat orally every 6 hr), ketoconazole (50 mg/cat orally every 12–24 hr), or itraconazole (5–10 mg/kg orally every 12–24 hr) may be considered for systemic candidiasis.

8. Do cats develop protothecosis, mucormycosis, or pythiosis?

Pythium insidiosum is a water mold associated with GI tract disease in dogs, primarily along the Gulf Coast. Infection of cats is rare. Infection with *Mucor* spp. fungi occurs in cats as a systemic disease. Protothecosis is a disseminated disease in dogs caused by the algae *Prototheca zopfii* and *P. wickerhamii*. Bloody diarrhea is a common manifestation. To date, only cutaneous protothecosis has been reported in cats.

BIBLIOGRAPHY

1. Baker R, Lumsden JH: Color Atlas of Cytology of the Dog and Cat. St. Louis, Mosby, 2000, p 23.
2. Blischok D, Bender H: What is your diagnosis—15-year old male domestic shorthair cat. Vet Clin Pathol 25:114.
3. Clinkenbeard KD, Wolf AM, Cowell RL, et al: Feline disseminated histoplasmosis. Compend Cont Educ Pract Vet 11:1223–1233.
4. Guilford WG, Strombeck DR: Gastrointestinal tract infections, parasites, and toxicoses. In Strombeck's Small Animal Gastroenterology. Philadelphia, W.B. Saunders, 1996, p 424.
5. Hodges RD, Legendre AM, Adams LG, et al: Itraconazole for the treatment of histoplasmosis in cats. J Vet Intern Med 8:409–413.
6. Lappin MR: Protozoal and miscellaneous infections. In Ettinger SJ, Feldman EC (eds): Textbook of Veterinary Internal Medicine. Philadelphia, W.B. Saunders, 2000, pp 408–412.
7. Sherding RG, Burrows, CF: Diarrhea. In Anderson NV (ed): Veterinary Gastroenterology. Philadelphia, Lea & Febiger, 1992, pp 445–449.
8. Taboada J: Systemic mycoses. In Ettinger SJ, Feldman EC (ed): Textbook of Veterinary Internal Medicine. Philadelphia, W.B. Saunders, 2000, pp 462–465.
9. Wolf AM: Histoplasmosis. In Greene CE (ed): Infectious Diseases of the Dog and Cat. Philadelphia, W.B. Saunders, 1998, pp 378–383.

23. INFLAMMATORY BOWEL DISEASE

Alice J. Johns, D.V.M.

1. Define inflammatory bowel disease.

Inflammatory bowel disease (IBD) is a group of idiopathic, chronic gastrointestinal (GI) tract disorders characterized by infiltration of the lamina propria by inflammatory cells. The cellular infiltrate may be lymphocytes, plasma cells, eosinophils, neutrophils, macrophages, or combinations of these.

2. What causes IBD?

The cause of IBD is probably multifactoral. It appears to involve host hypersensitivity responses to antigens (food, bacterial, or self) within the bowel lumen or mucosa. Genetic and psychosocial factors also may be involved. Increased permeability allows luminal antigens to cross the mucosa, leading to inflammation and further mucosal damage, which in turn further increase permeability. Mucosal inflammation occurs in a diverse group of disorders, including bacterial, viral, protozoal, and parasitic infections, bacterial overgrowth, metabolic disease, neoplasia, pancreatitis, and cholangiohepatitis. These conditions should be excluded from the differential list before a cat is assumed to have IBD due to dietary hypersensitivity.

3. Describe the pathophysiology of IBD.

IBD is an abnormal mucosal immune response, which results in the recruitment of inflammatory cells to the intestine. The immune response itself leads to tissue destruction and impairment of digestive and absorptive capabilities. Damage results from the following factors:

- Arachidonic acid metabolites
- Proinflammatory cytokines
- Leukotrienes, produced in the lipoxygenase pathway, that act as chemotactic agents, increase vascular permeability, and induce smooth muscle contraction
- Prostaglandins from the cyclo-oxygenase pathway, which result in pain, vasodilation, increased vascular permeability, and increased secretion of water and electrolytes
- Platelet-activating factor, which is chemotactic and increases vascular permeability
- Interleukins. which regulate the mucosal immune system
- Oxygen-derived free radicals and nitric oxide, which damage the mucosa
- GI peptides, including substance P, vasoactive intestinal peptide, and somatostatin
- Clonal expansion of activated intestinal B and T lymphocytes.

4. Describe the typical signalment for cats with IBD.

There is no age, sex, or breed predilection, although purebred cats may be at increased risk for lymphocytic-plasmacytic enteritis. Although most affected cats are middle aged (6–8 years) or older, about one-third of the patients are 2 years old or younger. IBD has been diagnosed as early as 5 months of age.

5. What are the common clinical signs of IBD?

Chronic vomiting and diarrhea are the most common clinical signs and may occur alone or in combination. Vomiting often is not associated with eating and should be differentiated from regurgitation (see Chapter 26). Diarrhea may contain mucus or blood, indicating large bowel involvement. Anorexia, weight loss, lethargy, loss of litter training, abdominal pain, and hematemesis also may be seen. The clinical signs are generally intermittent or cyclical and reflect the predominant sites of disease. Clinical signs are similar among the various histologic forms. Symptoms vary from mild to severe. Exacerbations and spontaneous remissions are common.

6. What characteristic abnormalities are found on physical examination?

No physical examination findings are pathognomonic, but several findings may suggest IBD. Cranial abdominal discomfort may be present and is more noticeable in cats with concurrent pancreatitis. Intestinal bowel loops may be thickened. Cats with "triaditis"—the combination of inflammatory bowel disease, pancreatitis, and cholangiohepatitis—may be icteric and have a palpable liver. Many cats are ill kempt, and emaciation may be noted, particularly if malabsorption is occurring.

7. What are the primary differential diagnoses for IBD?

- Endocrine diseases (hyperthyroidism, exocrine pancreatic insufficiency)
- Food intolerance
- Bacterial enteritis (*Helicobacter* spp., *Salmonella* spp., *Campylobacter* spp., *Clostridium perfringens*, *Escherichia coli*; see Chapter 20)

- Parasites (helminths, cestodes, protozoans; see Chapter 19)
- Fungal enteritis (*Histoplasma capsulatum*; see Chapter 22)
- Neoplasia (lymphosarcoma, adenoma, adenocarcinoma; see Chapter 24)
- Viral enteritis (feline leukemia virus [FeLV], feline immunodeficiency virus [FIV], feline enteric coronavirus, feline panleukopenia; see Chapter 21)
- Obstruction

8. How is IBD diagnosed?

IBD is diagnosed by combining histologic evidence of inflammation with exclusion of other causes of GI inflammation. Baseline laboratory tests should include complete blood count (CBC), serum biochemical profile, FeLV antigen test, FIV antibody test, serum total T4 concentration (for cats at risk for hyperthyroidism), urinalysis, fecal parasite examination (zinc sulfate flotation and direct smear), fecal wet mount, *Cryptosporidium* spp. screening, rectal cytology, and survey abdominal radiographs (see Chapter 18). Fecal culture is indicated in cats with suspected bacterial enteritis (see Chapter 20).

9. What CBC abnormalities support the diagnosis of IBD?

The CBC may show increased eosinophils. However, parasitic diseases and hypoadrenocorticism also induce this abormormality. Microcytic anemia may develop if IBD is severe and results in iron deficiency due to chronic blood loss. Plasma protein concentration decreases if protein-losing enteropathy is present.

10. How do serum biochemical abnormalities aid in the diagnosis of IBD?

The primary benefit of serum biochemical testing is to exclude other causes of vomiting and diarrhea. Panhypoproteinemia is consistent with protein-losing enteropathy, which may occur with some forms of IBD. Some cats (25%) with lymphocytic-plasmacytic enteritis are reported to have mildly increased serum alanine transferase (ALT), aspartate transferase (AST), and alkaline phosphatase (ALP) activities. Liver function tests are usually normal; in some cats, however, histologic examination of the liver reveals periportal inflammatory infiltrates. Because the pancreatic and biliary ducts are shared in cats and empty into the duodenum, IBD may result in concurrent pancreatitis and cholangiohepatitis (see Chapters 29 and 36). This syndrome has been called "triaditis" and may explain serum biochemical evidence of hepatic and pancreatic involvement. Triaditis may be due to translocation of bacteria from the diseased GI tract into the portal circulation. Cobalamin, folate, and vitamin K levels may be decreased as a result of malabsorption.

11. What is the diagnostic benefit of imaging procedures?

Survey and contrast films of the abdomen have a low likelihood of showing abnormalities (masses or increased small intestinal diameter). Barium studies may show flocculation of barium contrast material, irregular mucosal-barium interface, delayed transit time, or persistent adherence of barium to mucosa. Ultrasound may show small intestinal abnormalities, including altered echogenicity, small intestinal wall thickening, or poor small intestinal wall definition. However, results of imaging procedures are not specific for IBD and are used primarily to exclude other causes of vomiting or diarrhea.

12. How should tissues be obtained for histologic evaluation?

Endoscopically obtained or full-thickness surgical biopsies may be used for histologic evaluation. Endoscopic mucosal biopsy is less invasive than surgery but provides small samples (usually 2.8 mm in diameter at most) that include mucosa only. Samples are easily obtained from the stomach, duodenum, rectum, and colon; the jejunum and ileum are less commonly sampled. Samples often have crush artifact, which makes histologic characterization difficult. Because only mucosa is obtained, deeper inflammation or neoplasia may be missed, and it is difficult to document the presence of lymphangectasia. It is important to obtain samples even if the mucosal surface appears normal. Multiple samples should be obtained from each site. In dogs, duodenal aspirates are performed to assess for *Giardia* spp. and bacterial overgrowth. In cats, however, *Giardia* spp. reside more distally in the small bowel, and normal cats have extremely variable numbers of bacteria in the duodenum. Thus the diagnostic benefit of these tests is limited. If gastritis is suspected, samples should be collected from the cardia and placed on a urea slant to assess for the presence of urease activity, which supports the diagnosis of helicobacteriosis (see Chapter 20).

If endoscopic biopsies are nondiagnostic in a cat with clinical signs of IBD and other causes of vomiting and diarrhea have been ruled out, surgical, full-thickness biopsies are warranted. Surgery has the additional benefit of allowing visualization and biopsy of the pancreas and liver in cats with suspected triaditis. Because endoscopically obtained biopsies are occasionally falsely negative, require specialized equipment, and limit testing to the mucosal surface, exploratory laparotomy may be the preferred procedure for clients with limited budgets.

13. In what forms does IBD occur?

IBD is classified by the area of the GI tract that is affected and the predominant type of inflammatory cell:

Lymphocytic-plasmacytic enterocolitis is the most common type of IBD diagnosed in cats. The lamina propria is infiltrated with lymphocytes and plasma cells. The disease may progress to diffuse intestinal lymphoma.

Eosinophilic enterocolitis and hypereosinophilic syndrome are rare forms of IBD characterized by diffuse or focal infiltration of mature eosinophils into one or more layers of the intestinal tract. Usually they are accompanied by peripheral eosinophilia. Although eosinophilic enterocolitis is confined to the GI tract, hypereosinophilic syndrome may involve the liver, spleen, lymph nodes, bone marrow, lung, pancreas, adrenal glands, or skin. Hypereosinophilic syndrome responds poorly to glucocorticoids, is considered a preneoplastic condition, and has a high mortality rate.

Regional granulomatous enterocolitis is less common. It is characterized by transmural granulomatous inflammation, usually of the ileum and colon, that causes stenosing, mass-like thickening of a region of bowel wall. Regional lymph nodes and adjacent mesentery also may be involved.

Other rare forms (all treated as lymphocytic-plasmacytic IBD) include neutrophilic (suppurative) colitis, granulomatous colitis, histiocytic colitis, necrotic colitis, and angiopathic colitis with vasculitis and ischemic ulcers.

14. How is IBD treated?

The basic concepts of treatment are to remove the antigenic source of inflammation and then suppress the cell-mediated inflammatory response in the GI tract. The goals are remission of clinical signs, control with dietary management, and use of metronidazole and/or prednisolone. Relapses often occur and require drug therapy. Severe and refractory IBD may require the use of potent immunosuppressive drugs. Some cats require indefinite drug administration for control.

15. Describe dietary management of IBD.

The diet should contain a single, highly digestible, novel protein (one that the cat has not eaten before) and reduced amounts of food additives. It also should be gluten-free; use rice or potato as a carbohydrate source. High-fat diets should be avoided. If colitis is present, consider high-fiber diets containing either insoluble (cellulose) or soluble (psyllium) fiber. When a homemade diet is used for initial treatment, many cats find baby rice cereal more palatable than cooked white rice. Some people advocate a "sacrificial protein" for the first 6 weeks of treatment, on the theory that the cat is more likely to develop dietary sensitivity during the time that the gut is inflamed. Protein hydrolysates have reduced molecular weights (< 10,000 daltons) that should decrease antigenicity.

Commercially Available Hypoallergenic Diets

Lamb	Venison
Hill's Prescription Diet D/D (canned)	Innovative Veterinary Diets (canned or dry)
Innovative Veterinary Diets (dry or canned)	Waltham Select Protein (canned)
Iams Eukanuba Response Formula (canned)	Duck
Rabbit	Innovative Veterinary Diets (dry)
Innovative Veterinary Diets (canned)	Hydrolyzed proteins
Nature's Recipe Rabbit (canned)	Hills Prescription Diet Z/D (dry)

Hill's Pet Nutrition, Topeka, KS; Innovative Veterinary Diet, Nature's Recipe Co., Newport, KY; Iams Company, Dayton, OH; Waltham USA, Vernon, CA.

16. What dietary supplements are commonly recommended?
Various nutritional deficiencies secondary to IBD require supplementation. In addition, some nutritional supplements may have anti-inflammatory effects or promote healing of the intestinal tract. Controlled studies of these supplements for treatment of feline IBD are lacking.
- Vitamin B12 (cobalamine) and folate concentrations are often reduced by malabsorption.
- Vitamin K deficiency due to malabsorption of fats may be severe enough to cause bleeding and abnormal hemostasis.
- N-acetyl glucosamine has shown promise in the treatment of inflammatory disorders, including IBD, colitis and Crohn's disease in people.
- Glutamine can be supplemented as an energy source for mucosal cells of the digestive tract.
- Vitamin C scavenges free radicals, enhances immune function, has anti-inflammatory properties, and may reduce stress.
- *Lactobacillus acidophilus* is a probiotic that may help to restore normal intestinal flora.
- Dimethylglycine modulates production of lymphocytes and antibodies. It is theorized to decrease the allergic response.
- Proanthocyanidin complex is a bioflavinoid that theoretically works with vitamin C to reduce inflammation, strengthen capillaries, scavenge free radicals, and improve immune function. Antiviral activity also has been proposed.
- Vitamin E, vitamin A, and selenium are antioxidants that may protect cells from free oxygen radical-induced damage.
- Zinc is thought to potentiate immune system response and enhance healing.

Dietary Supplements for Management of IBD

SUPPLEMENT	PROPOSED DOSE
Cobalamine	125–250 mg/wk SC or IM for 6–8 weeks
Dimethylglycine	50–250 mg/cat PO, indefinitely
Folate	0.5 mg/day PO for 1 month
Glutamine	250–5000 mg/cat PO, indefinitely
N-acetyl glucosamine	250–1500 mg/cat PO, indefinitely
Lactobacillus acidophilus	50–500 million microorganisms/cat PO, until stool returns to normal consistency
Proanthocyanidin complex	10–200 mg/cat PO, indefinitely
Selenium	15 µg/day PO, indefinitely
Vitamin A	1000–5000 IU/day PO as beta carotine, indefinitely
Vitamin C	250–300 mg/cat PO, indefinitely.
Vitamin E	200 IU/day PO as alpha tocopherol daily, indefinitely.
Zinc	7.5 mg/day PO, indefinitely

SC = subcutaneously, IM = intramuscularly, PO = orally.

17. What drugs are used to manage IBD?

DRUG	PROPOSED DOSE
Chlorambucil	2 mg PO every other day or 2 mg/ M²/day for 7 days; then 1 mg/M²/day for 7 days; then taper to lowest effective maintenance dose
Cyclophosphamide	50 mg/M² PO 4 times/wk; during remission, use chlorambucil
Cyclosporine	0.5–8.5 mg/kg PO every 12–24 hr, indefinitely
Methylprednisolone	10–20 mg/cat IM every 2 wk until controlled; then as needed
Metronidazole	10–20 mg/kg PO every 8–12 hr for 2–4 wk; then gradually taper off over 1–2 mo
Prednisolone	1–2 mg/kg PO every 12–24 hr for 2–4 wk; then reduce dose by half every 2 weeks until lowest effective maintenance dose is found.
Azathioprine	0.3 mg/kg PO every 48 hr, indefinitely.
Sulfasalazine	10–20 mg/kg PO every 24 hr for 7–10 days

PO = orally, IM = intramuscularly.

18. Describe the effects of metronidazole.

This antibiotic is one of the antiprotozoal drugs of choice for *Giardia* spp. in cats. Because it has an excellent anaerobic spectrum, it may aid in the treatment of secondary bacterial overgrowth. It is proposed to inhibit cell-mediated immunity and to alter neutrophil chemotaxis and thus may be an effective adjunct to glucocorticoids. Side effects include salivation (due to bad taste), anorexia, vomiting, central nervous system abnormalities (seizures), and neutropenia.

19. Discuss the role of glucocorticoids.

Prednisolone is used most frequently, but if the cat cannot or will not take oral medications, methylprednisolone can be used. Control seems to be more difficult with parenteral depository glucocorticoids. Transdermal dosing of prednisolone also may be helpful when oral drugs cannot be administered. Glucocorticoids should not be prescribed until the diagnosis of IBD is confirmed by histology. Common side effects include polyuria, polydipsia, polyphagia, skin disease, weight gain, and type 2 diabetes mellitus (see Chapter 54).

20. How does azathioprine work?

The mechanism of immunosuppression has not been determined, but it is thought to depend on several factors. Azathioprine antagonizes purine metabolism, resulting in inhibition of RNA, DNA synthesis, and mitosis. Incorporation into nucleic acids may cause chromosome breaks, and inhibition of coenzyme function may disrupt cellular metabolism. Azathioprine has a greater effect on cellular immunity and delayed hypersensitivity than on humoral antibody responses. It is thought to take at least 1–3 weeks to become fully effective, and clinical response may require 6 weeks. It is used most often in cases of IBD that cannot be controlled by diet modifications and glucocorticoids or in cats that glucocorticoids make ill. Side effects may include bone marrow suppression, pancreatitis, hepatic damage, and anorexia. CBC should be monitored once or twice weekly for 10–14 days after starting, then monthly.

21. What is the mechanism of action of sulfasalazine?

The mechanism of action is not known. It is thought that after colonic bacteria cleave sulfasalazine into sulfapyridine and 5-aminosalicylic acid (5-ASA), the antibacterial (sulfapyridine) and anti-inflammatory (5-ASA) activity modify the course of the disease. Levels of both drugs are higher in the colon when the compound is used than with separate administration. Dosing in cats may be difficult without compounding. Primary side effects include anorexia, vomiting, and anemia; in dogs sulfasalazine has induced keratoconjunctivitis sicca.

22. How do cyclophosphamide and chlorambucil work?

The metabolites of **cyclophosphamide** act as alkylating agents, interfering with DNA replication, RNA transcription and replication, and nucleic acid function. The phosphorylating activity of cyclophosphamide also enhances its cytotoxic properties. The mechanism of action for its immunosuppressive activity on T-cells and antibody production is unknown. The drug is associated with bone marrow suppression and hemorrhagic cystitis (rarely). It should not be used over the long term. If it is effective during the induction phase, the related drug chlorambucil should be used for chronic management.

The mechanism of action of **chlorambucil** is cross-linking with cellular DNA. It is cytotoxic and cell cycle-nonspecific. Side effects include myelosuppression, resulting in anemia, leukopenia, and thrombocytopenia. It can also result in anorexia, vomiting, and diarrhea. A complete blood count with platelets should be done weekly until the cat is stable, then every other week.

23. Describe the mechanism of action of cyclosporine.

The mechanism of action is impedance of calcium-dependent signal transduction in the cytosol of lymphocytes. Cyclosporine stimulates secretion of transforming growth factor beta, which inhibits interleukin 2-stimulated T-cell proliferation and generation of antigen-specific cytotoxic lymphocytes. The primary side effects in people and dogs include inappetence, GI irritation, and gingival hyperplasia. Blood levels should be measured 24–48 hours after starting therapy to ensure adequate levels and periodically during therapy. The goal is a 12-hour whole-blood trough level of 250–500 ng/ml. Gelatin capsules may be needed for administration because of the unpleasant taste.

24. What is the prognosis for cats with IBD?

The prognosis depends on the form of IBD. In general, although the condition cannot be cured, the prognosis for control is good.

BIBLIOGRAPHY

1. Davenport DJ, Remillard RL, Simpson KW, et al: Gastrointestinal and exocrine pancreatic disease. In Hand MS, Thatcher CD, Remillard RL, Roudebush P (eds): Small Animal Clinic Nutrition, 4th ed. Marceline, MO, Mark Morris Institute, 2000, pp 757–763.
2. Diehl KJ: Enteritis, lymphocytic-plasmacytic. In Tilley LP, Smith FWK (eds): The Five Minute Veterinary Consult, Canine and Feline. Baltimore, Williams & Wilkins, 1997, pp 554–555.
3. Dimski DS: Therapy of inflammatory bowel disease. In Kirk RW, Bonagura JD (eds): Current Veterinary Therapy XII—Small Animal Practice. Philadelphia, W.B. Saunders, 1995, pp 723–727.
4. Jergens AE: Inflammatory bowel disease. In August JR (ed): Consultations in Feline Internal Medicine, vol. 2. Philadelphia, W.B. Saunders, 1994, pp 75–81.
5. Jergens AE: Inflammatory bowel disease. Vet Clin North Am Small Animal Pract 29:501–521, 1999.
6. Kendall RV: Therapeutic nutrition for the cat, dog, and horse. In Schoen AM, Wynn SG (eds): Complementary and Alternative Veterinary Medicine: Principles and Practice. St. Louis, Mosby, 1998, pp 5, 61, 64, 121-122.
7. Leib MS, Matz ME: Diseases of the large intestine. In Ettinger SJ, Feldman EC (eds): Textbook of Veterinary Internal Medicine, 4th ed. Philadelphia, W.B. Saunders, 1995, pp 1241–1247.
8. Marks SL, Fascetti AJ: Nutritional management of diarrheal diseases. In Bonagura JD (ed): Current Veterinary Therapy XIII—Small Animal Practice. Philadelphia, W.B. Saunders, 2000, pp 654–655.
9. Meyer DJ, Twedt DC: Effect of extrahepatic disease on the liver. In Bonagura JD (ed): Current Veterinary Therapy XIII—Small Animal Practice. Philadelphia, W.B.Saunders, 2000, pp 668–671.
10. Plumb DC: Veterinary Drug Handbook, 3rd ed. Ames, IA, Iowa State University Press, 1999.
11. Sherding RG, Johnson SE: Diseases of the intestines. In Birchard SJ, Sherding RJ (eds): Saunders Manual of Small Animal Practice. Philadelphia, W.B. Saunders, 1994, pp 704–709.
12. Sherk M: IBD: A misleading misnomer (inflammatory digestive tract syndrome). In Proceedings of the 16th Annual ACVIM Forum, San Diego, CA, 1998, pp 537–539.
13. Williams DA: Cobalamin and folate in feline malabsorption. Proceedings of the 16th Annual ACVIM Forum, San Diego, CA, 1998, pp 534–536.

24. NEOPLASIA AND OTHER FORMS OF INTESTINAL OBSTRUCTION

Kim Selting, D.V.M.

1. List the possible clinical signs of intestinal neoplasia and/or obstruction (partial or complete) in cats.
- Vomiting
- Anorexia/inappetence
- Gagging/dysphagia (linear foreign body anchored in the mouth)
- Weight loss/cachexia
- Diarrhea
- Tenesmus (with lesion in colon or ileum)
- Hematochezia (colon or rectum); melena (small intestine)
- Lack of stool/constipation
- Dehydration
- Lethargy/malaise
- Ascites and/or carcinomatosis
- Central nervous system (CNS) signs and icterus
- Palpable abdominal mass (approximately 50% of cases)
- Rectal prolapse of ileocecal lymphoma mass

2. Which clinical findings are most common?
In most reports, vomiting, anorexia, and weight loss are by far the most common signs, although the order of their prevalence varies. Clinical signs do not necessarily correlate with the location of the tumor in the gastrointestinal (GI) tract with the exception of tenesmus and hematochezia, which occur with colonic or rectal disease. Palpating an abdominal mass is a consistent finding but depends on the practitioner's level of palpation skill. The rest of the clinical findings are less common. Duration of clinical signs before diagnosis can range from days to months. Many cases are treated for clinical signs conservatively before relapse and definitive diagnosis. CNS signs, icterus, and other polysystemic signs may occur in cats with feline infectious peritonitis (see Chapter 38).

3. What are the most common differential diagnoses for intestinal obstruction?
Intestinal neoplasia, foreign body, and intussusception are common causes of intestinal obstruction in cats. Lymphoma is the most common neoplasm. Despite repeated references in current texts to mast cell tumor as the second most common feline GI neoplasm, no current studies focus on this disease. Adenocarcinoma is the most common nonlymphatic/nonhematopoietic neoplasm. Intestinal obstruction due to adenocarcinoma results from an annular ring of tissue created by the solitary tumor. Lymphoma and mast cell tumors may be discrete or diffuse.

Uncommonly diagnosed GI tract tumors include lipoma, leiomyosarcoma, leiomyoma, globule leukocyte tumor, granulated round cell tumor, fibrosarcoma, carcinoid, osteosarcoma, ganglioneuroma, gastric extramedullary plasmacytoma, and granulated round cell tumor.

Intussusception most commonly occurs in the ileocecocolic region. Predisposing causes include parasites, foreign body, previous abdominal surgery, viral enteritis, and mural lesions. Many cases, however, are idiopathic.

Trichobezoar, volvulus, intestinal torsion, incarceration of bowel in a hernia, adhesions, stricture, intramural abscess, granuloma or hematoma, congenital malformations, and feline infectious peritonitis (FIP) are less common causes of GI obstruction. Trichobezoars may form in part because of a lack of interdigestive migrating myoelectric complexes in cats.

4. How does FIP cause obstructive disease?

Noneffusive FIP can create solitary mural intestinal inflammatory lesions. In one study, this presentation predominated in approximately 20% of cats with histopathologically documented FIP. Histologically, the intestine is markedly thickened; multifocal pyogranulomas extend through the wall with areas of necrosis and fibrosis. Presence of coronavirus was confirmed by immunohistochemical staining of the tissues (New York State Veterinary Diagnostic Laboratory, Ithaca, NY). In the 26 cats reported in the study, 76% of obstructions occurred in the colon or at the ileocecocolic junction. Ragdolls and Himalayans may have been overrepresented, but reported numbers are small. Half of the cats were < 1 year of age, 11 of 26 were 1–6 years old, and only 2 of 26 were 11 years old. Most cats died of the disease within 9 months. A few cats had effusions at surgery, but the fluid was not typical for effusive FIP (see Chapter 38).

5. What hematologic abnormalities may be seen in cats with intestinal obstruction?

Hematologic abnormalities are common but generally not specific for any one disease:

Complete blood cell count. Leukocytosis with or without left shift, monocytosis, and lymphopenia have been detected in some cats. Eosinophilia, basophilia, and thrombocytosis were detected in a cat with lymphoma. Anemia may result from chronic disease, GI blood loss (anemia may be microcytic because of iron deficiency in chronic cases), or bone marrow involvement (feline leukemia virus [FeLV]).

Serum biochemical panel. Panhypoproteinemia may result from GI blood loss. In some cats, hyperglobulinemia results from chronic inflammatory disease, FIP, or neoplasia. Hyperglycemia, increased activities of liver enzymes, and hypercholesterolemia may occur. Hypochloremic metabolic alkalosis may be seen with pyloric outflow tract obstruction.

Serology tests. FeLV serum antigen tests are usually negative with adenocarcinoma and occasionally positive with lymphoma. Positive coronavirus titers indicate only exposure to a coronavirus, not FIP (see Chapter 38).

Serum electrophoresis. Monoclonal gammopathy is most consistent with plasmacytoid neoplasia but is occasionally detected in cats with FIP.

6. What imaging studies may be helpful in evaluating intestinal obstruction?

Plain radiographs may reveal a mass effect, fluid-filled stomach, or intestinal obstructive pattern characterized by gas-filled loops of bowel. Thoracic radiographs rarely reveal metastasis, but findings consistent with aspiration pneumonia may be present.

Positive contrast radiographs are used to confirm partial or complete obstruction.

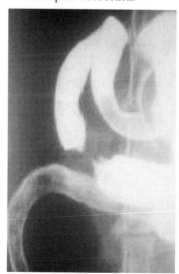

Barium series in a cat with adenocarcinoma of the small intestine. (Courtesy of Dr. David Twedt, Colorado State University.)

Ultrasound may be used to document masses localized to the GI tract, thickened bowel loops, enlarged mesenteric lymph nodes, abnormal peristalsis, and intussusceptions. In addition, tissue aspirates for cytology also can be guided by ultrasound.

Endoscopy/colonoscopy can be used to visualize mass lesions and to obtain biopsies, depending on the location of the abnormality. Biopsies should be done in all patients because diffuse, microscopic disease may be detected on histopathology. Adenocarcinoma may look like stricture or fibrous tissue rather than a mass lesion.

7. What other diagnostic techniques may be helpful?
- Exploratory laparotomy is used to confirm and relieve obstructive disease and to obtain tissue for definitive diagnosis.
- Cytology obtained before surgery or intraoperatively can help to make a definite diagnosis, especially of lymphoma. Aspiration cytology is unreliable for adenocarcinoma.
- Histology and immunohistochemistry are used to confirm the diagnosis of neoplasia and FIP.

8. How are intestinal obstructions treated?
For most intestinal obstructions, surgery is the mainstay of treatment. Some foreign bodies in the pyloric outflow tract can be removed via endoscopy, but disease in other regions requires surgery. If an intussusception is documented, it should be reduced if the intestine is viable and the primary disease treatable (e.g., foreign body). If the primary disease is neoplasia or the intestine is not viable, resection and anastomosis are indicated. Enteroplication should be considered because the recurrence rate for intussusceptions is as high as 27%. When adenocarcinoma is detected, surgery is the primary treatment (see question 14). When lymphosarcoma is detected, chemotherapy should be used as the primary treatment if possible (see question 18). Most trichobezoars are found in the proximal jejunum to distal ileum.

9. What preventive methods are used after surgical removal?
- Administration of emollient laxatives (use petroleum-based products, not mineral oil, to avoid lipid aspiration pneumonia)
- Attempts to prevent overgrooming (brush frequently, control fleas, and address behavioral problems)
- Shaving long hair
- Administration of prokinetic drugs (e.g., metoclopramide)

10. What are adenocarcinomas? How common are they?
Adenocarcinomas are malignant tumors of glandular epithelium that originate from the crypts of Lieberkuhn. They are the most common nonlymphoid neoplasia, accounting for 25–30% of all GI neoplasms. Osseous or chondroid metaplasia occurs in some cases. In one study, luminal stricture occurred in 12 of 44 cats.

11. Describe the typical signalment of cats with adenocarcinoma.
Adenocarcinomas occur most commonly in middle-aged cats (mean age = 8–11 years, range = 2–17 years). Siamese are overrepresented, accounting for 71% of cases (8 times the incidence in other breeds). The disease is more common in females than males.

12. Where are most adenocarcinomas located?
Adenocarcinomas may occur in either the small or large intestine. Up to 70% occur in the small intestine, especially the jejunum. The tumor is uncommon in the duodenum.

13. How does metastasis occur? What are the most common sites?
Adenocarcinomas spread via the lymphatic system. If metastasis occurs, the mesenteric nodes are the most common site (50%), followed by carcinomatosis (29%), lung, and liver.

14. What treatment is recommended for adenocarcinoma?

Surgical resection and anastomosis are the treatment of choice. In one study, administration of adriamycin (1 mg/kg intravenously every 3 weeks for 5–6 treatments) improved median survival time for colonic adenocarcinoma.

15. Describe the prognosis for cats with adenocarcinoma.

Prognosis varies among studies. A major limitation is the small number of reported cases. Notable findings of several studies include:

- In the study by Birchard, survival after surgery was 7 days (range = 1–13 day) vs. 3 days without surgery.
- In the study by Kosovsky, cats that lived for > 2 weeks after surgery had a mean survival time of 15 months.
- In the study by Cribb, the mean survival time after resection and anastamosis was 2.5 months with a range of 0–24 months.
- In the study by Turk, the mean survival time after surgery was 5 weeks; the median survival time was 20 weeks with a range of 2 days to 2 years.
- Kosovsky reported survival times of 4.5 and 28 months in two cats that survived surgery but with carcinomatosis.
- The presence of metastasis is prognostic. According to Cribb, the postoperative mean survival times for cats with and without metastasis were 5 months and 10 months, respectively.
- Histologic type may be prognostic as in humans. According to Cribb, the mean survival times for tubular, undifferentiated, and mucinous types were 11, 4, and 4 months, respectively.

16. What causes intestinal lymphosarcoma?

Most intestinal lymphosarcomas are of T-cell origin. Feline coronavirus-associated cell membrane antigen (FOCMA) may be causative after exposure to FeLV.

17. Describe the presentation of intestinal lymphosarcoma.

- The median age is 12 years (range = 3–18 years).
- Discrete and diffuse lymphosarcomas occur with equal frequency in the small intestine.
- Fewer cases occur in the large intestine.
- Affected cats can be either FeLV-positive or FeLV-negative.
- Approximately 13% of feline lymphosarcomas are exclusively in the GI tract.
- Approximately 40% of feline lymphosarcomas metastasize to extra-GI sites.
- Lymphoblastic lymphosarcoma (59%) is more likely than lymphocytic lymphosarcoma (24%) to present with an abdominal mass.

18. How are intestinal lymphosarcomas treated?

Recommended treatment is discussed in Chapter 68. Recently, the combination of prednisolone with chlorambucil was reported.

19. Discuss the prognosis for cats with lymphosarcoma.

- The most consistent prognostic factor is response to therapy. Duration of first remission also correlates directly with survival.
- A positive FeLV serologic test is a negative prognostic indicator in some studies.
- Anatomic location does not predict response rate or survival time.
- Survival ranges from 2–2000+ days. The mean survival time ranges from 50 days to 23 months. Survival time is probably prolonged in a subset of cats.
- Histologic grade may be prognostic. In one study, the complete remission rates and median survival times for lymphoblastic lymphosarcoma were 18% and 2.7 months, respectively; the corresponding values for lymphocytic lymphosarcoma were 69% and 22.8 months.

20. How does colonic neoplasia differ from neoplasia in other areas of the GI tract?

Colonic neoplasia accounts for 10–15% of GI neoplasms and <1% of all feline neoplasms. The mean age for diagnosis of colonic cancer is 12.5 years, and the median age is 13 years, which is comparable to neoplasia in other areas of the GI tract. Adenocarcinoma is most common, followed by lymphosarcoma and then by mast cell tumors. A few cases of neuroendocrine carcinoma have been reported. Treatment combines surgery and chemotherapy, as discussed for adenocarcinoma and lymphoma of the small intestine.

21. Summarize the prognosis for cats with colonic neoplasia.

PROGNOSTIC FACTOR	ADENOCARCINOMA	LYMPHOSARCOMA	MAST CELL TUMOR
Received chemotherapy	Doxorubicin with, MST = 280 days without, MST = 56 days	Not prognostic	All 4 cats in study treated with prednisone
Type of surgery Subtotal colectomy Mass resection Biopsy	MST = 138 days MST = 68 days MST = 10 days	Surgery not prognostic, but 1 cat lived 1355 days	All had surgery, but numbers too small for assessment
Metastasis	With: MST = 49 days Without: MST = 259 days	Not evaluated	Not evaluated MST = 199 days for 4 cats

MST = median survival time.

BIBLIOGRAPHY

1. Barrand KR, Scudmore CL: Intestinal leiomyosarcoma in a cat. J Small Anim Pract 40: 216–219, 1999.
2. Barrs VR, Beatty JA, Tisdall PLC, et al: Intestinal obstruction by trichobezoars in five cats. J Feline Med Surg 1:199–207, 1999.
3. Bedford PN: Partial intestinal obstruction due to colonic adenocarcinoma in a cat. Can Vet J 39:769–771, 1998.
4. Birchard SJ, Couto CG, Johnson S: Nonlymphoid intestinal neoplasia in 32 dogs and 14 cats. J Am Anim Hosp Assoc 22:533–537, 1986.
5. Cribb AE: Feline gastrointestinal adenocarcinoma: A review and retrospective study. Can Vet J 29:709–712, 1988.
6. Demetriou JL, Welsh EM: Rectal prolapse of an ileocecal neoplasm associated with intussusception in a cat. J Feline Med Surg 1:253–256, 1999.
7. Fondacaro JV, Richter KP, Carpenter JL, et al: Feline gastrointestinal lymphoma: 67 cases (1988–1996). Eur J Comp Gastroenterol 4:5–11, 1999.
8. Gabor LJ, Malik R, Canfield PJ: Clinical and anatomical features of lymphosarcoma in 118 cats. Aust Vet J 76:725–732, 1998.
9. Harvey CJ, Lopez GW, Hendrick MJ: An uncommon intestinal manifestation of feline infectious peritonitis: 26 cases (1986–1993). J Am Vet Med Assoc 209:1117–1120, 1996.
10. Kosovsky JE, Matthiesen DT, Patnaik AK: Small intestinal adenocarcinoma in cats: 32 cases (1978–1985). J Am Vet Med Assoc 192:233–235, 1988.
11. McEntee MF, Horton S, Blue J, et al: Granulated round cell tumor of cats. Vet Pathol 30:195–203, 1993.
12. Slawienski MJ, Mauldin GE, Mauldin GN, et al: Malignant colonic neoplasia in cats: 46 cases (1990–1996). J Am Vet Med Assoc 211:878–881, 1997.
13. Turk MAM, Gallina AM, Russell TS: Nonhematopoietic gastrointestinal neoplasia in cats: A retrospective study of 44 cases. Vet Pathol 18:614–620, 1981.
14. Thorn CE, Aubert I: Abdominal mass aspirate from a cat with eosinophilia and basophilia. Vet Clin Pathol 28:139–141, 1999.
15. Zikes CD, Spielman B, Shapiro W, et al: Gastric extramedullary plasmacytoma in a cat. J Vet Intern Med 12:381–383, 1998.

25. SECONDARY GASTROINTESTINAL DISEASES

Craig B. Webb, Ph.D., D.V.M.

1. Define secondary gastrointestinal disease.
Secondary gastrointestinal (GI) diseases are disorders that do not directly involve structures of the primary GI tract (oral cavity, esophagus, stomach, small and large intestines) but manifest, at least in part, with vomiting and diarrhea.

2. What are the secondary GI differentials for vomiting and diarrhea?
Inflammatory, infectious, metabolic, endocrine, and neurologic diseases of organs outside the gastrointestinal tract can result in vomiting or diarrhea.

Common Secondary Gastrointestinal Causes of Vomiting and Diarrhea

Inflammation	**Infection**
Pancreatitis	Viral
Cholangiohepatitis	Feline infectious peritonitis
Nephritis	Feline leukemia virus
Peritonitis	Feline immunodeficiency virus
Encephalitis	Bacterial
Steatitis	Pyelonephritis
Metabolic/endocrine disorders	Cystitis
Diabetic ketoacidosis	Pyometra
Hyperthyroidism	Cholangiohepatitis
Hypokalemia	Heartworm disease
Hypoadrenocorticism	**Neoplasia**
Uremia (renal failure)	Pancreatic
Urinary tract obstruction	Hepatic
Bile duct obstruction	Central nervous system
Congestive heart failure	**Neurologic disorders**
Exocrine pancreatic insufficiency	Vestibular disease
Drugs/toxins	Encephalitis
Antibiotics	Hydrocephalus
Chemotherapeutics	Trauma
Digoxin	Psychogenic
Ethylene glycol	
Heavy metals	
Plants	

3. What are the common inflammatory and infectious causes of secondary GI disease?
Hepatic or pancreatic neoplasia, pancreatitis, peritonitis, cholangiohepatitis, bile duct obstruction, steatitis, pyelonephritis, heartworm disease, pyometra, and septicemia.

4. What are the common metabolic and endocrine causes of secondary GI disease?
Hepatic lipidosis, lipemia, uremia, hypokalemia, hypercalcemia, urinary tract obstruction, hyperthyroidism, diabetic ketoacidosis, and hypoadrenocorticism.

5. What primary neurologic disorders are associated with secondary vomiting?
Vestibular disease, dysautonomia, central nervous system neoplasia, encephalitis, hydrocephalus, and psychogenic disorders.

6. Besides vomiting and/or diarrhea, what are the common presenting signs in cats with secondary GI disease?

Most of the historical and chief complaints for cats with secondary GI disease are nonspecific. Examples include thin body condition, anorexia, polyphagia (i.e., hyperthyroidism or diabetes mellitus), polyuria, polydipsia, weakness, lethargy, hyperactivity (i.e., hyperthyroidism), and weight loss.

7. What mechanisms cause vomiting in secondary GI diseases?

Vomiting from secondary GI diseases can be induced by afferent impulses to the emetic center, stimulation of the chemoreceptor trigger zone (CRTZ), and altered GI motility.

8. How do secondary GI diseases stimulate the emetic center?

The emetic center is located in the reticular formation in the lateral medullary region of the brain. Within the reticular formation, the nucleus of the solitary tract receives convergent input from the vagus nerve, area postrema, and vestibular and limbic systems. Sources of neural input to the emetic center include afferents from the GI tract, abdominal viscera, heart, vestibular system, CRTZ, and higher brain centers. Within the abdomen, the liver, pancreas, urinary tract, internal genitalia, and abdominal mesentery provide input to the brainstem emetic center. Afferent fibers from the abdomen travel to the emetic center in the medulla via the vagal and sympathetic nerve fibers.

9. What are other potential causes of vomiting in secondary GI diseases?

Fluid and electrolyte imbalances (i.e., hypokalemia, hyponatremia, hypercalcemia) and acidosis (i.e., renal failure, diabetic ketoacidosis) often occur with systemic diseases. These conditions may alter GI motility or stimulate the CRTZ. Endocrine disease also may produce metabolic abnormalities that stimulate the CRTZ. The CRTZ is on the floor of the fourth ventricle—specifically, the area postrema. The area postrema is located on the dorsal surface of the medulla oblongata, as part of the floor of the fourth ventricle, and lacks the usual blood-brain diffusion barrier. In this position, the CRTZ can monitor chemical levels in both blood and cerebrospinal fluid, making it susceptible to many stimuli.

10. What is the initial diagnostic plan for assessment of secondary causes of GI symptoms?

Complete blood cell count, serum biochemical panel, urinalysis, and plain abdominal radiographs are often used to assess for secondary causes of GI tract signs. Most renal, hepatic, pancreatic, and endocrine diseases produce abnormalities that are evident on these tests.

11. What pancreatic diseases result in secondary GI disease?

Vomiting, inappetence, weight loss, and, occasionally, diarrhea can result from pancreatitis (see Chapter 36). Small bowel diarrhea, polyphagia, and failure to thrive result from exocrine pancreatic insufficiency (EPI).

12. What chemistry panel abnormalities may suggest pancreatitis in cats?

Elevated activities of the liver enzymes (alkaline phosphatase [ALP], alanine aminotransferase [ALT]), elevated total bilirubin, and azotemia are common. Hypocalcemia and hypoproteinemia occur in some cats. Histologically confirmed cases of feline pancreatitis may have serum amylase and lipase activities that are above normal, normal, or below normal; therefore, these tests are not often helpful.

13. What other diagnostic procedures are used to diagnose pancreatitis?

In some cats with pancreatitis, radiographs reveal a decrease in serosal detail in the cranial abdomen, displacement of the pyloric antrum and duodenum, and dilated, gas-filled loops of intestine, especially the duodenum. Ultrasonographic findings of pancreatitis include hypoechoic pancreatic parenchyma, dilated pancreatic ducts, hyperechoic peripancreatic fat, and a mild peritoneal effusion. An assay for feline trypsin-like immunoreactivity (fTLI) has been developed and may prove to be a more specific marker of the disease. Several studies have found significantly elevated fTLI levels in cats with pancreatitis, although one recent report found a poor association between fTLI levels and pancreatic histopathology (see Chapter 36).

14. What is the most common cause of EPI in cats?
Chronic pancreatitis is the most common cause of exocrine pancreatic insufficiency in cats. Other causes include pancreatic fluke infestation, pancreatic adenocarcinoma, and possibly congenital conditions and idiopathic acinar atrophy.

15. Describe the most common presentation of EPI. How is it diagnosed?
As with dogs, the most common presenting complaints for cats with EPI are polyphagia, weight loss, diarrhea, and vomiting, with an oily, unkempt haircoat. Patients often produce large volumes of soft, pale, malodorous stool. Increased neutral fats may be found on Sudan staining of feces from cats with EPI, but a more sensitive test is the recently developed assay for fTLI. Significantly decreased fTLI levels are found in cats with EPI.

16. Which hepatic diseases most commonly result in secondary GI tract disease?
Hepatic lipidosis, cholangiohepatitis/cholangitis complex, feline infectious peritonitis, and hepatic neoplasia (see Chapters 29, 30, 31, and 38).

17. What is "triaditis"?
Triaditis refers to concurrent liver (hepatic lipidosis, cholangiohepatitis), pancreatic (pancreatitis), and intestinal disease (inflammatory bowel disease) in cats exhibiting symptoms of primary GI disease (see Chapter 29).

18. What is the anatomic explanation for concurrent cholangiohepatitis in cats with pancreatitis?
In cats, the common bile duct and main pancreatic duct conjoin before entering the duodenum at the major duodenal papilla. Acute suppurative cholangiohepatitis probably is caused by an ascending infection from the GI tract to the biliary tree through the bile duct. This ascension also may affect the pancreas.

19. Which endocrine diseases most commonly cause GI signs and symptoms?
Diabetic ketoacidosis, hyperthyroidism, and hypoadrenocorticism can induce vomiting or diarrhea.

20. What are the common historical complaints and physical examination findings?
The most common **historical sign** of hyperthyroidism is weight loss; other presenting complaints include polyphagia or anorexia, vomiting, hyperactivity, polyuria and polydipsia, diarrhea, and muscle weakness (see Chapter 53). **Physical examination findings** include a palpably enlarged thyroid gland, thin body condition, tachycardia, and cardiac murmur. Most cats are older.

21. What are the most common serum chemistry abnormalities in cats with hyperthyroidism?
Hyperthyroidism is the number-one cause of elevated liver enzyme activities (ALT, ALP, and aspartate aminotransferase) in cats. Most patients have increased total T4 concentrations. Less common biochemical abnormalities include elevated blood urea nitrogen, creatinine, blood glucose, and packed cell volume.

22. Why do hyperthyroid cats have diarrhea?
Approximately 45% of hyperthyroid cats have diarrhea. Although the exact cause is unknown, the most likely candidates are a thyroid hormone-induced increase in GI motility and a decrease in GI transit time. Increased enterocyte levels of cyclic adenosine monophosphate,

relative deficiency of trypsin secretion by the pancreas, intestinal mucosal edema, and polyphagia are also potential contributing factors.

23. What causes emesis in hyperthyroid cats?

There are several possible, but still unproven, causes of vomiting in cats with hyperthyroidism. Proposed mechanisms include gastric hypoacidity, hypergastrinemia, superficial gastritis, and esophageal dysfunction. Thyroid hormone may act directly on the CRTZ.

24. What historical, physical examination, or serum biochemistry panel findings may help to distinguish between cats with or without diabetic ketoacidosis (DKA)?

Anorexia or decreased appetite is more common in cases of DKA (see Chapter 56). Decreased activity, weakness, thin body condition, and vomiting are also more common in cats with DKA. Elevated liver enzymes, azotemia, and electrolyte abnormalities (hypokalemia, hyponatremia, and hypochloremia) are more frequent and more significant in cats with DKA.

25. What diseases most commonly accompany DKA?

Hyperthyroidism, inflammatory bowel disease, eosinophilic granuloma complex, urinary tract infection, and pancreatitis.

26. What historical, physical examination, and chemistry panel findings lead to inclusion of hypoadrenocorticism on a list of differentials for vomiting cats?

In addition to vomiting, owners may report lethargy, anorexia, weight loss, and polyuria (see Chapter 55). Physical examination may reveal dehydration, hypothermia, prolonged capillary refill time, weak pulses, and sinus bradycardia. Hyponatremia and hyperkalemia should be seen on a chemistry panel. The diagnosis can be confirmed with an adrenocorticotropic hormone stimulation test.

27. What are possible explanations for vomiting and diarrhea in cats with hypoadrenocorticism?

As in dogs, the cause of these symptoms remains unclear. Physiologic levels of cortisol act as a trophic factor for the gastrointestinal mucosa. Without that input, there is a decrease in mucosal blood flow. Gastric motility is also decreased in hypoadrenocorticism because of electrolyte imbalances and inhibition of gastric contractions by elevated levels of corticotropin-releasing factor (CRF).

28. What are the most common presenting clinical signs in cats with heartworm disease?

Vomiting is one of the most frequently reported presenting complaints in cats subsequently diagnosed with heartworm disease (see Chapter 10). Other common symptoms include coughing, dyspnea, lethargy, anorexia, and weight loss. Vomiting episodes may be intermittent and unpredictable (i.e., not necessarily related to food ingestion).

29. What causes emesis in cats with heartworm disease?

Although the mechanism is unknown, one possible pathway involves the release of inflammatory mediators from diseased lungs that interact with receptors in the CRTZ.

30. What other feline cardiac diseases may be associated with vomiting?

In cases of feline cardiomyopathy (restrictive, dilated, hypertrophic, or idiopathic), vomiting may proceed cardiopulmonary signs (e.g., dyspnea, cough, lethargy) by 1–3 days.

31. Which classes of drugs are currently used as antiemetics in feline veterinary medicine?

Antiemetics agents include alpha$_2$-adrenergic antagonists (e.g., chlorpromazine, prochlorperazine), D$_2$-dopaminergic antagonists (e.g., metoclopramide), histaminergic antagonists (e.g., meclizine, diphenhydramine), and 5-HT$_3$-receptor antagonists (e.g., ondansetron, metoclopramide).

32. Is antiemetic therapy for cats different from antiemetic therapy for dogs?

Lesions in the CRTZ of dogs can abolish vomiting in response to oral emetic agents in almost 80% of trials, whereas similar lesions in cats abolish emesis to the same agents in only 30% of trials. Various explanations are under investigation, including differences in neurotransmitter receptor type, location, and sensitivity.

33. What is the role of metoclopramide as an antiemetic in cats?

Metoclopramide, a D_2-dopamine receptor antagonist, is a highly effective, centrally acting antiemetic in dogs. Research suggests that D_2-dopamine receptors are much less important in centrally mediated emesis in cats; therefore, metoclopramide is significantly less effective as a central antiemetic agent. As a prokinetic, metoclopramide acts peripherally as a 5-HT_4 receptor agonist. However, the ability of metoclopramide to enhance gastric emptying of solids (compared to liquids) is questionable.

34. How effective are antihistamines for motion sickness in cats?

Although antihistamines are useful for the treatment of motion sickness in dogs, histamine receptors have not been demonstrated in the CRTZ of cats, making antihistamine therapy much less effective for motion sickness. Research suggests that 5-HT_{1A} receptor agonists (e.g., buspirone) suppress vomiting secondary to motion sickness in cats.

35. Ondansetron is one of the newest antiemetics in veterinary medicine. What is its mechanism of action? In what circumstance does it seem particularly effective?

Ondansetron, a 5-HT_3 receptor antagonist, appears to be particularly effective in the control of chemotherapy-induced emesis. As with other antiemetics, the receptor location and mode of action may be different for cats (central) and dogs (peripheral).

BIBLIOGRAPHY

1. Andrews PLR, Naylor RJ, Joss RA: Neuropharmacology of emesis and its relevance to anti-emetic therapy. Support Care Cancer 6:197–203, 1998
2. Atkins CE, DeFrancesco TC, Coats JR et al: Heartworm infection in cats: 50 cases (1985–1997). J Am Vet Med Assoc 217:355–358, 2000.
3. Broussard JD, Peterson ME, Fox PR: Changes in clinical and laboratory findings in cats with hyperthyroidism from 1983–1993. J Am Vet Med Assoc 206:302–305, 1995.
4. Crenshaw KL, Peterson ME: Pretreatment clinical and laboratory evaluation of cats with diabetes mellitus: 104 cases (1992–1994). J Am Vet Med Assoc 209:943–949, 1996.
5. Dillon R: Clinical significance of feline heartworm disease. Vet Clin North Am Small Animal Pract 28:1547–1565, 1998.
6. Guilford, WG, Center SA, Strombeck DR, et al (ed): Strombeck's Small Animal Gastroenterology, 3rd ed. Philadelphia, W.B. Saunders, 1996, pp 256–260.
7. Hall JA, Washabau RJ: Diagnosis and treatment of gastric motility disorders. Vet Clin North Am Small Anim Pract 29:377–395, 1999.
8. King GL: Animal models in the study of vomiting. Can J Physiol Pharmacol 68:260, 1990.
9. Miller AD: Central mechanisms of vomiting. Digest Dis Sci 44:39S–43S, 1999.
10. Peterson ME, Greco DS, Orth DN: Primary hypoadrenocorticism in ten cats. J Vet Intern Med 3:55–58, 1989.
11. Rosenthal FD, Jones C, Lewis SI: Thyrotoxic vomiting. BMJ 2:209–211, 1976.
12. Shaker EH, Zawie DA, Garvey MS, et al: Suppurative cholangiohepatitis in a cat. J Am Animal Hosp Assoc 27:148–150, 1991.
13. Sleisenger,MH (ed): Gastrointestinal Disease: Pathophysiology, Diagnosis, and Management. Philadelphia, W.B. Saunders, 1993, pp 509–523.
14. Steiner JM, Williams DA: Feline exocrine pancreatic disorders. Vet Clin North Am Small Anim Pract 29:551–575, 1999.
15. Steiner JM, Williams DA: Feline pancreatitis. Comp Cont Educ Pract Vet 19:590–601, 1997.
16. Swift NC, Marks SL, MacLachlan NJ, et al: Evaluation of serum feline trypsin-like immunoreactivity for the diagnosis of pancreatitis in cats. J Am Vet Med Assoc 217:37–42, 2000.
17. Washabau RJ, Elie MS: Antiemetic therapy. In Bonagura JD, Kirk RW (eds): Current Veterinary Therapy XII. Philadelphia, W.B. Saunders, 1995, pp 679–684.

26. REGURGITATION

Donald S. Westfall, D.V.M.

1. Define regurgitation, dysphagia, and vomiting.

Regurgitation is the passive expulsion of food or fluid from the oral cavity, pharyngeal cavity, or esophagus. **Dysphagia** is regurgitation of oral or pharyngeal origin. **Vomiting** is the forceful ejection of stomach and proximal duodenal contents through the mouth. Input into the vestibular system, vagal nerve, chemoreceptor trigger zone, or emetic center can induce vomiting. Localized diseases usually cause regurgitation of an esophageal origin, although many of these diseases have systemic consequences. Esophageal diseases are relatively rare in cats compared with dogs.

2. What pathophysiologic mechanisms can lead to esophageal regurgitation?

Regurgitation can be caused by local obstruction to the passage of esophageal contents, obstruction at the level of the lower esophageal sphincter, or decreased esophageal peristaltic activity.

Differential Diagnoses of Regurgitation in Cats

Obstructive causes–esophagus	Obstructive/structural causes
Foreign bodies	Hiatal hernia
Neoplasia	Gastroesophageal intussusception
Intraluminal	Gastric neoplasia
Squamous cell carcinoma	Pyloric stenosis
Sarcoma	
Extraluminal	**Decreased esophageal peristalsis**
Mediastinal lymphoma	Congenital idiopathic megaesophagus (Siamese cats)
Thymoma	Acquired idiopathic megaesophagus
Heart-based tumors	Acquired megaesophagus
Lung tumors	Esophagitis
Strictures	Chronic obstructive esophageal disease
Doxycycline-associated	Systemic neuromuscular disease
NSAID-associated (not reported	Feline dysautonomia (Key-Gaskell syndrome)
in cats to date)	Myasthenia gravis
Gastroesophageal reflux	Lead toxicity
Idiopathic	Polymyositis
Postanesthetic	Polymyopathies
Vascular ring anomaly	Polyneuropathies
Persistent right aortic arch (most common)	

NSAID = nonsteroidal anti-inflammatory drug.

3. What local esophageal obstructions lead to regurgitation?

Local esophageal obstruction can result from foreign bodies (bones, toys), intra- or extraluminal neoplasia (Fig. 1), esophageal strictures (Figs. 1 and 2), or vascular ring anomalies (persistent right aortic arch).

4. Describe the pathophysiology of esophageal stricture formation.

Benign esophageal strictures result from esophageal irritation and cause dysphagia and regurgitation. Specific causes include esophageal trauma secondary to foreign body ingestion, gastroesophageal reflux leading to esophagitis (idiopathic or postanesthetic), chronic vomiting, and substances that damage the esophageal mucosa. There have been numerous reports of

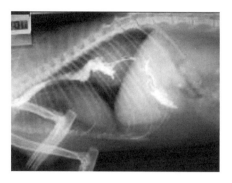

Figure 1. Lateral barium contrast radiograph from a cat with esophageal squamous cell carcinoma.

tablet-associated esophageal strictures in humans and cats. In humans, nonsteroidal anti-inflammatory drugs as well as other medications, including tetracycline antibiotics such as doxycycline, are most common.The Colorado State University Veterinary Teaching Hospital (CSU-VTH) has documented 7 cats with doxycycline tablet-induced esophageal strictures. The proposed mechanism is failure of adequate esophageal propagation of the tablet into the stomach, leading to esophageal retention, focal esophagitis, and subsequent esophageal stricture formation from the caustic nature of the antibiotic.

5. How do you prevent esophageal stricture formation during treatment with doxycycline?
   Cats do not successfully propagate tablets given routinely (dry) through the esophagus into the stomach, as documented by fluoroscopic evaluation of barium tablet administration. Typically, the tablets remain lodged in the esophagus for ≥ 180 seconds, which can lead to esophageal trauma and, possibly, esophageal stricture formation. Conversely, when cats are given tablets followed by 6 ml of water, tablets easily pass into the stomach within 30 seconds. Based on these results, CSU-VTH recommends that all cats be given 6 ml of water after tablet administration, particularly when prescribing doxycycline and NSAIDs.

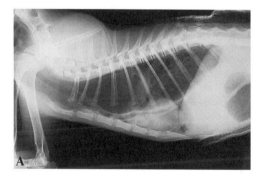

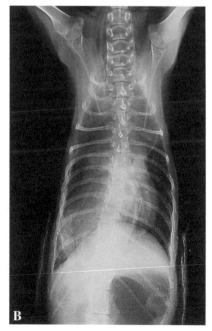

Figure 2. Lateral *(A)* and ventrodorsal *(B)* thoracic radiograph of a cat with suspected congenital mega-esophagus.

6. What structural abnormalities or obstructions at the level of the lower esophageal sphincter (LES) lead to regurgitation?

Diseases affecting the LES include hiatal hernias, gastroesophageal intussusception, gastric neoplasia, and pyloric stenosis. Hiatal hernias are protrusions of the distal esophagus or proximal stomach through the esophageal hiatus of the diaphragm into the thorax. Gastroesophageal intussusceptions are prolapses of the stomach into the lumen of the distal esophagus. Hiatal hernias and gastroesophageal intussusception are rare in the cat. Esophageal diverticula also are associated with regurgitation in cats.

7. What is the normal peristaltic activity of the feline esophagus?

The proximal two-thirds of the feline esophagus is composed of striated muscle; the lower third, which leads to the LES, is composed of smooth muscle. Innervation of both striated and smooth muscle and the LES is via the vagus nerve and its branches. Coordination of swallowing involves three stages: oropharyngeal, esophageal, and gastroesophageal. A bolus of food or liquid is formed in the oropharyngeal stage; this bolus is perpetuated through the upper esophageal sphincter. The esophageal stage transports the bolus through most of the esophagus via a primary peristaltic wave, which is initiated by swallowing. Additional primary peristaltic waves or secondary peristaltic waves transport any residual volume. The gastroesophageal stage involves transport of the bolus through the LES. Normally, mechanical, neural, and hormonal factors allow relaxation of the LES. LES pressure is maintained between boluses to prevent esophageal reflux.

8. What causes decreased esophageal peristaltic activity?

Primary idiopathic congenital megaesophagus can occur in cats, but is rare compared with dogs (see Fig. 1). Familial congenital megaesophagus and a gastric emptying disorder occur in Siamese cats. Acquired megaesophagus may be either idiopathic or secondary. Idiopathic acquired megaesophagus is diagnosed by excluding all other known causes of megaesophagus. Secondary causes include esophagitis, chronic obstructive lesions, and systemic neuromuscular diseases. Esophagitis of any cause (reflux esophagitis due to esophageal reflux through the LES, chemical injury, drugs, trauma, or foreign body ingestion) can lead to esophageal motility disorders. Any metabolic, endocrine, or systemic disease with neuromuscular manifestations can theoretically affect the esophagus. Examples include feline dysautonomia (Key-Gaskell syndrome), myasthenia gravis, lead toxicity, polymyositis, polymyopathies, and polyneuropathies. To the author's knowledge, megaesophagus associated with hypoadrenocorticism, systemic lupus erythematosus, and hypothyroidism has not been documented in cats.

9. How can signalment help to rank the differential list?

Signalment can give hints as to the underlying cause of regurgitation in many cases. For example, the incidence of esophageal neoplasia (squamous cell carcinoma) in younger cats is lower than in older cats. Mediastinal masses associated with lymphoma are more common in younger cats, wheras thymoma is more common in older cats. Younger cats may be more likely to ingest foreign bodies than older cats. Typically, regurgitation associated with a persistent right aortic arch manifests just after weaning.

10. How can the history help to rank the differential list?

Systemic illnesses leading to muscle weakness and regurgitation often are associated with concurrent medical problems. A history of doxycycline administration should alert the clinician to the possibility of tablet-associated esophageal stricture. Likewise, a history of esophageal trauma (such as foreign body ingestion) or postanesthetic esophageal reflux should result in a high index of suspicion for esophageal stricture. An acute onset of clinical signs is most consistent with foreign body ingestion; a more insidious course suggests other causes. Timing of the regurgitation after eating also helps to localize the cause of regurgitation. For example, regurgitation immediately after ingestion of food implies a problem in the proximal esophagus or oropharynx, whereas delayed regurgitation implies a problem in the distal esophagus. Regurgitation of both solids and liquids implies a more complete obstruction.

11. Outline a diagnostic plan to determine the cause of regurgitation.

If systemic illness is present, complete blood cell count, serum bichemical panel, and urinalysis should be performed to search for underlying systemic illness that may lead to muscle weakness and esophageal hypomotility. The most useful information often is obtained by performing barium contrast radiography (see Fig. 2). It is important to obtain a radiograph immediately after administering the contrast material to ensure a diagnostic study if the source of regurgitation is located proximally. You should use both solid (food mixed with barium) and liquid barium in performing a study to identify the source of regurgitation. Fluoroscopy can be used as an adjunct procedure to identify abnormalities in primary and secondary contractions. Manometry and esophageal scintigraphy also have been used to evaluate esophageal motility in cases of megaesophagus. If a localized problem is identified (such as a stricture), endoscopy can obtain more useful information, such as exact location, extent of disease, and pathogenesis of the disease process. For example, esophagitis due to esophageal reflux may be diagnosed by visualizing diffuse ulceration at the distal portion of the esophagus and by documenting a dilated LES. Barium contrast radiography, fluoroscopy, and endoscopy are also useful in diagnosis of hiatal hernias or gastroesophageal intussusceptions.

12. What treatment options are available for regurgitation?

The treatment of regurgitation depends largely on the underlying cause. Localized obstructions such as neoplasia, vascular ring anomalies, and esophageal strictures are best treated with local therapy. Extraluminal compression of the esophagus with mediastinal lymphoma is best treated with chemotherapy, whereas thymoma is a surgical disease. Intraluminal masses such as squamous cell carcinoma are best treated with surgery followed by chemotherapy. A persistent right aortic arch is best treated with surgery (thoracotomy or thoracoscopy). Esophageal strictures can be managed with endoscopy and balloon dilatation or bougienage. The author prefers balloon dilatation. Esophagitis is treated with sucralfate in a liquid suspension ($\frac{1}{4}$ gm crushed and mixed with 6 ml of water orally every 8 hours or 1.0–2.5 ml of 100 mg/ml commercially available suspension orally every 12hr), which acts as a diffusion barrier to promote mucosal ulcer healing and an antacid (H_2 blocker or proton pump inhibitor). The author prefers famotidine (0.5–1.0 mg/kg orally or intravenously every 24 hours) or omeprazole (0.7 mg/kg orally every 24 hours). Omeprazole is available only in a 20-mg sustained-release capsule. For administration to cats, mix the contents of the capsule in a strip of melted butter in foil and freeze. The appropriate dose is easily administered by sectioning the butter/omeprazole mixture. For example, a 5.7-kg cat should receive 4.0 mg of omeprazole, which is equivalent to one-fifth of the butter-mixed strip of medication. If the underlying cause is esophageal reflux, further therapy can be aimed at promoting LES tone and gastric emptying. Metoclopramide (0.2–0.4 mg/kg orally every 8 hours) or cisapride (0.1–0.5 mg/kg orally every 8 hours) is used most frequently. The author prefers cisapride, which is more potent than metoclopramide at the LES and is superior at promoting gastric emptying. Systemic diseases should be treated specifically.

BIBLIOGRAPHY

 1. Graham JP, Lipman AH, Newell SM, et al: Esophageal transit of capsules in clinically normal cats. Am J Vet Res 61:655–657, 2000.
 2. Hoenig M, Mahaffey MB, Parnell PG, et al: Megaesophagus in two cats. J Am Vet Med Assoc 196:763–765, 1990.
 3. Johnson JR: Diseases of the esophagus. In Scherding RG (ed): The Cat Diseases and Clinical Management, 2nd ed. New York, Churchill Livingstone, 1994, pp 1153–1179.
 4. Joseph RJ, Carrillo JM, Lennon VA: Myasthenia gravis in the cat. J Vet Int Med 2:75–79, 1988.
 5. Matz ME: Regurgitation: Diagnosis and management. In August JR (ed): Consultations in Feline Internal Medicine, 2nd ed. Philadelphia, W.B. Saunders, 1994, pp 65–73.
 6. Mears EA, Jenkins CC: Canine and feline megaesophagus. Comp Cont Educ Small Anim Pract 19:313–326, 1997.

7. Melendez LD, Twedt DC, Weyrauch EA, et al: Conservative therapy using balloon dilation for intramural, inflammatory esophageal strictures in dogs and cats: A retrospective study of 23 cases (1987–1997). Eur J Comp Gastroenterol 3:31–36, 1998.
8. Melendez LD, Twedt DC: Esophageal strictures secondary to doxycycline administration in 4 cats. Fel Pract 28:10–12, 2000.
9. Moses L, Harpster NK, Beck KA, et al: Esophageal motility dysfunction in cats: A study of 44 cases. J Am Anim Hosp Assoc 36:309–312, 2000.
10. Patterson CJ: Suspected cases of feline dysautonomia. Vet Rec 134:123, 1994.
11. Prymak C, Saunders HM, Washbau RJ: Hiatal hernia repair by restoration and stabilization of normal anatomy:An evaluation in four dogs and one cat. Vet Surg 18:386–391, 1989.
12. Symonds HW, Mc Williams P, Thompson H, et al: A cluster of cases of feline dysautonomia (Key-Gaskell syndrome) in a closed colony of cats. Vet Rec 136:353–355, 1995.
13. Weyrauch EA, Willard MD: Esophagitis and benign esophageal strictures. Comp Cont Educ Small Anim Pract 20:203–212, 1998.

27. CONSTIPATION, OBSTIPATION, AND MEGACOLON

Elyse M. Kent, D.V.M.

1. What differentiates constipation from obstipation?

Constipation is defined as the infrequent or difficult evacuation of feces. It may be acute or chronic and does not imply a permanent loss of function. **Obstipation** is intractable or refractory constipation that has failed to resolve after several courses of medical and dietary therapy. It implies a permanent loss of function.

2. Define dyschezia, tenesmus, and megacolon.

Dyschezia, a term applied to some cats with constipation, refers to difficult or painful evacuation of feces. Cats with constipation or obstipation may exhibit **tenesmus**, which is defined as painful or ineffective straining during defecation. Recurring episodes of either constipation or obstipation may culminate in **megacolon**, which is defined as chronic constipation with a marked increase in the diameter of the colon.

3. What are the two pathologic mechanisms by which megacolon can develop?

Megacolon can develop by hypertrophy or dilation. Hypertrophic megacolon results from obstructive lesions (e.g., malunion of pelvic fractures causing narrowing of the pelvic canal, foreign bodies, tumors) and may progress to dilated megacolon. If unchecked, dilated megacolon is the end-stage result of colonic dysfunction. Cats with idiopathic dilated megacolon have permanent loss of colonic function and frequently also have loss of colonic structure. Colonic dilation disrupts the coordinated motility patterns of the distal colon and rectum that allow fecal storage. Dilation also interferes with the large migrating contractions of the colon and rectum that lead to the defecation reflex.

4. What causes megacolon?

The list of differential diagnoses includes neuromuscular, pharmacologic, obstructive, dietary, environmental, metabolic-endocrine, behavioral, and idiopathic causes. Most cases are orthopedic, neurologic, or idiopathic in origin. More than 60% of the cases are idiopathic. Spinal cord or pelvic nerve injuries account for about 6% of cases. About 5% of all cases occur in Manx cats as a result of congenital sacral and caudal vertebral defects with malformations of the caudal spinal cord and cauda equina.

Causes of Constipation

Dietary: bones or foreign material mixed with feces

Environmental: decreased exercise, dirty litter box or change in type of litter, change of location or schedule, hospitalization, introduction of new pets

Traumatic: fractured pelvis or hip, dislocated hip, bite wound, or abscess in perineal area

Obstructive: anal stricture, rectal foreign body or tumor, pseudocoprostasis (hair pasted over anus), healed pelvic fracture causing a narrowed pelvic canal

Neuromuscular: spinal cord disease or congenital spinal anomaly (Manx cat), paraplegia, central nervous system dysfunction, dysautonomia, idiopathic megacolon (colonic smooth muscle dysfunction)

Metabolic-endocrine: hypokalemia, dehydration, generalized debility, muscle weakness secondary to another disease

Pharmacologic: antihistamines, anticholinergics, diurectics, barium sulfate

---

5. **What anatomic or physiologic alterations cause colonic dysfunction in cats with idiopathic megacolon?**

Colonic smooth muscle function appears to be impaired in cats with idiopathic megacolon. In one study, megacolonic smooth muscle developed less isometric stress compared with healthy controls in response to neurotransmitters (acetylcholine, substance P, and cholecystokinin), membrane depolarization (potassium chloride), and electrical field stimulation. These changes were observed in both longitudinal and circular smooth muscle in the proximal and distal colon. Megacolon probably results from a disturbance in the activation of smooth muscle myofilaments. Smooth muscle cells and myenteric neurons appear histologically normal.

6. **What are the clinical findings of megacolon?**

Cats with megacolon typically present with a history of fecal obstruction and show signs including dyschezia, depression, anorexia, and vomiting. A small amount of liquid feces (possibly containing mucus or blood) may ooze around a central colonic or rectal fecal mass. Abdominal palpation reveals a large amount of abnormally firm feces in an enlarged colon. Other signs suggestive of spinal cord or pelvic injury may be present, including decreased tone and sensation of the tail, decreased or absent anal tone, atonic bladder with urinary incontinence, and paraparesis or paraplegia.

7. **Describe the minimal diagnostic plan for cats with obstipation or suspected megacolon.**

1. Complete blood count, serum biochemical panel, and urinalysis should be evaluated. Although changes in laboratory parameters are unlikely to be found, dehydration and hypokalemia may be observed occasionally.

2. Digital rectal palpation should be performed, preferably in an anesthetized cat.

3. Abdominal radiographs should be made in all recurrent cases (Fig. 1). Possible predisposing factors such as radiopaque foreign material, intra- or extraluminal colonic masses, pelvic fractures, and spinal canal abnormalities may be seen on radiographs. However, radiographic features cannot differentiate between constipation, obstipation, and idiopathic megacolon in some cases.

8. **What additional studies may be ordered?**

1. Abdominal ultrasound, proctoscopy, and colonoscopy are used to define mass lesions, inflammatory lesions, strictures, or diverticula in greater detail.

2. Barium enemas are helpful in delineating masses, strictures, or tumors if colonoscopy is not available.

3. Cerebrospinal fluid taps, myelograms, computed tomography, or magnetic resonance imaging should be considered (when financially practical) if the cat has neurologic signs.

4. If masses or lymphadenopathy is suspected, fine-needle aspiration with cytology and abdominal radiographs are recommended. Colonic impaction may be confused with gastrointestinal lymphoma. Masses or enlarged mesenteric lymph nodes are often difficult to differentiate

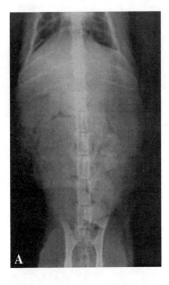

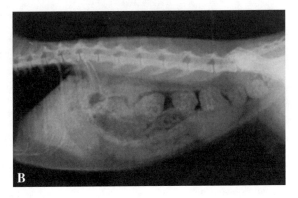

Figure 1.   Abdominal radiographs of a cat with constipation. *A,* Ventrodorsal view. *B,* Lateral view.

from impacted feces by palpation of the abdomen alone. Megacolon is identified radiographically by extreme dilation of the colon on survey radiographs (Fig. 2). Obstructive lesions causing secondary megacolon (e.g., tumors, strictures, or old pelvic fractures) may be visible on survey abdominal radiographs after multiple enemas, anesthesia, and manual removal of the fecal mass.

9. How should the first episode of constipation be managed?

A solitary episode of constipation may resolve spontaneously. However, most practitioners administer an enema to provide immediate relief of discomfort. Warm water enemas are most often used, but dilute diocytl sodium succinate (DSS; 10% in warm water) is also effective as an emollient enema. Several other types of enema solutions are commonly used, such as mineral oil,

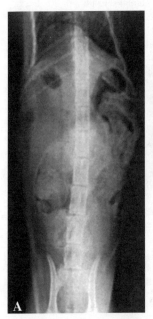

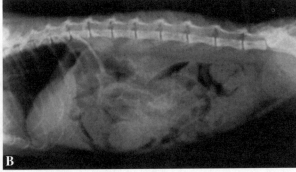

Figure 2.   Abdominal radiographs of a cat with idiopathic megacolon. *A,* Ventrodorsal view. *B,* Lateral view

mild soap (without hexachlorophene, which is potentially neurotoxic), warm isotonic saline, or lactulose. The volume of DSS, mineral oil, or lactulose in an enema solution should not exceed 5–10 ml/cat. It is safest to use a well-lubricated, 10–12-French soft red rubber catheter or feeding tube attached to a 60-ml syringe to administer an enema. The soft tube can be "threaded" inward gently to reduce mucosal trauma. Do *not* mix DSS and mineral oil in an enema solution because DSS increases mucosal absorption of mineral oil. A single episode of constipation does not warrant management at home other than observation of defecation by the owner in an effort to detect any signs of recurrent constipation. Sodium phosphate enemas (prepackaged enemas for humans) are contraindicated in cats because they induce hypernatremia, hyperphosphatemia, and hypocalcemia that may be life-threatening.

10. What therapy is used for recurrent episodes of constipation or idiopathic megacolon?
    1. Mild-to-moderate fecal impaction that recurs requires initial relief of the impaction by enemas and manual evacuation in the hospital. The dangers of having clients administer enemas to cats at home include the possibility of perforation of the rectum or colon (too much intraluminal pressure) and owner injury due to poor restraint techniques.
    2. Take steps to improve both fecal hydration and bulk at home. Advise owners to increase fiber content in the cat's diet through fiber-enriched food or fiber supplements (cellulose, methylcellulose, psyllium, bran, pumpkin). Fiber helps to prevent constipation by increasing fecal water content, decreasing intestinal transit time, and increasing the frequency of defecation. All cats must be well hydrated before initiating fiber supplementation to maximize therapeutic effects and prevent exacerbation of impaction by mixing of dry fiber with dry feces. Premeasured doses of powdered psyllium are available in capsule form and as chewable treats (tablets). Bran can be added to food but is not palatable to most cats. Canned pumpkin is somewhat palatable when added to food.
    3. Periodic enemas may be administered intermittently if a cat shows signs of impaction or if no bowel movements are observed over several days.
    4. Various types of laxatives are recommended, and each should be used singly or in combination to effect in a given patient.
    5. Colonic prokinetic drugs or motility agents (ranitidine, cisapride, nizatidine) help to stimulate colonic propulsive motility, some via stimulation of colonic smooth muscle.

11. Describe the various types of laxatives and their indications.
    Emollient laxatives (e.g., DSS), lubricant laxatives (e.g., mineral oil or petrolatum), stimulant laxatives (e.g., bisacodyl), saline laxatives (e.g., magnesium citrate), and hyperosmotic laxatives (lactulose) are effective in some patients. Bisacodyl is classified as a stimulant laxative and tends to work well in most cats. It is available over the counter and produces its effect by stimulating colonic smooth muscle and the myenteric plexus to cause peristaltic contractions. Bisacodyl is often the laxative of choice, combined with fiber, for control of mild-to-moderate constipation. Hyperosmotic laxatives (e.g., lactulose) are effective alone in some cats or in combination with increased fiber and possibly additional laxatives. Osmotic and emollient laxatives are irritating to colonic mucosa and should not be used before endoscopic procedures. Mineral oil and flavored petrolatum are helpful only in the mildest cases of constipation. Chronic use of lubricant laxatives may lead to malabsorption of fat-soluble vitamins. Mineral oil must be administered orally with caution because it can cause "lipid-aspiration pneumonia" if it is aspirated.

12. What prokinetic drugs are available?
    Oral cisapride has been the author's choice for the past several years but currently is not available because of toxicity in humans. Ranitidine and nizatidine (H_2 receptor antagonists) stimulate motility by increasing the amount of acetylcholine available to bind smooth muscle muscarinic cholinergic receptors. Erythromycin stimulates colonic motility in dogs but has no such effect in cats. The prokinetic effect of metoclopramide is seen only in the proximal gastrointestinal tract, not in the colon.

13. Summarize the medical therapy for feline constipation and obstipation.

DRUG CLASSIFICATION AND EXAMPLE	DOSE
Enemas	
Warm tap water	5–10 ml/kg
Warm isotonic saline	5–10 ml/kg
Dioctyl sodium sulfosuccinate	5–10 ml/cat
Dioctyl sodium sulfosuccinate	250 mg (12 ml) given per rectum as needed (prepackaged)
Mineral oil	5–10 ml/cat
Lactulose	5–10 ml/cat
Oral laxatives	
Bulk laxatives	
Psyllium	1–4 tsp mixed with food every 12–24 hr
Canned pumpkin	1–4 tbsp mixed with food every 24 hr
Coarse wheat bran	1–2 tbsp mixed with food every 24 hr
Emollient laxatives	
Dioctyl sodium sulfosuccinate	50 mg/cat orally every 24 hr
Dioctyl calcium sulfosuccinate	50 mg/cat orally every 12–24 hr as needed
Lubricant laxatives	
Mineral oil	10–25 ml/cat orally every 24 hr
Petrolatum	1–5 ml/cat orally every 24 hr
Hyperosmotic laxative	
Lactulose	0.5 ml/kg orally every 8–12 hr as needed
Stimulant laxative	
Bisacodyl	5 mg/cat orally every 24 hr
Prokinetic agents	
Ranitidine	1.0–2.0 mg/kg orally every 8–12 hr
Nizatidine	2.5–5.0 mg/kg orally every 24 hr

Modified from Washabau RJ, Hasler AH: Constipation, obstipation, and megacolon. In August JR (ed): Consultations in Feline Internal Medicine, vol. 3. Philadelphia, W.B. Saunders, 1996, pp 104–111, with permission.

14. How should severe, protracted cases of fecal impaction be managed?

Most cats with severe, protracted fecal impaction need to be hospitalized to correct fluid and electrolyte abnormalities and to allow sufficient time for repeated enemas and multiple manual evacuations of feces. Fecal concretions can be removed digitally with a well-lubricated, gloved, hooked index finger or with sponge forceps. General anesthesia is required for manual evacuation in most cases. Rapid administration of an enema may induce vomiting, even in an anesthetized cat. To prevent aspiration of vomitus, place the head in a "nose-down" position and intubate the cat with an inflated cuff on the endotracheal tube. Sometimes it is helpful to instill 40–60 ml of warm water or dilute DSS (10% solution) and subsequently "knead" the hard feces through the abdominal wall and then "milk" the softened feces toward the rectum and anus before attempting to grasp or pull out the feces. Be as gentle as possible while breaking down and removing fecal concretions. Some colonic and rectal mucosal bleeding is common during this procedure. In the most severely impacted patients, alternating enemas and manual fecal evacuation are best performed over 1–3 days.

15. Describe the home medical management of severe cases of fecal impaction.
- Fiber (preferably in diet)
- Hyperosmotic (lactulose) or stimulant laxative (bisacodyl)
- Prokinetic agent (ranitidine or others)
- Close monitoring for frequency and consistency of bowel movements

Evaluate the status of the cat and palpate for fecal concretions twice monthly at the start of the medical management program to assess success or failure of therapy.

16. Summarize the approach to management of constipation in cats.

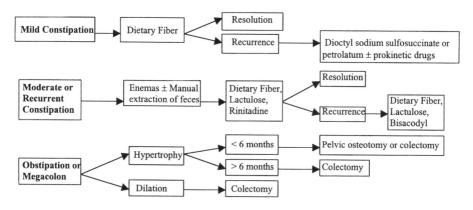

Figure 3.   Therapeutic approach to constipated cats. (Adapted from Washabau RJ, Hasler AH: Constipation, obstipation, and megacolon. In August JR (ed): Consultations in Feline Internal Medicine, vol. 3. Philadelphia, W.B. Saunders, 1996, pp 104–111, with permission.)

17. When should a colectomy be recommended?

Colectomy should be considered in any cat suffering from obstipation or idiopathic megacolon that is unresponsive to medical therapy. The objective of the surgery is to remove all of the colon, except for a short distal segment necessary to reestablish intestinal continuity (Fig. 4). Preservation of the ileocolic valve is controversial because the valve minimizes access of colonic bacteria to the small intestine. Removal of the ileocolic valve may lead to bacterial overgrowth in the small intestine along with steatorrhea and deconjugation of bile salts.

After surgery, most cats initially exhibit tenesmus and have dark, tarry stools. The diarrhea gradually changes to soft, formed stool over 6–8 weeks. Occasionally, cats produce semiformed feces permanently. Studies have indicated that enteric function is similar in normal cats and cats that have had a colectomy. The most common complication of colectomy is constipation. Usually, the constipation can be easily managed by a high-fiber diet, laxatives, and DSS.

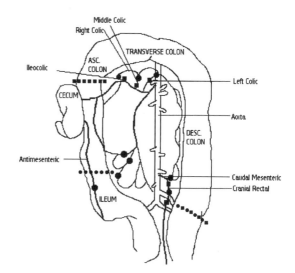

Figure 4.   Partial colectomy. Vascular ligations and level of resection with (1) preservation of the ileocolic valve, or colocolostomy *(squares)* and (2) removal of the ileocolic valve and part of the ileum, or ileocolostomy *(circles).*

18. What is the prognosis for cats with chronic constipation or megacolon?
The prognosis is guarded for cats receiving medical treatment alone. Therapeutic success or failure depends on the severity and stage of disease at first presentation and client compliance in persisting with ongoing therapy at home. The prognosis for patients treated with subtotal colectomy is good. As soon as it is evident that colonic dysfunction is irreversible, colectomy is the treatment of choice. Owners perceive the long-term results of colectomy as good to excellent. Most clients say that the cat's personality improves postoperatively and that behavior returns to what it was before the onset of constipation.

BIBLIOGRAPHY

1. Burrows CF: Constipation and megacolon. In August JR (ed): Consultations in Feline Internal Medicine, vol 2. Philadelphia, W.B. Saunders, 1994, pp 445–449.
2. Gregory CR, Guilford WG, Berry CR, et al: Enteric function in cats after subtotal colectomy for treatment of megacolon. Vet Surg 19:216–220, 1990.
3. Hilsenroth R: Medical therapy for diseases of gastronintestinal motility in cats. Feline Pract 27:24, 1999.
4. Holt D, Johnston DE: Idiopathic megacolon in cats. Compend Cont Educ Pract Vet 13:1411–1416, 1991.
5. Rosin E: Megacolon in cats—the role of colectomy. Vet Clin North Am Small Anim Pract 23:587–593, 1993.
6. Washabau RJ, Hall JA: Diagnosis and management of gastrointestinal motility disorders in dogs and cats. Compend Cont Educ Pract Vet 19:730–734, 1997.
7. Washabau RJ, Hasler AH: Constipation, obstipation, and megacolon. In August JR (ed): Consultations in Feline Internal Medicine, vol. 3. Philadelphia, W.B. Saunders, 1996, pp 104–111.
8. Washabau RJ, Stalis IH: Alterations in colonic smooth muscle function in cats with megacolon. Am J Vet Res 57:580–587, 1996.
9. Washabau RJ, Holt D: Pathogenesis, diagnosis and therapy of feline idiopathic megacolon. Vet Clin North Am Small Anim Pract 29:589–601, 1999.
10. Washabau RJ, Holt D: Feline constipation and idiopathic megacolon. In Bonagura JD (ed): Kirk's Current Veterinary Therapy XIII, Small Animal Practice. Philadelphia, W.B. Saunders, 2000, pp 648–652.
11. Zoran DL: Diet and drugs: The keys to managing feline colonic disease. Compend Cont Educ Pract Vet 21:744–747, 1999.

28. HYPERBILIRUBINEMIA AND ICTERUS: INITIAL DIAGNOSTIC APPROACH

Michael R. Lappin, D.V.M., Ph.D.

1. Define hyperbilirubinemia and icterus.
Hyperbilirubinemia is defined as serum total bilirubin concentrations greater than the normal range. When hyperbilirubinemia is severe enough, a characteristic yellowing of tissues known as **icterus** can be detected on physical examination. Icterus generally is detected when serum bilirubin concentrations are > 2 mg/dl and is most evident on the sclera and mucous membranes. After serum bilirubin concentrations normalize, it may take days for icterus to resolve.

2. What causes hyperbilirubinemia?
Hyperbilirubinemia can be grouped into prehepatic, hepatic, and posthepatic causes. Hemolysis of red blood cells is the cause of prehepatic hyperbilirubinemia (see Chapter 72). Multiple primary hepatic diseases result in hyperbilirubinemia. In approximately 90% of cases, one of the following is found to be the cause; hepatic lipidosis, cholangiohepatitis/cholangitis syndrome, feline infectious peritonitis virus, or feline leukemia-associated hepatic lymphoma. Posthepatic hyperbilirubinemia can result from intrahepatic cholestasis or extrahepatic bile duct

obstruction. Extrahepatic bile duct obstruction generally results from biliary tract neoplasia, pancreatitis, or duodenal disease.

Primary Differential Diagnoses for Hyperbilirubinemia and Icterus

Prehepatic
  Haemobartonella felis
  FeLV-associated immune-mediated hemolytic anemia
  Cytauxzoon felis
  Vaccine-induced, drug-induced, or idiopathic immune-mediated hemolytic anemia

Hepatic
  Bacterial cholangiohepatitis (suppurative)
  Immune-mediated cholangiohepatitis (nonsuppurative)
  Hepatic lipidosis (idiopathic or associated with diabetes mellitus)
  FeLV-associated lymphosarcoma
  Feline infectious peritonitis
  Toxoplasma gondii
  Hepatic abscessation
  Hepatotoxins (acetaminophen)
  Epithelial neoplasia
  Hyperthyroidism

Posthepatic
  Bile duct neoplasia
  Pancreatitis
  Duodenal disease
  Cholelithiasis
  Platynosomum concinnum (liver fluke, Florida and Hawaii)

FeLV = feline leukemia virus.

3. How can the signalment help to rank the differential list?
Young cats are more likely to have congenital liver diseases such as portosystemic shunts; old cats are more likely to have hepatic neoplasia. Effusive feline infectious peritonitis (FIP) is more common in young cats than old cats. Hyperthyroidism is more common in older cats.

4. How can the history help to rank the differential list?
Cats with toxoplasmosis have a history of hunting, particularly mice. Cats with haemobartonellosis often have a history of exposure to *Ctenocephalides* spp. or other cats. Cats with cytauxzoonosis come from the southern states and may have a history of *Dermacentor* tick infestation. Cats with pancreatitis often have vomiting, weight loss, and an intermittent, vague history. Cats with FIP generally have polysystemic disease. Cats with idiopathic lipidosis are often previously obese and have had recent stressful events in their lives.

5. How can the physical examination help to rank the differential list?
Most cats with prehepatic disease have pale mucus membranes and elevated heart and respiratory rates. Hepatic neoplasia generally results in hepatomegaly. In addition, cats with acute hepatic or posthepatic diseases often have hepatomegaly. The liver may become smaller with chronicity if inflammation leads to fibrosis and cirrhosis. Cats with FIP or toxoplasmosis may have conconcurrent uveitis. Fever is detected in many cats with bacterial hepatic diseases, FIP, toxoplasmosis, haemobartonellosis, and pancreatitis. Splenomegaly is commonly palpated in cats with icterus due to lymphoma, mastocytosis, and haemobartonellosis.

6. Describe the initial diagnostic plan for most cats with icterus.
Packed cell volume is assessed immediately to determine whether prehepatic icterus is likely. Complete blood count, serum biochemical panel, urinalysis, feline leukemia virus antigen

test, feline immunodeficiency virus antibody test, and total T4 concentration (cats > 5 years old) are indicated for the initial assessment of icteric cats. Fecal flotation or sedimentation should be included in areas endemic for liver flukes. Urinalysis is important; normal cats do not have bilirubinuria. Hemolysis of red blood cells due to traumatic collection may cause false increases in bilirubin concentrations on many blood chemistry machines. If serum bilirubin is elevated but urine bilirubin is negative, the serum result is probably a laboratory error.

7. How do patterns of hepatic enzyme activities aid in the ranking of differential diagnoses?

Differences in hepatic enzyme activities have some predictive value. In general, cats with lipidosis generally have greater activities of alkaline phosphatase (ALP) than alanine aminotransferase (ALT), whereas cats with the cholangiohepatitis/cholangitis complex generally have greater activities of ALT (see Chapter 29). Cats with lipidosis generally have increased ALP activity but normal gamma-glutamyl transferase (GGT) activity (see Chapter 30).

8. Can routine biochemical testing document posthepatic diseases?

No serum biochemical test can document posthepatic disease. However, if the magnitude of the hyperbilirubinemia is great (> 10 mg/dl) but clinical signs are minimal, posthepatic disease is likely. If bilirubin but not urobilinogen is present in urine, posthepatic disease is likely. The serum total T4 concentration is usually elevated in cats with hyperthyroidism.

9. Is measurement of serum bile acids indicated in cats with hyperbilirubinemia or icterus?

Measurement of pre- and postprandial bile acids is indicated only in the evaluation of cats with suspected hepatic disease that have normal serum bilirubin concentrations.

10. How do imaging techniques aid in the ranking of differential diagnoses?

Abdominal radiographs can be used to confirm hepatic size, to distinguish between diffuse or focal disease, to assess peritoneal effusions, and to assess evidence of pancreatitis. Hepatic and pancreatic ultrasound exams are beneficial for evaluating parenchymal tissues and assessing peritoneal fluid, bile duct obstruction, and gallbladder abnormalities. If peritoneal effusion is present, abdominal pericentesis is indicated. Ultrasound also can be used to guide aspirates or biopsies of hepatic tissues.

11. When are hepatic aspirates or biopsies indicated? What techniques should be used?

Hepatic aspirates or biopsies can be obtained percutaneously on the basis of landmarks or palpation or with ultrasound guidance, by laparoscopy, or by exploratory laparotomy. If the liver is enlarged, percutaneous biopsy by palpation or ultrasound guidance is generally easy. If the liver is small, laparoscopy or laparotomy is a safer technique. Laparotomy should be performed if extrahepatic bile duct obstruction caused by something other than pancreatitis is suspected. Activated clotting time (ACT) and platelet estimate should be performed in all hyperbilirubinemic cats before hepatic aspiration or biopsy.

Icteric cats with cholestatic liver disease develop vitamin K absence and subsequently decreased concentrations of active factors II, VII, IX, and X. If the ACT is prolonged, administer vitamin K_1 (1 mg/kg subcutaneously) and recheck in 12 hours. Cats with coagulation problems due to decreased factor production from hepatic insufficiency do not respond to vitamin K treatment. Hepatic aspiration can lead to a definitive diagnosis of hepatic lymphoma and mastocytosis and a presumptive diagnosis of hepatic lipidosis. Hepatic biopsy is the optimal procedure for all other hepatic diseases. Biopsies for histopathologic evaluation, aerobic culture, anaerobic culture, and antimicrobial susceptibility should be performed. If the bile or gallbladder wall appears thickened on ultrasonic evaluation, bile should be aspirated for culture.

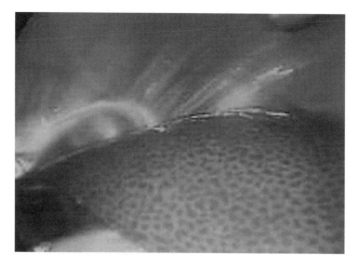

Laparoscopic appearance of lymphocytic-plasmacytic hepatitis in a cat.

12. Describe the initial treatment plan for icteric cats.

Intravenous fluids as supportive care are indicated in most cats, particularly if dehydration is occurring. The primary disease should then be treated.

BIBLIOGRAPHY

1. Bunch SE: Clinical manifestations of hepatobiliary disease. In Nelson RW, Couto GC (eds): Small Animal Internal Medicine, 2nd ed. Philadelphia, Mosby, 1998, pp 476–486.
2. Weiss DJ, Armstrong PJ, Gagne JM: Feline cholangiohepatitis. In Bonagura JD (ed): Current Veterinary Therapy. Philadelphia, W.B. Saunders, 2000, pp 672–674.

29. CHOLANGITIS/CHOLANGIOHEPATITIS COMPLEX

Margie Scherk, D.V.M.

1. Define cholangitis and cholangiohepatitis.

Cholangitis is inflammation of the biliary tract. **Cholangiohepatitis** refers to inflammation of the peribiliary hepatocytes as well as the biliary tract. The biliary tract is composed of the bile canaliculi, collecting ducts, bile duct, and gallbladder. When both conditions are present, the term **cholangitis/cholangiohepatitis complex** (CCHC) is often used.

2. What is unique about the anatomy of the feline biliary tree? Why is it significant?

In cats, the pancreatic duct enters the common bile duct before it opens into the duodenum. When disease (e.g., inflammation, infection, neoplasia, stasis) is present in the small bowel, it may ascend into the common bile duct and from there affect the pancreas and the rest of the biliary tree. Similarly, disease in the biliary tree or pancreas may affect the other two regions. This scenario is termed **triaditis**.

3. What are the most common forms of CCHC?

The most common forms are suppurative and nonsuppurative. Histologically, neutrophils are the predominant cell infiltrate in the suppurative form, whereas lymphocytes and plasma cells are the predominant cell infiltrate in the nonsuppurative form.

4. How is a diagnosis of CCHC made clinically?

The clinical presentation includes a vague history of inappetence, anorexia, and lethargy as well as possible nausea, vomiting, diarrhea, and weight loss. The signs may have a chronic intermittent occurrence. Physical examination may reveal signs of dehydration, weight loss, muscle wasting, icterus, salivation, palpable liver margins, and cranial abdominal tenderness or firmness. Suppurative and nonsuppurative CCHC cannot be differentiated on the basis of history and physical examination alone; both forms may or may not present with an elevated temperature.

5. What minimal database should be performed to help make the diagnosis of CCHC?

Complete blood cell count, serum biochemical panel, urinalysis, and blood pressure evaluation are indicated initially. These tests help to differentiate CCHC from other conditions but cannot be used for definitive diagnosis. An inflammatory leukogram increases the likelihood of a suppurative condition. As with any chronic, inflammatory condition, nonregenerative anemia and hyperglobulinemia may be present. Hepatic disease may change red cell morphology, resulting in the presence of schistocytes, blister cells, elliptocytes, acanthocytes, or keratocytes. If hepatic insufficiency develops from chronic inflammation, red blood cell microcytosis and thrombocytosis may be present.

Cats with CCHC often have hyperbilirubinemia and bilirubinuria, but these findings do not differentiate the conditions from other hepatic, prehepatic or posthepatic causes of icterus. In patients with bilirubinuria, lack of urobilinogen should increase suspicion of extrahepatic bile duct obstruction. Serum alkaline phosphatase (ALP), alanine transferase (ALT), and gamma glutamyl transferase (GGT) may be increased to varying degrees but do not distinguish between suppurative and nonsuppurative CCHC. Cats with hepatic lipidosis usually have markedly increased ALP activity compared with ALT activity and normal GGT activity (see Chapter 30). In contrast, cats with CCHC usually have ALP and ALT increases of equal magnitude, or the increase is greater in ALT than ALP; GGT activity is usually increased as well.

Some patients may have chronic CCHC, resulting in decreased functional liver mass; therefore, increases in ALT, ALP, GGT or bilirubin may not occur. There may be variable changes in albumin, glucose, blood urea nitrogen, and cholesterol. If you believe that liver disease is possible, a liver function test is indicated. The combination of pre- and postprandial serum bile acid measurement is used most frequently to assess liver function.

6. What further tests help to make a definitive diagnosis of CCHC?

Ultrasound of the abdomen is ideal before obtaining biopsies of the liver. It allows determination of the extent of the disease process and determines whether the disease is focal or generalized, which helps you advise the client about the best biopsy method and which tissues should be sampled. Ultrasound also allows visualization of the pancreas and may indicate whether the duodenum is involved. Hepatic fine-needle aspiration (FNA) can lead to a definitive diagnosis of hepatic lymphoma and mastocytosis and a presumptive diagnosis of hepatic lipidosis. Hepatic biopsy is the optimal procedure for all other hepatic diseases, including CCHC (see Chapter 28).

7. Why is hepatic biopsy preferred over FNA for CCHC?

If you were blind-folded and told to sample an apple pie with a drinking straw, the sample sucked up through the straw would be limited; you would get mush and liquid that tastes of apples. With FNA, you are restricted in what you harvest, and the limited sample is mutilated by the aspiration action and slide preparation. On the other hand, if you were to take a full-thickness piece of pie, you would recognize the crust, chunks of apples, apple-tasting mush, and cheddar cheese. Some types of cells do not exfoliate readily (e.g., mesenchymal neoplasias such as fibrosarcoma). With FNA you get only a cytologic diagnosis of whatever cells are sampled easily and may not see a real picture of the underlying disease process. In addition, orientation of the cellular reaction within tissue is critical in differentiating what role neutrophils or lymphocytes play. For example, peribiliary inflammation and periportal inflammation define different disease processes and may indicate different therapy and different prognosis.

8. What hepatic biopsy techniques are preferred for CCHC?

Before the liver is aspirated or biopsied, a platelet count and factor function test or a PIVKA (protein induced by vitamin K absence or antagonism) test should be performed (see Chapter 71). Hepatic tissue can be obtained percutaneously using landmarks or with ultrasound guidance via laparoscopy or laparotomy. Percutaneous techniques usually use Tru-cut needles, which obtain tissues of superior quality compared with FNA, but often result in the collection of small, broken samples compared with wedge biopsies. They do not allow direct visualization of the liver and do not contribute to hemostasis. With laparoscopy, part of the hepatic parenchyma can be visualized, large biopsies can be made, the pancreas can be biopsied (if indicated), and hemostasis can be applied (if required). However, special equipment is required. Surgically obtained biopsies have many advantages. The entire biliary tree can be examined, the gallbladder can be palpated, expressed, and aspirated for culture and sensitivity, and both the duodenum and pancreas can be biopsied in cases of suspected triaditis. Tissue obtained through biopsy should be submitted for histopathologic evaluation as well as aerobic and anaerobic bacterial culture and antimicrobial susceptibility.

9. How do suppurative and nonsuppurative CCHC differ histologically?

Changes associated with suppurative CCHC include infiltrates of nondegenerate and degenerate neutrophils within dilated intrahepatic bile ducts, canaliculi, and hepatic parenchyma. The adjacent tissues (duct lining) have varying degrees of fibrosis, but usually it is minimal. In cases with suppurative cholangitis, *Escherichia coli, Clostridium* spp., *Bacteroides* spp., *Actinomyces* spp., and alpha-hemolytic *Streptococcus* spp. are often cultured. Nonsuppurative CCHC has aggregates of inflammatory cells (lymphocytes, plasma cells, eosinophils, and some neutrophils) in portal regions and around the bile ducts. Fibrosis also may be present.

10. How is suppurative CCHC treated?

Wherever possible, underlying or concurrent problems, such as inflammatory bowel disease, pancreatitis, liver flukes, or hepatic lipidosis, should be identified and treated. Suppurative CCHC requires appropriate antimicrobial therapy. If a culture of liver tissue or bile was obtained, choice of antimicrobial should be based on the sensitivity profile. While awaiting culture results or if treating empirically, choose an antibiotic that concentrates in the liver and biliary system and is tolerated by cats and that the client will be able to administer. Therapy is required for a minimum of 6–8 weeks and perhaps as long as 6 months. Appropriate choices include penicillins (ampicillin, amoxicillin, or amoxicillin-clavulanate), first- or second-generation cephalosporins, or a fluoroquinolone. Because anaerobic bacteria are often present, penicillins, cephalosporins, or metronidazole often is used in combination with fluoroquinolones, particularly if evidence of sepsis exists. Metronidazole also may be beneficial for its immune-modulating properties, particularly if inflammatory bowel disease exists concurrently. Glucocorticoids should be avoided except in cats that fail to respond to antimicrobial therapy.

11. What diet is recommended for nonsuppurative CCHC? ?

Lymphocytic/plasmacytic disorders like nonsuppurative CCHC require elimination of allergens, wherever possible, as well as modulation of the immune response. Thus, an enteric bland diet, which has limited antigens and low residue and is calorie-dense, is advisable once the patient is eating well. Some diets may include omega-6 and omega-3 fatty acids in a 5:1 ratio, which has an anti-inflammatory effect. Protein restriction is not required unless the patient is encephalopathic. The fact that the cat is eating is more important than what the cat eats (see Chapter 62).

12. What drugs are used to treat nonsuppurative CCHC?

Glucocorticoids, such as prednisone or prednisolone, are the cornerstone of therapy of lymphocytic/plasmacytic disorders in cats. Prednisolone may be more effective because it requires less hepatic biotransformation than prednisone. As with inflammatory bowel disease, it is important to start with a high enough dose to suppress the inflammatory response. Prednisone and prednisolone, 2–4 mg/kg orally every 12 hours for 1 month or until clinical remission is achieved—are commonly used. The dose is then tapered to 0.5 mg/kg orally every 48 hours over 2–3 months, if possible (see Chapter 23).

Metronidazole often is used concurrently for its anaerobic bacterial spectrum as well as its immune-modulating properties. At oral doses of 7.5 mg/kg every 12 hours, it can be used for long periods (months) in conjunction with glucocorticoids. Higher doses should be avoided because metronidazole is metabolized in the liver and has the potential for hepatotoxicity.

Cats with sclerosing CCHS do not respond to prednisolone, metronidazole, and ursodeoxycholic acid alone; thus, adjunctive therapies such as methotrexate may be tried. Although treatment with chlorambucil or azathioprine has not been helpful in sclerotic cases, both agents may be tried as alternatives or adjunctive therapies in nonsclerotic nonsuppurative CCHC when prednisolone, metronidazole, and ursodeoxycholic acid do not achieve clinical improvement.

Drugs Used in the Management of CCHC

DRUG	STARTING DOSES
Amoxicillin	11–22 mg/kg PO every 8–12 hr
Amoxicillin/clavulanate	15 mg/kg PO every 8 hr
Ampicillin	20–40 mg/kg PO every 8 hr
Azathioprine	0.3 mg/kg PO every 48 hr
Cefoxitin	30 mg/kg IV every 6–8 hr
Cephalexin	22–35 mg/kg PO every 12 hr
Chlorambucil	2 mg/cat PO every 48 hr
Enrofloxacin	5–20 mg/kg PO or IM every 24 hr
Methorexate	0.13 mg/cat every 12 hr × 3 doses, repeated once weekly
Metronidazole	7.5–10 mg/kg PO every 12 hr
Prednisolone	2–4 mg/kg PO every 12 hr
Taurine	250 mg/cat PO every 12–24hr
Ursodeoxycholic acid	15 mg/kg PO every 24 hr
Vitamin B1 (thiamine)	5–50 mg/cat PO every 24 hr
Vitamin B12 (cobalamin)	50–100 μ/cat PO every 24 hr
Vitamin E	100–200 IU/day PO
Vitamin K$_1$	0.5–1.0 mg/kg SC every 24 hr for 3–4 days; then once weekly

PO = orally, IV = intravenously, IM = intramuscularly, SC = subcutaneously.

13. What treatments are used for both suppurative and nonsuppurative forms of CCHC?

- Supportive care
- Subcutaneous administration of vitamin K$_1$
- Water-soluble vitamin B complex
- Ursodeoxycholic acid
- Vitamin E

14. What are the essential elements of supportive care?

Supportive care includes fluid therapy to normalize electrolytes and acid base imbalances as well as to re-hydrate and correct hypovolemia. Inappetant cats are generally hypokalemic, which should be corrected. Nutritional support cannot be overemphasized (see Chapter 62). Placement of a feeding tube may be necessary. Cats require approximately 60–80 kcal/kg/day. If a cat is vomiting and antiemetic therapy is ineffective, feeding of smaller meals more frequently over the 24-hour period, continuous trickle feeding through a feeding tube, or total parenteral nutrition may be required.

15. Why is subcutaneous vitamin K_1 recommended?

Vitamin K is absorbed in the small bowel and recycled in the liver. Cats with liver diseases are often inappetent and do not ingest vitamin K. Because of the severe cholestasis in cats with CCHC, fat-soluble vitamins, including vitamin K, are not readily absorbed. In addition, cats with CCHC may have altered mucosal permeability due to bacterial colonization and may have decreased or absent vitamin K epoxidase activity in the liver.

16. What is the role of water-soluble vitamin B complex?

Addition of a water-soluble vitamin B complex to intravenous fluids or daily oral administration is recommended because B vitamins are minimally stored and inappetence reduces their availability. In addition, cats with liver failure and polyuria lose water-soluble vitamins in the urine. Cobalamin deficiency may play a role in hepatic lipidosis; lipidosis often occurs concurrently with CCHC (see Chapter 30). Cervical ventroflexion may indicate a deficiency in thiamine, which is easily corrected.

17. Discuss the effects of ursodeoxycholic acid.

Ursodeoxycholic acid (Actigall, Ciba-Geigy) is a therapeutic bile acid used to alleviate sludged bile as well as to ease bile flow in swollen hepatocytes or narrowed canaliculi. It carries IgA and is believed to have hepatoprotective effects. It should be used in cats with hepatic lipidosis or inflammatory liver diseases. It is contraindicated in complete bile duct obstruction; be sure to check for the presence of urobilinogen. In cats administered ursodeoxycholic acid, taurine supplementation is advised for conjugation.

18. Why is vitamin E supplementation recommended?

Because of its antioxidative properties.

19. What is the most serious complication of CCHC?

Severe, chronic CCHC can lead to hepatic insufficiency, which may result in hepatic encephalopathy. Treatment of this condition is described in Chapter 35.

20. How is therapeutic response evaluated?

The client's perception and observations of the cat are helpful, although subjective. Physical examinations help to assess hydration weight gain and overall condition as well as to evaluate previously noted abnormalities. However, because it is unlikely that the disease "started" exactly when the client first noticed it and because some degree of illness most likely preceded the first observable signs, evaluation of previously abnormal serum biochemistries (liver enzymes, liver function tests) is recommended. Ultrasound or repeat evaluation of liver biopsies is ideal.

21. What is the prognosis for cats with CCHC?

The prognosis for cats with CCHC depends on the extent of histopathologic changes, presence of fibrosis or cirrhosis, and concurrent disorders. Most cats with suppurative CCHC recover fully. Most cats with nonsuppurative CCHC recover clinically but have ongoing lymphocytic/plasmacytic inflammation that must be controlled to avoid development of hepatic insufficiency and hepatic encephalopathy.

BIBLIOGRAPHY

1. Center SA: The feline cholangitis/cholangiohepatitis syndrome. In Proceedings of the 15th Annual Meeting of the American College of Veterinary Internal Medicine, Lakewood, CO, ACVIM, 1997, pp 409–412.
2. Weiss DJ, Armstrong PJ, Gagne JM: Feline cholangiohepatitis. In Bonagura JD (ed): Current Veterinary Therapy XIII. Philadelphia, W.B. Saunders, 2000, pp 672–674.
3. Willard MD, Weeks BR, Johnson M: Fine-needle aspirate cytology suggesting hepatic lipidosis in four cats with infiltrative hepatic disease. J Feline Med Surg 1:215–220, 1999.

30. HEPATIC LIPIDOSIS

Michelle L. Berry, D.V.M.

1. Define hepatic lipidosis.

Hepatic lipidosis (HL), one of the most common hepatobiliary disorders of domestic cats in North America, is defined as a clinical syndrome in which at least 50% of hepatocellular cytosol is displaced by triglyceride (TG).

2. What causes HL?

Abnormal fat accumulation in hepatocytes may occur for various reasons. It has been associated with endocrine conditions, nutritional and metabolic derangements, and some forms of hepatic disease. As free fatty acids (FFAs) are introduced to the liver, they can be (1) esterified into TG, packaged as very low density lipoproteins (VLDL), and exported from the liver, (2) esterified into TG and stored in the hepatocytes, or (3) undergo beta oxidation and be utilized as energy. Any condition that decreases VLDL synthesis or export or overwhelms the ability to oxidize FFAs for energy results in increased TG storage. Specific causes include obesity, imbalanced caloric intake, poor nutrition, hepatotoxins, systemic diseases, and idiopathic disease (approximately 50%).

3. Describe the typical history of a cat with HL.

Typically the owner notes weight loss, lethargy, and anorexia. Feline HL occurs twice as often in females as males. Cats that are obese may be predisposed. The anorexia usually occurs for at least 2 weeks, and weight loss often exceeds 25% of original body weight. The cat may have a history of vomiting, diarrhea, or constipation.

4. What physical examination findings are typical in cats with HL?

Icterus, hepatomegaly, and dehydration often are detected on physical examination. The cat may exhibit signs of hepatic encephalopathy (HE), such as ptyalism or other neurologic signs, but they are generally uncommon. Other findings consistent with a primary disease process inducing anorexia may be found (see Chapter 62).

5. What are the differential diagnoses for cats with these findings?

Because icterus is the main clinical presentation with specific diagnoses, the primary differentials include all causes of prehepatic, hepatic, and posthepatic hyperbilirubinemia (see Chapter 28). Because hepatomegaly is common, hepatic and posthepatic causes are higher on the differential list than prehepatic causes.

6. Describe the initial diagnostic plan for a cat with suspected HL.

Packed cell volume should be assessed immediately to eliminate prehepatic causes of hyperbilirubinemia. Complete blood count (CBC) and serum biochemisty profile, including electrolytes, urinalysis, feline leukemia virus antigen test, and feline immunodeficiency virus antibody test, are indicated. In cats older than 5 years, total T4 concentration should be determined as well. A search for underlying diseases should be undertaken, as indicated by other historical and physical examination findings. Disorders associated with feline HL are listed in the table below.

Disorders Associated with Hepatic Lipidosis in Cats

DISEASE	PROPOSED MECHANISMS
Diabetes mellitus	Increased lipolysis of adipose tissue
Intestinal bacterial overgrowth and inflammatory bowel disease	Formation of endotoxins, impaired gut absorption of nutrients, formation of toxic bile acids

Table continued on following page

Disorders Associated with Hepatic Lipidosis in Cats (Continued)

DISEASE	PROPOSED MECHANISMS
Anorexia	Increased mobilization of FFA, decreased protein; any illness with associated anorexia can precipitate HL
Carnitine deficiency	Decreased fatty acid beta-oxidation
Poor nutrition	Insufficient protein
Cholangiohepatitis	Anorexia, liver dysfunction
Chronic parenteral carbohydrate	Increased hepatic synthesis of triglycerides, blocking of beta infusion oxidation of fatty acids
Hepatotoxins (various)	Impaired oxidation of fatty acids, assembly of VLDL, and export of VLDL

FFA = free fatty acids, HL = hepatic lipidosis, VLDL = very low density lipoprotein.

7. Is there a typical pattern of hepatic enzymes in HL?

In most cats with HL, alkaline phosphatase (ALP) activity is higher than alanine transferase (ALT) activity; gamma-glutamyl transferase activity is usually normal. Approximately 80% of cats have a twofold or more increase in ALP activity; 55% have a fivefold or more increase.

8. What other abnormalities are often identified on CBC and serum biochemistry profile?

CBC often reveals a mild anemia, which may be regenerative or nonregenerative. Poikilocytosis is common. The leukogram may be helpful because cats with idiopathic HL usually do not have an inflammatory leukogram, whereas cats with underlying disease leading to HL often do.

Serum biochemisty profile changes often reflect cholestasis with hyperbilirubinemia. Some cats may have a low albumin concentration with a normal globulin concentration. Additional inconsistent findings include hypercholesterolemia, decreased blood urea nitrogen, and hyperglycemia.

Serum electrolyte concentrations are variable. Approximately 30% of cats with HL have hypokalemia, which is significantly related to failure to survive.

9. What additional diagnostic tests should be performed?

Abdominal radiography is rarely helpful in supporting a diagnosis of HL. Hepatomegaly may be detected, but usually it is recognized on abdominal palpation during the physical examination. Abdominal ultrasound in the hands of an experienced ultrasonographer can provide valuable information about the cause of liver dysfunction. Cats with HL have diffuse hyperechoic parenchyma. Findings consistent with bile duct obstruction or cholangitis/cholangiohepatitis, such as gallbladder wall thickening or bile duct thickening, increase suspicion of other underlying disorders.

10. How is HL definitely diagnosed?

Liver tissue must be evaluated microscopically to arrive at a definitive diagnosis of HL. This goal can be achieved with fine-needle aspirate and cytology or biopsy and histology. Because liver disease commonly results in coagulopathies, coagulation tests should be performed before aspiration or biopsy. An activated clotting time (ACT), prothrombin time (PT), or activated partial thromboplastin time (APTT) may help to identify cats with increased risk of bleeding. A test for proteins induced by vitamin K absence or antagonism (PIVKA) also may be valuable.

Ultrasound-guided percutaneous fine-needle aspiration may be sufficient for a diagnosis of HL, but it also may miss other underlying hepatic diseases. If an underlying liver disease is suspected, hepatic biopsy should be performed (see Chapter 29).

11. Why are cats with liver disease predisposed to bleeding tendencies?

Because normal liver function and regular flow of bile is necessary to absorb fat-soluble vitamins such as vitamin K, cats with abnormal liver function or cholestasis may have a decreased amount of vitamin K available to activate clotting factors II, VII, IX, and X. The other primary mechanism is decrease in hepatic production of clotting factors.

12. What should you do if the PT or APTT is prolonged?

The patient should be treated with subcutaneous administration of vitamin K_1 at 5 mg/cat. You should wait 12 hours before biopsy is performed. This therapy should treat vitamin K deficiency effectively but does not correct clotting factor deficiency secondary to liver insufficiency. In cats suspected of having a clotting factor deficiency, fresh frozen plasma or fresh whole blood should be given before biopsy to provide necessary clotting factors. All cats should be blood-typed or cross-matched before biopsy in case bleeding occurs. Many clinicians prefer to treat cats with liver dysfunction with vitamin K_1 regardless of coagulation status before biopsy because side effects are minimal.

13. Describe the initial treatment plan for HL.

Fluid therapy should be initiated immediately to replenish fluid losses and normalize acid-base status. Normal saline (0.9% sodium chloride) or other polyionic isotonic solutions are appropriate. Because hypokalemia is common, 20 mEq of potassisum chloride should be added per liter of fluid for maintenance. If hypokalemia is present, more aggressive potassium supplementation may be warranted. Dextrose should not be added to the fluids unless hypoglycemia has been identified because excessive carbohydrates stimulate hepatic synthesis of triglycerides and block oxidation of fatty acids, further exacerbating the lipidosis. Because the liver metabolizes lactate to produce bicarbonate, fluids with lactate added as a buffer (i.e., lactated Ringer's solution) should be avoided in patients with liver dysfunction, especially cats with HL.

Aggressive nutritional management is the cornerstone of effective HL therapy. Sufficient protein must be provided because cats catabolize a set amount of protein for energy to be used for hepatic triglyceride clearance.

14. What is the best way to provide nutritional support?

Gastrostomy tubes provide the easiest, most reliable method of long-term alimentation. A self-retaining, 14–20-French catheter with a reinforced mushroom tip (Bardex self-retaining catheter, Bard Urological Division, Murray Hill, NJ) is commonly used. Some clinicians use esophagostomy tubes with success (see Chapter 62). Pharyngostomy tubes are poorly tolerated by cats and should be avoided.

15. When should a gastrostomy tube be placed?

A gastrostomy tube should be placed as soon as possible. If the cat needs to be stabilized before anesthesia for tube placement, a nasoesophageal or nasogastric tube can be placed to deliver nutrition. Because of the small size of these tubes, a liquid diet must be used. A commercial feline liquid diet (CliniCare Feline Maintenance, Pet Ag Inc., Hampshire, IL) is often sufficient for short-term nutritional support. Because liquid formulations do not provide adequate protein, they are not recommended for long-term nutritional therapy. Force feeding by the oral route, while successful in some cats, is generally unreliable and not recommended. It is difficult to ensure proper caloric intake, and cats may develop a food aversion because of oral forced feeding.

16. What should you do if the cat shows signs of hepatic encephalopathy (HE)?

Cats showing overt signs of HE should be evaluated for conditions known to precipitate HE, such as gastrointestinal bleeding, hypokalemia, alkalosis, systemic infection, azotemia, and constipation.

17. How is HE treated?

Treatment is aimed at decreasing production and absorption of alimentary-derived toxins. The most often implicated toxin associated with HE is ammonia, a breakdown product of protein. Cats presenting with signs of HE should be treated with warm cleansing enemas of normal saline to evacuate the colon. Cleansing should be followed with retention enemas containing lactulose (5–10 ml diluted 1:3 with warm water) or neomycin.

Hypokalemia should be treated by addition of potassium chloride to intravenous fluids. Delivery of potassium chloride should not exceed a rate of 0.5 mEq/kg/hr.

Once the signs abate, the cat can be managed with a diet containing decreased protein and oral lactulose (see Chapter 35). Oral antibiotics, such as amoxicillin, neomycin, or metronidazole, may be beneficial.

18. How should a cat be fed with a gastrostomy tube?

Twenty-four to 36 hours after placement, feeding can begin. Initially, 5 ml of warm water is instilled into the tube. If it is tolerated with no signs of nausea or vomiting, small amounts of food may be given. Caloric requirements should be calculated for each cat. The following formula is commonly used:

$$\text{Estimated caloric needs} = 1.5 \times [30 \times \text{body wt (kg)} + 70]$$

At first, small amounts of food should be given. Caloric requirements usually are introduced in thirds. On the first day, one-third of the nutritional requirement is given, divided into separate feedings every 4–6 hours. As the cat adjusts to the introduction of food, volumes are increased gradually in thirds until full caloric requirements are received. After full caloric requirements are met, the frequency of feeding can be reduced gradually until the cat is fed every 8 hours. Before each feeding, the tube should be aspirated to quantify residual stomach contents. If the amount aspirated is > 20% of the previous feeding, the scheduled feeding should be skipped and therapy with a prokinetic drug, such as metoclopramide (0.2–0.5 mg/kg every 8 hr), should be initiated. Always return the aspirated fluid to the cat to avoid potential acid-base and/or electrolyte imbalances.

Typical Gastrostomy or Esophagostomy Feeding Plan for 4-kg Cat with Hepatic Lipidosis

- Estimated caloric needs = 1.5 × [(30 × 4) + 70] = 285 kcal/day
- Blenderize food with enough water to make 1 kcal/ml
- Strain the blenderized mixture twice and refrigerate
- Warm the amount of mixture to room temperature or slightly warmer before feeding

Day 1

24 hours after tube placement, instill 5 ml of warm water in tube. If no vomiting or signs of nausea occur, proceed with feeding. If vomiting or signs of nausea occur, initiate parenteral metoclopramide therapy.

- Offer wet food orally before feeding through the tube. Do not force the cat to eat.
- Before administering food, aspirate the tube. If > 5 ml of fluid is retrieved, skip the feeding. Give the aspirated fluid back through the tube. Initiate metoclopramide therapy. Give 16 ml of blenderized food mixture through the tube over 20–30 minute. If the cat vomits during feeding, stop. Flush the tube with 5 ml of warm water, and wait until next feeding. If the cat tolerates the feeding, finish the 16 ml, and flush the tube with 5 ml warm water. Repeat every 4 hours for the first 24 hours.
- Subsequent feedings throughout the day. Before administering food, aspirate tube. If > 5 ml is aspirated during the first day, skip the feeding. Give the aspirated fluid back through the tube. Initiate metoclopramide therapy.

Day 2

If the cat has been tolerating the feedings, increase daily total amount to two-thirds of total requirements. If the food is 1 kcal/ml, the total daily amount increases to 188 ml, given as 31 ml every 4 hours. If aspirate is > 6 ml before feeding, skip the feeding and wait until the next scheduled feeding.

Day 3

If the cat has been tolerating the feedings, increase daily total amount to full caloric requirements. If the food is 1 kcal/ml, the total daily amount increases to 285 ml, given as 48 ml every 4 hours. If aspirate is > 10 ml before feeding, skip the feeding and wait until the next scheduled feeding.

After full caloric requirements are being given

As the cat does better with the feedings, decrease the frequency to every 6 hours for a few days, then every 8 hours. For example, if the cat is fed every 6 hours at full caloric requirements, a total of 71 ml is given at each feeding. If the cat is fed every 8 hours at full caloric requirements, a total of 95 ml is given at each feeding.

19. What kind of food should be fed?

A balanced commercial feline diet is the best choice because it contains all of the necessary protein and amino acids for cats. Canned food should be blenderized with water to form a slurry that can be given through the tube with ease. If a homemade diet is used, ensure that adequate amounts of arginine and taurine are provided.

20. What should be done if the cat vomits?

Vomiting is a common complication in cats with feeding tubes. If vomiting occurs, prokinetic drugs such as metoclopramide should be used. In the hospital, metoclopramide can be given parenterally via subcutaneous injection or in a continuous-rate infusion with intravenous fluids. Alternatively, the medications may be given via the gastrostomy or esophagostomy tube 30 minutes before tube-feeding. Protracted vomiting may signify other underlying disorders, such as worsening hepatic disease, pancreatitis, or tube problems (e.g., cellulitis or sepsis), and should be investigated.

21. How should the tube be managed at home?

Give specific written instructions for tube feeding and care at home. Instruct the owner to inspect the exit sight daily for exudate or irritation, and call if there is any concern. Tube clogging is a common problem and usually can be alleviated with a flush of warm water. For more difficult clogs, about 5-6 ml of a carbonated beverage can be instilled in the tube. Wait 5–10 minutes, then try flushing again. Before each feeding, the owner should offer the cat a tasty variety of food to stimulate normal eating. Once the cat is eating spontaneously, tube feedings can be decreased gradually until the cat is eating all of the nutritional requirements orally. At that time, tube removal should be considered.

22. How long should the gastrostomy tube stay in the cat?

Because all cats are different, the time varies on an individual basis. Many cats require tube feeding for 4–6 weeks. For appropriate healing, the tube should not be removed before 2 weeks after placement. Some clinicians remove the tube when the cat is ingesting all nutritional requirements with no supplementation from the tube for at least 2 weeks. The cat should gain weight (if needed) or maintain current weight with oral feeding. A serum biochemistry profile should reveal normal hepatic enzyme activities and normal total bilirubin.

23. Are additional dietary supplements needed for cats with HL?

Some clinicians prefer to supplement the diets of cats with HL. A list of the most commonly used supplements and their suspected benefit is included in the table below. To date, no scientific evidence indicates that these supplements are necessary or beneficial.

Nutritional Supplements for Cats with Hepatic Lipidosis

Arginine	May be essential for formation of certain apoproteins. Cats can develop hepatic encephalopathy if fed a diet low in arginine. An oral dose of 1 gm/cat every 24 hr has been recommended.
Taurine	Taurine is essential in cats for conjugation of bile acids, among other activities. Because cholestasis may occur with HL, cats may deplete taurine stores. An oral dose of 250–500 mg/cat every 12 hr has been recommended.
Carnitine	Carnitine may help to increase fatty acid beta-oxidation. An oral dose of 250–500 mg/cat every 24 hr has been recommended.
Thiamine	Supplementation may be needed in anorectic cats. An oral dose of 50–100 mg/cat every 24 hr has been recommended.
Vitamin K_1	Normal liver function and flow of bile are necessary for absorption of fat-soluble vitamins such as vitamin K. Vitamin K is necessary for activation of clotting factors II, VII, IX, and X. An oral dose of 5 mg/cat every 12 hr for 2–3 days, then every 3 days, is recommended.

Table continued on following page

Nutritional Supplements for Cats with Hepatic Lipidosis (Continued)

Vitamin E	This fat-soluble vitamin has antioxidant properties. An oral dose of 20–100 mg beta tocopherol/cat every 24 hr is recommended.
Zinc	Low levels of zinc have been documented in humans with liver insufficiency. Low levels of zinc are suspected to cause signs of hepatic encephalopathy; therefore, zinc is supplemented by some clinicians. An oral dose of 7–10 mg/cat every 24 hr has been recommended.

24. What is the prognosis for cats with hepatic lipidosis?

Identification of underlying causes followed by appropriate and aggressive treatment has improved the prognosis for cats with hepatic lipidosis. Cats that receive the necessary therapy have a > 60% chance at survival, regardless of whether there is an underlying cause or the lipidosis is idiopathic.

BIBLIOGRAPHY

1. Center SA: Hepatic lipidosis. In Guilford WG, Center SA, Strombeck DR, et al (eds): Strombeck's Small Animal Gastroenterology, 3rd ed. Philadelphia, W.B. Saunders, 1996, pp 766–782.
2. Cornelius LM, Bartges JW, Miller CC: CVT Update: Therapy for Hepatic Lipidosis. In Bonagura JD (ed): Kirk's Current Veterinary Therapy XIII, Small Animal Practice. Philadelphia, W.B. Saunders, 2000, pp 686–690.
3. Roudebush P, Davenport DJ, Dimski DS: Hepatobiliary disease. In Hand MS, Thatcher CD, Remillard RL, Roudebush P (eds): Small Animal Clinical Nutrition, 4th ed. Topeka, KS, Mark Morris Institute, 2000, pp 826–827.

31. HEPATIC NEOPLASIA

Timothy M. Fan, D.V.M.

1. What is the difference between a primary hepatic neoplasm and a secondary or metastatic hepatic neoplasm?

A **primary** hepatic neoplasm is a tumor that originates from the hepatic parenchyma or associated structures, whereas a **secondary** or metastatic hepatic neoplasm arises from another source and spreads or invades into the liver parenchyma as a consequence of disease progression.

2. Name the most common malignant primary hepatic neoplasms of the feline liver.

The most common primary feline hepatic neoplasms may be of epithelial or nonepithelial origin. Hepatobiliary epithelial neoplasms include hepatocellular adenocarcinoma, biliary duct carcinoma, and biliary duct adenoma. Hepatobiliary nonepithelial neoplasms include hemangiosarcoma, fibrosarcoma, and leiomyosarcoma.

3. What are the most common metastatic hepatic neoplasms in cats?

Lymphosarcoma, infiltrative mast cell tumors, pancreatic carcinoma, intestinal carcinoma, and carcinoids are the most common metastatic neoplasms affecting the feline liver. The term **visceral mastocytosis** describes infiltrative mast cell tumors involving the internal organs, such as the liver and intestines. Most metastatic hepatic neoplasms are characterized by diffuse infiltration of the liver, resulting in generalized hepatomegaly.

4. Which are more common, primary hepatic neoplasms or metastatic hepatic neoplasms?

Metastatic neoplasms of the liver are more common than primary hepatic neoplasms. Hepatic lymphosarcoma and visceral mastocytoma typically cause generalized hepatomegaly;

however, metastatic pancreatic or intestinal carcinoma generally produces multiple discrete nodules involving more than one liver lobe. The most common primary hepatic neoplasm of epithelial origin in cats is bile duct adenoma, followed by bile duct adenocarcinoma.

5. What are the common clinical manifestations of hepatobiliary neoplasia?

Most affected cats are presented for vague nonspecific signs of illness, including anorexia, vomiting, diarrhea, weight loss, and lethargy. Some are overtly icteric. Icterus associated with feline hepatic neoplasia is caused most commonly by intrahepatic biliary duct occlusion, resulting in posthepatic hyperbilirubinemia. In extreme cases, advanced neoplastic infiltration may compromise liver function, resulting in hepatic icterus. A minority of cats with hepatobiliary neoplasia have peritoneal effusion. Potential causes of peritoneal effusion include increased vascular permeability due to the release of inflammatory cytokines, occlusion of hepatic lymphatics from neoplastic infiltration, and decreased oncotic pressure secondary to hypoalbuminemia.

6. Name common hematologic and biochemical abnormalities that may be supportive of hepatobiliary neoplasia.

Hematologic abnormalities may include nonregenerative anemia and leukocytosis. Degree of leukocytosis can be variable and should not be automatically attributed to infectious causes of hepatic disease. Profound leukocytosis (> 80,000 cells/μl) can be a paraneoplastic syndrome associated with neoplastic production and release of granulocyte colony-stimulating factor. Biochemical abnormalities may include increased serum activities of alanine aminotransferase (ALT), aspartate aminotransferase (AST), gamma-glutamyl transferase (GGT), and alkaline phosphatase (ALP), hyperbilirubinemia, and abnormal coagulation tests. The absence of biochemical abnormalities does not exclude the possibility of hepatobiliary neoplasia. If hepatic function is severely compromised by advanced neoplastic disease, biochemical abnormalities associated with liver failure, such as hypoalbuminemia, hypoglycemia, low blood urea nitrogen, and hypocholesterolemia, may be identified.

7. Describe potential radiographic and sonographic findings associated with hepatobiliary neoplasia.

Abdominal radiographs may identify diffuse hepatomegaly or a cranial abdominal mass effect. Significant abdominal effusion may impede visualization of normal anatomic structures because of diminished radiographic contrast and detail. Sonographically, primary and metastatic hepatobiliary neoplasms may produce variable patterns of echogenicity. Diffuse hepatomegaly, a solitary hepatic mass, or multiple hepatic nodules may be identified, depending on the location and type of hepatobiliary neoplasm. Imaging studies are helpful in supporting the diagnosis of hepatobiliary neoplasia; however, definitive diagnosis is based on cytologic or histologic findings.

8. How is a liver biopsy obtained in cats?

Definitive diagnosis of hepatic neoplasms other than lymphosarcoma and mastocytosis traditionally requires a liver biopsy for histologic evaluation. Methods for obtaining an adequate amount of tissue include percutaneous ultrasound-guided liver biopsy, laparoscopic biopsy, or exploratory laparotomy with biopsy. Risk for hemorrhage is greatest with percutaneous, ultrasound-guided liver biopsy; this technique also yields the smallest amounts of tissue. During exploratory laparotomy, large biopsies can be taken and hemorrhage can be controlled, but general anesthesia is required and there is risk of poor wound healing in severely affected patients. Percutaneous ultrasound-guided and laparoscopy-obtained biopsies have the benefits of not requiring a significant surgical incision, and both techniques can be performed with sedation. Although histopathologic evaluation is the only definitive method for diagnosing some malignancies, cytologic confirmation of malignancy can be obtained by fine-needle aspiration of the liver or, in some cases, evaluation of peritoneal effusions and can be performed instead of biopsy for the benefit of compromised patients.

9. How can surgery aid in the treatment of hepatic neoplasia?

Surgical resection may prove to be curative in dealing with solitary primary hepatocellular adenocarcinomas or adenomas. In general, primary tumors affecting one or two lobes should be excised by hepatic lobectomy. Unfortunately, most epithelial and nonepithelial hepatobiliary neoplasms involve multiple liver lobes, precluding complete surgical excision. Surgical resection of biliary duct adenocarcinomas is rarely curative because of anatomic limitations for complete surgical resection, as well as the aggressive metastatic behavior of the tumor. Approximately 75% of hepatobiliary adenocarcinomas at time of diagnosis have already metastasized to the lungs, regional lymph nodes, and intestinal serosa.

10. When should I use systemic chemotherapy in the treatment of hepatic neoplasia?

Systemic chemotherapy should be considered as a primary therapeutic modality for hepatic lymphosarcoma or visceral mastocytoma. Systemic chemotherapy should be recommended in an adjunctive setting for the control of micrometastatic disease after surgical debulking of primary hepatobiliary neoplasms. At this point in veterinary oncology, the effective use of radiation therapy or immunotherapy for the treatment of hepatobiliary neoplasia remains poorly explored.

11. How successful is systemic chemotherapy in the treatment of hepatobiliary neoplasms?

In general, when treating hepatobiliary neoplasms with systemic chemotherapy, response rates, remission duration, and survival times remain disappointing. One postulated explanation for the poorer response rates concerns the expression of P-glycoprotein by hepatocytes. For a chemotherapeutic agent to be effective in killing a tumor cell, several requirements must be met, including a high enough concentration of the agent within the tumor cell to induce apoptosis (programmed cell death). Certain tumor cells protect themselves from reaching this lethal threshold concentration by upregulating an intrinsic cellular efflux pump known as P-glycoprotein. Activation of P-glycoprotein enhances the ability of tumor cells to export chemotherapeutic agents, thereby circumventing cellular death. Normal tissues involved with xenobiotic metabolism and excretion, such as the liver and kidney, have higher inherent expressions of P-glycoprotein. Neoplasms originating from the liver or kidney tend to express very high levels of P-glycoprotein, making them more resistant to the effects of systemic chemotherapy.

12. In treating an icteric cat with systemic chemotherapy for hepatobiliary lymphosarcoma, which chemotherapy drugs should be used with caution?

Most traditional chemotherapeutic regimens for the treatment of lymphosarcoma include the use of adriamycin, vincristine, cyclophosphamide, prednisone, and L-asparaginase (See Chapter 68). Both adriamycin and vincristine rely on hepatobiliary excretion and at the very least should be dose-reduced, if not completely avoided, in the treatment of icteric patients. If the patient does not have evidence of icterus, standard dosing of adriamycin and vincristine may be recommended. Cyclophosphamide and prednisone are prodrugs requiring hepatic transformation to their respective active metabolites, 4-hydroxycyclophosphamide and prednisolone. There are no contraindications for the use of cyclophosphamide or prednisone in icteric cats, but if hyperbilirubinemia is secondary to synthetic liver failure, biotransformation of cyclophosphamide or prednisone to its active metabolite may be incomplete. L-asparaginase degrades endogenous L-asparagine to L-aspartic acid and ammonia, depriving malignant lymphoid cells of necessary L-asparagine for rapid protein synthesis and growth. There have been no reported contraindications for the use of L-asparaginase in the treatment of feline hepatic lymphosarcoma, but hyperammonemia with subsequent hepatic encephalopathy has been reported in humans treated with L-asparaginase.

13. What is visceral mastocytosis? How can you manage the clinical signs associated with visceral mast cell degranulation?

Visceral mastocytosis describes the diffuse infiltration of neoplastic mast cells within a visceral organ. Visceral mastocytosis may affect the liver, spleen, or intestines. Systemic signs of illness are caused not only by neoplastic infiltration into organ sites but also by mast cell degranulation. Mast cells contain numerous cytoplasmic granules that are released by immuno-logic (IgE or complement-mediated) and nonimmunologic (temperature, pressure, drug expo-sure) mechanisms. The process of cytoplasmic granule release is termed degranulation. One major component responsible for many of the clinical signs associated with mast cell degranula-tion is histamine. Histamine can activate H_2 receptors on the parietal cell, resulting in excessive hydrochloric acid production and subsequent vomiting, anorexia, melena, and gastric ulceration. In addition, histamine can activate H_1 receptors found on vascular endothelium, resulting in pro-found vasodilation and increased capillary membrane permeability. The use of an H_1 blocker (diphenhydramine) and an H_2 blocker (famotidine, ranitidine, or cimetidine) may ameliorate sys-temic signs attributed to mast cell degranulation.

14. What chemotherapeutic protocol is used for visceral mastocytosis?

Visceral mastocytosis tends to be a highly aggressive disease, with common involvement of the intestine, liver, and spleen. Even with multiorgan involvement, splenectomy has proved to be beneficial in prolonging survival times of cats. The use of systemic chemotherapy should be viewed at best as palliative, with a low probability of providing a definitive cure for systemic vis-ceral mastocytosis. Adjunctive medical therapies with histamine blockers (diphenhydramine and famotidine) should be implemented in attempts to improve quality of life scores. Effective chemotherapy protocols for the treatment of visceral mastocytosis in cats have yet to be critically evaluated in a prospective manner. The concurrent use of lomustine and prednisone provides a relatively cost-effective and rational means of treating visceral mastocytosis. If hematologically tolerable, lomustine may be dosed at 60 mg/m² by mouth every 21 days, and prednisone may be dosed at 20 mg/m² by mouth daily. Vinblastine and cyclophosphamide used together or as single agents also may be effective in treating visceral mastocytosis.

BIBLIOGRAPHY

1. Alexander RW, Kock RA: Primary hepatic carcinoid (APUD cell carcinoma) in the cat. J Small Anim Pract 23:767, 1982.
2. Carr BI, Flickinger JC, Lotze MT: Hepatobiliary cancers. In Devita VT (ed): Cancer: Principles and Practice of Oncology, 5th ed. Philadelphia, Lippincott-Raven, 1997, pp 1087–1114.
3. Day DG: Diseases of the liver. In Sherding RG (ed): The Cat: Diseases and Clinical Management, 2nd ed. Philadelphia, W.B. Saunders, 1994, pp 1297–1340.
4. Feeney DA, Johnston GR, Hardy RM: Two-dimensional, gray-scale ultrasonography for assessment of hepatic and splenic neoplasia in the dog and cat. J Am Vet Med Assoc 184:68–81, 1984.
5. Feldman BF, Strafuss AC, Gabbert N: Bile duct carcinoma in the cat: Three case reports. Feline Pract 6:33, 1976.
6. Fondacaro JV, Guilpin VO, Powers BE, et al: Diagnostic correlation of liver aspiration cytology with histopathology in dogs and cats with liver disease. In Proceedings of the 17th Annual Veterinary Medical Forum, June 10–13, 1999, p 719.
7. Lawrence HJ, Erb HN, Harvey HJ: Nonlymphomatous hepatobiliary masses in cats: 41 cases (1972 to 1991). Vet Surg 23:365–368, 1994.
8. Morrison WB: Primary cancers and cancer-like lesions of the liver, biliary epithelium, and exocrine pan-creas. In Morrison WB (ed): Cancer in Dogs and Cats: Medical and Surgical Management. Philadelphia, Lippincott Williams & Wilkins, 1998, pp 559–568.
9. Patnaik AK: A morphologic and immunocytochemical study of hepatic neoplasms in cats. Vet Pathol 29:405–415, 1992.
10. Post G, Patnaik AK: Nonhematopoietic hepatic neoplasms in cats: 21 cases (1983–1988). J Am Vet Med Assoc 201:1080–1082, 1992.
11. Scavelli TD, Patnaik AK, Mehlhaff CJ, et al: Hemangiosarcoma in the cat: Retrospective evaluation of 31 surgical cases. J Am Vet Med Assoc 187: 817, 1985.
12. Straw RC: Hepatic tumors. In Withrow SJ, MacEwen GE (eds): Small Animal Clinical Oncology, 2nd ed. Philadelphia, W.B. Saunders, 1996, pp 248–252.
13. Strombeck DR, Guilford GW: Hepatic neoplasms. In Guilford GW (ed): Strombeck's Small Animal Gastroenterology, 3rd ed. Philadelphia, W.B. Saunders, 1996, pp 847–859.
14. Trout NJ, Berg RJ, et al: Surgical treatment of hepatobiliary cystadenomas in cats: Five cases (1988–1993). J Am Vet Med Assoc 206:505–507, 1995.

32. HEPATIC INFECTIONS

Timothy M. Fan, D.V.M.

1. What infectious agents are associated with hepatic disease in cats?

Infectious causes of hepatic disease include viruses (feline infectious peritonitis, feline leukemia virus), parasites (*Toxocara cati, Platynosomum concinnum, Toxoplama gondii, Cytauxzoon felis*), bacteria (suppurative cholangitis/cholangiohepatitis complex), and fungi (*Mucor* spp., *Aspergillus* spp).

2. What is the most common hepatic infection?

The bacterial cholangitis/cholangiohepatitis complex is most common (see Chapter 29).

3. Which protozoans are associated with hepatic infections?

At least four different protozoal organisms have been associated with hepatic infections: *Toxoplasma gondii*; a coccidia-like organism from the protozoan family Eimeriidae; a protozoan parasite similar to *Hepatozoon canis*; and *Cytauxzoon felis* (see Chapter 75). *T. gondii* is the most frequently encountered protozoan parasite causing cholangitis/cholangiohepatitis.

4. How does hyperbilirubinemia due to toxoplasmosis develop?

Cats are infected by *T. gondii* by ingestion of sporulated oocysts or tissue cysts or transplacentally or lactationally from primary infection of the queen. Clinical toxoplasmosis is most severe in transplacentally infected or neonatally infected kittens; the type and severity of clinical illness depend on the degree and localization of tissue injury. The organism infects the gastrointestinal epithelium and disseminates through the blood. Intracellular replication of *T. gondii* tachyzoites results in destruction of infected cells and necrosis. Replication is common in hepatocytes and the pancreas and can result in hyperbilirubinemia from either hepatic disease or pancreatic disease. Hepatic disease seems to be uncommon in chronically infected cats. Clinical signs in acutely infected cats include anorexia, depression, fever, abdominal distension, crying, dyspnea, central nervous system signs, icterus, and death.

5. How is hepatic toxoplasmosis diagnosed?

A diagnosis of *T. gondii* infection can be made by various testing procedures. Tachyzoites may be detected cytologically in various tissues and body fluids (pleural and peritoneal effusions) during acute infection. Fecal examination for *T. gondii* oocysts may be beneficial 1–2 weeks after initial exposure. Serologic testing has become the most practical and accepted means of diagnosing *T. gondii* infection. Serologic evidence of recent or active infection consists of high IgM titers, or a fourfold or greater increase in IgG titers. However, these findings document only recent infection, not clinical disease due to infection.

6. How is hepatic toxoplasmosis treated?

Drugs attempted for the treatment of acute extraintestinal toxoplasmosis include clindamycin (10–12.5 mg/kg orally every 8–12 hr), pyrimethamine (0.25–0.5 mg/kg orally every 12 hr), and trimethoprim-sulfonamide (15 mg/kg orally every 12 hr). If pyrimethamine is used, it is generally combined with one of the other drugs; it is rarely given to cats because of the high incidence of side effects.

7. How does *Cytauxzoon felis* cause hyperbilirubinemia?

Cytauxzoon felis results in severe disease in most infected domestic cats (see Chapter 75). Hyperbilirubinemia in infected cats is probably due to two mechanisms: (1) red blood cell destruction from the piroplasm stage and (2) hepatic dysfunction or cholestasis from hepatic infiltration by schizont-infected macrophages.

8. What trematode parasites cause hyperbilirubinemia in cats?

The liver fluke, *Platynosomum concinnum*, has been reported to infect cats in tropical to semitropical climates. Infestation with this trematode is uncommon but has been reported in cats living in or with a history of travel to Hawaii, Florida, Polynesia, Malaysia, New Guinea, Australia, Nigeria, Brazil, Bahamas, and Puerto Rico. Other species of trematodes that have been identified in the livers of cats include *Amphimerus pseudoflineus, Opisthorcus tenuicollis,* and *Metorchus conjunctus*; infestation with these species is rare.

Platynosomum concinnum requires two intermediate hosts to complete its life cycle: a land snail and a reptile (gecko, lizard, or skink) or amphibian (toad). Embryonated eggs are ingested by the land snail and hatch within the snail's intestinal tract. The miracidia then penetrate the host's tissues and transform into sporocysts. The second intermediate host ingests oocysts shed by the snail, and the cat becomes infected when it ingests an infected second intermediate host. Infective flukes migrate up the common bile duct into the gallbladder and bile ducts.

Although most cats are subclinically infected, some cats with a high, chronic fluke burden may manifest weight loss, vomiting, diarrhea, icterus, and hepatomegaly ("lizard poisoning"). The presence of the flukes within the biliary system incites an inflammatory process that eventually may lead to bile duct fibrosis and biliary epithelial hyperplasia.

9. How are liver fluke infections diagnosed?

Diagnosis of *P. concinnum* can be difficult because most cats are subclinically infected. Identification of the parasite by fecal examination has poor sensitivity because of the small number and variable morphology of *P. concinnum* eggs. Observe for the double-operculated eggs after fecal sedimentation. Cholecystocentesis is a more definitive means of diagnosing *P. concinnum* infection in cats; however, given the invasive nature of the procedure, it should be reserved for cases in which the index of suspicion for fluke infestation is high and the cat is clinically symptomatic.

10. How are liver fluke infections treated?

Effective treatment of *P. concinnum* infection remains poorly defined. Current recommendations are to administer albendazole (50 mg/kg/day) until fluke eggs disappear from feces or fenbendazole (50 mg/kg orally every 12 hr) for 5 consecutive days. Albendazole may cause bone marrow toxicity in cats treated for more than 5 consecutive days; therefore, the risk-benefit ratio must be considered with chronic administration of albendazole.

11. Is toxocariasis a common cause of liver disease in cats?

Toxocara cati migrates through the liver of cats after ingestion of larvated eggs or infected transport hosts (see Chapter 19). However, clinical findings consistent with liver disease are usually not detected.

12. What are the clinical findings of liver disease due to feline infectious peritonitis?

Feline infectious peritonitis (FIP) is thought to result from infection by a mutated variant of the universally prevalent feline enteric coronavirus (FECV). FIP can manifest as either effusive (wet) or noneffusive (dry), depending on predominant type (humoral or cell-mediated) and efficacy of the host's immune response (see Chapter 38). Hyperbilirubinemia has been associated most commonly with the noneffusive form of FIP. A primary mechanism for hyperbilirubinemia due to FIP is the formation of perivascular pyogranulomas within the hepatic parenchyma and bile duct system severe enough to cause either synthetic liver failure, intrahepatic biliary obstruction, or extrahepatic biliary obstruction. In addition, the hyperbilirubinemia associated with FIP can result from hepatic lipidosis induced by anorexia. The definitive diagnosis of hepatic involvement with the FIP virus requires a liver biopsy to document the characteristic lesions and to perform immunohistochemistry. Classical lesions include perivascular infiltration (arterioles and venules) of proliferating macrophages, lymphocytes, plasma cells, and neutrophils. Treatment responses are variable and prognosis is guarded.

13. How does feline leukemia virus infection result in hyperbilirubinemia?

Feline leukemia virus (FeLV) is the other principal viral cause of hepatic disease in cats. Although FeLV infection may cause multisystemic illness, the mechanism for liver disease usually is not associated with synthetic liver failure but rather with FeLV-induced malignant cell transformation leading to the development of hepatic lymphosarcoma. Hepatic lymphosarcoma causes hyperbilirubinemia as a result of malignant lymphocyte invasion into the hepatic parenchyma with subsequent intrahepatic cholestasis (see Chapters 24 and 31). Other mechanisms for FeLV associated hyperbilirubinemia include:

- Direct viral induction of hemolytic anemia and subsequent hyperbilirubinemia (see Chapter 76).
- Induction of immunosuppression and subsequent predisposition to *H. felis*-associated hemolytic anemia (see Chapter 75), FIP, or toxoplasmosis.
- Induction of anorexia and subsequent hepatic lipidosis

14. What are the clinical findings of liver disease associated with fungal infection?

Cats with systemic fungal disease are occasionally presented for evaluation of clinical findings consistent with hepatic disease. Anorexia, wasting, lethargy, diarrhea, and icterus are the most common clinical manifestations. In one report, *Mucor* spp. and *Aspergillus* spp. were the two reported isolates. A presumptive diagnosis is based on cytologic or histopathologic evidence of fungal infection; definitive diagnosis is based on culture. In the one large case series, all cats were diagnosed on necropsy; therefore, definitive treatment recommendations cannot be made.

BIBLIOGRAPHY

1. Addie DD, Jarrett O: Feline coronavirus infection. In Greene CE (ed): Infectious Diseases of the Dog and Cat, 2nd ed. Philadelphia, W.B. Saunders, 1998, pp 58–69.
2. Bielsa LM, Greiner EC: Liver flukes *(Platynosomum concinnum)* in cats. J Am Anim Hosp Assoc 21:269–274, 1985.
3. Center SA: Hepatobiliary infections. In Greene CE (ed): Infectious Diseases of the Dog and Cat, 2nd ed. Philadelphia, W.B. Saunders, 1998, pp 615–625.
4. Center SA: Diseases of the gallbladder and biliary tree. In Stombeck DR (ed): Stombeck's Small Animal Gastroenterology, 3rd ed. Philadelphia, W.B. Saunders, 1996, pp 860–888.
5. Chock E, Wolfe BM, Matolo NM: Acute suppurative cholangitis. Surg Clin North Am 61:885–892, 1981.
6. Cotter SM: Feline viral neoplasia. In Greene CE (ed): Infectious Diseases of the Dog and Cat, 2nd ed. Philadelphia, W.B. Saunders, 1998, pp 71–84.
7. Dubey JP, Carpenter JL: Histologically confirmed clinical toxoplasmosis in cats: 100 cases. J Am Vet Med Assoc 203:1556–1566, 1993.
8. Dubey JP, Lappin MR, Thulliez P: Diagnosis of induced toxoplasmosis in neonatal cats. J Am Vet Med Assoc 207:179–185, 1995.
9. Dubey JP, Zajac A, Osofshy SA, et al: Acute primary toxoplasmic hepatitis in an adult cat shedding Toxoplasma gondii oocysts. J Am Vet Med Assoc 197:1616–1618, 1990.
10. Ewing GO: Granulomatous cholangiohepatitis in a cat due to a protozoan parasite resembling *Hepatozoon canis*. Feline Pract 7:37–39, 1977.
11. Hirsch VM, Doige CE. Suppurative cholangitis in cats. J Am Vet Med Assoc 182:1223–1226, 1983.
12. Hitt HE: Liver fluke infection in South Florida cats. Feline Pract 11:26–29, 1981.
13. Jorgensen LS, Pentlarge VW, Flanders JA, et al: Recurrent cholelithiasis in a cat. Comp Cont Educ Pract Vet 9:265–267, 1987.
14. Neufeld JL, Brandt RW: Cholangiohepatitis in a cat associated with a coccidia-like organism. Can Vet J 15:156–159, 1974.
15. Ossent P: Systemic aspergillosis and mucormycosis in 23 cats. Vet Rec 120:330–333, 1987.
16. Shaker EH, Zawie DA, Garvey MS, et al: Suppurative cholangiohepatitis in a cat. J Am Anim Hosp Assoc 27:148–151, 1991.
17. Smart ME, Downey RS, Stockdale PHG: Toxoplasmosis in a cat associated with cholangitis and progressive pancreatitis. Can Vet J 14:313–316, 1973.
18. Taylor D, Perri SF: Experimental infection of cats with the liver fluke *Platynosomum concinnum*. Am J Vet Res 38:51–54, 1977.

33. BILIARY DISEASES

Lynda Melendez, D.V.M., M.S.

1. Which diseases typically affect the biliary system of cats?
Inflammatory diseases such as cholecystitis, choledochitis, and cholangiohepatitis/cholangitis complex (CHCC) occur, as do obstructive processes, *Platynosomum concinnum* infestation (see Chapter 32), and neoplastic disorders. Other than CHCC (see Chapter 29), most of these conditions are uncommon in cats.

2. What clinical signs are seen in cats with biliary disorders?
As with most liver diseases, the clinical signs of biliary disorders are often nonspecific. Cats can be subclinically affected for quite some time. Anorexia, lethargy, vomiting, fever, and varying degrees of icterus may be seen. If the condition is subacute or chronic, weight loss also may be detected. Some cats may exhibit signs of abdominal pain, but this can be difficult to assess. With severe cholestatic disease, acholic feces may be noted. If rupture of the bile duct or gallbladder has occurred or if concurrent hepatic disease has resulted in increased portal pressure or severe hypoalbuminemia, abdominal effusion may be present and detected on physical examination.

3. Which laboratory tests are helpful in diagnosing biliary tract disease in cats?
In icteric cats or cats with other signs that may be attributed to the liver, gastrointestinal system, or pancreas, a complete blood count (CBC), serum biochemistry panel, and urinalysis should be performed.

4. Describe the typical CBC findings.
CBC findings are often variable. Septic inflammation of the biliary tract often results in a neutrophilia with or without an increase in the number of band neutrophils in circulation. A stress leukogram also may be found. Cats with liver fluke infestation often have eosinophilia. With chronic disease, nonregenerative anemia may be present as a result of chronic inflammation or gastrointestinal blood loss.

5. What abnormalities may be seen on the serum biochemistry panel?
The serum biochemistry panel reveals an increase in the activities of cholestatic liver enzymes alkaline phosphatase (ALP) and gamma-glutamyl transferase (GGT) along with varying degrees of hyperbilirubinemia. If cholestasis is severe or concurrent liver disease is present, serum concentrations of hepatocellular enzymes alanine transferase (ALT) and aspartate transferase (AST) also are elevated. Hypercholesterolemia is usually associated with bile duct obstruction.

6. What does urinalysis reveal?
Urinalysis reveals bilirubinuria and, in cases of complete bile duct obstruction, lack of urobilinogen.

7. What other biochemical tests may be useful?
Coagulation times should be assessed in cats with hyperbiliubinemia or other clinical evidence of cholestasis. Because bile is necessary for the absorption of fat-soluble vitamins, cats with chronic cholestatic disease often have prolonged clotting times secondary to vitamin K deficiency. Fluid analysis should be performed in any cat with abdominal effusion.

8. Which imaging techniques can assist in the diagnosis of biliary tract disease?
Abdominal radiographs are often nonspecific but may reveal mineralized densities within the biliary tree, representing either dystrophic mineralization from chronic inflammation or cholelithiasis. Hepatomegaly or a mass in the region of the gallbladder, liver or pancreas may be

evident. Gas within the biliary system or parenchyma of the liver is diagnostic for emphysematous cholecystitis or a hepatic abscess caused by gas-forming bacteria such as *Clostridium* spp. This problem is recognized most frequently in diabetic patients or patients who have a disease process resulting in ischemia of the liver and/or gallbladder.

In the hands of a skilled ultrasonographer, **abdominal ultrasound** is more reliable than radiographs for evaluating the biliary structures and finding both radiodense and radiolucent stones. The gallbladder wall can be evaluated for thickness and irregularities as well as the presence of polyps or other discrete masses. Common bile duct enlargement can be recognized with ultrasound, and the region surrounding the common bile duct (e.g., pancreatic region, hepatic parenchyma, intestines) can be evaluated as well. In some cases, small amounts of abdominal effusion may be detected and aspirated for evaluation. Bile can be collected via ultrasound-guided fine-needle aspiration for cytology, anaerobic culture, aerobic culture, and antimicrobial susceptibility testing. Hepatic **nuclear scintigraphy** using technetium-labeled organic anions that are excreted in the bile can be used to help diagnose bile duct occlusion, gallbladder malfunction, and small-volume bile leakage into the peritoneal cavity.

9. What causes cholecystitis and choledochitis?

Cholecystitis (inflammation of the gallbladder) and choledochitis (inflammation of the common bile duct) are uncommon as primary diseases in cats. They generally are the sequelae of other inflammatory or infectious disease processes affecting the liver, duodenum, and/or pancreas. Because the feline common bile duct forms an anastomosis with the pancreatic duct before emptying into the proximal duodenum, pancreatic and intestinal diseases can cause the extension of inflammation up the biliary system to the gallbladder. Reflux of duodenal juices often introduces gastrointestinal flora into the biliary system, resulting in septic inflammation. Other disease processes that result in prolonged anorexia, which may cause bile stasis and sludging, also can result in inflammation or infection of the biliary system.

10. How are cholecystitis and choledochitis diagnosed?

Clinical signs are consistent with any cholestatic disease in cats. Abdominal ultrasound may show a thickened irregular gallbladder wall or dilated, tortuous common bile duct with varying degrees of bile sludging and stasis. With emphysematous cholecystitis, gas accumulation within the gallbladder may be evident on plain abdominal radiographs. Severe necrotizing cholecystitis may result in biliary rupture and bile peritonitis. Because cholecystitis and choledochitis in cats are often secondary to another disease process, every effort should be made to identify underlying or coexisting problems. Surgical biopsies are the best method for diagnosis of cholecystitis and choledochitis; abdominal exploratory surgery also provides the opportunity to evaluate for underlying disease. A portion of the gallbladder wall or a sample of bile should be submitted for anaerobic culture, aerobic culture, and antimicrobial susceptibility testing. With severe disease, cholecystectomy or biliary diversion procedures may be necessary.

11. Describe the treatment of cholecystitis and choledochitis.

Treatment should be directed primarily at any underlying condition. Fluid and electrolyte balance and nutritional support should be addressed. Colloidal support should be instituted for patients with hypoalbuminemia. While you are waiting for culture and sensitivity results, a broad-spectrum antibiotic regimen should be implemented. The author prefers ampicillin (22 mg/kg intravenously every 8 hr) combined with a fluorinated quinolone (enrofloxacin, 2.5–5 mg/kg intravenously every 12–24 hr). Vitamin K_1 (2.5 mg/kg subcutaneously or intramuscularly, divided every 12 hr) should be administered to all patients with evidence of chronic cholestatic disease and/or increased coagulation times, especially before going to surgery.

12. How common is cholelithiasis in cats?

Cholelithiasis (gallstone formation) is uncommon in cats. Although it has been associated with CHCC as well as cholecystitis, in many cats it is an incidental finding. The exact cause of cholelithiasis is unknown, but bile stasis and abnormal composition of bile are thought to contribute. Only about 50% of choleliths are radiodense, making abdominal ultrasound better for diagnosis than plain or contrast films. For cats with mild clinical signs, medical treatment with ursodeoxycholic acid (10–15 mg/kg orally every 24 hr) can be attempted for dissolution. Clinically ill cats with cholecystitis or bile duct occlusion should be explored surgically. A portion of the gallbladder and a sample of bile or a stone should be submitted for anaerobic culture, aerobic culture, and antimicrobial susceptibility testing. Long-term antibiotic therapy should be guided by susceptibility results. In the short term, broad-spectrum antibiotic coverage should be initiated as described in question 11.

13. What causes extrahepatic bile duct obstruction (EHBDO) in cats?

Pancreatitis, masses involving the common bile duct, cholelithiasis, and trematode infestation may cause EHBDO in cats. Other causes include extrinsic compression from regional lymph nodes and pancreatic masses, stricture formation as a sequela to severe inflammation, blunt trauma, or previous bile duct surgery, polycystic liver disease, and choledochitis. Diagnosis of EHBDO is based on clinical signs, biochemistry abnormalities, and confirmation with abdominal ultrasound, nuclear scintigraphy, and/or exploratory surgery. Treatment is aimed at identifying and correcting the underlying cause. In some cases, rerouting of the biliary system is required.

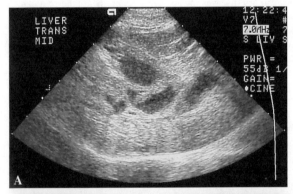

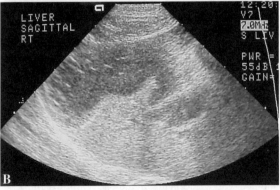

Distended bile ducts *(A)* and distended gallbladder and bile ducts *(B)* in a cat with EHBDO.

14. What causes bile peritonitis?

Leakage of bile into the abdominal cavity may result from traumatic rupture of the biliary system. Any disease process that interferes with the integrity of the gallbladder wall or biliary tree also may result in bile leakage (e.g., necrotizing cholecystitis, neoplasia). Iatrogenic damage to the biliary system may occur during surgery or percutaneous hepatic biopsy or aspiration. A small amount of sterile bile leaking into the peritoneal cavity is usually benign. Because bile is caustic, however, a large amount of bile accumulation or a continuous leak leads to an inflammatory response and subsequent abdominal effusion. Slow leakage of bile into the abdomen from a small defect may result in the loculation of fluid by the omentum (focal bile peritonitis) and be an incidental finding during abdominal ultrasound or exploratory laparotomy in evaluating an icteric patient. A large accumulation of bile results in diffuse abdominal effusion, which is usually evident on physical examination. Because marked inflammation of the peritoneal cavity can compromise the integrity of the intestinal wall, animals with diffuse bile peritonitis are at an increased risk of developing sepsis secondary to bacterial translocation from the gastrointestinal tract.

15. How is bile peritonitis diagnosed?
Diagnosis is based on analysis of the abdominal effusion. The fluid is often turbid and golden-brown or golden-green. Cytology reveals a marked inflammatory reaction containing many neutrophils and macrophages with intra- and extracellular particles of bile. Sepsis also can be determined from cytology. However, a sample of fluid should be submitted for culture and sensitivity to help direct long-term antibiotic therapy. The clinician also may compare concentrations of bilirubin in the fluid to serum bilirubin concentrations (with bile peritonitis, abdominal fluid has a markedly higher concentration of bilirubin).

16. How is bile peritonitis treated?
The patient should be fully assessed with CBC, serum biochemistry panel, and coagulation status in an attempt to identify any underlying or coexisting problems. Hypovolemic patients should be stabilized with adequate fluid therapy, and endotoxic shock should be addressed. Close attention should be given to electrolyte status. For patients with hypoalbuminemia or coagulation disorders, fresh or fresh frozen plasma should be administered. Once the animal is stabilized, surgical correction of the bile leakage is necessary. Collection of abdominal fluid in the area closest to the bile leak for cytologic evaluation and Gram stain for initial antimicrobial therapy as well as submission for culture and sensitivity for long–term antimicrobial therapy should be performed. Once the leak is repaired, copious lavage of the abdominal cavity with warm, physiologic saline should be done until the abdomen is free of bile-stained fluid.

17. What causes hepatobiliary cysts?
Hepatobiliary cysts may be congenital or acquired. Congenital cysts may be single or multiple and are thought to arise from embryonic bile ducts that lack communication with the biliary system. Polycystic disease often affects both the liver and the kidneys. Often the cysts affecting the liver are discovered incidentally during evaluation of a cat with evidence of renal insufficiency. Acquired cysts are usually solitary and may result from recent trauma, inflammation, or neoplasia. Although most cysts are incidental findings, they may become apparent if large enough to cause abdominal distention, impingement on normal surrounding tissues, or impaired movement of the diaphragm.

18. How are hepatobiliary cysts treated?
When a cat becomes symptomatic for an enlarged cyst, two options are available. The cyst can be aspirated with ultrasound guidance to relieve pressure. Fluid analysis should be performed to rule out other causes of fluid accumulation. The other option is surgical removal, which is performed if the cyst is causing biliary obstruction or if aspiration of the cyst has to be repeated multiple times to decrease pressure on neighboring structures.

BIBLIOGRAPHY

1. Center SA: Diseases of the gallbladder and biliary tree. In Strombeck's Small Animal Gastroenterology. 3rd ed. Philadelphia, W.B. Saunders, 1996, pp 860–888.
2. Day DG: Diseases of the liver. In Sherding RG (ed): The Cat: Diseases and Clinical Management, 2nd ed. New York, Churchill Livingstone, 1994, pp 1297–1340.
3. Tams TR: Hepatobiliary parasites. In Sherding RG (ed): The Cat: Diseases and Clinical Management, 2nd ed. New York, Churchill Livingstone, 1994, pp 607–611.

34. DRUG-INDUCED HEPATIC DISEASE

Marcella D. Ridgway, V.M.D., M.S.

1. Define drug-induced hepatopathy.
Any abnormality of liver function or structure resulting from the action of a drug or its metabolites on liver cells may be termed drug-induced hepatopathy. Lesions may be obvious, such as massive hepatic necrosis, or minute, such as changes in hepatocellular plasma membrane permeability that allow increased levels of cytosolic enzymes to leak into the systemic circulation.

2. What types of hepatic disease result from adverse drug reactions?
Adverse drug reactions produce either acute or chronic hepatic disease. Acute hepatic disease is more common and is associated histologically with hepatocellular necrosis. Acute disease may range from mild and inconsequential to massive hepatic necrosis and fulminant hepatic failure. Medications that cause acute hepatic disease also can cause chronic hepatic disease if the acute disease is mild and undetected while drug administration is continued. Chronic hepatic disease is associated histologically with mild degenerative changes and hepatic lipidosis.

3. Which drugs have been implicated in causing hepatic disease in the cat?
Hepatotoxicity of individual drugs varies significantly among species. Agents known to be hepatotoxic in other species cannot be assumed to be hepatotoxic in cats. Likewise, agents may cause hepatic injury in cats but not in other species. Drugs associated with acute hepatic disease (hepatocellular necrosis), chronic hepatic disease, or cholestasis are listed below. For drugs with no reported hepatotoxicity in cats, a high index of suspicion should be maintained for drugs with known hepatotoxicity in other species and drugs metabolized by the liver.

Acute hepatic necrosis
Acetaminophen
Aspirin
Diazepam
Iron-containing supplements
Glipizide
Griseofulvin
Ketamine
Ketoconazole
Methimazole
Phenazopyridine
Propylthiouracil
Tetracycline
Thiacetarsamide
Tiletamine/zolazepam

Chronic hepatic disease
Anabolic steroids
Corticosteroids
Colchicine
Megestrol acetate
Tetracycline
Valproic acid

Cholestasis
Erythromycin
Methyltestosterone
Trimethoprim-sulfa

4. Describe the mechanisms by which drugs cause acute hepatic disease.
Acute hepatic injury may be caused by a direct toxic effect of the drug or its metabolites on the hepatocyte, producing a predictable dose-dependent effect (acetaminophen, thiacetarsamide), or by idiosyncratic drug reactions, which occur unpredictably in a small number of cats exposed to a particular drug (diazepam, griseofulvin, glipizide, methimazole, others). Idiosyncratic drug reactions probably result from preexisting abnormalities of drug-metabolizing pathways, which are due to genetic differences or previous hepatic injury. Individual differences in drug metabolism may result in an inability to metabolize the drug to a nontoxic form or in transformation of a normally nontoxic drug to a toxic form via an atypical metabolic pathway. Most drug-related hepatotoxicities are due

to idiosyncratic reactions. In either direct toxicity or idiosyncratic reactions, the toxic form of the drug, usually a metabolite, causes cell damage by oxidative injury, depletion of intracellular compounds or binding cellular components, resulting in impaired cell function or cell death. The hepatocyte is usually the affected cell, although biliary epithelium may be affected concurrently. Chronic hepatic disease may result from continued administration of drugs that cause mild acute hepatic injury or with use of medications that alter metabolic pathways but do not usually cause hepatocellular necrosis. Tetracycline impairs fat mobilization by the liver by inhibiting synthesis of apoprotein or interfering with dispersal of very-low-density lipoprotein, leading to accumulation of triglycerides and hepatic lipidosis. Corticosteroids increase mobilization of free fatty acids to the liver by increasing lipolysis of peripheral fat stores; this process may result in hepatic lipidosis if hepatic fat metabolism is already compromised by anorexia or other abnormalities.

5. How frequently do drug-induced diseases occur?

The true incidence of drug-induced hepatic disease is unknown. Clinical signs and laboratory test results are nonspecific and do not differentiate drug-induced from other causes of hepatic disease. Consequently, drugs known to have hepatotoxic potential may be wrongly blamed for hepatic disease in a patient receiving the medication and subsequently found to have evidence of hepatic injury. This error may delay determination of an accurate diagnosis and lead to overestimation of the prevalence of drug-related hepatopathy. Conversely, failure to recognize the potential hepatotoxicity of a drug may delay measures to minimize exposure and the amount of resulting hepatic damage and also lead to underestimation of the prevalence of drug-related hepatopathy. Although the overall incidence of drug-induced hepatic disease is uncertain, severe drug-associated hepatotoxicity is uncommon.

6. What determines the severity of hepatic disease resulting from drug administration?

The degree of hepatic damage caused by a drug may range from mild degenerative changes and hepatic lipidosis to massive hepatic necrosis. Dose of the medication, route of administration, frequency and duration of administration, and physiologic condition of the individual animal affect the degree of liver damage. Administration of drugs at high doses, at greater frequency, or for longer periods or failure to recognize the onset of hepatic damage early in the course of therapy (i.e., greater total amount of drug to which a cat is exposed) may result in more severe hepatic injury if an adverse drug reaction occurs. Oral administration may potentiate hepatotoxicity because hepatocytes are exposed first and at higher drug concentrations via portal blood flow. Likewise, drugs undergoing enterohepatic circulation may have enhanced potential for hepatotoxicity. Host-related factors govern the response of an individual animal to a particular medication and the tendency to develop drug-associated hepatopathy.

7. What host factors may predispose to drug-induced hepatic disease?

Host factors such as age, sex, individual genetic constitution, nutrition, disease status, and prior or concomitant use of other medications can affect the likelihood and severity of drug-induced hepatic disease. Reduced protein binding in very young animals may alter the hepatotoxic potential of highly protein-bound agents. The rate of metabolism of some drugs may be decreased in younger animals because of lower hepatic enzyme activities. Older animals are more likely to have preexisting disease and alterations in hepatic blood flow that affect rates of drug metabolism and ability to compensate for hepatic injury. Females may be predisposed to drug-induced hepatic disease because of higher drug-metabolizing hepatic enzyme activities and increased capacity to generate toxic metabolites. Genetic make-up is important in determining hepatic enzyme activities, and inherited enzyme defects may significantly alter drug metabolizing capacity.

8. How may preexisting disease influence the hepatotoxic potential of a drug?

Malnutrition, especially protein deficiency, adversely affects hepatic enzyme and protein carrier systems and is of great significance in cats, which depend on dietary protein intake to meet energy as well as protein requirements. Any condition that alters hepatic blood flow, including cardiovascular disease, portosystemic shunting, and even dehydration, also alters drug metabolism by the liver. In animals with preexisting liver disease, reduced populations of functional liver cells as well as architectural changes and acquired portosystemic shunting limit the capacity of the liver to metabolize drugs and compromise its ability to compensate for additional hepatic damage. Cholestasis increases the toxic potential of drugs normally excreted in bile. Concurrent exposure to other medications that share high levels of protein binding or utilize the same carrier or enzyme systems can influence the hepatotoxicity of a drug. Many drugs and chemicals are metabolized via cytochrome P450 enzyme systems; prior administration of agents metabolized via this system may induce increases in P450 enzyme activities and result in increased capacity to metabolize other drugs, enhancing hepatotoxicity of drugs biotransformed by the P450 enzyme system to more toxic forms.

9. What species differences in metabolism may predispose cats to drug-induced hepatotoxicity?

Cats are true carnivores and have higher protein requirements than most other species. Energy is derived largely from dietary protein and fat rather than carbohydrate, and the cat has high levels of hepatic enzymes that deaminate amino acids for energy production. Metabolic adaptation or downregulation of these enzyme systems to compensate for changes in dietary protein does not occur; cats are unable to curtail metabolism of proteins for energy in the face of decreased protein intake. If dietary protein intake is inadequate, cats rapidly become deficient in important cellular proteins, including carrier proteins and enzymes that are necessary components of drug metabolic pathways. Another species variation affecting drug metabolism in cats is a relative deficiency of glucuronyl transferase, which mediates conjugation of various drugs to glucuronide for elimination. The inability to form glucuronide conjugates predisposes cats to toxicity with drugs dependent on glucuronide conjugation, such as aspirin, acetaminophen, morphine, and phenols. Some of these agents, such as aspirin, may be administered safely by increasing dosing intervals. Others, such as acetaminophen and phenolic compounds, should not be used at all in cats, yet exposure may occur when uninformed owners administer acetaminophen or apply phenolic dermal preparations (keratolytics, coal tar products, hexachlorophene) to their pets.

10. What clinical signs are associated with drug-induced hepatopathy in cats?

Clinical manifestations range from subclinical to chronic disease to acute hepatic failure. Subclinical mild acute hepatic injury may remain undetected unless serum chemistry profiles are obtained. In patients with clinical disease, presenting signs are nonspecific but may suggest hepatic disease. The severity of signs varies with the severity of the hepatic damage. Clinical signs consistent with drug-induced hepatic disease include depression, anorexia, ptyalism, vomiting, weakness, jaundice, and, less commonly, fever, hepatomegaly, cranial abdominal pain, and diarrhea. In severe cases, hemorrhage or petechiation may be noted, and neurologic signs of hepatic encephalopathy may be present. Ascites may develop but is relatively uncommon in cats. Most cases of drug-induced hepatopathy are mild and present with vague signs of lethargy and anorexia with or without vomiting or jaundice.

11. What laboratory findings are consistent with drug-induced hepatopathy?

Laboratory abnormalities reflect hepatic injury and are nonspecific for drug-induced vs. other causes of hepatic disease. Elevations in alanine aminotransferase (ALT) and aspartate aminotransferase (AST) activities are the most consistent finding. Serum alkaline phosphatase and gamma-glutamyl transferase activities also may be increased. Bilirubinuria and hyperbilirubinemia occur more commonly in cats than in dogs. Abnormalities in hepatic function tests (serum bile acid and ammonia testing) and reduced levels of hepatic synthetic products (glucose, albumin, cholesterol) are seen in more severe cases and roughly parallel the severity of the hepatic damage. Clotting factor deficiencies may arise as a result of synthetic failure or disseminated intravascular coagulation secondary to severe hepatic insult; coagulation profiles should be assessed before liver aspirate or biopsy procedures are performed. Electrolyte imbalances (hypokalemia, hyponatremia) and acid–base disturbances (metabolic acidosis) may occur. Patients with hepatic encephalopathy may develop respiratory alkalosis and hypophosphatemia. Complete blood count may show mild nonregenerative anemia, reduced platelet numbers, and either neutrophilia or neutropenia.

12. How is drug-induced hepatopathy diagnosed?

Because no clinical signs, laboratory profiles, or histopathologic changes are pathognomonic for drug-induced hepatic disease, diagnosis depends largely on recognition of the hepatotoxic potential of therapeutic agents, historical association of exposure to a drug coincidental with onset of hepatic disease, and diagnostic evaluation to rule out other causes of hepatic disease. Drug-induced hepatopathy should be considered as a differential in all cases of hepatic disease. A presumptive diagnosis of drug-induced hepatopathy may be based on the following findings:

- History of drug exposure
- Clinical signs and/or laboratory abnormalities consistent with hepatic damage due to administration of the drug
- Resolution of clinical signs and laboratory abnormalities (within a few days to a few weeks) when drug administration is discontinued.

Liver biopsy may help to rule out other potential causes of hepatic disease, but histopathologic changes seen in cases of adverse drug reactions are nonspecific and not diagnostic of drug-induced hepatopathy. Often, if a patient improves after withdrawal of the drug, a biopsy is not performed. Definitive diagnosis by resuming administration of the implicated drug and evaluating for recurrence of hepatic disease is usually contraindicated.

13. How are cats with drug-induced hepatic disease treated?

Immediate withdrawal of the drug is indicated in all patients with suspected drug-induced hepatopathy. With the exception of acetaminophen, phenol, or iron toxicity, there are no specific treatments or antidotes to counteract the effects of hepatotoxic drugs. Treatment, therefore, is directed at limiting exposure to the drug and providing supportive care proportionate to the level of hepatic dysfunction. In subclinical cases, identified only by elevations of hepatic transaminases, simply discontinuing the drug may be sufficient. In clinical cases, additional measures of general supportive treatment for acute hepatic disease are initiated and may include intravenous fluids, electrolyte supplementation, correction of acid–base status, glucose supplementation, antibiotics, and management of coagulopathies and hepatic encephalopathy. Use of medications that affect cytochrome P450 enzyme activity are best avoided. Cats showing clinical signs of hepatic disease usually require aggressive nutritional support to meet caloric and protein needs.

14. What additional treatments are available for specific therapy of hepatic disease caused by acetaminophen, phenol, or iron toxicity?

In addition to general supportive care, cats with acetaminophen-induced hepatic necrosis are treated with N-acetylcysteine to help to restore hepatic glutathione, which is depleted rapidly in cats exposed to acetaminophen or phenacetin. When given within the first 8–10 hours after exposure, N-acetylcysteine may limit formation of toxic metabolites. A 5% solution is administered initially at an intravenous or oral loading dose of 140 mg/kg, followed by 5–7 additional treatments of 70 mg/kg intravenously or orally every 4 hours. Treatment with N-acetylcysteine is also used in cases of phenol intoxication to limit hepatic injury, which occurs within the first 12–24 hours of phenol exposure. Iron toxicity is treated with desferroxamine, which chelates iron and enhances urinary excretion. Desferroxamine is administered by constant-rate infusion of 15 mg/kg/hr intravenously or 40 mg/kg intramuscularly every 4–8 hours until serum iron levels drop below 300 µl/dl.

15. Describe the main characteristics of diazepam-associated hepatic disease.

Severe acute hepatic necrosis and failure occur sporadically in cats treated with routine doses of diazepam prescribed for behavioral or micturition problems. Diazepam-associated hepatotoxicity is most likely due to an idiosyncratic drug reaction, occurring in only a few of the cats receiving the medication, and requires no prior sensitization. Affected cats show anorexia, lethargy, and ataxia within 4 days of starting therapy and jaundice within 11 days. Marked elevations of serum ALT and AST activities are consistently found; hypoglycemia, hypocholesterolemia, and abnormal coagulation tests also may be present. Most affected cats die of fulminant hepatic failure. Because of this hepatotoxic potential, cats placed on diazepam should be monitored for increases in ALT and AST. If hepatic enzyme abnormalities arise, drug therapy should be suspended and supportive care provided.

16. What is the prognosis for recovery from drug-induced hepatic disease?

Clinical outcome depends on the extent of hepatic damage. In most cases, the degree of liver injury is mild; with discontinuation of the drug and supportive therapy, complete recovery is likely. The liver has tremendous regenerative capacity. Even in severe cases, recovery of adequate hepatic function is possible if the patient can be supported through the initial period of acute hepatic necrosis and if the liver retains the ability to regenerate (adequate remaining cell populations and intact reticular framework). However, most cats that develop acute fulminant hepatic failure do not survive.

17. Are drug-induced hepatic diseases preventable?

Awareness of potential hepatotoxicity and predisposing factors as well as early detection of hepatic injury are key to selecting therapeutic agents and preventing clinically significant hepatic disease. Patients receiving drugs with hepatotoxic potential should be monitored for evidence of hepatic injury on serum chemistry profiles. Baseline chemistry values should be determined before treatment to serve as a reference point for monitoring and to help identify preexisting disease conditions. Avoid exceeding recommended dosing levels and frequency, and limit duration of therapy to the minimum required for effectiveness. Maintaining an index of suspicion of drugs as potential hepatotoxins and early evaluation of patients that develop clinical signs after receiving any drug for evidence of hepatic injury help to limit the degree of liver damage.

BIBLIOGRAPHY

1. Bunch SE: Acute hepatic disorders and systemic disorders that involve the liver. In Ettinger SJ, Feldman EC (eds): Textbook of Veterinary Internal Medicine Volume, vol. 2, 5th ed. Philadelphia, W.B. Saunders, 2000, pp 1326–1340.
2. Bunch SE: Hepatotoxicity associated with pharmacologic agents in dogs and cats. Vet Clin North Am Small Anim Pract 23:659–670, 1993.
3. Center SA: Acute hepatic injury: Hepatic necrosis and fulminant hepatic failure. In Guilford WG, Center SA, Strombeck DR, et al (eds): Strombeck's Small Animal Gastroenterology, 3rd ed. Philadelphia, W.B. Saunders, 1996, pp 654–704.
4. Center SA: Hepatic Lipidosis. In August JR: Consultations in Feline Internal Medicine 2. Philadelphia, W.B. Saunders Co., 1994, pp 87–101.
5. Center SA, Elston TH, Rowland PH, et al: Fulminant hepatic failure associated with oral administration of diazepam in 11 cats. J Am Vet Med Assoc 209:618–625, 1996.
6. Hooser SB: Hepatotoxins. In Bonagura JD (ed): Kirk's Current Veterinary Therapy XIII Small Animal Practice. Philadelphia, W.B. Saunders, 2000, pp 217–219.
7. Johnson SE: Diseases of the liver. In Ettinger SJ, Feldman EC(eds): Textbook of Veterinary Internal Medicine Volume, vol. 2, 4th ed. Philadelphia, W.B. Saunders., 1995, pp 1313–1326.
8. Kaufman AC, Greene CE: Increased alanine transaminase activity associated with tetracycline administration in a cat. J Am Vet Med Assoc 202:628–630, 1993.
9. Nelson RW, et al: Effect of an orally administered sulfonylurea, glipizide, for treatment of diabetes mellitus in cats. J Am Vet Med Assoc 203:821–827, 1993.
10. Papich MG, Davis LE: Drugs and the liver. Vet Clin North Am Small Anim Pract 15:77–95, 1985.
11. Peterson ME, Kintzer PP, Hurvitz AI: Methimazole treatment of 262 cats with hyperthyroidism. J Vet Intern Med 2:150–157, 1988.
12. Wilke JR: Idiosyncrasies of drug metabolism in cats: Effect on pharmacotherapeutics in feline practice. Vet Clin North Am 14:1345–1354, 1984.

35. PORTOSYSTEMIC SHUNTS

Margo L. Mehl, D.V.M.

1. Define portosystemic shunt.

A portosystemic shunt (PSS) is an abnormal vascular communication between the portal venous system and the systemic venous system. The portal system normally drains blood from the abdominal viscera to the liver for removal of toxins. A PSS diverts normal portal blood flow around the liver and directly into systemic circulation.

2. What is the difference between intrahepatic and extrahepatic portosystemic shunts?

The ductus venosus is a normal fetal structure that allows umbilical venous blood to bypass the liver; during gestation or shortly thereafter, it is stimulated to close. Intrahepatic shunts occur more commonly in dogs than cats and typically are congenital, singular shunts that represent failed closure of the ductus venosus. Extrahepatic shunts may be congenital or acquired. In cats, extrahepatic shunts are more common than intrahepatic shunts, and most shunt vessels arise from the left gastric vein and empty into the abdominal vena cava.

3. What is the difference between congenital and acquired portosystemic shunts?

A congenital shunt is present at birth and usually remains as a single intra- or extrahepatic shunt. An acquired shunt results from sustained portal hypertension, most often secondary to chronic liver disease. Most acquired shunts are multiple and extrahepatic; they are rare in cats.

4. Are portosystemic shunts hereditary?

Portosystemic shunts have not proven to be hereditary. However, they are recognized more frequently in male cats of mixed breeding (approximately 70%) that are < 3 years of age. Of the remaining 30% of purebred cats, 23% are of Himalayan and Persian breeds. Acquired PSS results from chronic liver disease and therefore can occur in any breed.

5. What are the common clinical findings of portosystemic shunts?

Physical examination findings and clinical abnormalities associated with PSS usually result from central nervous system disease, liver insufficiency, or urinary tract disease. Affected animals are usually thin and undersized. Ptyalism is the most frequently reported clinical sign in cats. In addition, copper-colored irises have been reported in cats with PSS.

Clinical Signs Associated with Portosystemic Shunt

Central nervous system		
Behavior changes	Deafness	Pacing
Blindness	Aggression	Ataxia
Seizures	Stupor/coma	Weakness
Dementia	Tremors	Disorientation
Liver insufficiency		
Anorexia	Lethargy	Diarrhea
Depression	Polydipsia	Ptyalism
Polyuria	Pica	Nausea
Weight loss	Stunted growth	Vomiting
Urinary system		
Hematuria	Stranguria	
Pollakiuria	Urethral obstruction	

6. Why do patients with portosystemic shunts have decreased liver function?

Portal venous blood supplies 50% of oxygen delivery to the liver and contains hepatotrophic (liver-supportive) growth factors such as insulin. These factors are necessary for hepatocyte growth and function. When a substantial PSS is present, these growth factors bypass the liver, resulting in atrophy, atresia, hypoplasia, and dysfunction. Hepatic hypertrophy, hyperplasia, regeneration, and glycogen storage are impaired.

7. Define hepatic encephalopathy.

Hepatic encephalopathy (HE) is abnormal mentation and neurologic function induced by absorbed intestinal toxins that have not been removed by the liver. To date, the exact mechanism of HE is not clear. HE is believed to result from diversion of portal blood flow around the liver, allowing ammonia, encephalotoxins, and endotoxins into systemic circulation. These toxins directly affect the cerebral cortex.

8. What findings of routine bloodwork and urinalysis support a diagnosis of PSS?

Laboratory findings are often nonspecific. The most common abnormalities include microcytic anemia, low blood urea nitrogen, hypoalbuminemia, hypoglycemia, hypocholesterolemia, and mild-to-moderate elevations in alanine aminotransferse (ALT) and alkaline phosphatase (ALP) activities. In any patient with a typical history, supportive clinical findings, and presence of ammonium biurate crystalluria, further liver function testing is recommended.

Laboratory Abnormalities Associated with Portosystemic Shunt

Hematologic findings	
Anemia	Neutrophilic leukocytosis
Microcytosis	Poikilocytosis
Hypochromasia	Target cell formation
Serum biochemical panel	
Low blood urea nitrogen	Hyperammonemia
Increased alkaline phosphatase	Increased alanine aminostransferase
Hypoglycemia	Hypocholesterolemia
Hypoproteinemia	Hypernatremia
Hyperchloremia	Hypokalemia
Urinalysis	
Isosthenuria	Ammonium biurate crystalluria
Hematuria	

9. How is PSS diagnosed?

Liver insufficiency is suggested by the combination of history, physical examination findings, and both hematologic and serum biochemical abnormalities. Results of pre- and postprandial measurements of serum bile acid concentration and ammonium tolerance tests are more sensitive than serum biochemical tests for detecting hepatic dysfunction but are not specific for PSS.

10. What imaging modalities are used to diagnose PSS?

Various imaging modalities are used to determine the extent and location of PSS. Abdominal radiographs often detect a small liver. Ultrasonograhy is a noninvasive way to evaluate liver architecture and vessels but is highly operator-dependent. Ultrasound also can be used intraoperatively to locate an intrahepatic PSS. Nuclear scintigraphy is a sensitive and specific technique to detect PSS but is not consistent in differentiating intra- and extrahepatic shunts. Angiography can be used to visualize the portal venous system, diagnose a shunt, and determine its location. Laparoscopy may allow visualization of an extrahepatic PSS. Most patients with PSS undergo exploratory laparotomy for diagnosis, determination of location, and potential surgical correction.

Imaging Modalities Used in the Diagnosis of Portosystemic Shunt

TECHNIQUE	SUPPORTIVE FINDINGS	DISADVANTAGES
Radiology	Microhepatica Renomegaly	Not specific
Ultrasonography	Microhepatica Undetectable portal or hepatic veins	Highly operator-dependent, less sensitive for extrahepatic shunts
Nuclear scintigraphy	Initially greater fraction of radio-activity in heart than in liver	Unable to determine location of shunt Unable to distinguish between single and multiple shunts
Angiography	Visualization of portal blood flow	Invasive, requires general anesthesia
Laparoscopy	Direct viewing of extrahepatic shunting vessel or lack thereof and obtaining of liver biopsy	Unable to see within liver parenchyma or to perform surgical correction

11. What differential diagnoses should be considered?

Other differential diagnoses refer to the organ system affected; gastrointestinal system, central nervous system, or urinary tract. Typical examples include liver failure due to other causes (hepatotoxins, infection, autoimmune disorder, neoplasia, or lipidosis), congenital urea cycle enzyme deficiency, other hepatic vascular disorders, and other causes of seizures in young animals.

12. How are most cases of PSS managed?

A combination of medical and surgical management is often used. The goal of medical management is to prevent the production and slow the absorption of central nervous system toxins produced by bacteria in the intestinal tract. Medical management alone has been successful in supporting some cases for more than 2 years. However, surgery should be performed, if possible, to redirect portal blood flow to the liver and potentially reverse hepatic atrophy and alleviate clinical signs. If surgery is performed, medical management typically is continued for 2–4 weeks beyond the resolution of clinical signs. Medical management includes a high-carbohydrate, low-protein diet to reduce the dietary source of ammonia, cathartics to decrease ammonia production and absorption, colonic pH modifiers to trap NH_4^+ in the colon, and oral antibiotics to reduce urease-producing intestinal bacteria.

Long-term Medical Management of Portosystemic Shunt and Hepatic Insufficiency

Dietary modifications

The goals of dietary modifications are to decrease the amount of protein available for ammonia production, increase fiber concentration, and promote fecal nitrogen excretion. Diets with protein requirements of at least 16% to 30% protein on a dry matter basis with easily digestible carbohydrate sources should be used. Diets used for the management of renal insufficiency (see Chapter 40) may be effective.

Oral antibiotics

Oral antibiotics are administered to decrease numbers of urease-producing bacteria in gastrointestinal tract. Urease-producing bacteria hydrolyze urea to ammonia in the intestine, thereby causing high ammonia levels.
   • Neomycin, 10–20 mg/kg orally every 8–12 hr
   • Metronidazole, 7.5 mg/kg orally every 8 hr
   • Ampicillin, 22–33 mg/kg orally every 8hr

Cathartics

Lactulose is a disaccharide that is converted in the colon to organic acids that lower colonic pH, resulting in conversion of NH_3 to NH_4^+, which is not as readily absorbed. In addition, lactulose increases intestinal transit time, thereby decreasing time for production and absorption of toxins. Dosage is empirical, starting with 0.25–0.5 ml/kg orally every 8–12 hr.

13. What considerations must be given to drug therapy and anesthetic use in patients with PSS?

In selecting anesthetic agents, hepatic metabolism, cardiovascular effects, and effects of the anesthetic agent on portal venous and hepatic arterial blood flow need to be considered. Barbiturates, acepromazine, and diazepam should be avoided because they are highly protein-bound and require liver metabolism. In addition, halothane is potentially hepatotoxic and should not be used. Isoflurane is the anesthetic agent of choice for induction and maintenance but has been reported to produce hypotension in some cases. An alternative for induction is fentanyl in small boluses (0.01–0.03 mg/kg intravenously) or as a constant-rate infusion (0.7 μg/kg/hr). However, narcotics can result in prolonged recovery time and may require administration of naloxone (0.02–0.04 mg/kg intravenously) as a reversal agent.

14. What parameters should be monitored postoperatively in cats with PSS?

Postoperatively cats should be monitored closely for signs of portal hypertension, including diarrhea, vomiting, distention of the abdomen or ascites, and abdominal pain as well as hypovolemia. Blood glucose should be monitored postoperatively. Cats with PSS also require close monitoring for seizures, which have been reported to occur up to 3 days postoperatively.

15. What are the complications of PSS?

The primary complications of medical management relate to progressive worsening of clinical disease associated with liver atrophy. Complications of preoperative anesthesia may include hypotension, hypothermia, and hypoglycemia. Portal hypertension during or after surgery, hemorrhage at liver biopsy site or during dissection, postsurgical sepsis, seizures, and recurrence of clinical signs are also possible. The most common complication after PSS ligation is abdominal distention, which may not need treatment if it is the only clinical abnormality.

16. What are the most common signs of postoperative portal hypertension? How should it be treated?

Clinical signs associated with portal hypertension include cardiovascular collapse, severe abdominal pain and distention, and delayed recovery from anesthesia. If clinical signs of portal hypertension occur after surgery, the patient requires supportive care and immediate surgical intervention to remove the ligature.

17. How is hepatic encephalopathy treated?

High-protein meals, constipation, infection, gastrointestinal hemorrhage, hypovolemia, hypokalemia, alkalosis, and hypoglycemia exacerbate neurologic signs in animals with PSS. Treatment, therefore, is aimed at correcting fluid deficits and electrolyte and or acid–base abnormalities, minimizing formation and absorption of ammonia and other toxins, and treating seizures. Administration of 0.9% sodium chloride with potassium supplementation helps to correct metabolic alkalosis and hypokalemia. Lactulose and either neomycin or metronidazole should be administered to conscious animals to increase intestinal transit time and to trap ammonium ions in the bowel. In comatose cats, lactulose or 10% povidone-iodine enemas should be given. Cats with seizures at the time of presentation should be treated parenterally to stop seizure activity.

18. What is the prognosis for a patient with PSS?

Although several different patterns of abnormal portosystemic vasculature connections have been described in dogs, the most common anomaly in cats is a single extrahepatic shunt. A single extrahepatic shunt in canine patients carries a good prognosis with surgical correction, but in cats this does not appear to be the case. Because of postoperative complications and decreased ability of the liver to accommodate the increased hepatic blood flow, the prognosis for PSS with surgery is less favorable in cats than in dogs.

BIBLIOGRAPHY

1. Holt D: Critical care management of the portosystemic shunt patient. Comp Cont Educ Pract Vet 16:879–889, 1994.
2. Holt DE, Schellin CG, Saunders MH, et al: Correction of ultrasonographic findings with surgical, porto-graphic, and necropsy findings in dogs and cats with portosystemic shunts: 63 cases (1987–1993). J Am Vet Med Assoc 207:1190–1193, 1995.
3. Koblik PD, Hornorf WJ: Transcolonic sodium pertechnetate Tc 99m scintigraphy for diagnosis of macrovascular portosystemic shunts in dogs, cats, and potbellied pigs: 176 cases (1988–1992). J Am Vet Med Assoc 207:729–732, 1995.
4. Lamb CR, Forester-van Hijfte MA, White RN, et al: Ultrasonographic diagnosis of congenital portosys-temic shunt in 14 cats. J Small Anim Pract 37:205–209, 1996.
5. Leveille-Webster CR: Disease of the hepatobiliary system. In Morgan RV (ed): Handbook of Small Animal Practice, 3rd ed. Philadelphia, W.B. Saunders, 1997, pp 383–401.
6. Martin RA: Congenital portosystemic shunts in the dog and cat. Vet Clin North Am 23:609–623, 1993.
7. Moon M: Diagnostic imaging of portosystemic shunts. Semin Vet Med Surg (Small Animal) 5:120–126, 1990.
8. Payne JT, Martin RA, Constantinescu GM: The anatomy and embryology of portosystemic shunts in dogs and cats. Semin Vet Med Surg (Small Animal) 5:76–82, 1990.
9. Swalec TK, Besser TE: Evaluation of leukocytosis, bacteremia, and portal vein partial oxygen tension in clinically normal dogs and dogs with portosystemic shunts. J Am Vet Med Assoc 211:715–718, 1997.
10. Swalec T, Karen M, Rawlings CA: Surgical techniques for extravascular occlusion of intrahepatic shunts. Comp Cont Educ Prac Vet 8:745–754, 1996.
11. Swalec T, Karen M, Seguin B, et al: Surgical approaches to single extrahepatic portosystemic shunts. Comp Cont Educ Prac Vet 20:593–601, 1998.
12. VanGundy TE, Boothe HW, Wolf A: Results of surgical management of feline portosystemic shunts. J Amr Anim Hosp Assoc 26:5–62, 1990.
13. Vogt JC, Krahwinkel DJ, Bright RM, et al: Gradual occlusion of extrahepatic portosystemic shunts in dogs and cats using the ameroid constrictor. Vet Surg 25:495–502, 1996.
14. White RN, Trower ND, McEvoy FJ, et al: A method for controlling portal pressure after attenuation of intrahepatic portacaval shunts. Vet Surg 25:407–413, 1996.
15. Whiting PG, Peterson SL: Portosystemic shunts. In Slatter (ed): Textbook of Small Animal Surgery, vol. 1, 2nd ed. Philadelphia, W.B. Saunders, 1993, pp 660–677.

36. PANCREATIC DISEASE

Margie Scherk, D.V.M.

1. Which pancreatic diseases occur in cats?

For years, feline pancreatic diseases were assumed to be similar to those in dogs. Currently, it appears that pancreatic disorders are quite different in cats. Overall, acute septicemic pancreatitis and exocrine pancreatic insufficiency (EPI) are much less common in cats than in dogs. Chronic nonsuppurative and suppurative pancreatitis are the most common forms. The most common pancreatic neoplasms include primary pancreatic adenocarcinoma as well as metastatic lymphosarcoma and mast cell tumor. Pancreatic abscesses are occasionally found. *Toxoplasma gondii, Eurytrema procyonis* (liver fluke), feline infectious peritonitis, feline parvovirus, and herpesvirus 1 can infect the pancreas. However, more than 90% of cases of feline pancreatitis are idiopathic.

2. What forms of pancreatitis are seen in cats?

Both acute and chronic pancreatitis are reported. Although both can be mild or severe, acute cases tend to be more severe than chronic cases. Mild pancreatitis generally results in minimal clinical signs, minimal necrosis, and low mortality rates In severe pancreatitis (necrotizing, hemmorhagic), extensive pancreatic necrosis and multiple-organ involvement with or without organ failure lead to a poor prognosis. Fortunately, this form is rare in cats.

Pancreatitis in cats is usually either suppurative (neutrophilic) or nonsuppurative (lympho-cytic/plasmacytic or eosinophilic). These disorders may be discrete or occur in conjunction with idiopathic inflammatory bowel disease, cholangitis/cholangiohepatitis complex, or both (triaditis). See Chapters 23 and 29 for a further discussion of triaditis.

3. What are the clinical findings of pancreatitis?

Presenting complaints are vague and may include lethargy, inappetence, weight loss, vomiting, diarrhea, abdominal pain, and ataxia. On physical examination, dehydration, hypothermia, weight loss, lethargy, icterus, and abdominal pain, which may be localized to the right anterior quadrant, are often detected. Pleural and peritoneal effusion rarely occur but can result in abdominal distention or dyspnea.

4. What is the initial diagnostic plan for cats with suspected pancreatitis?

Complete blood cell count with differential, serum biochemical panel, urinalysis, and blood pressure evaluation are usually performed in sick cats but do not show pathognomonic changes for pancreatic disease. An inflammatory leukogram, which indicates inflammation, infection, or an immune-mediated process, may be present, depending on the form of pancreatitis and degree of chronicity. In addition, mild, nonregenerative anemia (anemia of chronic disease) and hyperproteinemia occur in some cats with chronic inflammation. Changes in liver enzyme activities and other serum biochemical abnormalities vary, depending on predisposing diseases and presence of cholangiohepatitis.

5. Can imaging techniques aid in the diagnosis of pancreatitis?

Abdominal radiographs may show decreased serosal detail in the right anterior quadrant and bunching of small bowel loops in cases of acute pancreatitis. Sonographic evaluation of the pancreas by an experienced ultrasonographer may help to identify pancreatic changes, to interpret active inflammation or fibrosis of the pancreas, and to note other changes in adjacent viscera. Ultrasound may detect small amounts of fluid, which can aspirated for fluid analysis.

6. Are concurrent disorders common?

Many cats with pancreatitis have other diseases. Hepatic lipidosis, cholangitis/cholangiohepatitis, idiopathic inflammatory bowel disease, enteritis, diabetes mellitus, and vitamin K_1-responsive coagulopathy are common. Cats with hepatic lipidosis and pancreatitis have a poorer prognosis than cats with lipidosis alone.

7. Are serum amylase and lipase concentrations predictive of pancreatitis?

Not really. Amylase is a nonspecific gastrointestinal (GI) enzyme in cats; it may be elevated because of disease in other parts of the GI tract. In addition, amylase is excreted by the kidneys; decreased renal clearance (dehydration, concurrent renal disease) causes elevations of serum amylase. Thus, increased amylase activity does not correlate with the presence of pancreatic inflammation. Lipase is similar to amylase, but an elevated level is usually significant. The pancreas should be assessed with other tests, such as ultrasound or serum trypsin-like immunoreactivity (TLI). Unfortunately, many cats with pancreatitis have normal amylase and lipase activities.

8. Can abdominal effusion aid in the diagnosis of pancreatitis?

If abdominal effusion is present, routine cytologic evaluation should be performed. Most effusions are nonseptic suppurative exudates with increased protein concentrations and a mixture of degenerate neutrophils, nondegenerate neutrophils, and macrophages. It has been proposed that if lipase or amylase activities are greater in abdominal effusion than in serum, pancreatitis is present.

9. How does serum TLI aid in the diagnosis of pancreatic diseases?

Theoretically, serum TLI concentrations increase with inflammatory diseases of the pancreas and are decreased with EPI. However, serum TLI frequently fails to correlate with presence of chronic pancreatitis in cats.

10. How can suppurative and nonsuppurative pancreatitis be differentiated?

Histopathologic evaluation of pancreatic tissues is the only way to confirm and classify pancreatitis. Because triaditis is common, liver and small intestinal biopsies are often obtained at the same time (see Chapters 23 and 29). Pancreatic biopsies can be obtained via laparotomy or laparoscopy. The pancreas should be isolated gently, and 3–4-mm wedge samples should be taken from abnormal-appearing areas or from both left and right poles of the pancreas with small, sharp scissors such as iris scissors. Overall, laparoscopy-obtained biopsies are less invasive, but the areas of the pancreas that can be sampled are limited.

11. How is the pain associated with pancreatitis treated?

Regardless of the type, pancreatitis is painful. Use an opioid such as oxymorphone, hydromorphone, or morphine. Butorphanol is less effective for visceral analgesia. If the patient appears to benefit from a test dose of opioid, consider application of a transdermal fentanyl patch (Duragesic, Janssen Phamaceutical, Titusville, NJ). Analgesia is required for a number of days, and the continuous release by a transdermal patch avoids peak and trough levels of opioid. Do not make patients show you that they are in pain.

Analgesics Used in the Treatment of Pancreatitis

GENERIC NAME	TRADE NAME	DOSE
Butorphanol	Torbugesic	0.1–0.8 mg/kg every 4 hr IV, IM, SQ
Hydromorphone	Dilaudid	0.08–0.2 mg/kg every 4 hr IV, IM, SQ
Morphine	Morphine sulfate	0.1–0.4 mg/kg every 4hr IV, IM, SQ
Oxymorphone	Numorphan	0.025–0.1 mg/kg every 4 hr IV, IM, SQ

IV = intravenously, IM = intramuscularly, SQ = subcutaneously.

12. What antiemitics should be used?

Antiemetics should be used as indicated clinically; in cats with concurrent hepatic dysfunction, doses should be reduced accordingly. Antiemetics commonly used in the cat include metoclopramide and clorpromazine. Each has its side effects. Central nervous system sedation, frenzied behavior, or disorientation may be associated with metoclopramide, and chlorpromazine has a hypotensive effect. While costly, ondansentron is quite beneficial in the patient with intractable vomiting.

Antiemetics Used in the Treatment of Pancreatitis

GENERIC NAME	TRADE NAME	DOSE
Chlorpromazine	Thorazine, Largactil	0.5 mg/kg every 8hr IM
Prochlorpromazine	Compazine	0.1 mg/kg every 6 hr IM
Diphenhydramine	Benadryl	2.0–4.0 mg/kg every 8hr PO
		2.0 mg/kg every 8 hr IM
Dimenhydrinate	Dramamine	8.0 mg/kg every 8 hr PO
Prochlorpromazine + isopropamide	Darbazine	0.5–0.8 mg/kg every 12 hr IM, SQ
Metoclopramide	Reglan	1–2 mg/kg constant-rate IV infusion over 24 hr
Ondansentron	Zofran	0.1–0.15 mg/kg slow IV push every 6–12 hr, as needed

IM = intramuscularly, PO = orally, SQ = subcutaneously, IV = intravenous.
Adapted from Ogilvie G: Presentation at the Fall Meeting of the American Association of Feline Practitioners, 1997, with permission.

13. Describe the approach to nutritional support in cats with pancreatitis.

Nutritional support is critical even in the acute phase. In acute pancreatitis, total or partial parenteral nutrition may be required. If exploratory laparotomy for biopsies and lavage is performed, jejunal and gastric feeding tubes should be placed. Jejunal feeding should be given during the acute phase (see Chapter 62) because stimulation of pancreatic secretion is less likely than with use of a gastrostomy tube.

14. What other nonspecific treatments are used for acute pancreatitis?
- Fluid therapy with appropriate electrolyte adjustments and water-soluble vitamins is essential.
- If hypoalbuminemia develops, colloid support is indicated.
- Dopamine administered at a constant-rate infusion of 3 µg/kg/min improved pancreatic perfusion in a model of alcoholic pancreatitis in cats.

15. How is suppurative pancreatitis treated?
A quinolone combined with a penicillin or metronidazole should be administered empirically while you wait for bacterial culture and antimicrobial susceptibility results. Antimicrobial choices are then based on the results and administered for at least 6–8 weeks.

16. How is nonsuppurative pancreatitis treated?
1. **Prednisolone or another glucocorticoid** is the cornerstone of therapy for lymphocytic/plasmacytic disorders in cats. As with inflammatory bowel disease, it is important to start with a high enough dose to suppress the inflammatory response. A reasonable starting dose of prednisolone is 2–4 mg/kg orally every 12 hours for 1 month or until clinical remission occurs. The dose is then tapered to once every 48 hours for 2–3 months (see Chapter 23).

2. Metronidazole can be used concurrently for its anaerobic spectrum as well as its immune-modulating properties. At oral doses of 10 mg/kg every 12 hours, it can be used for long periods (months).

3. With lymphocytic/plasmacytic disorders, it is best to eliminate allergens whenever possible as well as to modulate immune response. Thus, an **enteric bland diet**, which has limited antigens and low residue and is calorie-dense, is recommended once the patient is eating well. Some of these diets may include omega-6 and omega-3 fatty acids in a 5:1 ratio, which has an anti-inflammatory effect. Protein restriction is not required unless the patient is encephalopathic. The fact that the cat eats is more important than what the cat eats (see Chapter 62).

17. Describe the treatment of pancreatitis induced by *Toxoplasma gondii*.
Pancreatitis induced by *T. gondii* is almost never documented on antemortem evaluation. Increasing IgG titers or high IgM titers suggest acute infection. The organism can be identified on histologic examination of pancreatic tissue. If it is suspected, clindamycin (10–12 mg/kg orally every12 hr) may be an effective treatment (see Chapter 36).

18. Describe the treatment of pancreatitis induced by *Eurytrema procyonis* and *Amphimerus pseudofelineus*.
E. procyonis may infest the pancreatic duct, whereas *A. pseudofelineus* may infest the pancreas itself. The diagnosis is made by finding the eggs on examination of fresh feces using formalin-ethyl sedimentation. Fenbendazole (30 mg/kg orally every 24 hr for 6 days) is recommended for treatment of E. procyonis; praziquantal has been used at a very high dose (40 mg/kg orally every 24 hr for 3 days) to treat *A. pseudofelineus*. *E. procyonis* may be considered when cats are exposed to raccoons or foxes.

19. How is therapeutic response monitored?
Cessation of vomiting and diarrhea are obvious signs of improvement. If lesions were initially present, repeat ultrasound examination can provide objective evidence of disease resolution. If CBC or biochemical abnormalities were present, resolution suggests improvement. Client and clinician evaluations are subjectively valuable; concrete assessments of body weight, muscle tone, coat condition, activity level, attitude, and appetite are also helpful.

20. What is the prognosis for cats with pancreatitis?
Prognosis depends on the type of pancreatitis as well as duration and severity. Many cats have chronic, low-grade smoldering pancreatitides and live long lives, but they do better with diagnosis and appropriate therapy.

21. Does chronic pancreatitis predispose to other clinical syndromes?

• Untreated nonsuppurative pancreatitis has the potential to develop into acute necrotizing pancreatitis.
• Type I diabetes mellitus may develop as a result of loss of beta cells.
• Exocrine pancreatic insufficiency (EPI) may result from loss of acinar tissue.
• Chronic lymphocytic plasmacytic inflammation may progress to small cell lymphoma in some patients (controversial).

22. Is EPI common in cats?

Congenital EPI is rare in cats compared with dogs. Occasionally EPI results from chronic pancreatitis.

23. Describe the clinical findings of EPI.

If active pancreatitis is not present, most cats have polyphagia with failure to thrive or weight loss and poor coats. The stool is often voluminous and may appear as undigested food; diarrhea may be present.

24. How is EPI diagnosed?

Increased neutral fats are present when stool is evaluated microscopically with Sudan IV stain. Fecal trypsin, as assessed by gel digestion, should be decreased, but this finding is not specific for EPI. Serum TLI concentrations should be decreased, but this parameter has not been used to assess large numbers of cats with EPI. Serum cobalamin and folate levels are expected to be subnormal in most cases.

25. How is EPI treated?

High-fat foods should be avoided. Pancreatic enzyme replacement is added to food to effect. Preincubation with the food for 15–30 minutes before feeding may be beneficial.

26. What is the prognosis for cats with pancreatic neoplasms?

The management and prognosis of pancreatic lymphosarcoma are similar to those described for alimenteric lymphosarcoma (see Chapter 24). Because there is no effective therapy for adenocarcinoma, the prognosis is guarded.

BIBLIOGRAPHY

1. Akol KG, Washabau RJ, Saunders HM, et al: Acute pancreatitis in cats with hepatic lipidosis. J Vet Intern Med 7:205–209, 1993.
2. Hill RC, Van Winkle TJ: Acute necrotizing pancreatitis and acute suppurative pancreatitis in the cat: A retrospective study of 40 cases (1976–1989). J Vet Intern Med 7:34–39, 1993.
3. Mathews KA: Pain assessment and general approach to management. Vet Clin North Am Small Animal Pract 30:729–755, 2000.
4. Parent C, Washabau RJ, Williams DA, et al: Serum trypsin-like immunoreactivity, amylase and lipase in the diagnosis of feline pancreatitis. Proceedings of 13th Annual Forum of the American College of Veterinary Internal Medicine, 1995.
5. Pascoe PJ: Opioid analgesics. Vet Clin North Am Small Animal Pract 30:757–772, 2000.
6. Steiner JM, Williams DA: Feline pancreatitis. Compend Contin Educ Pract Vet 19:590–603, 1997.
7. Steiner JM, Williams DA: Feline exocrine pancreatic disorders. Vet Clin North Am Small Anim Pract 29:551–575, 1999.
8. Stewart AF: Pancreatitis in dogs and cats: Cause, pathogenesis, diagnosis, and treatment. Compend Contin Educ Pract Vet 16:1423–1430, 1994.
9. Swift NC, Marks SL, MacLachlan NJ, et al: Evaluation of serum feline trypsin-like immunoreactivity for the diagnosis of pancreatitis in cats. J Am Vet Med Assoc 217:37–42, 2000.
10. Washabau R: The vomiting cat. Presented at the Waltham Feline Medicine Symposium, 1997.
11. Weiss DJ, Gagne JM, Armstrong PJ: Relationship between inflammatory hepatic disease and inflammatory bowel disease, pancreatitis, and nephritis in cats. J Am Vet Med Assoc 209:1114–1116, 1996.

37. ABDOMINAL DISTENTION AND ASCITES

Michael R. Lappin, D.V.M., Ph.D.

1. Define abdominal distention.
Abdominal distention is defined as a sudden or gradual increase in the size of the abdomen.

2. What causes abdominal distention?
Major differential groups include fluid accumulation, organomegaly, masses in the peritoneal cavity not involving organs (including obesity), and muscle weakness (usually associated with hyperadrenocorticism).

3. What are the principal fluid accumulations resulting in abdominal distention?
The most common abnormal fluid accumulations include blood, urine, ascites, exudates, and chyle (rare).

4. Define ascites.
Ascites is an abnormal accumulation of a transudate (low protein concentration) or modified transudate (high protein concentration) in the peritoneal cavity.

5. What are the primary differentials for hemoabdomen?
Organ or vessel ruptures are common causes of hemoabdomen and usually result from trauma, tumors, or torsions of the stomach and spleen. Although tumors (mainly of the liver and/or spleen) and trauma are possible causes of hemoabdomen in cats, torsions are extremely rare. The other major differential diagnosis for hemoabdomen is coagulopathy. Factor deficiencies such as those associated with warfarin toxicity are most common (see Chapter 71). Thrombocytopenia, platelet function abnormalities, vasculitis, and systemic arterial hypertension usually do not cause hemoabdomen.

6. What are the primary differentials for uroabdomen?
Uroabdomen results most commonly from rupture of the bladder due to trauma, neoplasia, or obstruction. Diseases associated with urine leakage from the kidneys, ureters, or urethra result in retroperitoneal leakage of fluid; if the peritoneum is also damaged, uroabdomen results.

7. What causes transudative ascites?
Transudates have low protein concentrations (< 2.5 gm/dl) and small numbers of cells (< 1000/µl). Abdominal effusions in this category are associated most commonly with decreased oncotic pressure due to hypoalbuminemia. Hypoalbuminemia is associated most frequently with renal loss, decreased hepatic production, gastrointestinal loss, starvation, and third spacing into tissues or body cavities. In rare cases, sustained portal hypertension from chronic liver diseases results in transudative ascites.

8. What causes ascites due to modified transudates?
Modified transudates have moderate protein concentrations (2.5–6.0 gm/dl) and moderate numbers of cells (250–20,000/µl). Right-sided congestive heart failure is a common cause in dogs but a rare cause in cats. Pericardial disease or obstruction of the caudal vena cava or hepatic vein can lead to vascular congestion of the liver and leakage of high-protein fluid from hepatic lymph vessels. In some cases, neoplasia, chyloperitoneum, and inflammatory diseases such as feline infectious peritonitis are classified as modified transudates based on cell and protein concentrations. However, other findings usually support the primary diagnosis. For example, neoplastic cells are often detected cytologically; triglycerides are elevated in chylous effusions.

9. What are the most common causes of exudative peritoneal effusion?

Exudates have high protein concentrations (> 3.5 gm/dl) and high numbers of cells (> 30,000/μl). Most cases result from infectious inflammatory diseases (feline infectious peritonitis [FIP], bacterial peritonitis from penetrating wounds, bowel rupture) or from diseases resulting in chemical irritation (pancreatitis, leakage of bile, leakage of urine).

10. What types of diseases result in organomegaly?

Organs can become enlarged when masses develop. Tumors, abscesses, granulomas, cysts, and hemotoma are the most common mass lesions. Congestion of the liver and spleen can cause organomegaly. Gastric or intestinal distention due to ileus, parasites, or obstructive diseases are other causes of organomegaly. Torsion of the stomach or spleen also may result in abdominal distention.

11. How is the initial differential list for abdominal distention determined?

Signalment, history, and physical examination are used initially. For example, young inbred cats from crowded environments most commonly develop effusive FIP; uveitis and fever may be detected. FIP, neoplasia and pancreatitis are the most likely causes of concurrent pleural effusion. Uroabdomen and hemoabdomen are commonly associated with trauma and are usually acute. Hypoalbuminemia associated with gastrointestinal (GI) loss is most often chronic and accompanied by a history of GI signs such as vomiting or diarrhea. Hypoalbuminemia associated with hepatic failure usually is chronic and has other signs, including hepatic encephalopathy and weight loss. Trauma, pancreatitis, exudates, and torsions usually have abdominal pain. A fluid wave can generally be balloted when abdominal distention is severe enough to be visible. Extreme abdominal distention with a fluid wave in a cat with minimal other clinical signs is more likely ascites than hemoperitoneum, uroabdomen, or exudates. Increased respiratory rate may result from diaphragmatic impingement. Polysystemic signs such as fever (exudates), pain (trauma, exudates), weakness (blood loss, heart failure), dermatologic changes (hyperadrenocorticism), and polyuria/polydipsia (hyperadrenocorticism) may help to differentiate causes of abdominal distention.

12. Describe the initial diagnostic plan for evaluating cats with abdominal distention.

Abdominal pericentesis is the logical first diagnostic procedure if a fluid wave is balloted. Because a large volume of fluid is required to result in abdominal distention, a single, midline aspirate is adequate. Four-quadrant abdominal pericentesis is indicated when a single midline tap is negative. It is better to use the linea alba for needle penetration because fewer sensory nerve endings are involved and, if a coagulopathy is present, hematomas are less likely to develop than if muscle is penetrated. Fluid should be placed onto a sterile swab and into transport media for possible culture and sensitivity and into an EDTA tube for fluid analysis; for cytologic assessment, it should be applied to a microscope slide in a thin smear. If the fluid is red, packed cell volume and total protein assessment should be performed and compared with peripheral blood to assess whether a vessel was hit or whether hemoabdomen exists. Remove only enough fluid for diagnostic testing and to relieve diaphragmatic impingement if dyspnea is present. If it is unclear whether fluid is present, abdominal radiographs should be taken.

13. What additional diagnostic tests are used for cats with organomegaly?

Additional tests depend on which organ is enlarged and the primary diseases suspected. For renal, splenic, and hepatic masses, complete blood count (CBC), serum biochemical panel, and urinalysis are usually performed. Ultrasound is often performed to evaluate enlarged parenchymal organs. Barium series are indicated if obstructive GI tract disease is suspected but cannot be confirmed by usual assessment of plain abdominal radiographs. Fecal examination is indicated in some animals, particularly kittens with possible toxocariasis. Laparoscopy or exploratory laparotomy can be used to evaluate enlarged organs and to obtain biopsies. Exploratory laparotomy should be performed if the mass can be excised.

14. Describe the additional diagnostic work-up for cats with transudates.

CBC, serum biochemical panel, and urinalysis should be performed to determine whether hypoalbuminemia is present and to assess for a site of potential loss. If hypoalbuminemia is present, assessment of serum globulin concentrations can be beneficial. Renal loss usually results in proteinuria with normal serum globulin concentrations. The further diagnostic plan usually includes the urine protein/creatinine ratio, renal ultrasound, and a search for potential causes of glomerulonephritis. Potential tests may include an antinuclear antibody titer, *Dirofilaria immitis* antigen and antibody testing, and renal biopsy. Decreased hepatic production of albumin usually has normal-to-increased serum globulin concentrations. Pre- and postprandial bile acid measurement, hepatic ultrasound, and hepatic biopsy are used for further assessment of hepatic diseases associated with transudative ascites. When GI diseases result in hypoalbuminemia, serum globulin concentrations are usually decreased as well. Rectal cytology, fecal examination, fecal fats, trypsin-like immunoreactivity, barium series, endoscopy, and exploratory laparotomy for biopsies are examples of tests used to evaluate causes of protein-losing enteropathies. If hypoalbuminemia is not present, the liver should be evaluated for potential causes of protracted portal hypertension by use of bile acid assessment, ultrasound, and, potentially, biopsy.

15. What additional diagnostic tests are used for cats with modified transudates?

Modified transduate should be examined cytologically to rule out neoplasia. If chyloperitoneum is suspected, triglyceride concentrations should be measured. Most cats with disease cranial to the liver have hepatomegaly. If cardiac tamponade is occurring, jugular pulses and jugular distention may be present; thoracic radiographs, cardiac ultrasound, and measurement of central venous pressure are indicated. If cardiac causes of the modified transudate are eliminated, CBC, serum biochemical panel, and urinalysis are indicated to evaluate other possible primary causes. Abdominal ultrasound, laparoscopy, or exploratory laparotomy often is needed to identify the primary cause.

16. Describe the additional diagnostic work-up for cats with exudates.

If an exudate is detected, CBC, serum biochemical panel, and urinalysis often are performed to evaluate for primary causes. Peritoneal effusion and serum lipase activities should be compared; the abdominal fluid lipase activity is usually greater if pancreatitis is present. If uroabdomen is suspected, creatinine and urea nitrogen concentrations in the abdominal fluid should be measured and compared with serum concentrations. Abdominal ultrasound often is indicated if a cytologic diagnosis cannot be made. If the exudate is septic or contains bile, immediate exploratory laparotomy is indicated. If the fluid has high protein concentration but only moderate increases in mature neutrophils and macrophages, FIP is likely. The albumin-to-globulin ratio of the fluid should be evaluated. Values < 0.4 suggest FIP, whereas values > 0.8 suggest that another disease is present.

17. What additional diagnostic tests are used for cats with hemoabdomen?

If trauma is not obvious, coagulopathy should be excluded by measuring an activated clotting time (or other factor tests, such as prothrombin time or activated partial thromboplastin time) and platelet count. Organ-associated bleeding is evaluated by ultrasound, laparoscopy, or exploratory laparotomy.

18. What additional diagnostic tests are used for cats with suspected myopathy associated with hyperadrenocorticism?

Exogenous glucocorticoid administration should be excluded by history. Naturally occurring hyperadrenocorticism is excluded by a combination of blood tests and imaging techniques (see Chapter 54).

19. How should abdominal distention be treated?

The treatment plan is based on the primary diagnosis. Palliative treatments include rest, delivery of oxygen, and therapeutic abdominal pericentesis to relieve diaphragmatic impingement.

BIBLIOGRAPHY

1. Cornelius LM: Abdominal distension. In Lorenz MD, Cornelius LM (eds); Small Animal Medical Diagnosis, 2nd ed. Philadelphia, J.B. Lippincott, 1993, pp 73–77.
2. Kruth SA: Abdominal distention, ascites, and peritonitis. In Ettinger JJ, Feldman EC (eds): Textbook of Veterinary Internal Medicine, 5th ed. Philadelphia, W.B. Saunders, 2000, pp 137–139.

38. FELINE INFECTIOUS PERITONITIS

Michelle L. Berry, D.V.M.

1. Define feline infectious peritonitis.

Feline infectious peritonitis (FIP) is a disseminated disease caused by feline coronaviruses (FCoV). Field strains of FCoV vary in disease-inducing potential. Some isolates cause FIP (feline infectious peritonitis virus [FIPV]), and some isolates cause a more localized gastrointestinal disturbance that often results in diarrhea (feline enteric coronavirus [FECV]). These two strains cannot be distinguished from one another morphologically or antigenically. FECV can mutate spontaneously in the host to become a FIP-inducing stain.

2. How do cats become infected with FCoV?

Cats usually become infected with FCoV by ingestion of virus, but inhalation may provide viral entrance. Because cats shed viral particles in feces, litterbox exposure and mutual grooming are probably the most important sources of infection. Cats living in multiple cat households or having exposure to multiple cats are at a greater risk of contracting FCoV and, as a result, FIP, in part because of higher levels of virus exposure and probably a higher level of stress.

3. Why is disease limited to enteric signs in some cats, whereas others develop FIP?

Both viral strain factors and host factors may play a role. FECV attaches to an enzyme in the intestinal brush border and replicates in enterocytes. This process causes the villous tips to slough, and diarrhea ensues, which usually is self-limiting. If the cat is exposed to FIPV or if FECV mutates to FIPV, the organism is able to replicate in enterocytes and macrophages. Disseminated infection can then occur. Genetic predispositions also are suspected. Host-derived immunity also may play a role in resistance to development of FIP.

4. Describe the typical presentation for a cat with FIP.

Cats with FIP can present for evaluation of many clinical syndromes. Anorexia is common, but some cats have a normal appetite. Ascites may be the only clinical sign. Historically, the cat is usually young, lives in a multicat household or cattery, and has been recently stressed with a new environment, surgery, or illness. The history may include diarrhea, lethargy, weight loss, or inappetence. Many cats present with a low-grade fever unresponsive to antibiotics. The clinical disease of FIP has two primary clinical forms, the effusive (wet) form and the noneffusive (dry) form. The most common historical and physical examination findings of noneffusive FIP relate to organomegaly and resultant organ failure. Hepatic, ocular, renal, alimenteric, and central nervous system dysfunction are common. Clinical manifestations of the effusive form relate to the development of body cavity effusions. A distended abdomen due to ascites and dyspnea and muffled heart and lung sounds due to pleural effusion are common. Although these distinctions are useful in diagnosing the disease and recognizing signs, they are not mutually exclusive; an individual cat can have manifestions of both forms. Some cats may initially have manifestations most consistent with the noneffusive form and later become effusive or vice versa.

Clinical Abnormalities Suggestive of Feline Infectious Peritonitis

Signalment and history

Cats < 3 years of age or > 10 years of age
Purebred cat
Purchase from a crowded cat environment
Previous history of gastrointestinal or upper respiratory disease
Serologic evidence of infection by feline leukemia virus
Nonspecific signs of anorexia, weight loss, or depression
Seizures, nystagmus, or ataxia
Acute, fulminant course in cats with effusive disease
Chronic, intermittent course in cats with noneffusive disease

Physical examination

Fever
Weight loss
Pale mucous membranes with or without petechiae
Dyspnea with a restrictive breathing pattern
Muffled heart or lung sounds
Abdominal distention with a fluid wave with or without scrotal swelling
Icterus with or without hepatomegaly
Chorioretinitis or iridocyclitis
Multifocal neurologic abnormalities
Irregularly marginated kidneys with or without renomegaly
Mesenteric lymphadenopathy
Splenomegaly

Clinicopathologic abnormalities

Nonregenerative anemia
Neutrophilic leukocytosis with or without a left shift
Lymphopenia
Hyperglobulinemia characterized as a polyclonal gammopathy with increases in $alpha_2$ and
    gammaglobulins; rare monoclonal gammopathies
Nonseptic, pyogranulomatous exudate in pleural space, peritoneal cavity, or pericardial
    space
Increased protein concentrations and neutrophilic pleocytosis in cerebrospinal fluid
Positive coronavirus antibody titer
Pyogranulomatous or granulomatous inflammation in perivascular location on histologic
    examination of tissues
Positive results of immunofluorescence or polymerase chain reaction performed on pleural
    or peritoneal exudate

---

5. What are the neurologic manifestations of FIP?

Some studies estimate that 12–35% of cats with FIP have neurologic signs. These numbers vary widely among institutions and possibly are affected by a skewed population. Some cats may show only central neurologic signs. The most common neurologic signs associated with FIP are ataxia, followed by nystagmus and seizures. Other neurologic signs depend on the location of the granuloma or whether the virus is causing meningitis.

6. What are the most common ocular manifestations of FIP?

Uveitis can be detected in cats with either form of disease, but it is thought to be more common in cats with noneffusive FIP. The most common ocular sign in FIP is iritis, which manifests as a color change (see Chapter 67). Keratic precipitates also may be seen because large numbers of inflammatory cells settle on the back of the cornea. Chorioretinitis due to vasculitis is recognized in some affected cats.

7. Why do effusions form in some cases of FIP?

When the organism is disseminating in infected macrophages, the body responds with antibody production, resulting in complement activation. It is hypothesized that the combination of viral particles or antigens bind to antibody, resulting in complement fixation and circulating immune complexes, which attach to blood vessels and cause severe vasculitis. It is also possible that complement is fixed to immune complexes in tissues. Vasculitis results in leakage of high protein fluids from affected organs; common sites of leakage are the peritoneum, kidney, and uvea. Exudation of fluid and plasma proteins occurs primarily in body cavities, resulting in ascites and pleural effusion. Cats developing the effusive form of disease may have poor cell-mediated immune responses.

8. Describe the pathophysiology of the noneffusive form of FIP.

It is hypothesized that the noneffusive form of FIP occurs in cats that are capable of mounting a partial cell-mediated immune response that does not totally contain the infection. Effusion may be less likely because less virus is available for the formation of immune complexes, resulting in less severe vasculitis. When circulating or tissue-associated immune complexes fix complement, neutrophils and macrophages are attracted to the involved organs and pyogranulomatous inflammation develops. Pyogranulomatous inflammation may become severe enough to cause organ dysfunction or failure.

9. At what age are cats more likely to develop FIP?

FIP is said to be a disease of the very young and the very old. Newborn kittens usually are protected by maternal antibodies that last for the first few weeks of life. As maternal antibody protection fades, the kittens are susceptible to infection. The most common age range for cats with FIP is 3 months to 3 years. Another peak in susceptibility occurs in cats older than 10 years, presumably because of an age-related decline in immune responses.

10. What is the relation between FIP and feline leukemia virus?

Previously it was believed that feline leukemia virus (FeLV) compromised the immune system and facilitated development of FIP. If this were true, it seems likely that the dramatic decrease in the incidence of FeLV would be accompanied by a parallel decrease in the incidence of FIP. Because the incidence of FIP has remained the same despite a decrease in the incidence of FeLV, the correlation between the two viruses is much weaker than once imagined.

11. How is FIP diagnosed?

Histology of affected tissues is considered the only way to reach an indisputable diagnosis of FIP. Immunohistochemical staining of tissues allows identification of viral antigen associated with inflammation and therefore provides a specific diagnosis.

12. How can effusions be used to aid in the diagnosis of FIP?

If the cat has ascites or pleural effusion, centesis and fluid analysis are valuable diagnostic tools. Typically the fluid is pale yellow and has increased viscosity. Evaluation of protein content yields a total protein > 3.5 gm/dl, over 50% of which is composed of gammaglobulins. Cytology of the fluid reveals an exudate with cellularity (< 5000 cells/μl) consisting primarily of nondegenerative neutrophils. In rare cases, the effusion is pink and chylous. With a combination of the above protein content, globulin predominance, and cytology, the positive predictive value for diagnosis of FIP based on fluid analysis is > 90%. In addition, the albumin-to-globulin ratio of the effusion is usually < 0.8; a ratio < 0.45 is usually predictive of effusive FIP. Documentation of coronaviral RNA by reverse transcriptase polymerase chain reaction (see question 15) supports the diagnosis of effusive FIP.

13. Can noneffusive FIP be diagnosed without obtaining tissue?

Clinicians strive to arrive at a diagnosis with less invasive methods because of the patient's often compromised condition. The noninvasive approach to diagnosis can prove to be difficult.

Currently no single test of serum or effusion fluid can give a definitive diagnosis of FIP; there-fore, the clinician must rely on careful history and observation, thorough physical examination, and multiple diagnostic tests. If the history and physical examination are suggestive of FIP, diagnostic tests can aid in confirmation.

Cats with clinical signs consistent with FIP and the combination of lymphopenia ($< 1.5 \times$ 103 cells/µl), FCoV antibody titer $> 1:160$, and hyperglobulinemia (> 5.1 gm/dl) have an 88.9% probability of having FIP. If the cat has clinical signs of FIP but does not have all three of the above diagnostic criteria, there is a 98.8% probability that the cat does *not* have FIP. Therefore, these tests can be quite helpful in excluding the diagnosis of FIP.

In cats with neurologic FIP, cerebrospinal fluid (CSF) analysis can provide helpful informa-tion to aid in diagnosis. CSF analysis in cats with neurologic FIP usually reveals increased protein concentrations and neutrophilic pleocytosis. Detection of coronavirus antibodies in CSF has not correlated consistently with a diagnosis of FIP and does not seem to correlate with serum titers.

14. What kind of serologic tests are available? How reliable are they in diagnosing FIP?

No available serologic test can differentiate between strains of FCoV. A positive test result reveals that the cat has been exposed to a coronavirus but does not predict that the cat will de-velop FIP. One study reported that cats with high coronavirus antibody titers had only a 38.9% probability of having FIP. In addition, cats that have been vaccinated for FIP can become seropositive. Although negative titers strongly suggest that the cat does not have FIP, some stud-ies have reported negative antibody titers in cats with histologically confirmed FIP. A possible explanation is that, with widespread immune complex formation, the antibody may be bound in the complex and prevented from reacting in the test. Alternatively, the cat may have had fulmi-nant FIP and died before mounting a humoral response. For these reasons, clinicians are urged not to rely on serology as a single diagnostic test. Many cats have been euthanized because of misconceptions about the validity of serologic tests as the sole determinant of disease.

15. What other tests are available for FIP?

Reverse transcriptase polymerase chain reaction (RT-PCR) test is available. Because coron-aviruses are RNA viruses, reverse transcriptase is used first to convert RNA to DNA. The DNA is then amplified in the polymerase chain reaction. Positive results of this test on whole blood may sup-port the diagnosis of FIP in a clinically ill, seronegative cat. However, as with serologic tests, RT-PCR does not distinguish between FCoV strains; a positive test indicates only exposure to a coronavirus. In one study, cats with enteric coronavirus infections were just as likely to be PCR-pos-itive as cats with FIP. In addition, false positives and false negatives have been reported. Whether RT-PCR performed on aqueous humor or CSF aids in the diagnosis of FIP is currently unknown.

16. What is the prognosis for cats with FIP?

Clinical FIP is almost always a fatal disease with a mortality rate $> 95\%$. Cats with the effu-sive form of FIP usually progress more quickly and often die within 2 months of initial clinical signs. The noneffusive form may run a slower course; some cats live for months to years.

17. What treatment is recommended for FIP?

Because FIP is an immune complex disease, immunosuppression is the mainstay of treatment. High doses of glucocorticoids are commonly used for their immunosuppressive and antiinflamma-tory properties. Cytotoxic drugs such as cyclophosphamide and chlorambucil have been used in con-junction with glucocorticoids. Success is greater with noneffusive FIP. Cats with effusive FIP are thought to have poor immunity and heavy viral load; glucocorticoid administration may exacerbate disease. In addition, although these drugs are needed to help control the immune response associated with clinical FIP, they also may cause susceptibility to bacterial infections due to myelosuppression and general immunosuppression. Therefore, broad-spectrum antibiotic therapy may be necessary as a prophylactic treatment. Reasonable choices include amoxicillin and cefadroxil. If an infection is documented, antibiotic selection should be based on culture and sensitivity.

18. What other drugs are used for treatment of FIP?

Antiviral drugs and immune-modulating drugs have been evaluated for the treatment of FIP. Recombinant human interferon-alpha has been given to cats in experimental settings and has slowed progression of disease. For debilitated cats with the effusive form, recombinant human interferon-alpha at high doses has been recommended. For cats with the noneffusive form, lower doses have been recommended. To date, no antiviral drugs have proved effective that can be tolerated by cats without severe side effects.

Treatment Recommendations for Feline Infectious Peritonitis

DRUG	DOSE
Immunosuppressive drugs	
Prednisolone	2–4 mg/kg orally every 24 hr
Cyclophosphamide	200-300 mg/m^2 orally every 2–3 wk *or*
	2.2 mg/kg every 24 hr for 4 consecutive days each week
or	
Chlorambucil	20 mg/m^2 orally every 2–3 wk
Antibiotic therapy	
Amoxicillin/clavulanic acid	10–20 mg/kg orally every 12 hr
or	
Cefadroxil	20 mg/kg orally every 12 hr
Immune-modulating drugs	
Recombinant human interferon-alpha	
Effusive form	2×10^4 IU/kg intramuscularly or subcutaneously every 24 hr for up to 3 wk
Noneffusive form	30 IU orally every 24 hr for life

19. What measures should be taken to aid in prevention of FIP?

Prevention strategies should be based on the housing and exposure possibilities of each patient. Cats living in a single cat household need a much less rigid prevention protocol than cats in a cattery or multiple cat household.

20. What prevention strategies are appropriate for seronegative single cat households?

Seronegative cats living in a single cat household are at low risk for developing FIP (incidence = 1 in 5000). Prevention is aimed at limiting exposure to other cats. Any new cat to be introduced to this household should be seronegative 30 days before entrance. Optimally, new cats should be quarantined for 3 weeks, then retested before free access to the household is given. Kittens should be tested after 12 weeks of age to allow time for clearance of lactationally derived antibodies and to allow seroconversion if they have been naturally exposed.

21. What prevention strategies are appropriate for seronegative multiple cat households?

Prevention is geared toward the same goal as the single cat seronegative household—limiting exposure. New additions to the household should be seronegative 30 days before entrance and should be quarantined for 3 weeks, then retested before gaining access to other cats in the household. Kittens should be tested at 12 weeks of age. Fecal contamination should be minimized by keeping food away from litterboxes and cleaning litterboxes daily.

22. Describe the appropriate prevention strategies for seropositive multiple cat households.

Decreasing stress and fecal-oral contamination are main concerns. Care should be taken to decrease fecal contamination of food by keeping food bowls and litterboxes in separate areas. Litterboxes should be cleaned daily and disinfected with a 1:32 dilution of bleach weekly. There should be one litterbox for every 1 or 2 cats. Cats should be kept in stable groups of three or four to decrease stress. In boarding or rescue facilities, cats should be housed singly.

23. Describe the appropriate prevention strategies for catteries.

In catteries or other breeding colonies, cleanliness guidelines should be enforced without exception. The kitten room should be kept separate from other rooms in the cattery, and exposure to other cats should be eliminated. The room should be cleaned with 1:32 dilute bleach solution before the queen is introduced into the room before parturition. Seropositive queens should be separated from their kittens at 5 weeks to limit exposure to the kittens. Kittens that are seronegative at 12–14 weeks of age can be assumed to be FoCV-naive.

24. When should vaccination for FIP be used?

Vaccination with the commerically available intranasal FIP vaccine is not recommended for all cats. Because cats from one- or two-cat households have such a low risk for development of FIP, vaccination is not recommended. In multicat households where FCoV is enzootic, vaccination of resident or incoming seronegative cats potentially decreases the incidence of FIP. Vaccination in these settings has been shown to decrease the incidence only in cats that were seronegative before vaccination.

BIBLIOGRAPHY

1. Addie DD, Jarret O: Feline coronavirus infection. In Greene CE (ed): Infectious Diseases of the Dog and Cat, 2nd ed. Philadelphia, W.B. Saunders, 1998, pp 59–67.
2. Foley JE, Lapointe JM, Koblik P, et al: Diagnostic features of clinical neurologic feline infectious peritonitis. J Vet Intern Med 12:415–423, 1998
3. Gunn-Moore DA, Gruffydd-Jones TJ, Harbour DA: Detection of coronaviruses by culture and reverse transcriptase-polymerase chain reaction of blood samples from healthy cats and cats with clinical feline infectious peritonitis. Vet Microbiol 62:193–205, 1998.
4. McReynolds C, Macy D: Feline infectious peritonitis. Part I: Etiology and diagnosis. Comp Cont Educ Pract Vet 19:1007–1014, 1997.
5. McReynolds C, Macy D: Feline infectious peritonitis. Part II: Treatment and prevention. Comp Cont Educ Pract Vet 19:1111–1116, 1997.
6. Paltrinieri S, Parodi MC, Cammarata G, et al: In vivo diagnosis of feline infectious peritonitis by comparison of protein content, cytology, and direct immunofluorescence test on peritoneal and pleural effusions. J Vet Diagn Invest 11:358–361, 1999.
7. Polland AM, Vennema H, Foley JE, et al: Two related strains of feline infectious peritonitis virus isolated from immunocompromised cats infected with a feline enteric coronavirus. J Clin Microbiol 34:3180–3184, 1996.
8. Shelly SM, Scarlett-Kranz J, Blue JT: Protein electrophoresis on effusions from cats as a diagnostic test for feline infectiouis peritonitis. J Am Anim Hosp Assoc 24:495–500, 1988.
9. Sparkes AH, Gruffydd-Jones TJ, Harbour DA: Feline infectious peritonitis: A review of clinicopathological changes in 65 cases and a critical assessment of their diagnostic value. Vet Rec 129:202–212, 1991.
10. Sparkes AH, Gruffydd-Jones TJ, Harbour DA: An appraisal of the value of laboratory tests in the diagnosis of feline infectious peritonitis. J Am Anim Hosp Assoc 30:345–350, 1994.

III. Urinary Problems

Section Editor: India F. Lane, D.V.M., M.S.

39. POLYURIA AND POLYDIPSIA: OVERVIEW AND DIAGNOSTIC PLAN

Michael R. Lappin, D.V.M., Ph.D.

1. Define polyuria and polydipsia.

Polyuria is increased urine production, and **polydipsia** is increased water consumption. In dogs and cats, polydipsia is defined as water consumption > 100 ml/kg/24 hours; polyuria is defined as urine production > 50 ml/kg/24 hours. There are primary causes of each condition, but clinical manifestations of both occur in most affected cats. For example, cats with polydipsia urinate larger volumes to clear the body of excessive fluids; polyuric cats dehydrate themselves and drink excessively to compensate.

2. What diseases are commonly associated with polyuria and polydipsia?

The multiple causes of polyuria/polydipsia in cats can be grouped into four major categoriers: renal, endocrine, metabolic, and miscellaneous. By far, the most common causes of polyuria/polydipsia in cats are renal failure, diabetes mellitus, and hyperthyroidism.

Primary Causes of Polyuria and Polydipsia in Cats

Renal	**Metabolic**
Acute renal failure	Hepatic failure
Chronic renal failure	Hypercalcemia
Pyelonephritis	Hypocalcemia
Primary renal glycosuria (rare)	
Glomerulonephritis	**Miscellaneous**
Idiopathic or congenital nephrogenic diabetes insipidus	Gram-negative endotoxins
	Drugs
Endocrine	Hyperviscosity syndromes
Diabetes mellitus	Psychogenic polydipsia (rare)
Hyperthyroidism	
Hypoadrenocorticism (rare)	
Hyperadrenocorticism (rare)	
Central diabetes insipidus	

3. Describe the signalment most commonly associated with causes of polyuria/polydipsia.

Acute renal failure and pyelonephritis can occur in cats of any age. Chronic renal failure is most common in older cats; exceptions include breeds with congenital renal diseases (see Chapters 40 and 42). Endocrine and metabolic disorders are most common in older cats; an exception is hepatic insufficiency due to congenital liver disease. Breed associations are seen with some causes of polyuria/polydipsia. For example, Persian cats commonly have polycystic kidney disease, and Abyssinian cats commonly have amyloidosis. Pyometra is most common in intact female cats.

4. What historical findings are commonly associated with causes of polyuria/polydipsia?

Clients generally report excessive urine in the litterbox, inappropriate urination, increased water consumption, or clinical signs reflecting the primary problem. Water intake may be from unusual sources (e.g., tubs, sinks, toilets, plant water containers). Drugs and toxins (nephrotoxicants) often can be excluded by history. Cats with pyelonephritis or chronic renal failure may have had recurrent episodes of lower urinary tract disease preceding polyuria/polydipsia. Cats with hepatic insufficiency commonly have protracted history of doing poorly and may have had weight loss, anorexia, vomiting, or icterus consistent with hepatic disease. Cats with hypoadrenocorticism usually have a history of intermittent gastrointestinal signs as well as polyuria/polydipsia. Polyphagia with polydipsia/polyuria is most common in cats with hyperthyroidism or diabetes mellitus. Cats with hyperthyroidism or hyperadrenocorticism often have a history of aggression; hyperadrenocorticism is commonly associated with dermatologic problems.

5. What physical examination findings are most commonly associated with causes of polyuria/polydipsia?

Cats with polyuria/polydipsia associated with renal diseases may have several different physical examination abnormalities. For example, large kidneys occur with acute renal diseases, obstructive nephropathy, and lymphoma. Cats with chronic renal failure usually have small, irregularly marginated kidneys with evidence of weight loss and may have soft bones or retinal lesions. Thyroid nodules often can be palpated in the ventral cervical region of cats with hyperthyroidism. Cats with hepatic failure usually are thin and may have evidence of ascites, icterus, or neurologic dysfunction. The uterus may be palpated in cats with pyometra. Many cats with diabetes mellitus have palpable hepatomegaly. Most cats with hyperadrenocorticism have alopecia and thinning of the skin.

6. How can I confirm polyuria/polydipsia?

Performance of a 24-hour water consumption study at home is best for determining whether a cat has polydipsia/polyuria. All faucets should be turned off, and the toilet lids placed in the down position so that a single water source can be used to determine consumption. Normal cats should drink < 100 ml/kg/24 hr and urinate < 50 ml/kg/day. In the absence of an accurate quantitated water consumption measurement, dilute urine on a urinalysis is supportive of polyuria.

7. What is included in the initial diagnostic plan for cats with polyuria/polydipsia?

In cats with documented polyuria/polydipsia, the combination of complete blood cell count, serum biochemical panel, urinalysis, serum osmolality, and total T4 (cats older than 5 years) is a good initial diagnostic plan that proves or eliminates most differential diagnoses.

8. How does the urinalysis aid in the ranking of the differential diagnoses?

The urine specific gravity is usually < 1.035 in cats with polyuria/polydipsia. Proteinuria is usually detected in cats with glomerular or tubular lesions in the kidneys. In cats with diabetes mellitus, glycosuria with or without ketonuria is detected. Glucosuria may be detected with tubular disease such as primary renal glycosuria, but the cat is euglycemic. Ammonium biurate crystals may be detected in cats with hepatic insufficiency; other crystal types may be detected in cats with other forms of obstructive uropathy. Pyuria and bacteriuria are common in cats with pyelonephritis. Cats with hyperadrenocorticism may have bacteriuria without pyuria; excessive urinary cortisol lessens inflammation while promoting infections. Cats with central or nephrogenic diabetes insipidus have the lowest urine specific gravity measurements (e.g., 1.001–1.008).

9. How does the serum osmolality aid in the ranking of differential diagnoses?

Most cats either have polydipsia with compensatory polyuria or polyuria with compensatory polydipsia. Cats with primary polydipsia dilute the serum osmolality and urinate excessively to clear the extra volume. Cats with polyuria dehydrate, increasing serum osmolality and resulting in compensatory polydipsia. Serum osmolality values < 280 and > 310 are most consistent with polydipsia and polyuria, respectively. Because of chronicity and compensatory mechanisms, however, a normal serum osmolality is observed in most cases.

10. What specialized blood tests are commonly used in the diagnostic work-up of cats with polyuria/polydipsia?

Diabetes mellitus is confirmed in cats with hyperglycemia, glycosuria, and three of the following clinical signs: polyphagia, polyuria, polydipsia, and weight loss. A baseline fructosamine concentration usually is determined after diagnosis and is used to monitor therapy (see Chapter 56). Cats with hepatic insufficiency resulting in polyuria/polydipsia usually have low albumin, low blood urea nitrogen, low glucose, low cholesterol, and high bilirubin concentrations on routine blood chemistries. Pre- and postprandial serum bile acids can be used to document hepatic insufficiency in cases with questionable results (see Chapter 28). Measurement of multiple serum total T4 concentrations, a T3 suppression test, or a technecium scan may be required to confirm hyperthyroidism (see Chapter 53). The adrenocorticotropic stimulation test can be used to exclude hyperadrenocorticism and hypoadrenocorticism (see Chapters 54 and 55). Most cats with hypoadrenocorticism have elevated potassium and low sodium concentrations. Protein electrophoresis determines the type of gammopathy in cats with hyperviscosity syndromes.

11. How do imaging techniques aid in the diagnosis of polyuria/polydipsia?

Radiographs and ultrasound are commonly used to aid in the evaluation of hepatic, renal or uterine causes of polyuria/polydipsia. Thoracic and abdominal radiographs usually are reviewed in cats with hypercalcemia to assess for evidence of neoplasia. Nuclear scintigraphy can be used to document glomerular filtration rate or to confirm hyperthyroidism. Computed tomography or magnetic resonance imaging of the brain may be required to evaluate causes of central diabetes insipidus.

12. When should a water deprivation test be performed?

Other than idiopathic nephrogenic diabetes insipidus, central diabetes insipidus, and psychogenic polydipsia, most causes of PU/PD in cats can be excluded as described above. Because these conditions are rare in cats, water deprivation testing is almost never required.

BIBLIOGRAPHY

Grauer GF: Clinical manifestations of urinary disorders. In Nelson RW, Couto CG (eds): Small Animal Internal Medicine, 2nd ed. St. Louis, Mosby, 1998, pp 581–584.

40. ACUTE AND CHRONIC RENAL FAILURE

Helen Tuzio, D.V.M., M.S.

1. Define renal failure.

It is the inability of the kidneys to perform hemodynamic, filtration, and excretory functions, resulting in the accumulation of uremic toxins and deregulation of fluid, electrolyte, and acid–base balance. Clinically, it is defined as azotemia (elevated concentrations of blood urea nitrogen [BUN] or creatinine) and concurrent decrease in urine-concentrating ability (urine specific gravity [USG] < 1.040).

2. Define azotemia.

Azotemia is an excess of urea and other nitrogenous compounds in the blood. It results from increased protein catabolism or reduced excretion capabilities and may be divided into renal, prerenal, and postrenal causes.

3. What causes renal azotemia?

Renal azotemia, defined as persistent azotemia with suboptimal urine concentrating ability in the absence of nonrenal factors, is due to a functional loss of nephrons (at least 75%).

4. What causes prerenal azotemia?

Increases in blood urea nitrogen (BUN) occur with factors other than renal failure, including dehydration, high protein diet, starvation, fever, burns, blood loss (especially gastrointestinal ulceration), and glucocorticoid administration. Creatinine may be falsely elevated if the sample is hemolyzed. In these nonrenal causes of azotemia, urine specific gravity (USG) is usually > 1.040. The kidneys receive 25% of cardiac output and do not have collateral circulation. As a result, ischemia can occur whenever renal blood flow is reduced. One of the most common prerenal causes of kidney failure is prolonged anesthesia. Other common causes are diuretics, thromboembolism, malignant hypertension, trauma, and hemorrhage. Conditions such as hypotension, circulatory collapse, prolonged renal vasoconstriction, disseminated intravascular coagulation, shock, pancreatitis, hypoproteinemia, and heat stroke also can produce hypovolemia or hypoperfusion. If left untreated, ischemia from reduced blood flow can produce intrinsic renal damage and subsequent acute or chronic renal failure.

5. What causes postrenal azotemia?

Azotemia also can occur with urinary tract obstruction (mucous plugs, uroliths, neoplasia) and leakage of urine into tissues (ruptured bladder, ureter or urethra), which result in failure to excrete uremic waste.

6. How does acute renal failure differ from chronic renal failure?

Acute renal failure (ARF) usually is associated with a sudden onset of clinical signs, rapid (hours to days) increases in BUN and serum creatinine, and electrolyte and acid–base disturbances. All of these manifestations result from tubular dysfunction and reduction in glomerular filtration rate. **Chronic renal failure** (CRF) is a long-term condition caused by a decrease in the number of functioning nephrons that can last for months to years. ARF that persists for 2 weeks or longer is considered chronic.

7. Does it make a difference whether renal failure is acute or chronic?

Unlike CRF, ARF is potentially reversible, especially if diagnosed early and treated appropriately. However, if therapy is delayed, ARF can produce irreparable kidney damage and subsequent death of the patient.

8. What causes intrinsic renal failure?

Diseases that directly or indirectly affect the vasculature, glomeruli, tubular epithelium, or interstitium of the kidney cause intrinsic renal failure. Glomerulonephritis, pyelonephritis, feline infectious peritonitis, lymphoma, and nephrotoxicants (e.g., ethylene glycol, nonsteroidal anti-inflammatory drugs [NSAIDs], aminoglycosides) are common causes.

9. Describe the progression of ARF.

ARF progresses sequentially through three phases:
1. In the **initiation phase**, the parenchyma and tubular epithelium are injured.
2. In the **maintenance phase**, the damage to the epithelium becomes irreversible.
3. During the **recovery phase**, repair occurs and some or all of the renal function is regained.

The initiation phase may last from hours to days. If treatment is instituted before the patient enters the maintenance phase, further progression of the disease can be prevented.

10. How common is renal failure in cats?

A study completed at the University of Minnesota between 1980 and 1990 found an overall prevalence of 3.05%. However, this figure annually increased from 0.5% to 4.5% over the10-year period. Because detection techniques, client knowledge, and clinician awareness of renal disease have improved significantly since 1990, the prevalence of renal failure may be far greater today.

11. How does age affect the prevalence of renal failure?

The incidence of renal failure increases with advancing age. Studies of age distributions have shown that cats younger than 10 years account for 37% of cases; cats between 10 and 15 years old are 5 times more likely to have renal failure than cats of other age groups and account for 31% of cases; and 32% of cats older than 15 years are diagnosed with renal failure. Cats older than 15 years are 20 times more likely to have renal failure than other age groups. According to published reports, the mean age of cats with CRF is 12.6 years, whereas the mean age at diagnosis is 7.4 years.

12. What other factors may predispose to renal failure?

Factors leading to the development of CRF may be inherited or acquired. The tendency to develop polycystic renal disease, for instance, appears to be familial (see Chapter 42). A higher incidence of renal failure has been identified in Abyssinian, Burmese, Maine coon, Russian blue, and Siamese cats. Acute renal insults, if left untreated, can lead to CRF by irreparably damaging the renal parenchyma, resulting in loss of functional nephrons. However, ARF may not be recognized in some cases. A study of cats with primary renal disease found that chronic tubulointerstitial nephritis was the most common (70.4% of 47 cats) histopathologic finding. It has been suggested that chronic pyelonephritis or glomerulonephritis may be inciting factors for chronic nephritis, although the etiology is most often undetermined.

13. What are the chief complaints associated with ARF?

With ARF, the main signs noted by the owners are nonspecific; anorexia, listlessness, weakness, and vomiting are common complaints. In advanced renal failure, ataxia, dyspnea, syncope and seizures are possible. Patients with ARF generally have a history of illness of < 1 week and may have had exposure to nephrotoxicants, administration of medication, recent surgery, or blood loss.

14. Describe the chief complaints associated with CRF.

CRF is usually slow in onset; the owner usually notices a general decline over weeks to months. Some cases may exhibit the classic **uremic syndrome**, which is characterized by depression, anorexia, lethargy, and vomiting. Weight loss, halitosis, inappropriate urination, constipation, and increased shedding may occur. Occasionally, owners report sudden onset of blindness, or hematemesis. Polyuria and polydipsia occur but are not as common in cats as in dogs. Cats with CRF may decompensate and present in an acute uremic crisis at any time.

15. What physical examination abnormalities are common in cats with renal failure?

Common findings in most cats with renal failure are lethargy and evidence of dehydration. In moderate-to-severe cases, hypothermia, uremic breath, tachypnea, bleeding tendency, muscle fasciculations, and altered mental status may be noted. Tachycardia may be detected in dehydrated or hypovolemic patients, bradycardia may be detected in hyperkalemic patients with ARF, and other cardiac arrhythmias may arise from uremic myocarditis. Ocular abnormalities due to systemic hypertension include reduced pupillary light reflexes, tortuous retinal vessels, hyphema, anterior uveitis, glaucoma, retinal hemorrhage, retinal detachment, and papilledema.

16. Can physical examination findings distinguish ARF from CRF?

Cats with **ARF** are usually in good body condition with normal haircoat and body weight. Weakness, mental dullness, and seizure activity may be noted. Abdominal pain and enlarged kidneys may be found on palpation. Lameness, back pain, icterus, discolored urine, and dysuria may be present in cats with infectious causes. Body temperature is usually normal but may be low because of uremia or elevated because of infection or severe inflammation. Uremic stomatitis may develop with ARF or CRF.

Cats with **CRF** are usually unkempt on initial examination. Dehydration, significant weight loss, and muscle wasting may be evident. Oral ulceration, fetid breath, tongue discoloration, or sloughing may be observed. Fundic examination may reveal findings consistent with hypertension. Mucous membranes may be pale (from anemia) and dry (from dehydration) or moist from vomiting (due to uremic gastritis). Petechial or ecchymotic hemorrhages may be noted. Heart murmurs or arrhythmias may be found on thoracic auscultation. Small, irregularly marginated, nonpainful kidneys are typically found on abdominal palpation; however, conditions such as neoplasia, pyelonephritis, nepholithiasis, and polycystic renal disease may produce renomegaly.

17. What is included in the diagnostic plan for suspected renal failure?

The initial database generally includes complete blood count (CBC) with differential, serum biochemistry profile (which should include concentrations of urea nitrogen, creatinine, sodium, potassium, chloride, bicarbonate or total carbon dioxide, calcium, and phosphorus), complete urinalysis (urine collected before fluid therapy is initiated), urine culture and antimicrobial susceptibility, plain abdominal radiographs, arterial blood pressure, and, in cats older than 6 years, total T4 concentration. In cats allowed outdoors and cats with bilateral renomegaly, a serum feline leukemia virus antigen test and serum feline immunodeficiency virus antibody test should be performed because of the potential for renal lymphoma. Kits for measurement of ethylene glycol or its toxic metabolites should be used if indicated by history and laboratory findings. If bladder rupture is suspected, abdominocentesis and fluid analysis should be performed. The fluid typically has a creatinine concentration that exceeds the serum creatinine concentration.

18. How do results of the CBC and serum biochemical panel help to differentiate ARF from CRF?

Nonregenerative anemia is characteristic of CRF, whereas cats with ARF have normal or increased red blood cell count, hematocrit, and hemoglobin concentration. In some cases of ARF, regenerative anemia, thrombocytopenia, and stress or inflammatory leukogram may be noted. Hematocrit and total protein measurements are affected by hydration status.

Increased BUN, creatinine, and phosphorus concentrations occur in both ARF and CRF. Serum potassium levels are generally increased in ARF and decreased in CRF but tend to vary with the extent of vomiting and anorexia and the degree of acidosis. Serum bicarbonate concentrations decrease with severity of the renal failure, which results in metabolic acidosis; the most dramatic acidosis is usually seen in ARF. Serum calcium concentrations may be normal, increased, or decreased with renal failure. Acute ethylene glycol toxicity often induces hypocalcemia and hyperglycemia. Total serum calcium > 3.4 mmol/L (13.2 mg/dl) may induce ARF. Measurement of ionized calcium may aid in determining whether hypercalcemia is the cause or the result of renal failure. Most cats with CRF have ionized hypocalcemia, even though total calcium levels may be increased. Only ionized hypercalcemia promotes renal failure; if it is present, the cat should be evaluated for a primary cause of hypercalcemia (see Chapter 57).

19. What information is likely to be provided by urinalysis?

Cats with prerenal azotemia should have USG > 1.040; cats with renal azotemia have USG < 1.040. A decrease in urine concentrating ability may be the first indicator of impending renal failure. Although cats have the potential to develop azotemia before losing urine concentrating ability, this scenario is not common. In evaluating urine specific gravity, nonrenal causes of dilute urine (e.g., hyperthyroidism, diabetes mellitus, hypercalcemia, severe hepatic disease, diabetes insipidus, diuretics) must be kept in mind.

Proteinuria is common in uremic patients and generally indicates tubular or glomerular injury, although it can be caused by hematuria or inflammation (see Chapter 43). Urine sediment examination is imperative. In pyelonephritis, cellular casts and inflammatory cells may be observed and may be accompanied by bacteria or yeast. Granular or hyaline casts indicate active renal injury with possible epithelial necrosis. Presence of crystalluria may help to rank differential diagnoses.

20. How are imaging techniques used to evaluate cats with renal failure?

Intravenous urography may be beneficial in some cases (e.g., bladder rupture), but contrast studies are not recommended in ARF because of their hypertonicity and potential to create additional renal damage.

Detection of changes in renal parenchyma by use of **ultrasonography** may help to rank differential diagnoses. Hyperechoic renal cortices are the most common finding in ARF but also may be associated with other causes such as pyelonephritis, ethylene glycol toxicity, renal lymphoma, and pyogranulomatous nephritis secondary to feline infectious peritonitis (FIP). Focal lesions that may be detected include masses, cysts, abscesses, or hematomas. Dilation of renal pelves may indicate excessive diuresis, obstruction, or pyelonephritis. In cases of CRF, the typical ultrasonographic findings are increased echogenicity and reduced renal size. Irregular contours or renal mineralization may also be visualized. Ultrasound can be used to guide renal aspirates (lymphoma) or biopsies if indicated.

Nuclear scintigraphy can be used to estimate glomerular filtration rate of each kidney individually and to assess for obstructive disease of the ureters and pelves.

21. Is renal biopsy necessary?

Fine-needle aspiration of a kidney is usually sufficient for documentation of renal lymphoma. Renal biopsy is indicated primarily to assess excessive proteinuria (see Chapter 43), to document neoplasms other than lymphoma, to confirm noneffusive FIP, and to evaluate and determine a prognosis in cats with severe uremia, hyperkalemia, or oliguria that persists despite therapy. In cases of suspected ARF, evidence of intact tubular basement membranes and tubular regeneration indicates a good prognosis, whereas interstitial mineralization, disrupted basement membranes, and extensive tubular necrosis indicate a poor prognosis. Renal biopsy is contraindicated in most cats with CRF, including those with severe debilitation, anemia, one kidney, hydronephrosis, renal cysts, perirenal abscess, pyelonephritis, or coagulopathies, and should not be used indiscriminately. Histopathologic studies have shown that the most common finding in CRF is chronic generalized nephritis.

22. What causes the common complications of renal failure?

Because the kidneys have excretory, metabolic, and endocrine functions, patients in renal failure are at risk for various complications, including electrolyte, blood pressure, fluid, and acid–base disorders, which in turn may create neuromuscular, cardiovascular, respiratory, and immune system compromise.

23. List the most common complications of renal failure.
- Hypertension
- Peripheral neuropathy
- Uremic encephalopathy
- Uremic pneumonitis
- Platelet and leukocyte dysfunction
- Metabolic acidosis
- Hyperphosphatemia and renal secondary hyperparathyroidism

24. How common is hypertension? What are the consequences?

Hypertension is diagnosed in nearly two-thirds of cats with CRF (see Chapter 63 and questions 60–62). Encephalopathies and ocular abnormalities may result.

25. How common is peripheral polyneuropathy? What are the typical signs?

Peripheral polyneuropathy (abnormal motor responses) associated with uremia has been described in up to 65% of cats with CRF and generally is characterized by sensory changes and sluggish reflexes in the distal limbs.

26. What are the typical signs of uremic encephalopathy? When does it occur?

Uremic encephalopathy is characterized by confusion, ataxia, sluggishness, and disorientation. It occurs with decreased GFR and may be exacerbated by increased cerebral calcium concentration, systemic hypertension, and electrolyte abnormalities.

27. What are the typical signs of uremic pneumonitis?

Dyspnea and alveolar lung disease.

28. Describe the platelet and leukocyte dysfunction associated with renal failure.

Platelet and leukocyte dysfunction occurs in the presence of urea, resulting in bleeding diatheses and reduced cellular immunity.

29. Is metabolic acidosis common? What are its adverse effects?

A large number of cats with CRF develop metabolic acidosis. Chronic acidosis has a number of adverse effects:

- Reduction of cardiac output and hepatic and renal blood flow
- Induction of cardiac arrhythmias, directly or indirectly, by influencing serum potassium concentration
- Enhancement of protein catabolism and possible inhibition of protein synthesis, which cause anorexia, nausea, and vomiting, all of which increase the risk of malnutrition
- Promotion of bone demineralization
- Enhancement of potassium and taurine depletion.

30. What are the possible consequences of hyperphosphatemia?

Hyperphosphatemia alone has no clinical signs; however, it predisposes patients to metastatic calcification, primarily affecting the stomach, kidneys, myocardium, lung, and liver. It may be used as a prognostic indicator because phosphorus does not usually become elevated unless 85% of the nephrons are nonfunctional. As hyperphosphatemia develops, hypocalcemia causes a reduction in calcitriol and an increase in circulating parathyroid hormone (**renal secondary hyperparathyroidism**). This syndrome directly affects the bones, kidneys, brain, heart, smooth muscles, lungs, erythrocytes, lymphocytes, pancreas, adrenals, and testes. Results may be impaired function of platelets, cardiac muscle, and skeletal muscle, increased number and severity of infections due to immunodeficiency, mental fatigue, and lethargy. It can produce nephrocalcinosis, leading to further renal deterioration. Renal osteodystrophy with demineralization of bone and proliferation of connective tissue has been documented but is uncommon. The resulting skeletal decalcification and associated pathological fractures, "rubber jaw," and pain seem rare in cats. Renal secondary hyperparathyroidism is said to occur in 84% of cats with spontaneous CRF and 100% of cats with end-stage CRF.

31. What are the goals and management issues in ARF?

The goals of therapy should be to correct hemodynamic changes, fluid volume abnormalities, and biochemical irregularities; to eliminate uremic toxins; to supply adequate nutrition, and to allow repair of renal damage. Treatment recommendations are primarily supportive and need to be initiated as early as possible to improve the chance of recovery. The inciting cause of ARF should be identified and eliminated when possible, and therapy should be targeted to the sequelae of acute uremia.

The first step in therapy is to address the acute crisis; this principle applies to ARF, decompensated CRF, and acute-on-chronic renal failure. Life-threatening abnormalities (e.g., hyperkalemia, hypovolemia, metabolic acidosis) should be noted and controlled. Patients with ARF must be stabilized by return to normal renal function or establishment of compensated chronic renal failure, which can be treated conservatively.

32. Outline the primary treatment plan for cats with ARF.

Most cats with ARF are oliguric or anuric. A patient is considered oliguric if urine output is < 0.27–0.5 ml/kg/hr; after rehydration, output < 1–2 ml/kg/hr is still inadequate. Evidence suggests that the efficacy of treatments for the promotion of diuresis may be negligible if they are administered more than a few hours after initiation of ARF. The following general steps are recommended:

1. A jugular catheter should be placed to allow monitoring of central venous pressure and repeated blood sampling.

2. Placement of a urinary catheter should be considered to allow accurate measurement of urine production.

3. Fluids should be administered intravenously at a rate that corrects dehydration within the first 4–6 hours of therapy and induces diuresis.

4. If oliguria is persistent, mannitol is the initial treatment of choice to increase renal blood flow, reverse cellular swelling, increase solute excretion, and discharge tubular debris. Other options include hypertonic glucose and furosemide.

5. The patients should be monitored appropriately (see question 37).

Therapeutic Guidelines for Cats in Renal Failure

1. Rehydrate and reestablish fluid and electrolyte balance.
   Buffered, balanced electrolyte solution or 0.9% sodium chloride (NaCl); replacement volume administered within 4–6 hr

   Replacement volume (ml) = [BW (kg)] × [estimated deficit (%)] × 1000

   Maintain fluid and electrolyte balance.
   0.45% NaCl with 2.5% dextrose or buffered, balanced electrolyte solution; rate based on rate of loss

   Volume (ml) = [20 ml/kg/day] + [urinary + GI losses}

2. Promote urine production (primarily of concern in ARF).
   Rehydrate with fluids (see above)
   20% mannitol, 0.25–1.0 gm/kg, administered over 20 minutes; use only after rehydration
   Furosemide: 2–6 mg/kg IV every 6–8 hr; use in hydrated patient, alone or with mannitol

3. Reestablish potassium balance.
   Hyperkalemia
   K+ up to 6.0 mEq/L (fluid therapy)
   K+ 6–8 mEq/L (fluid therapy, diuresis); if persistent:
   Sodium bicarbonate, 0.5-2.0 mEq/kg IV over 30 min, or
   Regular insulin, 0.1–0.25 U/kg, + dextrose, 1–2 gm/U insulin IV
   K+ > 8.0 mEq/L: 10% calcium gluconate, 0.5–1.0 ml/kg IV over 15 min, + fluid therapy
   Hypokalemia: potassium chloride, 0.5 mEq/kg/hr by IV infusion (see table in question 52)
   Maintenance: potassium gluconate, 2–6 mEq/cat/day PO

4. Correct metabolic acidosis.
   Fluid therapy alone for mild-to-moderate cases
   If pH < 7.1, sodium bicarbonate, 0.5–2.0 mEq/kg IV over 60 min, + fluid therapy

5. Correct hyperphosphatemia.
   Limit dietary phosphorus
   Phosphate binders given with meals:
   Aluminum hydroxide, 30–100 mg/kg/d divided PO, or
   Calcium acetate, 20–30 mg/kg every 8 hr PO, alone or with aluminum-based binder

6. Control uremic gastroenteritis.
   Famotidine, 0.5 mg/kg/day PO, SC, or IM
   Metoclopramide, 0.2–0.5 mg/kg every 8 hr PO, SC, or IV if vomiting
   Sucralfate, 0.25–0.5 gm/cat every 8–12 hr PO if gastric or oral ulceration

7. Provide adequate nutrition.
   Meet energy requirements as fat or carbohydrates:

   RER (kcal/day) = 70 + [30 × (BW (kg) × 1.2)]

   Meet protein requirements:
   Minimal protein requirement = 3.8–4.4 g/kg/day, 20–25 % protein on ME basis
   B vitamins

8. Control hypertension.
   Amlodipine, 0.625–1.25 mg/cat/day PO

9. Correct anemia
   Monitor fluid therapy
   Erythropoietin, 50–100 U/kg SC 3 times/wk,+ iron dextran, 50–100 mg/day PO

10. Control hyperparathyroidism
    Calcitriol, 2.5–3.5 ng/kg every 24 hr PO, if serum phosphorus concentration ≤ 6.0 mg/dl
    May need to use in conjunction with dietary phosphorus restriction and intestinal phosphorus binders

BW = body weight, GI = gastrointestinal, ARC = acute renal failure, IV = intravenously, PO = orally, SC = subcutaneously, IM = intramuscularly, RER = renal energy requirement, ME = metabolizable energy.

33. How should fluids be replaced?

The replacement volume may be calculated using the clinical estimate of dehydration according to the formula in the preceding table. Ideally, the replacement fluid should resemble the type of fluid lost. In the absence of severe blood loss, buffered, balanced electrolyte solutions are used initially. If replacement of the fluid deficits does not result in diuresis (urine production > 1 ml/kg/hr), an additional fluid volume (equal to 3–5% body weight) may be administered to produce mild volume expansion and stimulate urine production. Use care in animals with a history of cardiovascular disease.

34. How is mannitol administered?

Administer mannitol as a slow intravenous (IV) bolus of 0.25–1.0 gm/kg. If significant diuresis is established within 60 minutes, mannitol administration may be continued for 24–48 hours either as intermittent intravenous boluses of 0.25–0.5 g/kg every 4–6 hours or as a constant-rate infusion at 1–2 mg/kg/min. If diuresis is inadequate 60 minutes after the initial IV bolus, an additional IV bolus of 0.25–0.5 g/kg may be administered with caution. Potential complications associated with volume overexpansion (e.g., pulmonary edema) are more likely to occur with a repeat bolus. The most favorable results are obtained when mannitol is administered early in the course of ARF.

35. Describe the roles of hypertonic glucose and furosemide.

Hypertonic glucose can be used in place of mannitol to increase urine production and supply metabolizable energy; however, it does not have many of the protective effects (vasodilation, free-radical scavenging) of mannitol. Solutions of 10–20% dextrose may be formulated and administered as a slow (over 1–2 hours) IV bolus of 25–50 ml/kg 2 or 3 times daily.

Furosemide may be used alone or with mannitol to promote urine formation and facilitate management of overhydration. Before it is used, the patient must receive adequate fluid replacement. Furosemide is dosed initially at 2–6 mg/kg IV. If diuresis occurs within 30 minutes, the dose may be repeated every 6–8 hours or may be given as a constant-rate infusion at 0.25–1.0 mg/kg/hr for 24–48 hours. If diuresis is not achieved within the first 30 minutes, the dose should be repeated.

36. Why is dopamine usually not recommended for cats?

Dopamine, although widely used with furosemide in dogs, is not strongly recommended for use in cats. Although the drug induces diuresis, it probably acts via alpha-adrenergic receptors; effective doses for cats may create deleterious pressor effects on the kidney that worsen the initial problem. If used, dopamine should be administered at 3 μg/kg/min as a constant-rate IV infusion.

37. How should the patient be monitored during diuresis?

Patients undergoing diuresis should be monitored closely by measuring urine output, body weight, packed cell volume, serum total protein and electrolyte concentrations, and central venous pressure. In addition, they should be observed for signs of overhydration, which include restlessness and tachycardia, chemosis, bronchovesicular sounds, or serous nasal discharge. Auscultation of crackles and wheezes is indicative of pulmonary edema.

38. What should be done once the dehydration is corrected?

Once fluid volume is restored and urine production is adequate, IV fluid diuresis is continued until azotemia, acidosis, and electrolyte abnormalities have stabilized during the maintenance and recovery periods. The fluid rate should be based on insensible, urinary, and gastrointestinal losses (ins and outs). Insensible losses (e.g., through respiration) may be calculated as 20 ml/kg/day. Urinary output should be measured and the gastrointestinal losses estimated by the volume of vomiting and diarrhea. Buffered, balanced electrolyte solutions or 0.45% sodium chloride with 2.5% dextrose should be used.

39. What type of potassium imbalance typically develops with ARF?

Hyperkalemia is the most common potassium disorder in cats with ARF. Severity varies greatly depending on the degree of anorexia and vomiting. Hyperkalemia has a direct effect on the mycocardium that can be life-threatening. If potassium concentrations are unknown, an electrocardiogram should be monitored. Mild hyperkalemia produces peaked T waves, short R waves, and prolonged P-R intervals. Moderate hyperkalemia produces bradycardia, flat P waves, prolonged Q-T intervals, and wide QRS complexes. Severe hyperkalemia causes sinoventricular rhythms and ventricular fibrillation and may induce cardiac arrest. Cats with ARF or urinary obstruction frequently become hypokalemic during and after diuresis, particularly if the fluids used are low in potassium, or after insulin administration for correction of acidosis.

40. How is hyperkalemia treated?

Use of 5% dextrose or 0.9% sodium chloride solutions has been suggested because both are potassium-free. However, they are not buffered and may worsen acidosis. Therefore, unless hyperkalemia exceeds 10 mEq/L, buffered, balanced electrolyte solutions are reasonable choices, even though they contain small concentrations of potassium. Mild hyperkalemia (< 6.0 mEq/L) or moderate hyperkalemia (6.0-8.0 mEq/L) generally resolves with initial fluid therapy. In refractory cases, furosemide may be used in addition to fluid therapy to promote potassium excretion.

41. What additional measures may be needed for severe hyperkalemia?

Severe hyperkalemia (> 8.0 mEq/L) needs to be addressed immediately because of its life-threatening electrocardiac and neuromuscular disturbances. Calcium gluconate (10% solution, dosed at 0.5–1.0 ml/kg) should be administered intravenously over 10–15 minutes to stabilize heart rhythm directly and immediately. Because calcium has no effect on the serum potassium concentration, the patient should be given bicarbonate or insulin and glucose, as described below, once the cardiotoxic effects of hyperkalemia have been controlled. If the patient develops arrhythmia, bradycardia, or hypotension, calcium administration should be stopped immediately.

If hyperkalemia remains uncontrolled despite diuresis, sodium bicarbonate (0.5–2.0 mEq/kg) may be administered intravenously over 20–30 minutes to increase the intracellular pH and force an exchange between intracellular hydrogen and extracellular potassium. Bicarbonate therapy should not be used in patients with metabolic alkalosis, volume overload, or hypocalcemia (often seen with urinary obstruction).

In patients that cannot be given sodium bicarbonate, glucose or insulin may be used to stimulate cellular uptake of potassium. Intravenous glucose (20%) alone may be administered at 1.5 g/kg. Alternatively, regular insulin (0.1–0.25 U/kg) may be administered intravenously with dextrose at 1–2 g/U of insulin. Monitor closely for hypoglycemia for several hours after insulin administration.

42. How is metabolic acidosis managed?

Mild-to-moderate metabolic acidosis generally responds to diuresis. More severe cases of acidosis (blood pH < 7.10 or total carbon dioxide [CO_2] < 10 mEq/L) should be treated with sodium bicarbonate. In acute patients, the dose can be calculated using one of the following formulas:

MEq bicarbonate = body weight (kg) $\times$ 0.3 $\times$ (desired bicarbonate – measured bicarbonate)

or

MEq bicarbonate = 20 – total CO_2

or

0.5–2 mEq/kg slow IV

Half of this dose should be given over 20–30 minutes; the remainder is mixed with IV fluids and administered over 2–4 hours. Bicarbonate therapy is usually conservative; the goal is to bring the serum pH to 7.2. Severely uremic patients may require ongoing bicarbonate supplementation up to 80–90 mEq/kg/day. Bicarbonate supplementation must be monitored closely because of potentially severe effects of rapid correction of acidemia (pulmonary and cerebral edema, hypertension, hypovolemia, hypokalemia, hypocalcemia, hypercapnia, and paradoxical cerebral acidosis).

43. How is intractable vomiting managed?

Oral ingestion should be avoided for approximately 24 hours. H_2 receptor antagonists such as cimetidine, ranitidine, or famotidine are administered parenterally to lessen uremic gastritis. Antiemetics may be administered parenterally by injection until the vomiting is controlled.

Metoclopramide is often used initially as constant-rate infusion because it promotes gastric empty-ing; uremia induces gastric stasis. Because it is excreted by the kidneys, however, this dose should be reduced by 50% in severely uremic animals. High doses may produce neurologic complications (altered behavior, disorientation). Cats with intractable vomiting unresponsive to metoclopramide may be given phenothiazine antiemetics (acepromazine, chlorpromazine, or prochlorpromazine), provided they are well hydrated and normotensive and can safely tolerate the side effects of vasodi-lation, hypotension, and sedation.

44. Summarize the drugs commonly used in the management of renal failure.

Drugs Commonly Used in the Management of Renal Failure

DRUG NAME	DOSE	COMMENTS
Acepromazine	0.01–0.05 mg/kg every 8–12 hr IM, SC	Used for vomiting; patient must be hy-drated and normotensive
Aluminum carbonate (Basalgel)	30–120 mg/kg/day divided, with meals	Phosphate binders; use with dietary phosphorus restriction, dose to effect; potential for aluminum toxicity; do not use with citrate salts
Aluminum hydroxide (Amphogel)	30–100 mg/kg/day divided, with meals	
Amlodipine (Norvasc)	0.625–1.25 mg/cat PO every 24 hr	Calcium channel blocker for systemic hypertension
Calcitriol, vitamin D	2.5–3.5 ng/kg every 24 hr PO Pulse dose at 20 ng/kg PO 2 times/wk	Give at night on empty stomach; dose should not exceed 6.6 ng/kg; not for use in patients with serum phosphorus > 6 mg/dl; use with caution if giving calcium-based phosphorus binders
Calcium acetate (PhosLo)	20–30 mg/kg every 8–12 hr PO, with meals	Most effective calcium-based phosphate-binding agent
Calcium carbonate (Tums)	30–50 mg/kg every 8 hr PO, with meals	Phosphate binder; use with dietary phosphorus restriction; dose to effect; potential for hypercalcemia
Calcium gluconate 10%	0.5–1.0 mg/kg IV over 10–15 min	Used for severe hyperkalemia; monitor patient for bradycardia, hypertension, cardiac arrhythmias, ECG disturbances
Calcium phosphate	0.5–2.0 mmol/kg/day PO	Used for hypophosphatemia
Chlorpromazine	0.2–0.5 mg/kg every 6–8 hr IM, SC	Used for vomiting; patient must be hy-drated and normotensive
Cimetidine (Tagamet)	5–10 mg/kg every 6–8 hr PO, IM, IV	H_2 receptor antagonist; give slowly if IV; administer at least 30 min apart from metoclopramide, sucralfate, antacids; various drug interactions; reduce dose in hepatic or renal disease (by 10–25% if patient is severely uremic)
Cyproheptadine	2 mg/cat PO every 12 hr	Appetite stimulant
Dextrose (10–20% solution)	25–50 ml/kg over 1–2hr IV and repeat every 8–12 hr	Osmotic diuretic; test urine for glucose, and continue to monitor urine output; adjust maintenance fluid therapy ad-ministered between boluses to supply total daily calculated requirements; dis-continue if glucosuria is not present or if urine output is not adequate after half of recommended dose is given

Table continued on following page

Drugs Commonly Used in the Management of Renal Failure (Continued)

DRUG NAME	DOSE	COMMENTS
Diazepam (Valium)	0.2–0.3 mg/kg every 12 hr SQ	Used as appetite stimulant; causes hypotension and hypovolemia that may exacerbate renal failure
Enalapril (Vasotec, Enacard)	0.25–0.5 mg/kg every 12–24 hr PO	Angiotensin-converting enzyme inhibitor for hypertension; may cause nausea
Erythropoietin (Epogen)	50–100 U/kg SC 3 times/wk	Start when hematocrit reaches 18%; administer with iron; decrease dose by 50% if hypertensive; increase dose interval when hematocrit reaches 35%
Ethanol 20%	5 ml/kg IV every 6hr for 30 hr, then every 8 hr for 30 hr	Used for ethylene glycol toxicity
Famotidine (Pepcid)	0.5 mg/kg every 24 hr PO, SC, IM	H_2 blocker for uremic gastropathy; may cause hemolysis if given IV; give at least 30 min apart from metoclopramide, sucralfate, antacids; renal excretion: reduce dose by 10–25% in debilitated patients with renal failure
Ferrous sulfate	50–100 mg/cat every 24 hr PO	Iron supplement
Furosemide (Lasix)	2–6 mg/kg every 6–8 hr IV; incrementally increase dose every 1 hr up to 6 mg/kg if urine output remains poor	Loop diuretic; may produce dehydration, hypokalemia, aminoglycoside toxicity
Glucose 20%	1.5 gm/kg IV	Used to treat hyperkalemia
Magnesium chloride Magnesium sulfate	0.75–1.0 mEq/kg every 24 hr IV for 3–5 days, mixed with 5% dextrose in water	Used for hypomagnesemia
Mannitol (10–25% solution)	0.25–1.0 gm/kg; give as slow IV bolus over 15–20 min; may repeat every 4–6 hr	Osmotic diuretic; may be given as CRI of 8–10% solution; may cause dehydration, cardiopulmonary insufficiency, overhydration, elevated central venous pressure, intracranial hemorrhage
Metoclopramide (Reglan)	0.2–0.5 mg/kg every 8 hr PO, SC, IV 1–2 mg/kg CRI	Antiemetic; acts at CRTZ; enhances gastric emptying and cimetidine absorption; avoid in epileptics and hypertensives, incompatible with calcium gluconate, ampicillin sodium, penicillin G potassium, sodium bicarbonate and other drugs; high doses may cause mental disturbances; contraindicated with GI bleeding; excreted by kidneys: reduce dose by 50% if patient is severely uremic
Nitroprusside (Nipride)	3–10 mg/kg/min IV	Vasodilator
Oxazepam (Serax)	0.2–0.4 mg/kg every 12 hr PO	Appetite stimulant; causes hypotension and hypovolemia that may exacerbate renal failure
Potassium citrate (Urocit-K)	2–6 mEq/cat every 24 hr PO 40–60 mg/kg every 12 hr PO	Potassium supplement; may enhance intestinal absorption of aluminum

Table continued on following page

Drugs Commonly Used in the Management of Renal Failure (Continued)

DRUG NAME	DOSE	COMMENTS
Potassium gluconate (Kaon, Tumil-K)	2–6 mEq/cat every 24 hr PO	Potassium supplement
Potassium phosphate	0.01–0.03 mmol/kg/hr IV, mixed with 0.9% saline	Used to treat hypophosphatemia; check phosphorus levels every 6 hr
Prochlorperazine	0.1–0.5 mg/kg every 8–12 hr IM, SC	Used for vomiting; patient must be hydrated and normotensive
Ranitidine (Zantac)	2.5 mg/kg q12hr IV (administer slowly) 2-4mg/kg every 12 hr PO	H_2 antagonist; reduce dose in renal disease (by 50–75% if patient is debilitated)
Regular insulin	0.1–0.25 U/kg IV; with dextrose, 1–2 gm/U of insulin	Used to treat hyperkalemia
Sodium bicarbonate	0.5–2.0 mEq/kg IV over 20–30 min 5–10 mg/kg PO every 8–12 hr	Used to treat moderate hyperkalemia; tailor PO dose to individual
Sucralfate (Carafate)	0.25–0.5 gm/cat every 8–12 hr PO	GI protectant; give 30–60 min before administration of antacids or cimetidine; may cause constipation, impair absorption of other drugs

IV = intravenously, PO = orally, IM = intramuscularly, SC = subcutaneously, CRI = constant-rate infusion, CRTZ = chemoreceptor trigger zone, GI = gastrointestinal.

45. Why is nutrition important in ARF?

Maintaining adequate nutrition is mandatory in ARF to control muscle protein catabolism. Metabolic acidosis also serves as a major stimulus for catabolism in acute uremic patients, which, in turn, worsens azotemia, hyperkalemia, and hyperphosphatemia. Anorexia, nausea, vomiting, and uremic toxins worsen nutritional inadequacies that lead to muscle weakness, an impaired immune system, and delayed wound healing.

46. Describe a strategy for nutrition management in ARF.

Nutritional maintenance may be difficult in ARF patients due to persistent anorexia or vomiting as well as existing gastritis or gastrointestinal ulceration. There are no easy and reliable methods of assessing nutritional status, but weight loss, reduction in serum albumin or total protein, anemia, and muscle wasting are clinical indicators of poor nutrition. Once metabolic abnormalities associated with renal failure (dehydration, hypokalemia, anemia) have been corrected, and drug-associated (enalapril, antibiotics) anorexia been eliminated, uremic gastroenteritis should be considered and the patient treated accordingly, usually with an H_2 receptor antagonist and prokinetic agent.

Severely depleted animals may require periods of total parenteral nutrition, which is administered through a dedicated central intravenous catheter. Alternatively, peripheral parenteral nutrition with isotonic fluids may be used up to 5 days and then continued as a supplement to oral feeding. Appetite stimulants may be sufficient in animals that are anorexic but not vomiting. Inappetent cats unresponsive to appetite stimulants should be fed a nonrestricted diet or may require feeding via nasoesophageal, esophageal, or percutaneous gastric tube (see Chapter 62). See Chapter 50 and question 50 for a discussion of dietary recommendations.

47. How should patients with ARF be monitored?

Resolution of clinical signs, increase in appetite, and reversal of abnormal laboratory values are used to monitor response to therapy. Obviously, the patient with ARF needs to be monitored more closely than the patient with CRF. At minimum, urine output should be measured hourly, body weight and hematocrit 2 or 3 times/day, and BUN and creatinine once daily, at least in the initial phases of therapy. Ideally, potassium and blood gases should be assessed once or twice daily.

48. What are the key management issues in CRF?
- Maintaining adequate hydration
- Maintaining normal potassium concentrations
- Stabilizing azotemia
- Controlling metabolic acidosis
- Maintaining normal phosphorus concentrations
- Controlling uremic gastritis and ulcers
- Stabilizing anemia
- Controlling systemic hypertension

49. What fluid support is indicated for stable patients with CRF?
Because patients with CRF have obligatory polyuria, adequate fluid intake is extremely important to maintain fluid balance. Clear, fresh drinking water should always be available, canned foods should be fed, and tuna broth or other flavored liquids may be offered to increase fluid consumption. Prepared broths should be used with caution becaues of their high sodium content; milk should be used sparingly because of its high concentration of phosphate (0.029 mmol/ml).

If oral intake is insufficient, dehydration and renal hypoperfusion occur, possibly resulting in full uremic crisis and/or additional renal injury. Additional buffered, balanced electrolyte solutions can be given subcutaneously by the owner; the volume and frequency of administration are tailored to the individual patient's needs.

50. What diet should be fed to cats with CRF?
Diets designed for cats in renal failure usually have reduced protein, phosphorus, and sodium concentrations; higher potassium, vitamin B, and caloric content; and a neutral acid–base effect (see Chapter 50). Reduced protein intake minimizes hyperphosphatemia, hypertension, hypokalemia, and signs of uremia, but little evidence suggests that it alters the progression of the disease. Phosphorus restriction helps to minimize hyperphosphatemia and renal secondary hyperparathyroidism. Decreased sodium intake may help to control systemic hypertension. Vitamin B supplementation helps to restore supplies depleted by polyuria and anorexia. High caloric content helps to improve palatability and counter the effects of decreased food intake. Potassium supplementation helps to reduce the incidence of hypokalemia, to which cats with CRF are vulnerable.

51. What are the signs of hypokalemia in cats with CRF?
Hypokalemia is the most frequent electrolyte abnormality in cats with CRF. Hypokalemia causes generalized muscle weakness and cardiac rhythm disturbances, the hallmark sign being ventroflexion of the neck. In addition, hypokalemia reduces renal function, worsens dysfunction caused by metabolic acidosis, and causes polyuria as a result of nephrogenic diabetes insipidus (unresponsiveness to antidiuretic hormone) as well as weight loss and dull haircoat because it interferes with protein synthesis. Severe hypokalemia can cause death due to myocardial depression or paralysis of respiratory muscles.

52. Describe the management of hypokalemia.
Clinically stable cats with serum potassium concentrations < 4.0 mEq/L should be supplemented with oral potassium. Potassium gluconate is well tolerated by cats when administered orally at a dose of 2–6 mEq/cat/day. Potassium citrate (30 mg/lb/day, in divided doses every 8–12 hr orally) provides a beneficial alkalinizing side effect. Potassium chloride is an acidifier and not recommended. When serum potassium reaches 4.0 mEq/L, the oral dosage may be reduced to a maintenance level of 2 mEq/cat/day. Acidifying diets and diets low in magnesium should be avoided in cats with CRF because they promote hypokalemia.

Diuresis can potentiate hypokalemia. Oral potassium supplementation should be continued, if possible, and potassium should be added to fluids using the following formula:

Serum potassium concentration (mEq/L)	Potassium chloride/liter of fluid (mEq)
< 2.0	80
2.0–2.5	60
2.6–3.0	40
3.0–3.5	30
3.5–4.0	20

53. How should acid-base disturbances be treated?

For patients with moderate-to-severe acidosis (serum bicarbonate concentration ≤ 17 mEq/L), oral supplementation may be indicated. Sodium bicarbonate should be administered orally at 8–12 mg/kg every 8–12 hours; the final dose should be tailored to the individual. Alternatively, potassium citrate may be given orally (40–60 mg/kg every 12 hr); it has the benefit of aiding in the management of both acidosis and hypokalemia. Treatment of metabolic acidosis without concurrent treatment of hypokalemia may not be effective.

54. How is hyperphosphatemia treated?

Hyperphosphatemia should be controlled to prolong survival time and limit renal secondary hyperparathyroidism. Control is achieved by limiting dietary intake of phosphorus and administering phosphorus-binding agents. Although phosphorus-restricted diets are usually implemented when serum phosphate levels are elevated, evidence suggests that they should be started much earlier, because hyperparathyroidism may occur long before serum phosphate levels are affected. Because most dietary phosphorus is obtained from protein sources, reduced-protein diets are recommended (see Chapter 50).

55. When should phosphorus-binding agents be given?

When serum phosphorus concentrations remain elevated 2–4 weeks after implementing dietary restrictions, intestinal phosphorus-binding agents should be administered. They limit the absorption of phosphorus in the diet and inhibit resorption of phosphorus contained in saliva, bile, and intestinal fluids. Phosphorus-restricted diets should be used concurrently because there is less phosphorus to bind and reduced risk of toxic side effects when a lower dose can be used. Phosphate binders usually are dosed to effect based on serial blood measurement of phosphorus concentration; recommended dose ranges are intended simply to guide initial therapy.

56. Which phosphorus-binding agents are recommended?

Aluminum hydroxide, aluminum carbonate, or aluminum oxide is commonly used. Sucralfate, an aluminum relative given to many patients with CRF to treat gastrointestinal ulceration, also may be useful as a phosphorus-binding agent. Inappetence and constipation may result. Encephalopathies, microcytic anemia, and osteomalacia are toxic side-effects in humans but have not yet been documented in cats.

Calcium acetate, calcium carbonate, and calcium citrate avoid the risk of aluminum toxicity but may induce significant hypercalcemia. Calcium acetate is least likely to produce hypercalcemia and is a more effective binding agent than the others. Either calcium acetate or calcium carbonate may be combined with an aluminum-based binding agent to reduce the risks of aluminum toxicity and hypercalcemia. Calcium citrate should not be used with an aluminum-based phosphorus-binding agent. Serum calcium and phosphorus concentrations should be measured approximately 10–14 days after starting therapy and the dose adjusted accordingly.

57. How are the gastrointestinal side effects of uremia managed?

Uremic gastritis and ulcers cause inappetence, vomiting, and, in some cats, blood loss. H_2 receptor antagonists such as ranitidine, cimetidine, and famotidine can be adminstered parenterally until the cat is eating; at that point, they are administered orally. Because of renal clearance, ranitidine and famotidine doses should be reduced if the patient is severely ill. Many clinicians decrease the dosing frequency (in lieu of decreasing the dose) to every 48 or 72 hours. Gastric ulceration may be treated with the coating agent sucralfate. Oral ulcers can be treated with oral rinses of 0.1–0.2% chlorhexidine 3 or 4 times/day to reduce bacteria, prevent additional ulcer formation, and relieve discomfort. Very painful necrotic lesions may be treated with topical lidocaine. Metoclopramide can be given orally to improve gastric motility and lessen nausea.

58. Can the anemia of CRF be controlled?

- It is important to try to identify the cause of anemia and to control other potentiating problems.
- Uremia and gastric ulceration should be corrected first.
- Malnutrition, protein and vitamin deficiencies, and hyperphosphatemia can lead to anemia and should be corrected.
- Iron deficiency is fairly common in cats with CRF and may be treated with iron sulfate. Iron therapy also should be instituted in animals treated with recombinant erythropoietin.
- Transfusion with whole blood or packed red blood cells may be warranted in severely anemic patients with CRF, particularly those that are thought to be inappetent because of hypoxemia. This therapy is only used when necessary because of associated risks (i.e., transfusion reaction with multiple treatments, transfer of infectious agents), high cost, limited availability, and reduced life span of transfused cells in patients with uremia. Ideally, blood typing or cross-matching should be performed before transfusion to minimize complications. The target hematocrit should be at the low end of the normal range.

59. What strategies may be used to treat persistent anemia?

Persistent anemia (hematocrit < 20%) resulting in clinical signs such as weakness and inappetence often can be managed with recombinant human erythropoietin (rHuEPO). The usual starting dose is approximately 100 U/kg subcutaneously 3 times week. In hypertensive cats, a subcutaneous dose of 50 U/kg 3 times/week is suggested. The hematocrit should be monitored weekly and the dose adjusted accordingly. Resolution of the anemia usually takes 2–8 weeks. Because use of rHuEPO places a high demand on the body's iron stores, patients receiving hormone replacement therapy also should be given iron supplements. In addition to increased hematocrit, most treated cats exhibit improvements in appetite, energy, and body weight. The most common complications of rHuEPO administration are polycythemia and formation of anti-rHuEPO antibodies, resulting in refractory anemia. On rare occasions, cutaneous allergic reactions (which resolve when therapy is discontinued and often do not recur when therapy is reinstituted) and seizures (primarily in severely debilitated animals) have been noted.

60. When should systemic hypertension be treated?

Systolic pressure consistently exceeding 170 mmHg indicates systemic hypertension (see Chapter 63). Cats with systolic pressure > 200 mmHg can develop retinal detachment or neurologic signs and require immediate therapy. With acute retinal detachment or edema surrounding the optic disc, hospitalization and rapid reduction of blood pressure (15–20%) with intravenous sodium nitroprusside may be instituted.

61. Discuss the role of sodium restriction for chronic management of hypertension.

No conclusive studies document the effects of dietary sodium restriction on blood pressure in cats. Suggestions for the restriction of sodium have been extrapolated from studies in other (primarily human) species that link sodium with promotion of arterial hypertension. However, sodium restriction may result in prerenal azotemia by decreasing extracellular fluid volume. In addition, diets low in sodium may be less palatable. At this point inadequate data are available to suggest that sodium restriction is beneficial or harmful to cats. However, most renal diets are formulated with restricted sodium.

62. What drugs are used to control chronic hypertension?

The calcium channel antagonist amlodipine (0.625 mg/cat/day orally) is currently the drug of choice for systemic hypertension because of its ability to reduce blood pressure without causing fluid retention. Blood pressure measurements should be repeated every 2–4 weeks, with subsequent dosage adjustments, until systolic pressure is just below 170 mmHg. Hypotension accompanied by lethargy, weakness, or anorexia suggests that the dosage should be reduced, whereas a partial response to therapy suggests that the dosage may be increased.

If there is no response to a higher dose of amlodipine, a second drug should be added; angiotensin-converting enzyme inhibitors and beta antagonists are used most frequently (see Chapter 63). Patients undergoing hypertensive therapy also should be monitored closely for elevations in serum urea nitrogen and creatinine because hypotension can create prerenal azotemia and induce uremic crisis.

63. How common are drug interactions in cats with CRF?

Because of reduced renal clearance, changes in distribution, altered protein binding, and abnormal hepatic biotransformation, some medications may produce changes in therapeutic effects (both increased and decreased), resulting in increased incidence of adverse drug reactions in patients with CRF. In addition, some drugs are nephrotoxic even at normal doses and must be used with extreme care. Changes in binding capacity may promote toxicity of some drugs while lessening the therapeutic effect of other drugs administered within the normal dose range. Effects of reduced renal clearance must be taken into consideration before any therapy is changed.

Drugs Affected by Renal Failure

DRUG	PROBLEM	DOSE CHANGE
Amikacin	Nephrotoxic	Reduce dose interval*
Aminoglycoside antibiotics	Nephrotoxic	Avoid
Amoxicillin	Renal excretion	Use half dose or double dose interval in severely ill patients
Amphotericin B	Nephrotoxic	Reduce dose interval*
Ampicillin	Renal excretion	Use half dose or double dose interval
Antacids containing magnesium or phosphorus	Hypermagnesemia, hyperphosphatemia	Avoid
Carbenicillin	May promote acidosis, renal excretion	Use half dose or double dose interval
Cephalexin	Renal excretion	Reduce dose†
Cephalothin	Nephrotoxic (?), renal excretion, slow elimination	Reduce dose† or use half dose or double dose interval
Chloramphenicol	Partial renal excretion	Normal dose; avoid in advanced renal failure
Cimetidine	Increased binding, reduced renal clearance	Reduce dose by 10–25% in severe disease
Cis-platinum	Nephrotoxic	Contraindicated
Digoxin	Renal excretion	Reduce dose interval*
Doxycycline	Nephrotoxic (?), partial renal excretion	Normal dose
Enrofloxacin	Renal excretion	Reduce dose interval* or reduce dose†
Famotidine	Renal excretion	Reduce dose by 10–25% in severe disease
Furosemide	Nephrotoxic (?), renal excretion, hypokalemia	Normal dose
Gentamicin	Nephrotoxic, renal excretion	Reduce dose interval*
Glucocorticoids	May worsen proteinuria, increase BUN and protein catabolism	Avoid

Table continued on following page

Drugs Affected by Renal Failure (Continued)

DRUG	PROBLEM	DOSE CHANGE
Insulin	Slow elimination	
Kanamycin	Nephrotoxic, renal excretion	Reduce dose interval*
Methoxyflurane	Nephrotoxic	Avoid
Metoclopramide	Renal excretion	Reduce dose by 50% in severe disease
Neomycin	Nephrotoxic	Contraindicated in renal failure
Nitrofurantoin	Renal excretion, may promote acidosis	Contraindicated in renal failure
NSAIDs	Decreased binding	Avoid
Orbifloxacin	Renal excretion	Reduce dose interval* or reduce dose[†]
Penicillin	Renal excretion	Use half dose or double dose interval
Procainamide	Renal excretion	Use half dose or double dose interval
Propranolol	Slow to rapid renal clearance	Normal dose to start
Ranitidine	Renal excretion	Reduce dose by 50–75% in severe disease
Streptomycin	Nephrotoxic, renal excretion	Reduce dose[†]
Sulfonamides	Nephrotoxic	Reduce dose[†]
Tetracycline	Nephrotoxic, renal excretion, may increase BUN	Contraindicated
Tobramycin	Nephrotoxic, renal excretion	Reduce dose interval*
Trimethoprim-sulfamethoxazole	Nephrotoxic	Reduce dose,[†] avoid in advanced renal failure
Urinary acidifying agents (methanamine mandelate, nalidixic acid)	Promote acidosis	Avoid

* Normal interval × normal creatinine clearance/patient creatinine clearance *or* normal interval × patient creatinine/normal creatinine.
[†] Normal dose × patient creatinine clearance/normal creatinine clearance *or* normal dose × normal creatinine/patient creatinine.

64. How is the progress of a patient with renal failure monitored?

Once the cat is stabilized, evaluations should be performed 3 or 4 times/year. More frequent rechecks (every 2–4 weeks) are recommended when therapeutic alterations are made. Physical examination and serial blood and urine tests are the best methods of determining treatment response. Body weight, indirect blood pressure, packed cell volume and total protein, total carbon dioxide, and serum levels of BUN, creatinine, potassium, calcium (preferably ionized), and phosphorus should be measured; in addition, a complete urinalysis and urine culture should be performed.

65. Is dialysis available for cats?

Hemodialysis to remove uremic toxins is offered at a limited number of facilities across the nation. Hemodialysis is highly effective for ethylene glycol intoxication and for supporting renal function and reducing azotemia in both ARF and CRF. However, one study indicates that, although hemodialysis has proved effective and beneficial in ARF, complications and chronic debilitation limit its efficacy in CRF. Peritoneal dialysis is simpler to perform but is labor-intensive and requires a large owner and veterinarian commitment, including 24-hour facilities and care. Medical complications commonly encountered include peritonitis and hypoproteinemia.

66. When should dialysis be considered?

Dialysis should only be considered for short-term therapy in the following settings:

• Persistent oliguria despite appropriate fluid, diuretic, or vasodilator therapy

- Life-threatening electrolyte or acid–base disturbances that are nonresponsive to other treatments
- BUN > 100 mg/dl or serum creatinine > 10 mg/dl that is nonresponsive to other treatments
- Severe fluid overload, pulmonary edema, or congestive heart failure
- Acute poisoning or drug overdose
- Stabilization of renal transplant recipients before transplant or during episodes of acute rejection.

67. Is renal transplantation a viable option?

Renal transplantation can be considered if the patient is in early decompensation; has lost no more than 20% of healthy body weight; has no evidence of cardiac disease, urinary tract infection, or secondary illness; and is negative for feline retroviruses. In addition, the owner must be cooperative, able to medicate the recipient, willing to adopt the donor cat, and both willing and able to undertake the expense of surgery (estimated at $3000–$7000) and aftercare (which may be as high as several hundred dollars per month). Recipients must be placed on long-term immunosuppressive therapy (prednisolone and cyclosporine) postoperatively and monitored regularly. Researchers at the University of California College of Veterinary Medicine have reported a 79% survival rate in transplanted cats.

68. What is the prognosis for patients with ARF?

Prognosis depends on etiology and timely and aggressive administration of appropriate therapy. Cats with ARF due to prerenal or postrenal factors have an excellent prognosis if the inciting cause is removed before structural damage to the kidneys occurs. ARF due to infectious agents generally has a better chance of reversal than ARF due to nephrotoxic agents, although nephrotoxic ARF has a better prognosis than ischemic ARF. In general, polyuric renal failure has a better prognosis than oliguric or anuric renal failure. Magnitude of azotemia is not a good predictor of outcome. Cats that survive to the recovery phase frequently do not recover full renal function and should be observed for evidence of renal insufficiency or failure.

Studies have shown that hemodialysis has extended lives in severe cases of RF. In one study, 60% of cats with pyelonephritis or ethylene glycol toxicity that did not respond to conventional therapy recovered sufficiently that further dialysis was unnecessary, and 44% of cats with ethylene glycol toxicity, severe azotemia, and oliguria or anuria also survived with hemodialysis.

69. What is the prognosis for patients with CRF?

Because loss of renal function is permanent in CRF, prognosis depends on the extent or probability of abatement of clinical signs. Long-term prognosis should be based on a number of factors, including severity of clinical signs, likelihood of improving renal function, severity of impaired renal function, type and rate of progression of disease, and age of the patient.

Severity of clinical signs is usually a good short-term prognostic indicator, except in cases of acute-on-chronic renal failure when the patient may be in a temporary uremic state. Severity of renal dysfunction also may be useful in establishing long-term prognosis. Hydrated, well-fed cats with serum creatinine concentrations < 4.5 mg/dl typically fare rather well, whereas cats with concentrations > 10 mg/dl do not respond as favorably. Similarly, hyperphosphatemia is indicative of advanced disease and a guarded prognosis.

Many cats with CRF can be maintained with a good quality of life for months to years. However, CRF is a progressive disease, and no therapeutic strategies to date have been shown to alter markedly its progression in cats. The best method of predicting long-term prognosis is to assess progression and response to management with serial examinations and laboratory evaluations.

CONTROVERSIES

70. Can renal failure be prevented?

Potentially inciting factors should be avoided. Increasing natriuresis, urine volume, and solute excretion by saline diuresis before administration of nephrotoxic agents may help to prevent ARF.

Chronic metabolic acidosis due to acidifying diets may lead to bone demineralization as well as taurine and potassium depletion. Studies also suggest that hypokalemia may be a cause and not only a result of CRF in some cats.

Systemic hypertension may lead to chronic progression of renal failure. For the most part, it is unknown whether hypertensive cats with CRF develop systemic hypertension secondarily or whether chronic systemic hypertension causes CRF. Blood pressure measurement should be part of the yearly health assessment for middle-aged and geriatric cats.

71. Is calcitriol supplementation indicated?

Reduced calcitriol production may develop as renal tubular function declines, contributing to renal secondary hyperparathyroidism and increased levels of circulating parathyroid hormone. Calcitriol rapidly and effectively controls secondary hyperparathyroidism without requiring renal activation like other forms of vitamin D therapy. Some evidence suggests that calcitriol supplementation benefits patients with CRF; favorable results (improved appetite, brighter attitude, more active, longer life span) have been reported by clinicians. However, controlled clinical trials have not been conducted in cats.

72. When and how should calctriol administration be initiated?

Calcitriol administration may be initiated after dietary phosphorus restriction has been implemented and serum phosphorus is controlled (< 6 mg/dl). The recommended initial dose range is 1.5-3.5 ng/kg orally every 24 hours, but this recommendation should be amended for the individual patient, preferably not to exceed 6.6 ng/kg. Calcitriol is best administered at night on an empty stomach because of its propensity to increase intestinal absorption of both calcium and phosphorus. Calcitriol should be used with caution in patients receiving calcium–based phosphate binders, particularly calcium carbonate.

The onset of action and half-life of calcitriol are short ($\leq$ 24 hrs); BUN, creatinine, calcium, and phosphorus measurements should be evaluated 1 week after initiating calcitriol administration. Ideally, the concentration of calcium times phosphorus product should be between 42 and 50. If the product exceeds 60, calcitriol therapy should be discontinued. If hypercalcemia develops, calcium carbonate administration should be discontinued or replaced with an aluminum-based phosphorus-binding agent. If calcium carbonate is not administered, calcitriol treatment should be discontinued, then reinstituted at a lower dose when serum calcium levels return to normal.

73. Does magnesium imbalance occur in patients with renal failure?

Patients with CRF have the potential to be hypermagnesemic because the kidneys cannot excrete magnesium. Hypermagnesemia is not considered clinically significant unless it is accompanied by hypocalcemia. Magnesium-containing antacids are contraindicated.

More commonly, protein catabolism, peritoneal dialysis, use of diuretics, and aggressive fluid therapy produce abnormally low magnesium levels that may result in muscle weakness, tremors, and seizures. In addition, insufficient magnesium may leave the kidneys vulnerable to further insult, because magnesium may be renoprotective in some types of toxicity. If severe hypomagnesemia is documented ($\leq$ 1.2 mg/dl), supplementation should be administered intravenously by the addition of magnesium chloride or magnesium sulfate to 5% dextrose in water, using an initial dose of 0.75–1.0 mEq/kg/day for 3–5 days . In the case of life-threatening ventricular fibrillation, 0.15–0.3 mEq (50–100 mg) per kg may be added to a solution of 5% dextrose or 0.9% saline and administered intravenously over 5–15 minutes.

74. Are anabolic steroids indicated in anemic patients with CRF?

Anabolic steroids, once widely used, are no longer recommended because of their limited efficacy, prolonged onset of action, and adverse side effects. A recent study suggests that stanazolol can be hepatotoxic to cats. Although the effects may be reversed once therapy is discontinued, there still is no clear indication for the use of anabolic steroids in feline CRF.

75. When should diet therapy be instituted?

For reasons mentioned above, diet therapy should be instituted as soon as chronic renal disease is indicated. Patients are more likely to tolerate a change in diet before gastrointestinal effects of CRF occur, and early in renal disease it may be possible to control hyperparathyroidism by dietary intervention alone. However, protein restriction in patients whose serum creatinine concentration is < 5 mg/dl is controversial. Until we achieve a better understanding of the role of dietary protein in such patients, a reasonable compromise may be the gradual reduction of dietary protein in relation to the increase in serum creatinine. Morraillon suggests the following guidelines:

Serum Creatinine (mg/dl)	Dietary Protein (%DM)
3.5	25
4.0	19
4.5	14
5.0	10
5.5	7

76. Should fatty acid supplements be used?

Studies in people suggest that fatty acids may alter the progression of renal failure. However, human studies cannot be directly extrapolated to cats because, unlike in people, both linoleic and arachidonic acids are essential fatty acids in cats, and the conversion of one fatty acid to the other is limited. As a result, further studies of the benefits and risks of dietary supplementation with fatty acids are necessary before recommendations can be made.

BIBLIOGRAPHY

1. Barber PJ, Elliott J: Feline chronic renal failure: Calcium homeostasis in 80 cases diagnosed between 1992 and 1995. J Small Anim Pract 39:108–166, 1998.
2. Bartges JW, Willis AM, Polzin DJ: Hypertension and renal disease. Vet Clin North Amer Small Anim Prac 26:1331–1345, 1996.
3. Burkholder WJ: Dietary considerations for dogs and cats with renal disease. J Am Vet Med Assoc 216:1730–1734, 2000.
4. Cowgill LD, Elliott DA: Acute renal failure. In Ettinger SJ, Feldman EC (eds): Textbook of Veterinary Internal Medicine. Philadelphia, W.B. Saunders, 2000, pp 1615–1633.
5. Grooters AM, Duypers MD, Partington BP, et al: Renomegaly in dogs and cats. Part II: Diagnostic approach. Comp Cont Educ Pract Vet 19:1212–1229, 1997.
6. Harkin KR, Cowan LA, Andrews GA, et al: Hepatotoxicity of stanozolol in cats. J Am Vet Med Assoc 217:681–684, 2000.
7. Hurley KJ: Acute renal failure. Waltham FOCUS on the Urinary Tract. Presented at the 1998 British Small Animal Veterinary Association Conference. Waltham USA, Inc.. 1998, pp 7–17.
8. Lane IF, Grauer GF, Fettman MJ: Acute renal failure. Part I: Risk factors, prevention, and strategies for protection. Comp Cont Ed Pract Vet 16:15–29, 1994.
9. Lane IF, Grauer GF, Fettman MJ: Acute renal failure. Part II: Diagnosis, management, and prognosis. Comp Cont Educ Pract Vet 16:625–645, 1994.
10. Lulich JP, Osborne CA, O'Brien TD, et al: Feline renal failure: questions, answers, questions. Comp Cont Educ Pract Vet 14:127–152, 1992.
11. Macintire DK: Disorders of potassium, phosphorus, and magnesium in critical illness. Comp Cont Educ Pract Vet 19:41–48, 1997.
12. Nagode LA, Chew D, Podell M: Benefits of calcitriol therapy and serum phosphorus control in dogs and cats with chronic renal failure. Vet Clin North Amer Small Anim Prac 26:1293–1330, 1996.
13. Neel JA, Grindem CB: Understanding and evaluating renal function. Vet Med 95:555–565, 2000.
14. Norsworthy GD: Managing chronic renal failure in geriatric cats. Vet Med 95:11–18, 2000.
15. Polzin DJ, Osborne CA, Jacob F, et al: Chronic renal failure. In Ettinger SJ, Feldman EC (eds): Textbook of Veterinary Internal Medicine. Philadelphia, W.B. Saunders, 2000, pp 1634–1662.
16. Rubin SI: Chronic renal failure and its management and nephrolithiasis. Vet Clin North Am Small Anim Pract 27:1331–1354, 1997.
17. Sparkes AH: Diagnosis and management of chronic renal failure in cats. Waltham FOCUS on the Urinary Tract. Waltham USA, Inc., 1998, pp 25–31.

41. PYELONEPHRITIS

Helen Tuzio, D.V.M., M.S.

1. Define pyelonephritis.

Pyelonephritis refers to inflammation of the renal pelvis and parenchyma, especially the adjacent medulla, with potential extension into the cortex. The disease may be unilateral or bilateral, acute or chronic.

2. What causes pyelonephritis?

Pyelonephritis is a manifestation of bacterial infection of the kidneys. Usually bacteria ascend from the lower urinary tract, but they also may spread to the kidneys via the bloodstream (hematogenous route) from distant foci such as dental disease, bacterial endocarditis, or diskospondylitis. The most frequently implicated organisms include *Escherichia coli, Staphylococcus aureus, Streptococcus* spp., *Klebsiella pneumoniae, Pseudomonas aeruginosa, Enterobacter* spp., and *Proteus* spp. Rarely are anaerobes identified as the cause of urinary tract infections (UTIs).

3. What types of conditions predispose patients to pyelonephritis?

Normal voiding is a natural defense against UTI, effectively washing out bacteria from the urinary bladder. Therefore, disorders that decrease the frequency and/or volume of voided urine or that result in an increased urine residual volume (such as urethral stricture or urachal remnant) are predisposing factors. Damage to mucosal barriers of infection by uroliths, neoplasia, or even palpation leaves the patient susceptible to infection. Other anatomic anomalies, such as an ectopic ureteral termination, may allow ascending migration of bacteria.

Conditions that weaken the immune system, such as retroviral infection or hyperadrenocorticism, may predispose cats to pyelonephritis. Patients with diabetes mellitus generally have deficient immunity as well as a greater likelihood of lower UTI due to glucosuria. Conditions that result in dilute urine or extremes of urine pH reduce its antibacterial properties, making infection easier. Iatrogenic factors such as glucocorticoid administration, urinary catheterization, and surgical diversions (e.g., perineal urethrostomy) also predispose cats to kidney infection.

Other predisposing factors include decreased urine volume and decreasing frequency of voiding (from decreased water consumption or vomiting and diarrhea), voluntary retention of urine, vesicoureteral reflux, herniated bladder, and spinal diseases such as vertebral fractures, intervertebral disk disease, and spinal neoplasia.

4. What are the most commonly observed signs of pyelonephritis?

In the **acute form**, the most common signs are recent-onset lethargy, anorexia, fever, vomiting, and dehydration. Patients may demonstrate polyuria and polydipsia and have pain in the lumbar area. Signs of lower UTI (pollakiuria, strangiuria, dysuria, frank hematuria) also may be present.

The **chronic form** is subtle and may not be noticed by the owner. Patients may show weight loss or reduced appetite; some may be polydipsic and polyuric. Another common scenario suggesting upper UTI is a bacterial UTI that recurs when antibiotics are discontinued. In many cats, pyelonephritis is subclinical.

5. What may be found on physical examination?

Diagnosis usually is based on history, physical examination, and laboratory findings. In the **acute form**, fever and abdominal discomfort may be detected on physical examination. One or both kidneys may be enlarged or painful on palpation. Cats with the more subtle **chronic form** may have none of these physical indicators, and only a loss of weight may be noted.

6. What kind of laboratory tests should be done if pyelonephritis is suspected?
The minimum database should include complete blood count (CBC), serum biochemical panel, and urinalysis. In suspected cases, when the urine sediment is active or when the specific gravity is low (below 1.035), quantitative urine culture and sensitivity also should be performed.

7. What is typically found on urinalysis?
The simple and most sensitive diagnostic test of renal function, especially for diseases, such as pyelonephritis, that affect the medulla is a measure of the kidneys' concentrating ability, particularly in the face of dehydration or azotemia. The urine sample should be collected, preferably by cystocentesis, before drugs are administered. Urinalysis findings may include evidence of urinary tract inflammation (proteinuria, pyuria, and hematuria) as well as low specific gravity and bacteriuria. However, failure to detect bacteria in the sediment does not exclude the possibility of infection. Especially in patients with dilute urine, the sediment may be nonreactive.

8. When should urine be cultured?
In suspect cases or in cases of isosthenuria, the urine should be cultured qualitatively and quantitatively, even if no bacteria are observed in the sediment. Although ideally the culture should be initiated within 30 minutes of collection, the sample may be refrigerated for 6–8 hours before plating. Although the lower limit of bacterial growth in feline urine indicative of infection is thought to be lower than for dogs or people, the actual figure has yet to be determined. The consensus at present is that bacterial growth > 1000 bacteria/ml of sample collected by catheterization or any growth in a cystocentesis sample is indicative of UTI.

9. How is a kidney infection differentiated from a lower UTI?
The lower urinary tract is presumed to be involved in all cases of UTI, but in some cases it is difficult to determine whether the infection also involves the kidney(s) (see Chapter 46). In general, systemic signs such as fever, polyuria, polydipsia, depression, anorexia, vomiting, and dehydration are not seen with disorders limited to the bladder, urethra, or prostate. Granular casts (> 1/lpf), cellular casts, or renal epithelial cells in a urine sample help to localize the infection to the upper urinary tract; their absence, however, does not rule out the possibility of pyelonephritis. Upper UTI should be considered when infection recurs after initial therapy or when the infection is documented without concurrent lower urinary tract symptoms. In addition, a positive culture in dilute urine is suggestive of pyelonephritis.

Some cases of pyelonephritis are associated with concurrent changes in the hemogram and/or biochemistry referable to kidney disease. Hemogram (CBC and differential) abnormalities may include a neutrophilic leukocytosis with left shift (more likely in acute disease). The chronic form can result in a nonregenerative anemia. Serum biochemistry profile alterations observed during active infection may include azotemia and hyperphosphatemia, especially in patients with renal failure. Patients with azotemia typically have metabolic acidosis. In some cases serum biochemistry may be normal.

10. What other disorders may resemble pyelonephritis?
The nonspecific signs of systemic illness usually seen with pyelonephritis are also indicative of a myriad of other diseases, particularly those that affect both kidneys, such as polycystic kidney disease, feline infectious peritonitis, amyloidosis, bilateral hydronephrosis, renal lymphoma, and perinephric pseudocysts. Renomegaly may be identified in cases of hypertrophy, pyonephrosis, renal abscessation, and acute ureteral obstruction. Acute renal failure may resemble pyelonephritis but usually has a rapid onset. It is possible for a patient to have acute and/or chronic renal failure along with pyelonephritis (see Chapter 38).

11. What imaging tests help to confirm the diagnosis?
In some instances, imaging of the kidneys may be necessary to confirm the diagnosis or to identify predisposing factors. The normal feline kidney is 2.5–3.5 times the length of L2 on a

right lateral radiograph (3.0–4.3 cm on sonogram) and is located ventral to L1–L4 with the right kidney slightly cranial to the left. In cases of pyelonephritis, one or both kidneys may be enlarged, especially in the acute form of the disease. On abdominal ultrasound or excretory urogram, dilation of the renal pelvis(es) and ureter(s) may be seen. Incomplete filling of the diverticula may be evidence of an acute process, whereas blunting of the pelvic diverticula may be indicative of chronic pyelonephritis. A decrease in opacity of contrast media in the collecting system is suggestive of pyelonephritis, or good initial opacification may be followed by persistence of a dense nephrogram. Hyperechoic or asymmetrical cortices and hypoechoic or mixed echogenic renal pelves may be noted on abdominal ultrasound. However, diagnostic imaging is limited in that a normal study does not exclude the possibility of infection. In addition, neither imaging technique can quantify renal function or determine whether the disease process is reversible.

12. How is pyelonephritis treated?
Treatment consists of antibiotic administration to eradicate infection, correction of predisposing factors, and fluid therapy as needed. Animals that are acutely ill, anorexic, or azotemic benefit from intravenous fluid therapy and parental antibiotics until the systemic signs abate.

13. Which antibiotic should be administered?
The primary therapy consists of administration of the appropriate antimicrobial, based on urine culture and susceptibility results determined by minimum inhibitory concentration (MIC) of antimicrobials for the infecting organism. The preferred antibiotics are those that can penetrate the renal medulla, such as nitrofurantoin, trimethoprim, chloramphenicol, and enrofloxacin. The medication should be administered at the correct dosage for a minimum of 6–8 weeks. When the bacteria cannot be positively identified, penicillin should be used for gram-positive organisms; gram-negative organisms respond well to trimethoprim/sulfa or enrofloxacin. Because *Escherichia coli* is the most commonly isolated organism in feline UTI, patients with rods in the urine sediment may be treated with amoxicillin combined with clavulanic acid, trimethoprim-sulfa, or a quinolone until the sensitivity results are obtained. If cocci are identified, you may start the patient on ampicillin or amoxicillin while awaiting MIC results. In the absence of sensitivity testing, the following antibiotics are the drugs of choice for the most common infections: enrofloxacin for *E. coli* and *Klebsiella* spp.; amoxicillin-clavulanic acid for *Proteus* spp., *Staphylococcus* spp., and *Streptococcus* spp.; and tetracycline for *Enterobacter* spp. and *Pseudomonas* spp. Tetracyclines (except doxycycline) and aminoglycosides should be avoided in cases of renal insufficiency. In addition, the dosage of quinolones and cephalosporins should be reduced or the interval extended.

14. How are drug dosages adjusted in patients with renal failure?
1. Formula to adjust the dose of cephalosporins and quinolones:
Current dosage × (normal creatinine/patient's creatinine)
2. Formula to adjust the interval:
Current dosage × (patient's creatinine/normal creatinine)

15. How is the patient's progress monitored?
The urine should be cultured approximately 7–14 days after treatment is initiated to determine antimicrobial efficacy and then recultured 1 week after the therapeutic course is completed. If either culture is positive, a different antimicrobial should be selected (based on antimicrobial susceptibility testing) and the follow-up regimen repeated. If both cultures are negative, monthly cultures are recommended for several months to detect persistent infection. Ideally, the patient should not be considered recovered until three consecutive urine cultures are negative.

16. What causes "recurrent" UTIs?
A second episode may be due to **relapse** with the same infecting bacteria or to **reinfection** with a new strain of bacteria.

17. When does relapse usually occur? What are the typical causes?
Relapse usually occurs days to weeks after ending treatment and usually is caused by failure to clear the initial infection. Relapses are generally associated with a higher degree of antimicrobial resistance than original infections. The most common causes of relapse are as follows:
- Insufficient or inaccurate therapy
- Lack of owner compliance
- Failure to eliminate predisposing causes
- Impaired drug absorption from the gastrointestinal tract
- Bacterial sequestration or failure to multiply
- Mixed infections with only one pathogen eliminated by therapy
- Emergence of drug-resistant pathogens

18. When does reinfection occur? What are the typical causes?
Reinfection implies that the urinary tract again became infected after the initial infection was cleared. The time interval between reinfections is usually longer than that between relapses. Reinfections most frequently are due to the following causes:
- Failure or inability to relieve the predisposing factors
- Iatrogenic causes (catheterization)
- Sequelae to surgical techniques affecting host defenses (urethrostomy)

Reinfection with less invasive (opportunistic) bacteria, such as *Pseudomonas aeruginosa* or *Klebsiella pneumoniae*, usually suggests a compromised immune system.

19. What should be done for patients with frequent recurrences of UTI?
The first step should be a thorough effort to identify and eliminate predisposing factors, such as uroliths, anatomic defects, endocrinopathies, or other characteristics that interfere with the body's protective mechanism. Excretory urography and/or ultrasonography, if not previously performed, are recommended. In addition, a longer course of therapy (up to 6 months), should be instituted. If infection recurs after 6 months of full-course therapy, if reinfection occurs more than 4 times/year, or if predisposing factors are noncorrectable, suppressive therapy consisting of continuous low-dose administration of an antimicrobial should be initiated once the initial infection is cleared. Such patients usually do well on one-third to one-half the normal daily dose of antibiotic given once every 24 hours, preferably at night. Urine should be cultured monthly. If a positive culture is obtained, the patient is treated as though the infection were acute (full dose for 4–6 weeks) before returning to low-dose therapy; if the culture is negative, suppressive therapy should be continued. Most cases do well after 6 months of bacteria-free urine. However, in patients prone to reinfection, urine should be examined and cultured periodically, preferably at least 3 times/year.

20. What is the prognosis for cats with pyelonephritis?
The status of the host's defense mechanisms is the most important factor in assessing probable outcome of treatment for UTI. Pyelonephritis in both severe acute and chronic forms can lead to renal failure. Cats diagnosed early in the acute form and treated aggressively appear to do well. The prognosis is also good if predisposing factors are eliminated and treatment begun before the onset of endstage renal disease. Cats in which treatment is delayed or inadequate to eradicate infection often suffer permanent kidney damage and chronic renal failure.

CONTROVERSIES

21. What is the role of pyelocentesis and kidney biopsy in the diagnosis pyelonephritis?
Although culture of a pyelocentesis sample and histopathologic findings are necessary for definitive diagnosis of pyelonephritis, there are varying schools of thought about performing these procedures in the face of infection. Fine-needle aspiration can be performed with ultrasound guidance and may provide an ideal sample for culture of the upper urinary tract, but some

experts believe that renal sampling is contraindicated in cases of infection because of the potential for creating leakage into the abdomen and subsequent peritonitis. Renal biopsies also may contribute to progressive renal deterioration in cats. A good rule of thumb is that any cat with UTI and azotemia or dilute urine should be assumed to have pyelonephritis. With this principle in mind, few cases of UTI should require renal biopsy.

22. Are any adjunct treatments helpful in pyelonephritis?

Recent studies in rats treated with antibiotics have suggested that supplementation with vitamins A and E may help to decrease the extent of renal inflammation in acute bacterial pyelonephritis. However, these preliminary data have not yet been explored in cats.

23. In cats with unilateral disease, should the affected kidney be surgically removed?

Nephrectomy as a treatment for pyelonephritis is not recommended and rarely performed. It should be done only as a last resort, and only if (1) the diseased kidney appears grossly abnormal on excretory urogram; (2) the contralateral kidney appears normal on excretory urogram; and (3) the patient is not azotemic. Quantitative renal scintigraphy can be completed at referral centers to document individual kidney function before nephrectomy is performed.

BIBLIOGRAPHY

1. Barsanti JA: Genitourinary infections. In Greene CE (ed): Infectious Diseases of the Dog and Cat, 2nd ed. Philadelphia, W.B. Saunders, 1998, pp 626–646.
2. Bennett RT, Mazzaccaro RJ, Chopra N, et al: Suppression of renal inflammation with vitamins A and E in ascending pyelonephritis in rats. J Urol 161:1681–1684, 1999.
3. Cuypers M, Grooters AM, Williams J, et al: Renomegaly in dogs and cats. Part I: Differential diagnosis. Comp Cont Educ Pract Vet 19:1019–1032, 1997.
4. DiBartola SP: Renal diseases of the cat. Proceedings from the American Board of Veterinary Practitioners Symposium. Chicago, 1998, pp 197–214.
5. Feeney DA, Barber DL, Johnston GR, et al: The excretory urogram. Part II: Interpretation of abnormal findings. Compendium Collection: Renal Disease in Small Animal Practice. Trenton, NJ, Veterinary Learning Systems, 1994, pp 255–263.
6. Forrester SD, Lees GE: Diseases of the kidney and ureter. In Birchard SJ, Sherding RG (eds): Saunders Manual of Small Animal Practice. Philadelphia, W.B. Saunders, 1994, pp 807–808.
7. Grauer GF: Urinary disorders. In Nelson RW, Couto CG (eds): Manual of Small Animal Internal Medicine. St. Louis, Mosby, 1999, pp 355–408, 790.
8. Grauer GF: Complicated urinary tract infections. Scientific Proceedings of the American Animal Hospital Association, Chicago, 1998, pp 44–47.
9. Grooters AM, Cuypers M, Partington BP, et al: Renomegaly in dogs and cats. Part II: Diagnostic approach. Comp Cont Educ Small Anim Pract 19:1213–1229, 1997.
10. Lulich JP, Osborne CA, O'Brien TD, Polzin DJ: Feline renal failure: Questions, answers, questions. Comp Cont Educ Sm Anim Pract 14:127–152, 1992.
11. Osborne CA: Three steps to effective management of bacterial urinary tract infections: Diagnosis, diagnosis, and diagnosis. Comp Cont Educ Small Anim Pract 17:1233–1248, 1995.
12. Polzin DJ: Recurrent urinary tract infections. Scientific Proceedings of the American Animal Hospital Association, Seattle, WA, 1993, pp 461–464.
13. Rubin SI: The procedures that confirm and localize a urinary tract infection. Vet Med 85:352–364, 1990.
14. Senior DF: Bacterial urinary tract infections: Invasion, host defenses, and new approaches to prevention. Compendium Collection: Renal Disease in Small Animal Practice. Trenton, NJ, Veterinary Learning Systems, 1994, pp 160–168.

42. POLYCYSTIC KIDNEY DISEASE

Julie R. Fischer, D.V.M.

1. Define polycystic kidney disease.

Polycystic kidney disease (PKD) is an autosomal dominant condition that occurs most commonly in Persian and Persian crossbred cats, but it has been documented in many other breeds as well as in mixed-breed cats. Affected cats develop fluid-filled cysts in the renal parenchyma; cysts compress the normal renal tissue as they expand. The disease is progressive, and in most cats parenchymal compression and consequent interstitial nephritis eventually result in renal failure.

2. What historical findings support the diagnosis of PKD?

Because the clinical signs of PKD are due to renal failure, which may take years to develop, cats are usually subclinically affected and considered normal by their owners until the later stages of the disease. Once renal insufficiency or failure occurs, historical findings are the same as for other causes of chronic renal failure. Common examples include polyuria, polydipsia, inappetence, weight loss, vomiting, and weakness (see Chapter 40). Cats with PKD may be predisposed to develop urinary tract infections because the cysts can serve as a nidus for bacterial growth. Culture of cyst fluid may be necessary to document infection.

3. Describe the classic physical examination findings.

Cats with PKD may have renomegaly on physical examination. The kidneys usually have a palpably irregular surface and in severely affected cats can feel like small bunches of grapes. In the early stages of PKD, changes in renal structure are likely be the only abnormal physical examination finding. Physical examination performed in the late stages of the disease may reveal signs consistent with chronic renal failure; poor body condition, pallor, dehydration, and weakness are common. Uremic breath and oral ulceration are consistent with decompensated renal failure (see Chapter 40). Renal hemorrhages or retinal detachment may be seen in cats with concurrent systemic arterial hypertension.

4. What laboratory abnormalities are seen with PKD?

No blood or urine abnormalities are specific for PKD. The serum biochemical and urinalyses in an otherwise healthy cat are unremarkable before renal insufficiency occurs; afterward they are typical of this condition (see Chapter 40).

5. When should PKD be suspected?

Any Persian or Persian crossbred cat with historical, physical examination, or laboratory findings consistent with chronic renal failure or with persistent or recurrent bacterial urinary tract infection should be screened for PKD. In addition, any cat whose kidneys feel irregularly marginated on physical examination should be screened.

6. What is the best diagnostic test for PKD?

Ultrasonographic examination of the kidneys reliably detects PKD. The fluid-filled cysts are readily apparent as hypoechoic, usually spherical regions scattered through both kidneys. Cysts vary greatly in size (from < 1 mm to > 1 cm). Only a few cysts may be present, or cysts may occupy most of the renal parenchyma. Ultrasonography differentiates PKD from renal neoplasia and feline infectious peritonitis, both of which also can cause palpably irregular, lumpy kidneys. Excretory urography is also helpful in differentiating PKD from other causes of renomegaly. The nephrogram phase in a cat with PKD shows numerous, sharply demarcated radiolucencies in the

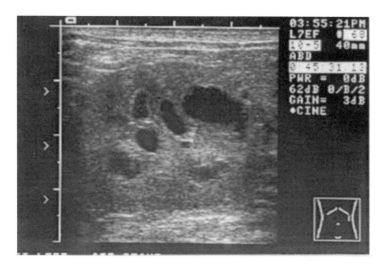

Longitudinal ultrasonographic image of the left kidney of a 4-year-old Persian cat with PKD. Note the multiple, varied, rounded, anechoic regions throughout the renal parenchyma. The other kidney was similarly affected. (Image courtesy of David S. Biller, D.V.M., Kansas State University.)

renal parenchyma, because the cysts do not fill with contrast media. Late in the disease, survey radiographs may detect bilateral renomegaly and irregular renal silhouettes.

7. What should I do if a client asks me to "screen" a cat for PKD?

If the cat is Persian or Persian crossbred, agree to it! Ultrasonographic examination can detect renal cysts noninvasively in kittens as young as 7 weeks of age. In one study, ultrasonographic findings in cats at least 36 weeks of age had a 91% sensitivity and 100% specificity for the detection of PKD. Sensitivity was 75% (but specificity was still 100%) in kittens 16 weeks of age or less. However, sensitivity and specificity are operator-dependent; experienced ultrasonographers should perform PKD screening examinations. A clinically normal cat of non-Persian breeding has a relatively low likelihood of having cystic renal disease (14% in one study), and, if present, the disease may not behave like PKD.

8. How can PKD affect the health of an affected cat?

PKD is a progressive disease. Cats with PKD develop renal insufficiency and eventual renal failure when cystic enlargement and interstitial nephritis destroy more than 67–75% of the renal parenchyma. Cats so affected should be treated like cats with chronic renal failure for any other reason (see Chapter 40). In addition, the cysts can become infected.

9. How are cyst infections diagnosed and treated?

Cyst infections may be difficult to diagnose and to clear. Cyst fluid can be aspirated with ultrasound guidance, and culture of the fluid gives the most solid basis for antimicrobial selection. If infected cysts are suspected or confirmed, lipid-soluble antimicrobials, which penetrate the cyst wall, should be used for therapy. Fluoroquinolones and potentiated sulfonamides have been shown to achieve excellent penetration into renal cysts in humans, and should be used for at least 4–6 weeks. Documented cyst infections should be treated as complicated urinary tract infections, with monitoring and reculturing as indicated (see Chapters 39 and 48).

10. How quickly does PKD progress?

The rate of progression to renal failure varies tremendously from cat to cat. Renal failure usually occurs between the ages of 3 and 10 years, with an average age at onset of 7 years. Occasionally, a cat will live a normal life span despite the presence of PKD.

11. What can be done to prevent PKD?

Because PKD is an autosomal dominant condition, it is theoretically possible to eliminate it from the Persian breed by careful screening and exclusion of affected cats from the breeding pool. Owners should be informed that PKD is heritable. Cats with PKD should be sterilized or otherwise prevented from reproducing.

BIBLIOGRAPHY

1. Biller DS, Chew DJ, DiBartola SJ: Polycystic kidney disease in a family of Persian cats. J Am Vet Med Assoc 196:1288–1290, 1990.
2. Biller DS, DiBartola SP: Familial renal disease in cats. In Bonagura JD, Kirk RW (eds): Current Veterinary Therapy XII. Philadelphia, W.B. Saunders, 1995, pp 977–979.
3. Biller DS, DiBartola SP, Eaton KA: Inheritance of polycystic kidney disease in Persian cats. J Hered 87:1–5, 1996.
4. DiBartola SP: Autosomal dominant polycystic kidney disease. In Proceedings of the 18th Annual Veterinary Medical Forum, Seattle, WA, 2000, pp 438–439.
5. Eaton KA, Biller DS, DiBartola SP, et al: Autosomal dominant polycystic kidney disease in Persian and Persian-cross cats. Vet Pathol 34:117–126, 1997.

43. FELINE GLOMERULAR DISEASES

Craig B. Webb, D.V.M., Ph.D.

1. What are the two major categories of glomerular disease?

Glomerulonephritis and amyloidosis.

2. How prevalent is glomerular disease in cats?

Confirmed cases of feline glomerular disease are rare. In two separate surveys of 160 and 333 sick cats, only one suspected case of glomerulonephritis was identified. One review of published reports of feline amyloidosis uncovered 20 cases over a 20-year time span. However, reports of glomerular disease in cats have increased in prevalence with the advent of electron microscopy and the ability to discern changes in basement membrane and podocyte foot process morphology.

3. Describe the pathogenesis of glomerulonephritis.

Glomerulonephritis results from one of two immunologic mechanisms: immune complex deposition or formation of antibodies to glomerular basement membrane components. Soluble, circulating antigen–antibody complexes may become localized in glomerular capillary walls, or in situ immune complexes may be formed in response to antigens within the glomerular basement membrane and capillary walls.

4. What glomerular changes result from immune complex deposition?

The glomerular response to immune complex deposition is glomerular cell proliferation and glomerular capillary wall thickening. Associated findings are cellular and mesangial matrix proliferation and glomerular basement membrane thickening.

5. Describe the pathologic progression of glomerulonephritis.

Antibody–antigen complexes within the glomerulus activate complement, stimulate platelet adhesion and aggregation, signal neutrophil infiltration, and activate the coagulation system. Complement activation triggers an inflammatory response, including the release of proteolytic and lysosomal enzymes by neutrophils, followed by fibrin deposition. Aggregated platelets release thromboxane, which further promotes inflammation.

6. What clinicopathological abnormalities are consistent with glomerulonephritis?

The hallmark abnormality of glomerulonephritis is proteinuria. In addition, an inactive urine sediment is usually present, and both hyaline and granular casts may be observed. Progression of the disease and response to treatment can be monitored by serial measurement of the urine protein:creatinine (UPC) ratio. Hypoalbuminemia and hypercholesterolemia may occur if nephrotic syndrome develops.

7. What is a normal UPC ratio?

A UPC ratio < 1 is considered by many to be normal. However, some clinicians consider a UPC > 0.5 significant in cats. A moderately elevated UPC ratio (i.e., > 1; < 20) is consistent with glomerulonephritis.

8. What nonspecific clinical findings are consistent with glomerulonephritis?

Nonspecific clinical findings associated with glomerulonephritis include anorexia, vomiting, weight loss, and lethargy; edema or ascites (rare in cats) secondary to hypoalbuminemia; azotemia; polyuria and polydipsia secondary to renal failure; hypertension; and hypercoagulability. Evidence of nephrotic syndrome (proteinuria, hypoalbuminemia, ascites or edema, and hypercholesterolemia) should alert the clinician to the possibility of glomerulonephritis. As glomerulonephritis is often secondary to another primary disease process, the clinical presentation may be dominated by the primary disease.

Primary Disease Processes That May Result in Secondary Feline Glomerular Disease

Bacterial pyoderma or chronic skin inflammation

Dental disease (e.g., chronic gingivitis)

Dirofilariasis

Ehrlichial infections

Endocarditis

Feline leukemia virus, feline immunodeficiency virus, feline infectious peritonitis, and associated conditions (e.g., lymphoma)

Immune-mediated diseases

Neoplasia

Pancreatitis

Pyometra

Systemic lupus erythematosus

9. Summarize the diagnostic plan for cats with suspected glomerulonephritis.

Complete cell count, serum biochemical panel, urinalysis with protein/creatinine ratio, and systemic blood pressure are recommended for all cats with glomerulonephritis. Renal ultrasound may be used to evaluate for morphologic renal diseases. Thoracic and abdominal radiographs may be used to evaluate for occult infections or neoplasia. Feline leukemia virus serum antigen test and feline immunodeficiency virus serum antibody test are indicated in most cases. Other specialized testing, such as serum coronavirus antibody titers, *Ehrlichia* spp. antibody titers, and *Dirofilaria immitis* serum antigen and antibody tests, are indicated in some cats.

10. How is glomerulonephritis diagnosed?

The definitive diagnosis of glomerulonephritis requires histologic examination of renal biopsy specimens.

11. How can renal tissues be collected? What are the risks?

Because of the availability of ultrasound and the potential for complications, it is no longer advisable to attempt biopsy of renal tissue "blindly." Ultrasound guidance or direct visualization with laparoscopy or exploratory laparotomy can be used to obtain samples of renal tissue. Excessive bleeding from the biopsy site is a potential complication, especially in animals that are hypertensive. Assessment of platelet count, activated clotting time or other clotting factor assessment, and arterial blood pressure is highly recommended before the procedure is performed. Laparoscopy offers the advantage of being able to apply direct pressure or Gel-foam to the biopsy site if persistent bleeding occurs.

12. What necropsy changes are seen with glomerulonephritis?

Any progressive destruction of nephrons results in gross and microscopic changes in the kidney that appear similar, regardless of the underlying cause. On gross inspection, kidneys are slightly smaller than normal, firm and pale, with irregular pitting and linear fibrosis.

13. Describe the histologic appearance of glomerulonephritis.

Histologic examination of renal tissue confirms medullary and glomerular deposition of eosinophilic hyaline material. In hematoxylin- and eosin-stained sections, glomerular capillary walls are diffusely thickened and intensely eosinophilic. Papillary necrosis, tubular dilatation, lymphocytic-plasmacytic cellular infiltration, and interstitial fibrosis also are seen. The glomerular walls are often thickened and eosinophilic. The periodic acid-Schiff stain is used to highlight small glomerular basement membrane projections consistent with immune complex deposition. Mesangial matrix and cell proliferation can be observed. Continued necrosis and glomerular atrophy lead to end-stage nephron destruction, scarring, fibrosis, and sclerosis.

14. What happens if glomerulonephritis is left untreated?

Without treatment, glomerulonephritis leads to irreversible damage from fibrin deposition and glomerulosclerosis. The loss of nephron function eventually leads to renal insufficiency and failure.

15. What are the treatment objectives for cats with glomerulonephritis?

The first objective of treatment is to identify and treat any underlying disease (i.e., removal of the offending antigen). Unfortunately, this goal is often impossible.

16. Are glucocorticoids appropriate for treatment of glomerular disease in cats?

Unless the primary disease process is a glucocorticoid-responsive condition, glucocorticoids are not recommended for the treatment of glomerular disease. Although cats are considered resistant to most side effects of long-term glucocorticoid use, treated dogs have demonstrated an increase in proteinuria and azotemia as well as loss of body condition. Elevated endogenous or exogenous glucocorticoid levels also predispose the animal to thromboembolic events. Other immunosuppressive drugs used to treat glomerular disease in dogs include azathioprine, chlorambucil, cyclophosphamide, and cyclosporine, but few controlled studies have investigated their efficacy in dogs. Several of these agents may be too toxic for use in cats (e.g., azathioprine).

17. What other treatments should be considered for glomerular disease in cats?

Thromboxane synthetase inhibitors, angiotensin-converting enzyme (ACE) inhibitors, prostaglandin analogs, leukotriene antagonists, and dietary omega-3 fatty acid supplements have been investigated for their ability to reduce glomerular inflammation and associated symptoms (e.g., proteinuria, hypertension). Antiplatelet therapy with low-dose aspirin is a mainstay of treatment for dogs with glomerular disease, but thromboembolic events secondary to glomerular disease are rare in cats. If edema or ascites is present, treatment may include a reduced sodium, protein-restricted diet in addition to an ACE inhibitor. For treatment of significant hypertension (systolic blood pressure > 170–180 mmHg), the calcium antagonist amlodipine (0.625 mg/cat once daily) is the drug of choice (see Chapter 63). Blood pressure should be rechecked at 2–4-week intervals at the start of therapy. The ACE inhibitor enalapril (0.25 mg/kg once daily) or a beta antagonist such as atenolol (6.25 mg/cat once daily) may be added if monotherapy is ineffective, but extreme caution and diligent follow-up are required to monitor for progressive azotemia and renal failure.

18. Define renal amyloidosis.
Amyloidosis is the deposition of fibrillar proteins in various tissues. These proteins assume a beta-pleated sheet configuration, which makes them insoluble and resistant to proteolysis. Amyloid impairs the function of the organ in which it is deposited. Renal amyloidoisis is usually secondary (reactive) to some infectious, inflammatory, or neoplastic disease process.

19. How does renal amyloidosis differ in cats and dogs?
Renal amyloidosis in cats is rare. Feline amyloidosis usually affects the medulla of the kidney, whereas in dogs renal amyloidosis is usually a glomerular disease. Amyloid deposit in the feline kidney results in medullary fibrosis and papillary necrosis. Unlike dogs, severe proteinuria is uncommon in cats because amyloid deposition is interstitial (sparing the glomeruli).

20. In what breed of cat does renal amyloidosis have a genetic basis?
Renal amyloidosis has been diagnosed in a number of related Abyssinian cats. The cats had marked medullary interstitial and glomerular amyloid deposition, interstitial fibrosis, and papillary necrosis. Siamese and Oriental shorthair breeds also have an increased incidence of amyloidosis.

21. What clinical and clinicopathologic abnormalities are associated with renal amyloidosis?
Cats are usually quite sick and often uremic, with nonregenerative anemia, hyperphosphatemia, metabolic acidosis, isosthenuria, and proteinuria. Concurrent amyloid deposits in the liver of Siamese and Oriental shorthair breeds may lead to hepatic rupture and severe, acute hemorrhage.

22. Describe the typical progression of renal amyloidosis.
Amyloid deposits interfere with the blood supply (vasa recta) to the renal medulla, resulting in papillary necrosis. The progressive loss of nephrons leads to renal failure and uremia. Feline amyloidosis carries a grave prognosis. Both dimethylsulfoxide (DMSO) and colchincine have been used to treat canine amyloidosis, but the results are equivocal, and similar studies have not been performed in feline amyloidosis. Both drugs may result in significant gastrointestinal side effects, and neither drug is likely to be of benefit once renal failure is established.

BIBLIOGRAPHY

1. Arthur JE, Lucke VM, Newby TJ, et al: The long-term prognosis of feline idiopathic membranous glomerulonephropathy. J Am Animal Hosp Assoc 22:731–737, 1986.
2. Blunden AS, Smith KC: Generalized amyloidosis and acute liver hemorrhage in four cats. J Small Anim Pract 33:566–570, 1992.
3. Boyce JT, DiBartola SP, Chew DJ, et al: Familial renal amyloidosis in Abyssinian cats. Vet Pathol 21:33–38, 1984.
4. Center SA, Smith CA, Wilkinson E, et al: Clinicopathologic, renal immunofluorescent, and light microscopic features of glomerulonephritis in the dog: 41 cases. J Am Vet Med Assoc 190:81–90, 1987.
5. Chew DJ, DiBartola SP, Boyce JT, et al: Renal amyloidosis in related Abyssinian cats. J Am Vet Med Assoc 181:139–142, 1982.
6. Glick AD, Horn RG, Holscher M: Characterization of feline glomerulonephritis associated with viral-induced hematopoietic neoplasms. Am J Pathol 92:321–332, 1978.
7. Grauer GF: CVT update: Canine glomerulonephritis In Bonagura J (ed): Kirk's Current Veterinary Therapy XIII (Small Animal Practice). Philadelphia, W.B. Saunders, 2000, pp 851–853.
8. Nash AS, Wright NG, Spencer AJ, et al: Membranous nephropathy in the cat: A clinical and pathological study. Vet Rec 105:71–77, 1979.
9. Osborne CA, Vernier RL: Glomerulonephritis in the dog and cat: A comparative review. J Am Anim Hosp Assoc 9:101–124, 1973.
10. Slauson DO, Lewis RM: Comparative pathology of glomerulonephritis in animals. Vet Pathol 16:135–164, 1979.

44. POLLAKIURIA: OVERVIEW AND DIAGNOSTIC PLAN

Michael R. Lappin, D.V.M., Ph.D.

1. Define pollakiuria, stranguria, and dysuria.

Pollakiuria is the passage of small amounts of urine frequently. **Stranguria** and **dysuria** are straining to urinate and difficulty with urination, respectively. These problems indicate inflammation or obstruction of the bladder or urethra and may or may not be accompanied by hematuria.

2. What are the major causes of pollakiuria?

Most causes of pollakiuria are local diseases of the bladder or urethra. In most cats, the cause of the disease is unknown. but uroliths, neoplasia, and infections occur in some (see Chapters 45–49). Extraluminal obstruction and neurologic causes also occur.

Primary Differential Diagnoses for Pollakiuria in Cats

Urinary tract disease	
Idiopathic or sterile (interstitial cystitis ?)	Viral infection (?)
Urolithiasis	Fungal infection
Neoplasia	Parasitic infestation
Bacterial infection	
Neurologic disease	
Extraluminal obstruction	

3. Define reflex dysynnergia.

Reflex dysynnergia (or detrusor-urethral dyssynergia) is a syndrome that develops when neurologic conditions result in a failure of coordination between detrusor contractions and urethral relaxation. It generally occurs with upper motor neuron lesions. In most cats, overt neurologic disease is noted on physical examination. Other types of functional urinary obstruction lead to incomplete emptying and are attributed to neurologic or nonneurologic disorders (see Chapter 49).

4. What signalment findings are commonly associated with causes of pollakiuria?

Lower urinary tract disorders can occur in cats of any age. Ranking of differential diagnoses varies with the signalment. For example, urate calculi are detected most frequently in young cats with portosystemic shunts and resultant hepatic insufficiency. Idiopathic cystitis most often starts in young adult cats. Bacterial urinary tract infections (UTIs) are rare in cats, but queens are more predisposed than toms because their urethra is shorter and has less muscular tone. Toms with perineal urethrostomy, however, are predisposed to bacterial UTIs compared with normal toms. Bacterial UTI and neoplasia become more common in older cats.

5. Describe the historical findings commonly associated with causes of pollakiuria.

Owners usually complain of inappropriate urination or excessive time in the litterbox. It can be difficult for the owner to differentiate stranguria from constipation. Depending on the cause of pollakiuria, hematuria also may be noted. In cases of total obstruction, vocalization or clinical signs of uremia (e.g., inappetence, depression, vomiting) also may be present.

6. What physical examination findings are commonly associated with causes of pollakiuria?

Cats with reflex dyssynergia often have decreased proprioception to the limbs, hyperactive reflexes, ataxia, and a variably distended, taut urinary bladder. Cats with idiopathic cystitis and infections commonly have small thickened bladders on palpation. Cats with inflammatory diseases generally urinate when minimal pressure is placed on the bladder. Blood may be noted in the urine or in the perineal region with some diseases. Occasionally, masses or calculi in the bladder can be palpated through the body wall. With complete obstruction, the urinary bladder is palpably distended. Extraluminal obstructive lesions and urethral calculi in the pelvic urethra can sometimes be detected by rectal palpation. The penis of toms with inflammatory disease or obstructive uropathy may be darker red in color than normal or may be inflamed.

7. Describe the initial diagnostic plan for cats with pollakiuria.

Urinalysis should be performed on urine collected by cystocentesis. It may be difficult to collect urine using this method because most affected cats maintain a small bladder or urinate immediately on gentle palpation. Mid-stream, free-catch urine or urine collected by catheterization may need to be evaluated. Abdominal radiographs also should be performed and evaluated for radiodense calculi. Because it is not always possible to estimate accurately the duration and frequency of clinical signs, abdominal radiographs are recommended in all cats with pollakiuria.

8. How does urinalysis aid in ranking of the differential diagnoses?

Hematuria is the most consistent finding with most causes of pollakiuria. Crystalluria may be detected in cases with calculi. Struvite (alkaline pH) and calcium oxalate (acidic pH) are the most common crystals (see Chapter 45). Pyuria and bacteriuria are detected in most cats with bacterial cystourethritis; aerobic infections are most common (see Chapter 48). Aerobic culture and antimicrobial susceptibility testing are indicated in cats with pyuria or elevated urine pH, whether or not bacteriuria is noted. Hematuria without significant pyuria or bacteriuria is the most common finding in cats with idiopathic cystitis (see Chapter 47).

9. What imaging techniques are most beneficial in the evaluation of cats with pollakiuria?

Because most uroliths in cats are radioopaque, abdominal radiographs are a useful screening technique. Ultrasound is effective for evaluation of cystic diseases, including masses, radiolucent uroliths, blood, and mineral debris; urine in the bladder serves as contrast. However, contrast urethrography is required to evaluate the urethra adequately.

10. Does endoscopy aid in the work-up of cases with pollakiuria?

Rigid cystoscopes can be used to evaluate the bladder lumen of queens or toms with perineal urethrostomies. Small flexible cystoscopes are available for use in other toms. Calculi, neoplasia, urachal remnants, ureteral orifices, and glomerulations consistent with interstitial cystitis can be visualized. In addition, the urethral lumen can be visualized. Unfortunately, most cats are too small for use of cystoscopes with biopsy sleeves.

BIBLIOGRAPHY

1. Grauer GF: Clinical manifestations of urinary tract disorders. In Nelson RW, Couto GC (eds): Small Animal Internal Medicine, 2nd ed. St. Louis, Mosby, 1998, pp 572–588.
2. Kalkstein TK, Kruger JK, Osborne CA: Feline idiopathic lower urinary tract disease. Part 1: Clinical manifestations. Comp Cont Educ Pract Vet 21:15–26, 1999.
3. Kalkstein TK, Kruger JK, Osborne CA: Feline idiopathic lower urinary tract disease. Part 2: Potential causes. Comp Cont Educ Pract Vet 21:148–154, 1999.
4. Kalkstein TK, Kruger JK, Osborne CA: Feline idiopathic lower urinary tract disease. Part 3: Diagnosis. Comp Cont Educ Pract Vet 21:387–394, 1999.
5. Kalkstein TK, Kruger JK, Osborne CA: Feline idiopathic lower urinary tract disease. Part 4: Therapeutic options. Comp Cont Educ Pract Vet 21:15–26, 1999.

45. URINARY CALCULI

Cynthia L. Bowlin, D.V.M.

1. What urinary calculi occur in cats?

Struvite (magnesium ammonium phosphate) urinary crystals, microcalculi, or uroliths are found in approximately 35% of affected cats. In contrast, 20 years ago approximately 80–90% of urinary calculi in cats were struvite. Calcium oxalate calculi are becoming increasingly common in cats and now account for more than 50% of calculi. Urate, calcium phosphate, silica, and cystine calculi also have been identified in cats but with much less frequency. Decreased water intake resulting in concentrated urine influences the saturation level of mineral components and promotes crystal and calculi formation. Thus, dry kibble diets may be associated with an increased incidence of calculi. Why some cats form calculi when others do not, even when the same diet and feeding practices are used, has yet to be determined.

2. What clinical signs suggest urinary calculi in cats?

Cystic calculi cause inflammation of the bladder and possibly the urethra. Inflammation may result in pollakiuria (increased frequency of urination), hematuria (blood in the urine), dysuria (difficult urination) and stranguria (straining to urinate). The other primary differential diagnoses are idiopathic cystitis and neoplasia; lower urinary tract inflammation is rarely caused by a primary bacterial infection in cats (see Chapter 44). With urate uroliths, clinical findings consistent with hepatic insufficiency may be present (see Chapter 35). If calcium oxalate uroliths are due to hypercalcemia, clinical signs of the primary disease may occur (see Chapter 57). Nepholiths are often subclinical unless concurrent lower urinary tract disease or obstructive uropathy resulting in azotemia is also present.

3. What factors influence formation of struvite calculi in cats?

Struvite calculi are detected most frequently in younger cats. Struvite calculi form primarily in the bladder, most often in neutral-to-alkaline urine (pH > 6.5), when the mineral components reach a saturation level that allows crystallization. Diets that provide adequate mineral components such as magnesium and phosphorous may influence struvite calculi formation. The decrease in the incidence of struvite calculi in the past two decades is attributed at least partially to the change in mineral composition and acidification of feline diets. In addition to the moisture content and alkalinizing potential of the diet, other dietary risk factors associated with struvite calculi formation include low-fat dry diets, high magnesium levels, and high phosphorous levels (see Chapter 50).

4. What factors influence formation of calcium oxalate calculi in cats?

Calcium oxalate calculi are seen most commonly in middle-aged to older cats. Acidifying diets and acidic urine may enhance formation of calcium oxalate calculi; an increased incidence has been noted since feline diets formulated to promote urine acidity have been widely fed. Calcium oxalate nepholiths are more common than struvite nepholiths and usually do not cause clinical signs until they pass or form in a ureter or the bladder. Other than moisture content and acidifying potential of the diet, dietary risk factors associated with calcium oxalate urolith formation in cats are feeding ad libitum, excessive vitamin D and C content, excessive calcium restriction, and low fiber levels in dry food. Epidemiologic studies have shown that overweight, 4–8-year-old, indoor cats of the Himalayan and Persian breeds that eat dry diets are most likely to have calcium oxalate urolithiasis.

5. What physical examination findings suggest urinary calculi?

Any cat with signs of lower urinary tract inflammation should be evaluated for calculi. Cats with cystic calculi may have palpably thickened bladder walls due to chronic irritation, but this

216

finding also occurs with other urinary tract diseases. If multiple, large calculi are present in the bladder, they may be palpated through the abdominal and bladder walls. If a large urinary bladder is present but difficult to express, cystic or urethral calculi are high on the differential list. Changes in renal size are variable, but the affected kidney is usually enlarged when obstruction is due to nephroliths. Discomfort on palpation of the bladder or kidneys is detected in some cats with urinary calculi.

6. Describe the initial diagnostic plan for documentation of urinary calculi.

Cats with clinical signs consistent with urinary tract disease should be assessed with urinalysis and abdominal radiographs (see Chapter 44). A urine sample should be obtained and examined immediately to ensure an accurate assessment of crystalluria. Crystal formation can readily occur in vitro (outside the cat) because of cooling or delayed analysis of the urine. In vivo crystalluria may or may not be clinically significant, but it does indicate oversaturation of minerals in the urine and suggests an increased risk for stone formation. If calcium oxalate or urate calculi are suspected, a serum biochemical panel should be performed to assess for hypercalcemia and hepatic disease, respectively.

7. How does imaging aid in the diagnosis of urinary calculi?

The most common urinary calculi of cats are radioopaque and readily seen on survey radiographs. However, small and radiolucent calculi (urate and cysteine) may be overlooked. Double-contrast cystography or ultrasonography should be performed if calculi or neoplasia are suspected but not documented by survey radiographs. Ultrasonographic evaluation of the lower urinary tract can be inaccurate if there is no urine in the bladder to act as contrast (a common occurrence in cats with pollakiuria). Contrast radiography has the advantage of screening the entire lower urinary tract and can be more accurate than ultrasound for quantifying the total number and location of calculi—particularly if calculi are located in the urethra, which is poorly imaged with ultrasound. Nuclear scintigraphy can be used to assess degree of obstruction associated with ureteroliths and nephroliths as well as function of the contralateral kidney if surgical removal is contemplated.

8. What are the treatment options for cystic calculi?

Treatment options for cystic calculi include medical dissolution (some calculi), voiding urohydropropulsion, and surgical removal via cystotomy. Treatment options for nephrolithiasis include medical dissolution (some calculi) and surgical removal by pyelotomy, nephrotomy, or nephrectomy.

9. Which calculi can be dissolved medically?

If struvite calculi are suspected, medical management can be considered. A specially formulated diet (Prescription Diet Feline S/D; Hills Pet Nutrition, Inc., Topeka, KS) has been shown to dissolve struvite calculi in the bladder after 1–3 months (see Chapter 50). If dissolution has not occurred after 3 months, other forms of management should be instituted. The advantages of this method are avoidance of a surgical procedure and easy administration if the cat will accept the new diet. The disadvantage of this method is that the cat often continues to be painful, dysuric, and pollakiuric until dissolution is complete. House soiling outside the litterbox can continue to be a problem for the owner. Because most nephroliths are calcium oxalate, medical dissolution is ineffective.

10. How is urohydropropulsion performed?

Lower urinary calculi of any type small enough to pass through the female urethra may be removed by urohydropropulsion. Voiding urohydropropulsion involves catheterizing an anesthetized or sedated cat, distending the bladder with saline, and then (while holding the cat in an upright position) applying manual pressure to the urinary bladder to "force" the fluid and, hopefully, the accompanying stones out through the urethra. Multiple catheterizations and expulsions may be necessary to remove the stones. If this method is successful, surgical intervention is avoided.

11. When is cystotomy indicated?

If medical management is not indicated or unsuccessful and if calculi are too large for uro-hydropropulsion, cystic calculi should be removed surgically. About 20–80% of surgeons leave one or more calculi in the bladder during surgical removal. Thus, postoperative radiographs are always indicated. Nephroliths may move into the bladder at any time; if they are present, the owner should be advised that cystic uroliths also may recur from this source. Cystic calculi can be an incidental finding in cats with no obvious clinical signs of urinary discomfort. Surgical intervention in subclinically affected cats is a decision best left to the clinician and owner, but regular monitoring for infection or change is indicated. Cystic calculi also may obstruct the urethra.

12. When is surgical management of nephroliths considered?

Pyelolithotomy or nephrotomy is generally performed only in cats with evidence of obstructive uropathy based on contrast studies, ultrasonic evaluation, or nuclear scintigraphy. Surgical procedures on the feline renal pelves have a large degree of postsurgical morbidity from urine leakage and ureteral scarring. Nephrectomy should be performed only if the affected kidney is considered nonfunctional and function of the contralateral kidney is adequate to control azotemia.

13. Define lithotripsy.

Lithotripsy is the breaking up of stones, usually with shock waves. Shock waves may be generated at the tip of an instrument placed directly on a stone (intracorporeal lithotripsy) or by an electrohydraulic or electromagnetic source outside the body and transmitted to the stone via a water interface (extracorporeal shock-wave lithotripsy [ESWL]).

14. Can lithotripsy be used to treat uroliths in cats?

Protocols for safely treating nephroliths in cats have not been determined. The feline kidney appears more sensitive than other species to potentially damaging effects of the shock waves. In addition, feline upper tract uroliths appear more difficult to fragment with ESWL than canine uroliths. However, attempts to fragment feline nephroliths and ureteroliths are limited; some types of ESWL may be effective and safe in cats. The procedure may be best considered for obstructive ureteroliths. Centers providing lithotripsy can be contacted for specific recommendations.

ESWL is not widely recommended for treatment of bladder stones because mobile stones can move out of the shock-wave path within the bladder lumen. Treatment may be considered for larger or multiple bladder stones and for patients that have had multiple surgeries, are poor surgical candidates, or are being treated concurrently for upper urinary tract stones. Multiple cystouroliths have been fragmented using ESWL in at least one cat; the composition of these stones, unfortunately, was not known.

15. What else can be done to aid in the management of urinary calculi?

Preventing recurrence of calculi is often more difficult than initial diagnosis and treatment. All calculi should undergo quantitative analysis to determine mineral composition, which aids in instituting a program to prevent reformation. At removal, bladder tissue and calculi should be submitted for bacterial culture and sensitivity. Appropriate long-term antibiotic therapy should be administered to eliminate infection, if present (see Chapter 48). Treatment of confirmed infection should continue for 2 weeks after medical dissolution is complete or 4 weeks after surgical removal. For susceptible cats with a history of urinary calculi formation, urine should be evaluated at least every 3–6 months to look for crystal formation, evaluate urine pH, and monitor urine concentration.

16. How can recurrence of urinary calculi be avoided?

Dietary management is the mainstay of preventative therapy (see Chapter 50). Increasing water intake to reduce urine specific gravity and urine saturation is also important in preventing calculi reformation. Canned food diets and flavored waters have been advocated for this purpose. Flavored waters (beef or chicken bouillon cubes, tuna water, or clam juice) should be used as a supplement and not in place of regular fresh water.

17. What specific recommendations may help to prevent struvite calculi?

A diet formulated to be low in magnesium and to create a urine pH around 6.5–6.8 is indicated to prevent recurrence of stuvite calculi. Treating and preventing struvite crystalluria and calculi formation, however, does not prevent recurrent episodes of idiopathic feline lower urinary tract disease (see Chapter 45).

18. What specificie recommendations may help to prevent calcium oxylate calculi?

Acidifying diets should be avoided and a more neutral urine pH (6.5–7.5) maintained. If urine pH remains below 6.5, potassium citrate (50–75 mg orally every 12 hr) can be used to raise urine pH. If a primary cause of hypercalcemia is identified, it should be corrected if possible (see Chapter 57).

19. What is the prognosis for cats with urinary calculi?

The prognosis for cats with cystic calculi is good. Because of difficulties associated with nephric and ureteral surgery in cats, the prognosis for nephroliths and ureteroliths is more guarded. Unfortunately, except for struvite uroliths, the chance for recurrence of other types of uroliths remains high despite the best preventive recommendations.

CONTROVERSIES

20. What is the ideal dietary regimen for cats?

We often talk about "acidifying diets" because in the past 15 or 20 year pet food manufacturers have reformulated cat foods to maintain a urine pH at 6.2 –6.5 for most cats. In fact, cats fed a diet exclusively of rats and mice maintain a urine pH around 6–6.2. A diet of corn, corn gluten, and meat byproducts creates a urine pH of about 7. By reformulating these foods to reduce urine pH, the pet food industry has simply corrected a problem that it created. Cats are true carnivores, but largely we continue to recommend and provide dry cereal grain diets, tweaked and supplemented in an attempt to meet the species' unique nutritional requirements. Worse yet, indoor, well-tended cats have been victims of the professional advise to feed one brand and only one brand ("Changing foods is bad"). In the author's opinion, probably the worse thing you can do for a cat, nutritionally or medically, is to feed one diet exclusively for years and years. Offering a commercially available feline diet, supplemented with various other meats, fish, grain products, fruits, and vegetables may help to reduce the incidence of urolithiasis and other disorders.

BIBLIOGRAPHY

1. Allen TA: Colloquium on urology. Fel Pract 25:5-32, 1997.
2. Buffington CAT, Chew DL, Kendall MS, et al: Clinical evaluation of cats with nonobstructive urinary tract diseases. J Am Vet Med Assoc 210:46-50, 1997.
3. Fossum TW: Surgery of the kidney and ureter. In Fossum TW (ed): Small Animal Surgery. St. Louis, MO, Mosby-Year Book, Inc., 1997, pp 461-480.
4. Grauer GF: Feline Lower Urinary Tract Inflammation. In Nelson RW, Couto CG (eds): Small Animal Internal Medicine, 2nd ed. Mosby, St. Louis, Mo, 1998, pp 650-657.
5. Lulich JP, Osborne CA: Voiding Urohydroprpulsion: A nonsurgical technique for removal of urocystoliths. In Bonagura JD, editor: Current Veterinary Therapy XII, Philadelphia, 1995, WB Saunders Co., pp 1003-1006.
6. Osborne CA, Kruger JM, Lulich JP, et al: Disorders of the feline lower urinary tract. In Osborne CA, Finco DR (eds): Canine and Feline Nephrology and Urology. Philadelphia, Williams and Wilkins, 1995, pp 665-674.
7. Osborne CA, Lulich JP, Thumchai R: Feline Calcium Oxalate Urolithiasis. In Bonagura JD, editor: Current Veterinary Therapy XII, Philadelphia, 1995, WB Saunders Co., pp 989-992.
8. Polzin DJ, Osborne CA: Dysuria, hematuria, pollakiuria, and urethral obstruction in cats. Proc Waltham Feline Medicine Symposium, Vernon, California, 1996, pp 29-32.
9. Thumchai R, Lulich JP, Osborne CA, et al: Epizoologic evaluation of urolithiasis in cats: 3498 cases (1982-1992). J Am Vet Med Assoc 208:547-551, 1996.

46. URINARY TRACT NEOPLASIA

Tammy Anderson, D.V.M.

1. How common are urinary tract neoplasms in cats?
Urinary tract neoplasms are rare in cats. Primary renal tumors reportedly constitute 1.6–2.5% of all neoplasms in cats. Primary bladder tumors account for > 1% of all reported neoplasms in cats.

2. Describe the biologic behavior of urinary tract neoplasms in cats.
Most urinary tract neoplasms in cats are malignant. Renal tumors most commonly metastasize to the lungs, liver, brain, and bone. Bladder tumors most commonly metastasize to the lungs, regional lymph nodes, kidney, and liver. The disease is often advanced at the time of diagnosis.

3. What clinical signs and physical examination findings are associated with upper urinary tract neoplasia?
Clinical signs often are nonspecific and include anorexia, weight loss, and lethargy. Abdominal distention may be present. Abdominal palpation may detect a mass or enlarged kidneys or elicit pain.

4. What laboratory findings are associated with upper urinary tract neoplasia?
Hematuria, proteinuria, and pyuria unassociated with lower urinary tract signs may be present. Anemia of chronic disease may be detected on complete blood count. Renal failure may or may not be evident. Lymphosarcoma, which often affects both kidneys, is the tumor type most likely to cause renal failure. Paraneoplastic syndromes are rare in cats, but polycythemia secondary to increased erythropoeitin production by a renal tumor has been reported. Hypertrophic osteopathy also has been reported in a cat with a renal papillary adenoma.

5. Describe the signalment of cats with renal neoplasia.
The mean age of cats with renal neoplasia exclusive of lymphosarcoma is 9 years. Males are slightly more likely to be affected. Cats with renal lymphosarcoma tend to be younger (median age = 6 years), and 50% of affected cats test positive for feline leukemia virus (FeLV).

6. What are the most common upper urinary tract neoplasms in cats?
Most renal tumors are primary and malignant. Lymphosarcoma is the most common upper urinary tract tumor in cats and often represents an extension of alimentary lymphosarcoma. Adenocarcinomas, adenomas, nephroblastomas, and other tumor types are less commonly reported. Primary ureteral tumors have not been reported in cats.

7. What other disorders should be considered in the differential diagnoses?
The differential diagnoses are based on clinical signs, physical examination findings, and laboratory results. Palpation of a mass may indicate neoplasia of other abdominal organs. Hematuria may be due to lower urinary tract disease, trauma, or coagulopathy. Pyuria and proteinuria may be due to lower urinary tract disease. Proteinuria also may be caused by a protein-losing nephropathy. Abdominal distention and pain may be due to ascites, peritonitis, or organomegaly. Enlarged kidneys may be secondary to ureteral obstruction, pyelonephritis, or renal pseudocysts.

8. What ancillary tests are recommended in cats with renal neoplasia?
Complete blood count, serum biochemistry panel, urinalysis, serum FeLV antigen test, and serum feline immunodeficiency virus (FIV) antibody test are recommended to determine the general health of the cat and aid in prognosis. Because most tumors are malignant, thoracic and

abdominal radiographs and abdominal ultrasound are indicated to detect metastatic disease. Before nephrectomy is performed, function of the contralateral kidney should be evaluated with an excretory urogram or glomerular filtration rate, as estimated by nuclear scintigraphy.

9. How are tumors of the upper urinary tract diagnosed?

Tumor type may be determined by fine-needle aspiration or biopsy. Fine-needle aspiration is especially useful in cases of lymphosarcoma because the cells easily exfoliate. Percutaneous (blind, ultrasound guided, or laparoscopy obtained) or surgical biopsies may be obtained. Laparoscopy has the benefits of allowing accurate biopsy site selection and hemorrhage control, if needed. Contraindications to renal biopsy include untreated coagulopathy, acute pyelonephritis, systemic arterial hypertension, and solitary kidney. Platelet count, activated clotting time (or other factor function test), and systemic arterial blood pressure should be assessed before biopsy.

10. What are the treatment options for upper urinary tract neoplasms in cats?

For tumors other than lymphosarcoma, surgical excision is the treatment of choice in cats with no evidence of metastatic disease and adequate function of the contralateral kidney. With the exception of lymphosarcoma, most tumor types respond poorly to chemotherapy. Lymphoma may be treated with various chemotherapy protocols. In Mooney's study, a protocol that included vincristine, L-asparaginase, prednisone, cyclophosphamide, methotrexate, and cytosine arabinoside, achieved a 61% complete remission rate.

11. Describe the prognosis for upper urinary tract neoplasms in cats.

In Mooney's study, the mean survival time was > 408 days, and the median survival time was 169 days. Azotemia and stage of lymphosarcoma have not been shown to be accurate predictors of prognosis; however, positive FeLV status affects survival negatively. Central nervous system signs are detected in 40% of cats dying of renal lymphoma.

12. What clinical signs and physical examination findings are most commonly associated with neoplasms of the lower urinary tract?

Clinical signs are typical of any lower urinary tract disease and include hematuria, dysuria, stranguria, and pollakiuria. Physical examination findings may include a palpably thickened bladder wall or thickened urethra. Painful and enlarged kidneys may be present in cats with ureteral or urethral obstruction. A mucoid urethral discharge also may be present.

13. What laboratory findings are associated with lower urinary tract disease?

Hematuria, proteinuria, and pyuria are common. Recurrent or unresponsive urinary tract infections also may occur. Azotemia and signs consistent with renal failure may be evident in cats with bilateral ureteral obstruction.

14. Describe the signalment of cats with bladder tumors.

Cats with bladder tumors tend to be older (average age = 9 years). Males are affected more often than females.

15. What are the most common lower urinary tract neoplasms in cats?

Most bladder tumors are primary and malignant. Transitional cell carcinoma is the most common tumor type; squamous cell carcinoma, adenocarcinoma, and others have been reported. At the time of diagnosis, 30–50% of lower urinary tract neoplasms have metastasized to the sublumbar lymph nodes, pelvic or lumbar vertebrae, or lungs.

16. How do bladder tumors differ in cats and dogs?

Bladder tumors in cats often originate in the apex of the bladder or are widespread in the bladder wall, whereas bladder tumors in dogs often involve the trigone region. This difference makes bladder tumors more amenable to surgery in cats than in dogs. In general, bladder tumors are less common in cats than in dogs.

17. What other disorders should be considered in the differential diagnoses for bladder disease in cats?

Differential diagnoses include other lower urinary tract diseases such as idiopathic feline lower urinary tract disease, cystic calculi, and bacterial urinary tract infection (see Chapter 44). Hematuria may be caused by trauma or coagulopathies.

18. How are tumors of the lower urinary tract diagnosed?

Mass lesions are documented by ultrasound or double-contrast cystourethrography. Cytology of urinary sediment or fine-needle aspiration of the tumor may help with diagnosis. Histopathology may be preferred because neoplastic cells often are difficult to differentiate from reactive transitional cells on cytologic evaluation. Biopsy samples may be obtained by cystoscopy or open surgery. There is a potential risk of tumor cell transplantation during surgery if the tumor is incised or manipulated with the same instruments that are used to close the surgical site. Therefore, changing surgical packs before closure is recommended.

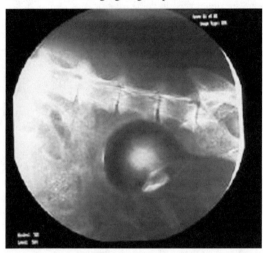

Double-contrast cystogram revealing a mass in the urinary bladder.

19. What ancillary tests are recommended in cats with lower urinary tract neoplasia?

Complete blood count, serum biochemical panel, urinalysis, serum FeLV antigen test, and serum FIV antibody test should be completed to evaluate the general health of the cat. Abdominal and thoracic radiographs and abdominal ultrasound are recommended to evaluate for metastasis. Contrast cystourethrography or ultrasound is useful to evaluate the extent of tumor. An excretory urogram is indicated if azotemia or renomegaly is present.

20. What are the treatment options for lower urinary tract neoplasms in cats?

Traditional chemotherapy protocols are generally not effective. Carboplatin has been suggested as a chemotherapeutic option in cats, although its efficacy is unknown. Radiation therapy is not recommended because of its significant side effects, including bladder or colon rupture, incontinence, and urinary fibrosis. Surgical resection may be considered if no metastasis is present and the mass does not involve the trigone. If the tumor is at the apex, up to 75–80% of the bladder may be removed. Surgical margins of at least 2 cm are recommended.

21. Does piroxicam work in cats?

Piroxicam, a nonsteroidal anti-inflammatory drug, has been used anecdotally for transitional cell carcinomas. Piroxicam should be used only in well-hydrated animals with normal renal function because it can be nephrotoxic. It is frequently combined with misoprostol because it may cause gastrointestinal ulceration in dogs and humans. The safety and efficacy of piroxicam in cats have not been evaluated. The drug has been administered at 0.3 mg/kg orally every 48–72 hours without side effects in some cats.

BIBLIOGRAPHY

1. Crow SE: Urinary tract neoplasms in dogs and cats. Comp Contin Educ Pract Vet 7:607–618, 1985.
2. Klausner JS, Caywood DD: Neoplasms of the urinary tract. In Osbourne CA, Finco DR (eds): Canine and Feline Nephrology and Urology. Philadelphia, Lippincott Williams & Wilkins, 1995, pp 903–916.
3. Mooney SC, Hayes AA, Matus RE, et al: Renal lymphoma in cats 28 cases (1977–1984). J Am Vet Med Assoc 191:1473–1477, 1987.
4. Morrison WB: Cancers of the urinary tract. In Morrison WB (ed): Cancer in Dogs and Cats: Medical and Surgical Management. Philadelphia, Lippincott Williams & Wilkins, 1998, pp 569–579.
5. Ogilvie GK, Moore AS: Tumors of the urinary tract. In Ogilvie GK, Moore AS (eds): Managing the Veterinary Cancer Patient: A Practice Manual. Trenton, NJ, Veterinary Learning Systems, 1995, pp 403–414.
6. Phillips BS: Bladder tumors in dogs and cats. Comp Contin Educ Pract Vet 21:540–547, 1999.
7. Schwartz PD, Greene RW, Patnaik AK: Urinary bladder tumors in the cat: A review of 27 cases. J Am Anim Hosp Assoc 21:237–245, 1985.

47. IDIOPATHIC LOWER URINARY TRACT DISEASE

Tina S. Kalkstein, D.V.M., M.A.

1. What are the signs of feline lower urinary tract disease?
Feline lower urinary tract diseases (LUTDs) manifest clinically with similar symptoms, regardless of cause. Hematuria, pollakiuria, dysuria, inappropriate urination, and/or urethral obstruction are the clinical signs associated with LUTD in cats (see Chapter 44).

2. What diseases affect the feline lower urinary tract?
Idiopathic LUTD is the most common cause of hematuria, dysuria, pollakiuria, inappropriate urination, and urethral obstruction in male and female cats. Other common causes of feline LUTD are urolithiasis and urethral plugs. Uncommon causes of LUTD in cats include infectious, iatrogenic, or traumatic disorders. Rarely, anatomic abnormalities (congenital or acquired), neoplasia, or neurologic disorders may affect the bladder and/or urethra of cats.

3. Define idiopathic LUTD.
Idiopathic LUTD is a diagnosis reserved for male and female cats with clinical signs of LUTD for which the specific cause cannot be determined after an appropriate and thorough diagnostic evaluation. The exact cause of idiopathic LUTD remains unknown, but various theories have been suggested, including bacterial and viral infections, autoimmune disease, urinary toxins, leaky bladder transitional epithelium, stress, neurogenic, and mast cell-mediated inflammation. Rather than one single cause, multiple factors probably interact to result in idiopathic LUTD.

4. Are crystals a cause of idiopathic LUTD?
Crystalluria naturally occurs in cats in the absence of clinical disease. In one study, the prevalence of crystalluria was not significantly different in cats with nonobstructive idiopathic LUTD and unaffected control cats. The signs of idiopathic LUTD also occur commonly in the absence of crystals on urine sediment exam. Together, these findings suggest that crystals are not the cause of idiopathic LUTD.

5. Is idiopathic LUTD of cats synonymous with interstitial cystitis in humans?

Interstitial cystitis refers to an idiopathic LUTD of humans that bears many clinical and diagnostic similarities to feline idiopathic LUTD. In addition, both disorders are characterized by an elusive cause and unknown effective therapy. Because of these similarities, it has been suggested that feline idiopathic LUTD and human interstital cystitis represent the same disease in different species. However, considering that the lower urinary tract of any species has a limited ability to react to a number of different diseases, the similarities between feline idiopathic LUTD and human interstitial cystitis may be coincidental. Future studies of both disorders may reveal significant differences or similarities between the human and feline diseases. Additional information is needed to define more clearly the relationship between the two disorders.

6. Are bacterial infections the cause of idiopathic LUTD?

Results of urine culture for aerobic bacteria and other less common bacterial organisms (e.g., anaerobes, mycoplasmas, ureaplasmas, spirochetes) are consistently negative in cats with idiopathic LUTD, supporting the conclusion that bacteria are not the cause. Using novel diagnostic techniques, however, recent research has identified bacteria and bacterial nucleic acid sequences in some humans with interstitial cystitis. These findings do not define a causative role for bacteria in the etiopathogenesis of human interstitial cystitis but have led to the development of new hypotheses about the role of bacteria in human interstitial cystitis. The new hypotheses suggest that in people with interstitial cystitis active infection may occur with atypical, difficult-to-culture, or nonculturable organisms or that, in the absence of active infection, bacterial products may stimulate pathology leading to clinically significant disease.

7. Can viruses be the cause of idiopathic LUTD?

In laboratory settings, viral agents can provoke feline LUTD. Recently, calicivirus and virus-like particles have been identified in the urine and urethral plugs, respectively, of cats with naturally occurring idiopathic LUTD. As with bacterial pathogens, these findings do not define a causal relationship. Furthermore, little evidence demonstrates that viruses cause naturally occurring feline idiopathic LUTD. Nonetheless, the new information about bacterial and viral pathogens reinforces the need to continue evaluation and development of more sensitive microbial detection methods. Armed with new information, researchers may be able to define more clearly the role of uropathogens in development of idiopathic LUTD.

8. Which cats get idiopathic LUTD?

The typical cat with nonobstructive idiopathic LUTD is a young to middle-aged male or female of any breed; however, any age can be affected. Obstructive idiopathic LUTD (idiopathic urethral obstruction) occurs primarily in male cats.

9. Describe the usual clinical course of idiopathic LUTD.

Most cats with idiopathic LUTD have acute, nonobstructive signs of a few days' duration. Fortunately, clinical signs resolve spontaneously within 3–7 days in most cats. Episodes of hematuria, dysuria, pollakiuria, and inappropriate urination may recur at unpredictable intervals but tend to decrease in severity and frequency as the cat ages.

Some cats present with frequently recurring episodes or a more prolonged duration of nonobstructive symptoms (weeks to months). Signs may eventually subside without therapy and recur unpredictably. Urethral obstruction may occur in male cats with or without a prior history of nonobstructive disease.

10. How is idiopathic LUTD diagnosed?

The clinical signs of idiopathic LUTD are identical to symptoms of other feline LUTDs. Because no diagnostic test is specific for idiopathic LUTD, the syndrome is diagnosed after a thorough evaluation in which other known causes of feline LUTD have been excluded. The choice of individual tests depends on several factors:

- Duration of clinical signs and frequency of recurrence
- Abnormalities identified on initial examination or diagnostic tests
- Presence of urethral obstruction or concurrent disease

11. Which diagnostic tests are recommended for cats presenting for the first time with acute nonobstructive LUTD?

Thorough history and physical examination. Prior episodes of LUTD should be noted, including episodes of urolithiasis or urethral obstruction that may have predisposed the cat to urethral stricture formation from a previously lodged urethral stone or iatrogenic causes (e.g., urethral catheter placement).

Survey abdominal radiographs should be obtained to rule out the presence of radiopaque uroliths and crystalline-matrix urethral plugs. The entire perineum should be included on the lateral radiographic view to evaluate the entire length of the urethra.

Urinalysis should be done to evaluate for chemical and sediment examination.

Cystocentesis should be performed to obtain a urine sample for aerobic culture.

12. Which diagnostic tests are recommended for cats with hematuria but no other signs of LUTD?

Diagnostic evaluation should include assessment of the upper urinary tract, reproductive tract, and coagulation cascade.

13. Which diagnostic tests are recommended for cats presenting with prolonged or recurrent episodes of LUTD?

In cats with prolonged or frequently recurring LUTD, a more thorough evaluation is indicated. In addition to the tests listed in question 11, diagnostic evaluation should include:

- Contrast cystourethrography to rule out radiolucent or small (< 3 mm) radiopaque uroliths, anatomic abnormalities, or neoplasia.
- Cystoscopy may be pursued if appropriate equipment is available to identify mass lesions, uroliths, or anatomic abnormalities. In clinical practice, however, high-quality contrast cystourethrography usually is sufficient.
- Complete blood count (CBC) and biochemistry profile may be indicated in some cats for exclusion of systemic illness and before anesthesia for contrast cystourethrography or cystoscopy.

14. Is ultrasound useful in the evaluation of cats with LUTD?

Ultrasound is a useful, noninvasive imaging technique to evaluate the urinary bladder and kidneys in cats. Ultrasound examination of a fully distended urinary bladder may identify radiolucent or radiopaque uroliths, mass lesions, echogenic urine sediment, and diffuse or focal mucosal irregularities. Significant limitations of sonographic exam of the lower urinary tract in cats with LUTD include (1) the need for a fully distended urinary bladder (many cats with pollakiuria have a contracted urinary bladder) and (2) the inability to evaluate the entire urethra (urethral lesions may be overlooked if ultrasound is used as an alternative to survey and contrast radiography).

15. Are cystotomy and biopsy indicated in the diagnostic evaluation of cats with LUTD?

Cystotomy and biopsy are not necessary to establish the diagnosis of idiopathic LUTD or most other feline LUTDs. Less invasive methods are sufficient.

16. What findings of CBC and serum biochemical profile are consistent with idiopathic LUTD?

CBC and serum biochemical profile are normal in cats with nonobstructive idiopathic LUTD in the absence of other illness. Cats with idiopathic urethral obstruction may have biochemical abnormalities such as postrenal azotemia, metabolic acidosis, and hyperkalemia.

17. What urinalysis and urine culture findings are common in cats with idiopathic LUTD?
    Common urinalysis findings include well-concentrated and acidic urine, hematuria, and usually the absence of pyuria or bacteriuria. False-positive reactions may occur on the leukocyte pad of urine dipsticks; microscopic urine sediment exam is imperative to evaluate for white blood cells in feline urine. In addition, the observation of bacteria in urine sediment is suggestive but not conclusive evidence of bacterial urinary tract infection. Bacteria may appear in urine samples via contamination during collection (common with catheter-obtained or voided samples because of commensal flora of the distal urethra) or storage. In addition, many components of urine sediment, such as fat droplets and cellular debris, appear morphologically similar to and may be mistaken for bacteria in unstained urine preparations. Urine cultures are negative in cats with idiopathic LUTD.

18. What imaging abnormalitites may be seen in cats with idiopathic LUTD?
    • Survey abdominal radiographs are usually normal in cats with idiopathic LUTD.
    • Double-contrast cystogram and retrograde positive contrast urethrogram may be normal or may expose bladder wall thickening, mucosal irregularities, vesicoureteral reflux, and/or vesicourachal diverticula.
    • Cystoscopy may reveal submucosal petechiae and increased vascularity.

19. Is an effective therapy for idiopathic LUTD available?
    An effective and safe therapy for idiopathic LUTD has not been identified. However, few therapies have been the subject of controlled clinical studies. At this time, only symptomatic therapy for idiopathic LUTD is available, and controversy surrounds most, if not all, of the recommended symptomatic therapeutics.

20. What therapies for idiopathic LUTD have been studied?
    Controlled studies have been performed to evaluate the efficacy of chloramphenicol, propantheline (an antispasmodic), subcutaneous fluid administration, and prednisolone. None of these therapeutics were effective in reducing the duration or severity of clinical signs in cats with nonobstructive idiopathic LUTD.

21. In the absence of an effective therapy, how are cats with idiopathic LUTD managed?
    Management protocols for cats with idiopathic LUTD should be based on the following:
    • Thorough diagnostic evaluation to exclude causes of feline LUTD with known effective and specific therapy
    • Client education about the self-limiting nature and short duration of symptoms in most cats and the lack of studies proving the efficacy of recommended therapies
    • Protocols to minimize risk factors associated with urethral obstruction
    • Protocols to prevent iatrogenic disease (e.g., urinary catheter complications such as stricture or infection, diet-induced uroliths or metabolic complications, adverse drug reactions)
    • Consideration of pharmacologic management of persistent or recurrent clinical signs

22. Is stress reduction helpful for cats with idiopathic LUTD?
    Stressful events such as extreme weather conditions, residential moves, diet change, and major holidays have been associated with recurrent episodes of LUTD in cats. Although it is unlikely that stress is a primary cause of idiopathic LUTD in cats, its etiopathogenic role is unclear. Stress-induced immune, endocrine, and inflammatory responses may induce or aggravate signs of idiopathic LUTD, regardless of the underlying cause. Potential stressful aspects of the cat's home environment should be identified and eliminated or at least minimized. Possible feline stressors may include changes or disruptions in the home population (people or other animals), diet, or feeding schedule; changes in litter type, location, or cleanliness; and lack of toys and hiding places.

23. Is amitriptyline helpful for cats with idiopathic LUTD?
    Amitriptyline has been recommended for the symptomatic relief of cats with acute and chronic forms of idiopathic LUTD. Amitriptyline is a tricyclic antidepressant and anxiolytic drug

with other potentially beneficial properties, including anticholinergic, antihistaminic, anti-alpha adrenergic, anti-inflammatory, and analgesic effects. The exact mechanism of action is unknown but may be related to the relief of neurogenic and mast cell-mediated inflammation. Ongoing studies are evaluating the safety and therapeutic value of amitriptyline in managing cats with idiopathic LUTD.

24. How should amitriptyline be used?
Dose, frequency, and duration of amitriptyline therapy are empirical. Dose recommendations range from 2.5–12.5 mg/cat orally every 24 hours at bedtime. The goal is to produce a mild calming effect. Adverse reactions may include urine retention, blood dyscrasias, and liver enzyme elevations. If amitriptyline is chosen for use in the symptomatic management of cats with idiopathic LUTD, caution should be exercised. Clients should be educated about its empirical use, and routine monitoring should include CBC and liver enzyme evaluation before commencing therapy as well as regularly during therapy (monthly at first, then every 3–6 months).

25. Are glycosaminoglycans helpful for cats with idiopathic LUTD?
The transitional epithelium of the urinary tract is lined by a layer of glycosaminoglycans (GAGs) that function to prevent microbial and crystal adherence to the bladder epithelium and minimize the movement of urine solutes and proteins through the bladder epithelium. One hypothesis in the pathogenesis of idiopathic LUTD suggests that cats with a deficient or defective GAG layer develop increased bladder wall permeability. Chronic exposure of the bladder epithelium to urine constituents may result in sensory nerve stimulation, mast cell activation, and/or induction of immune-mediated or neurogenic inflammation. Research has shown that some cats with idiopathic LUTD have increased bladder permeability, but it is not known whether this finding is a cause or an effect of idiopathic LUTD.

26. Which GAG has been used in cats?
Pentosan polysulfate sodium is a semisynthetic, low-molecular-weight heparin GAG analog used with some success in the management of human interstitial cystitis and recently considered for use in cats with idiopathic LUTD. The empirical dose of pentosan polysulfate for use in cats with idiopathic LUTD is 2–10 mg/kg orally every 12 hours. Adverse effects reported in humans include bleeding disorders, alopecia, abdominal pain, diarrhea, and nausea. The safety and efficacy of pentosan polysulfate or other GAG replacement therapy in feline idiopathic LUTD has not been reported.

27. Are antimicrobial agents helpful for cats with idiopathic LUTD?
Antibiotics are not recommended for the following reasons:
1. Bacterial urinary tract infections are rare (1-3%) in young to middle-aged cats with LUTD.
2. Urine cultures are negative in cats with idiopathic LUTD.
3. Antibacterial drugs are not beneficial to abacteriuric cats with LUTD.
4. Bacterial resistance may be induced by the arbitrary use of antibiotics

28. Are acidifying diets recommended for cats with idiopathic LUTD?
Acidifying diets are designed to minimize or prevent struvite crystals, struvite uroliths, or struvite crystalline matrix urethral plugs (see Chapter 50). Because crystals are not believed to be a cause of idiopathic LUTD and most cats with idiopathic LUTD have acidic urine without significant crystalluria, acidifying diets do not appear to offer a therapeutic advantage for most cats. However, some male cats with heavy crystalluria may benefit from dietary therapy designed to minimize crystalluria, crystalline matrix plug formation, and potential urethral obstruction.

29. How should an appropriate diet be selected?
Urine sediment and chemical examination should be used as a guide for the choice of an appropriate diet because not all male cats with idiopathic LUTD will benefit from an acidifying diet. For example, cats with acidic urine and heavy calcium oxalate crystalluria may develop calcium oxalate uroliths or calcium oxalate crystalline urethral plugs. An acceptable urine pH and sediment

composition should be defined, and follow-up urinalysis should be performed after a few weeks of consuming the new diet to evaluate the desired effect. Urinalyses should be evaluated at regular intervals to ensure maintenance of the desired effect or early recognition of adverse effects. Acidifying diets are contraindicated in immature cats and in the presence of disorders that may predispose cats to metabolic acidosis, such as renal or postrenal azotemia. New diets should be introduced gradually and should be fed for long periods to minimize stress related to diet change.

30. Are glucocorticoids useful in the symptomatic management of idiopathic LUTD?

Mononuclear inflammation is a common histopathologic finding in the urinary bladder of cats with idiopathic LUTD. The cause of the inflammation is unknown. Anti-inflammatory dosages of glucocorticoids have been used in attempts to decrease symptoms attributed to inflammation, such as hematuria and dysuria. A small (n = 12), double-blind, placebo controlled, pilot study of untreated cats with idiopathic LUTD has shown that prednisolone therapy at an anti-inflammatory dose (1 mg/kg orally every 12 hours for 10 days) did not minimize clinical signs compared with placebo. In cats treated with either prednisolone or placebo, clinical symptoms and urinalysis findings of hematuria and dysuria subsided within 2–5 days. Because glucocorticoids do not appear to produce a clinically favorable effect and are associated with clinically significant adverse effects, they are not recommended for use in cats with either obstructive or nonobstructive idiopathic LUTD.

31. How is obstructive idiopathic LUTD managed?

Cats with obstructive idiopathic LUTD should be managed like cats with any other cause of urinary obstruction. Urethral catheterization is necessary to relieve the obstruction in most cases. The priorities of management are to determine the presence and extent of metabolic derangements (e.g., postrenal azotemia, metabolic acidosis, hyperkalemia), to address these complications, and to relieve urethral obstruction. Intravenous access should be obtained as soon as possible to administer fluid therapy, other medications, and injectable anesthetic agents, if needed. The lower urinary tract should be evaluated radiographically before catheterization and flushing, if possible.

32. Is sedation or general anesthesia necessary in cats with urinary obstruction?

Sedation or general anesthesia is necessary in most male and female cats with urinary obstruction. However, severely depressed cats with postrenal azotemia may allow urethral manipulations with manual restraint, possibly including a small amount of topical anesthetic solution. Urinary obstruction is occasionally due to a distal penile urethral plug. In these cases, penile massage may facilitate expulsion of the plug and negate the need for sedation and catheterization altogether. This simple technique should be attempted in all obstructed male cats. In noncompliant cats, the risk of sedation or general anesthesia may be acceptable considering that iatrogenic trauma to or infection of the urinary tract may be an even greater risk.

33. Which sedative or anesthetic agents should be used?

Agents that do not undergo renal metabolism, such as short-acting barbiturates, diazepam, midazolam, propofol, or inhalation agents, are common choices. Combinations of ketamine and diazepam or midazolam also have been used. Because ketamine is metabolized and eliminated via the kidneys, however, intubation and maintenance with inhaled anesthestics should be strongly considered instead of additional doses if the initial dose of ketamine is unsuccessful. In uncooperative patients that are not good anesthetic risks at the time of presentation, careful decompressive cystocentesis can be performed to "buy time" for stabilization before anesthesia.

34. What types of catheters should be used?

The urethral lumen of most male and female cats is large enough to fit a 5-French catheter. Catheters of smaller diameter may be necessary in some cats, but they become kinked or plugged more easily than larger catheters, especially if they are maintained as an indwelling system. Polyvinyl chloride (red-rubber) catheters are preferred over polypropylene catheters because they are softer and more pliable and have been found to induce much less uroepithelial injury.

35. Describe the technique for catheter insertion.

Aseptic and nontraumatic technique with sterile aqueous lubricant should be used during all attempts to pass a urethral catheter. If the obstruction is within the distal urethra, short catheters such as a 1-inch, 22-gauge intravenous catheter with the needle removed, may be passed initially. Once the urethral catheter is advanced to the level of the obstruction, reverse flushing with 0.9% saline or lactated Ringer's solution is performed to dislodge, soften, or retropulse a urethral plug. Large volumes (several hundred milliliters) of lavage solutions are sometimes needed to manipulate the plug or move a urolith (if a urolith is present, the obstruction is not due to idiopathic disease). Physiologic solutions such as normal saline or lactated Ringer's solution are preferred over other solutions because they are isotonic and nonirritating to the mucosal membranes of the urinary tract. After relieving the obstruction, the bladder and urethra should be lavaged to remove cellular, proteinaceous, and/or crystalline debris. If the obstruction cannot be relieved, decompressive cystocentesis should be performed, and another attempt to pass a urethral catheter should be made at a later time rather than risk additional trauma to the urethra. Urethral catheterization may be unsuccessful in obstructive idiopathic LUTD because of a stubborn and firm urethral plug, urethral edema or spasm, blood clots. or sloughed mucosal fragments. Concurrent diseases may prevent easy catheterization. such as urolithiasis or an intraluminal, mural, or extramural mass.

36. What are the most common risks of urethral catheterization? How are they minimized?

The most common risks of urethral catheterization include iatrogenic trauma to and infection of the lower urinary tract. Iatrogenic trauma can be prevented or minimized with gentle technique, pliant catheters, copious amounts of lubricant, and use of sedation or anesthesia in uncooperative patients. The risk of infection can be minimized with the use of sterile materials (including sterile gloves, flush, and catheters), nontraumatic technique, minimal use of indwelling catheters, use of sterile, closed collection systems when indwelling catheters are deemed necessary, and removal of the catheter as soon as possible. The risk of infection increases with the duration of catheterization.

37. What are the indications for an indwelling catheter?

Not all cats with recent obstruction require an indwelling catheter. Indications for an indwelling urethral catheter after obstruction include a narrowed urethral lumen, persistent debris in the urinary tract, and detrusor atony. These findings are risk factors for reobstruction during the first few days after urethral patency is reestablished. Cats with severe postrenal azotemia as a consequence of obstructive idiopathic LUTD also may benefit from an indwelling catheter. Antibiotics and/or glucocorticoids should not be substituted for aseptic, nontraumatic technique and closed collection systems. Repeat obstruction occurs after catheter removal in some cats due to functional urethral spasm. See Chapter 49 for a discussion of pharmocologic agents that may be of benefit.

38. When should I consider a perineal urethrostomy?

Because of the increased risk for bacterial urinary tract infections (see Chapter 48), perineal urethrostomy is no longer routinely performed. However, if urethral scarring has resulted from multiple episodes of idiopathic LUTD or repeated urethral catheterization, surgery may be indicated. Perineal urethrostomy does not resolve idiopathic LUTD; it only lessens the odds of developing an obstructive uropathy.

39. What is the prognosis for cats with idiopathic LUTD?

The prognosis for most cats with idiopathic LUTD is good. The disease is usually self-limiting and of short duration. Symptoms may recur at unpredictable intervals but again subside in about 1 week without therapy. Only a small population of cats with idiopathic LUTD develop frequently recurring or persistent symptoms. However, as the cat ages, episodes tend to become less frequent and severe. Unfortunately, male cats with idiopathic LUTD are at increased risk of urethral obstruction due to the formation of urethral plugs. Recognition of certain risk factors for urethral obstruction in some male cats may help to prevent urethral obstruction but will not prevent nonobstructive episodes.

BIBLIOGRAPHY

1. Buffington, CAT, Chew DJ: CVT update: Idiopathic (interstitial) cystitis in cats. In Bonagura JD (ed): Kirk's Current Veterinary Therapy XIII (Small Animal Practice). Philadelphia, W.B. Saunders, 1999, pp 894–896.
2. Kalkstein TK, Kruger JK, Osborne CA: Feline idiopathic lower urinary tract disease. Part 1: Clinical manifestations. Comp Cont Educ Pract Vet 21:15–26, 1999.
3. Kalkstein TK, Kruger JK, Osborne CA: Feline idiopathic lower urinary tract disease. Part 2: Potential causes. Comp Cont Educ Pract Vet 21:148–154, 1999.
4. Kalkstein TK, Kruger JK, Osborne CA: Feline idiopathic lower urinary tract disease. Part 3: Diagnosis. Comp Cont Educ Prac Vet 21:387–394, 1999.
5. Kalkstein TK, Kruger JK, Osborne CA: Feline idiopathic lower urinary tract disease. Part 4: Therapeutic options. Comp Cont Educ Pract Vet 21:497–509, 1999.
6. Lees GE: Use and misuse of indwelling urethral catheters. Vet Clin North Am 26:499–505, 1996.
7. Osborne CA, Kruger JM, Lulich JP, et al: Prednisolone therapy of idiopathic feline lower urinary tract disease: A double-blind clinical study. Vet Clin North Am 26:563–570, 1996.

48. URINARY TRACT INFECTIONS

Laurie J. Blanco, D.V.M.

1. How common are bacterial urinary tract infections in cats?

Bacterial urinary tract infections are uncommon in young cats. In one prospective study of 141 young cats with lower urinary tract disease, the incidence of infections was < 2%. The mean age of the cats studied was 56.6 months. In one retrospective study, 25% (341 of 1380) of feline urine cultures submitted in a university hospital had positive bacterial urine cultures. The mean age of these cats was 8.2 years. In another retrospective study of cats older than 10 years of age with lower urinary tract disease, urinary tract infections were documented in 36 of 81 cats (45%).

2. Why are urinary tract infections so uncommon in young cats?

Many factors prevent bacterial colonization in the lower urinary tract of cats. One of the most important defenses is the normal flushing action of micturition. Normal flora that reside in the distal urethra and penis or vagina prevent colonization of pathogenic bacteria. In addition, the bladder mucosa has a layer of glycosaminoglycan (GAG) that is hypothesized to bind water and form a barrier to prevent contact of bacteria with the mucosa. Urine is also a relatively bacteriostatic medium. High osmolality, low pH, high urea concentration, and organic acids contribute to its bacteriostatic properties. The high urine osmolality of cats may be the major factor for the low incidence of infections. Finally, local and systemic immune responses also contribute to the prevention of urinary tract infections.

3. What are predisposing factors for developing an infection?

Any problem that disrupts the natural barriers of the urinary system predisposes cats to infections. Uroliths can create a nidus for bacterial infection. Cats with perineal urethrostomies are at a greater risk for introduction of bacteria than cats without perineal urethrostomies. Urinary catheters also disrupt the normal urethral barriers and introduce bacteria from the distal urethra and genital area. In a retrospective study of older cats with urinary tract infections, two-thirds of the cats had concurrent renal failure, and diagnoses in other cats included hyperthyroidism, feline immunodeficiency infection, feline leukemia virus infection, urinary incontinence, and neoplasia.

4. How can urinalysis help in the diagnosis of urinary tract infection?

A significant number of white blood cells in the sediment suggests an infection. Unfortunately, the leukocyte assay on urine dipsticks is highly unreliable for cat urine. Rod-shaped bacteria may be seen in the sediment if there are > 10,000 bacteria/ml. Cocci usually are not seen unless there are > 100,000 bacteria/ml. The absence of observable bacteria does not rule out an infection. Alkaline urine may be caused by urease-producing bacteria; however, many factors influence urine pH, and a high urine pH is not necessarily indicative of infection. The presence of white blood cell or bacterial casts indicates renal involvement. Although urinalysis results help to increase the suspicion for infection, urine culture is the gold standard for diagnosis of urinary tract infection.

5. What is considered significant bacteriuria in a urine culture?

Because the urinary bladder is considered sterile, any sample collected via cystocentesis should be devoid of bacteria unless there is contamination in vitro. Bacterial growth > 1,000 colony-forming units per milliliter (cfu/ml) in a urine sample obtained by cystocentesis or catheterization is considered significant. Because normal cats can have up to 100,000 cfu/ml on voided samples, this method of collection is not recommended if an infection is suspected.

6. What are the most common urinary pathogens in cats?

Escherichia spp., *Staphylococcus* spp., *Streptococcus* spp., *Proteus* spp., *Klebsiella* spp., *Pseudomonas* spp., and *Enterobacter* spp.

7. While you are waiting for urine culture results, what empiric therapy can be instituted?

Urinalysis with a sediment exam can be helpful for selecting empiric therapy. If the urine is alkaline, *Staphylococcus* or *Proteus* spp. are likely. Nearly 100% of *Staphylococcus* spp. and 80% of *Proteus* spp. are susceptible to beta-lactam antibiotics (penicillin, amoxicillin, or amoxicillin/clavulanic acid). If cocci are present in the sediment, one should suspect *Staphylococcus* or *Streptococcus* spp.; both are also susceptible to the beta-lactams. If rods are present, it can be more difficult to select an effective antibiotic because various rod-shaped bacteria have distinct susceptibility patterns. Because *Escherichia coli* is the most common rod-shaped bacteria in urinary tract infections, empirical treatment with a potentiated sulfa or quinolone is appropriate until susceptibility results are available.

8. What is the appropriate duration of antibiotic therapy?

In an uncomplicated lower urinary tract infection, 10–14 days of treatment is usually sufficient. In most cats, however, urinary tract infections are considered complicated (e.g, asssociated with a concurrent abnormality of the urinary tract or host defenses). The length of treatment depends on the type of host defense abnormality. If the abnormality can be corrected, the infection should be treated until the urinary tract has healed. If the abnormality cannot be corrected, treatment should extend 2–3 weeks after clinical signs have resolved. If signs recur soon after discontinuing treatment, the duration may need to be longer or daily preventive therapy may be necessary. Cats with pyelonephritis should be treated for at least 4–6 weeks (see Chapter 39).

9. Describe the ideal monitoring plan for cats with urinary tract infections.

Urine culture and sensitivity should be obtained via cystocentesis 3–5 days after starting antibiotic therapy. If the culture is positive, a different antibiotic should be selected based on susceptibility results. Another urine culture should be obtained 7–10 days after discontinuing antibiotic therapy. If this culture is positive, relapse or reinfection has occurred (see Chapter 39). If the posttreatment urine culture is negative, urinalyses and urine cultures can be monitored every 3–6 months.

BIBLIOGRAPHY

1. Bartges JW, Barsanti JA: Bacterial urinary tract infections in cats. In Bonagura JD (ed): Current Veterinary Therapy XIII (Small Animal Practice). Philadelphia, W.B. Saunders, 2000, pp 880–882.
2. Davidson AP, Ling GV, Stephens E, et al: Urinary tract infections in cats: A retrospective study, 1977–1989. Calif Vet 46:32–34, 1992.
3. Kruger JM, Osborne CA, Goyal SM, et al: Clinical evaluation of cats with lower urinary tract disease. J Am Vet Med Assoc 199:211–216, 1996.
4. Lees GE: Epidemiology of naturally occurring feline bacterial urinary tract infections. Vet Clin North Am 14:471–479, 1984.
5. Lees GE, Simpson RB, Green RA: Results of analysis and bacterial cultures of urine specimens obtained from clinically normal cats by three methods. J Am Vet Med Assoc 184:449–454, 1984.
6. Lees GE, Rogers KS: Treatment of urinary tract infections in dogs and cats. J Am Vet Med Assoc 189:648–652, 1986.

49. FUNCTIONAL URINARY OBSTRUCTION

Julie R. Fischer, D.V.M., and India F. Lane, D.V.M., M.S.

1. Define functional urinary obstruction.

Functional urinary obstruction refers to the inability to urinate because of excessive resistance in the bladder neck or urethra in the absence of an intraluminal or extraluminal anatomic obstruction. Normal elimination of urine requires coordinated relaxation of the bladder neck and urethra during detrusor contraction. In functional obstruction, the detrusor may contract, but inappropriate urethral or bladder neck contraction prevents effective or complete voiding of urine. Reflex dyssynergia, detrusor-sphincter dyssynergia, and urethrospasm also have been used to describe functional urinary obstruction in veterinary medicine.

2. What historical findings are common in cats with functional urinary obstruction?

Cats with functional urinary obstruction usually have a history of a predisposing medical condition, such as recent anatomic urethral obstruction or spinal injury. Idiopathic functional obstruction is rare in cats. If the condition is acute, owners may report straining (some think that the cat is constipated), vocalizing while voiding, and decreased amounts of urine in the litterbox. They may notice that the cat's abdomen is painful and may report nonspecific signs of illness, such as decreased food or water intake, lethargy, or hiding behavior. Cats with chronic partial obstruction may not be painful and may cease to strain. Overflow incontinence may develop, leading to a wet perineal area or urine scald. In hospitalized cats, persistent dysuria, stranguria, and distended urinary bladder are usually observed.

3. How should you focus the physical examination if functional urinary obstruction is suspected?

In the course of the physical examination, careful attention should be focused on the size and turgidity of the urinary bladder, external genitalia, and neurologic status.

4. What questions should be asked about the genitourinary system?

- Is the urinary bladder palpably enlarged? Is bladder tone soft or firm?
- Does the cat resent urinary bladder palpation?
- If the bladder is moderately enlarged, can urine be expressed with gentle, judicious pressure? Manual expression is somewhat difficult in a conscious, healthy male cat; however, it *is* possible to rupture a bladder with manual pressure, especially a diseased one. Be cautious!
- Is the abdomen distended (e.g. uroabdomen)?
- Is there evidence of self-trauma, swelling, urine scald, or inflammation of the external genitalia?

5. What questions should be asked to evaluate neurologic status?

- Are the cat's mentation and gait normal?
- Are hind limb reflexes normal?
- Does the cat have any areas of pain on firm palpation of the spinal column?
- Is tail carriage normal?
- Is perineal sensation intact? You should be able to elicit an anal "wink" with perineal stimulation, and there should be good anal tone when a rectal thermometer is passed.

6. What are common causes of functional urinary obstruction in cats?

Functional urinary obstruction in cats commonly occurs after a physical obstruction (usually a mucoprotein plug or stone) has been relieved by catheterization. Irritation caused by the physical obstruction and by the procedures required to remove the obstruction can result in a hypercontractile or "spastic" urethra. Spasm of the urethral musculature can be sufficient to prevent urine flow, despite repeated voiding attempts by the cat. In fact, repeated straining and increased sympathetic tone due to pain and irritation may stimulate further contraction of the urethra and bladder.

Injury to the spinal cord (most commonly from trauma, tumor, or disk disease) above the level of the sacral segments can disinhibit urethral sphincter reflexes and lead to continuous sphincter contraction. Cats with upper motor neuron bladders usually have firm bladders that are difficult to express manually. Sometimes even a cord lesion in the sacral region can produce dyssynergic voiding that mimics a suprasacral lesion. Prolonged bladder distention resulting from a neurologic lesion can lead to detrusor atony, which may further complicate management.

Less common causes of functional urinary obstruction include surgery or trauma of the caudal abdominal region, perineal region, or urogenital tract.

7. Do cats with functional urinary obstruction have characteristic laboratory abnormalities?

If a cat has had complete urinary obstruction for an extended period, azotemia, hyperkalemia, and metabolic acidosis may be detected. Hematuria, pyuria, or bacteriuria may be observed on urinalysis, reflecting bladder wall pathology, inflammation, or infection secondary to urine retention and urinary bladder distention. Because of these potential sequelae to partial or complete urinary obstruction, a minimal laboratory database should include complete blood count, serum biochemical profile with electrolytes, and urinalysis with sediment examination and culture. Serum feline leukemia antigen testing and feline immunodeficiency virus antibody testing are indicated if spinal cord compression is suspected in cats with no history of trauma; cats with spinal lymphoma often are infected with a retrovirus.

8. How is functional urinary obstruction diagnosed?

Functional urinary obstruction is characterized by a distended urinary bladder that is difficult to express and absence of anatomic obstruction. A cat that has just urinated should have minimal (a few milliliters) urine left in the bladder. The bladder should be small or nondetectable radiographically and on palpation. If the bladder is radiographically or palpably much larger than a small plum after voluntary urination, urethral catheterization is the next diagnostic and therapeutic step. A well-lubricated, 3.5-French polypropylene, red rubber, or silicone urinary catheter should pass relatively easily and smoothly through the urethra of a sedated or anesthetized male cat. Feel for areas of resistance or grittiness as you pass the catheter. Do not forget the curve in the male feline urethra; pulling the penis straight caudally should facilitate atraumatic catheterization. Female cats can be catheterized with the use of a tiny speculum or by passing the catheter along the floor of the vestibule.

9. Discuss the role of imaging modalities.

Survey radiography and abdominal ultrasonography can be helpful in ruling out the presence of small or mobile stones that are not detected via catheterization. A retrograde cystourethrogram can show urethral strictures and radiolucent stones. Urodynamic studies (such as urethral pressure profilometry, cystometrography, or electromyography) are available at selected referral institutions and are sometimes helpful in documenting detrusor and urethral muscle dysfunction in confusing cases.

10. What are the other common causes of voiding difficulty after relief of urethral obstruction?

Reobstruction (anatomic)
- Mucoproteinaceous urethral plug material
- Mobile urolith
- Blood clot
- Crystalline material

Detrusor atony

11. How should functional urinary obstruction be treated?

If the cat has a treatable cause of spinal trauma or urethral disease, management of these disorders is the most valuable component of treatment. Cats with spinal injury, postobstructive disorders, or idiopathic functional urinary obstruction may benefit from short- or long-term medication to provide urethral relaxation. The selective alpha-1 antagonists (e.g., prazosin, doxazosin, alfuzosin) have been shown to decrease urethral pressures in anesthetized male cats. Because of the greater percentage of skeletal muscle in the feline urethra compared with the canine urethra, skeletal muscle relaxants (diazepam, dantrolene) often are added to the therapeutic regimen. Bladder care and monitoring are important. The bladder should be kept relatively small (i.e., after micturition or expression it should be smaller than a small plum).

Most urethral relaxant medications are safe for long-term use. The exception is diazepam—long-term use is not recommended because of the possibility of idiopathic hepatic necrosis. If effective, the medications can be slowly tapered over a few weeks to determine continued need. Medications are usually tapered more quickly when urethral obstruction has been cleared.

Agents Used as Urethral Relaxants in Cats

DRUG	MECHANISM	RECOMMENDED DOSAGE	POSSIBLE ADVERSE EFFECTS	CONTRAINDICATIONS OR COMMENTS
Acepromazine	Skeletal muscle relaxation via neuroleptic effect Smooth muscle relaxation via alpha antagonism	Up to 0.1 mg/kg IV every 12–24 hr (doses as low as 0.02 mg/kg IV may be effective) 1.1–2.2 mg/kg PO every 12–24 hr	Hypotension Sedation Exacerbation of seizure disorder	Hypovolemia Cardiac disease Seizure disorder
Dantrolene	Skeletal muscle relaxation via direct effects	0.5–2.0 mg/kg PO every 8 hr 1.0 mg/kg IV	Weakness Hepatotoxicity	
Diazepam	Skeletal muscle relaxation via central effects (benzodiazepine)	0.2–0.5 mg/kg IV every 8 hr or PRN (doses as low as 0.1 mg/kg IV may be effective) 2.5–5.0 mg/cat PO every 8 hr or PRN	Sedation Paradoxic excitation Idiopathic hepatic necrosis (with PO use only) Polyphagia	Cardiopulmonary disease
Phenoxybenzamine	Smooth muscle relaxation via nonspecific alpha antagonism	1.25–7.5 mg/cat PO every 8–12 hr	Hypotension Tachycardia GI upset	Cardiac disease Hypovolemia Glaucoma Renal failure Diabetes mellitus (type II)
Prazosin	Smooth muscle relaxation via alpha-1 antagonism	0.25–0.5 mg/cat PO every 12–24 hr 0.03 mg/kg IV	Hypotension Mild sedation Ptyalism	Cardiac disease Renal failure
Alprazolam	Centrally acting anxiolytic benzodiazepine	0.125–0.25 mg/cat PO every 12 hr	As for diazepam, except idiopathic hepatic necrosis has not been documented	May be good alternative if oral therapy is needed

IV = intravenously, PO = orally, PRN = as needed.

12. What are the advantages and disadvantages of using an indwelling urinary catheter in functionally obstructed cats?

Cats that are functionally obstructed after relief of a mechanical obstruction usually require replacement of an indwelling urinary catheter for 1–3 days to maintain urine flow and prevent further urinary bladder damage. Unfortunately, urethral catheterization may contribute to urethral inflammation and spasm. The following suggestions may reduce the risk of creating or exacerbating functional urinary obstruction during indwelling urinary catheterization:

1. Use soft, nonirritating catheters for indwelling placement in the urethra. Less irritating catheter types include silicone, Teflon, and soft infant feeding-tubes. Polypropylene catheters (tom-cat catheters) are extremely irritating when left in contact with the bladder or urethral mucosa. The use of pharmacologic urethral relaxants during and after the period of catheterization should be considered (see table in preceding question). Diazepam and acepromazine also may have an anxiolytic effect, which reduces stranguria while the catheter is in place. Acepromazine is contraindicated in dehydrated or hypotensive patients.

2. Consider the one-time use of a nonsteroidal anti-inflammatory drug (NSAID), such as ketoprofen, at the time of catheterization or catheter removal. NSAIDs may be contraindicated in azotemic animals.

3. Ensure patency of the indwelling catheter at all times so that the urinary bladder remains empty and urine flows freely when the catheter is in place.

13. What is the prognosis for a cat with functional urinary obstruction?

Prognosis for functional urinary obstruction depends on the cause. The vast majority of cats who have postobstructive dysfunction recover normal urinary function if given adequate time and supportive care. Rarely do cats require longer than 1 week of in-hospital management in this scenario. Cats with suprasacral spinal injuries usually recover urinary function as they recover motor function to the limbs; recovery may be prolonged. Most cats with complete sacrococcygeal ("tail-pull") lesions never recover normal urinary function and may require lifelong treatment. Initially such cats usually have an easily expressed, lower motor neuron bladder, but sphincter hypertonicity eventually develops.

BIBLIOGRAPHY

1. Bartges JW, Finco DR, Polzin DJ, et al: Pathophysiology of urethral obstruction. Vet Clin North Am Small Anim Pract 26:255–264, 1996.
2. Fletcher TF: Applied anatomy and physiology of the feline lower urinary tract. Vet Clin North Am Small Anim Pract 26:181–196, 1996.
3. Frenier SL, Knowlen GG, Speth RC, et al: Urethral pressure response to alpha-adrenergic agonist and antagonist drugs in anesthetized male cats. Am J Vet Res 53:1161–1165, 1992.
4. Marks SL, Straeter-Knowled IM, Moore M, et al: Effects of acepromazine maleate and phenoxybenzamine on urethral pressure profiles of anesthetized, healthy, sexually intact male cats. Am J Vet Res 57:1497–1500, 1996.
5. Lane IF: Diagnosis and management of urinary retention. Vet Clin North Am Small Anim Pract 30:25–57, 2000.
6. Lane IF: Disorders of micturition. In Osborne CA, Finco DR (eds): Canine and Feline Nephrology and Urology, 2nd ed. Baltimore, Williams & Wilkins, 1995, pp 693–717.
7. Osborne CA, Kruger JM, Lulich JP, et al: Feline lower urinary tract diseases. In Ettinger SA, Feldman EC (eds): Textbook of Veterinary Internal Medicine. Philadelphia, W.B. Saunders, 2000, pp 1738–1739.
8. Straeter-Knowlen IM, Marks SI, Rishniw M, et al: Urethral pressure response to smooth and skeletal muscle relaxants in anesthetized, male cats with naturally acquired urethral obstruction. Am J Vet Res 56:919–923, 1995.

50. COMMON DIETARY QUESTIONS

Joseph W. Bartges, B.S., D.V.M., Ph.D., and India F. Lane, D.V.M., M.S.

1. How is a nutritional plan formulated?

A nutritional plan is formulated using a two-step iterative process:

1. **Assessment** of the animal (signalment, history, physical examination, laboratory results, and nutritional factors related to the life stage and/or disease process), diet (current diet), and feeding method (frequency and amount of meals).

2. Formulating and implementing a **feeding plan**, including selecting a diet formulated to meet the nutritional factors identified in the assessment process (the diet that the animal is currently consuming or a different diet) and providing the diet (meal feeding, free-choice feeding, tube feeding, or parenteral feeding). Included in the nutritional plan is a reassessment of the implemented feeding plan; changes are made as indicated by the two-step iterative process.

2. What urinary tract diseases may respond to dietary modification?

Most information about dietary considerations of dogs and cats with urinary tract disease is limited to chronic renal failure and urolithiasis; however, nutritional modification has a role in management of all diseases, including other urinary tract diseases. Dietary modification may favorably alter urine composition, thereby aiding in the treatment or prevention of urinary tract diseases (see table on following two pages).

3. What are the key features of dietary modification for specific diseases?

- Chronic renal failure: reduced protein, reduced phosphorous, alkalinization, and adequate potassium.
- Protein-losing nephropathy: reduced protein.
- Hypertension: reduced sodium.
- Struvite calculi: reduced protein, reduced phosphorous, reduced magnesium, acidification, and induction of diuresis.
- Calcium oxalate calculi: reduced protein, reduced sodium, adequate magnesium and phosphorous, and alkalinization; *or* increased fiber
- Urate calculi: reduced protein and alkalinization.
- Cystine calculi: reduced protein, reduced sodium, and alkalinization.
- Idiopathic lower urinary tract disease: reduced protein, reduced phosphorous, reduced magnesium, acidification, and induction of diuresis.

4. Define chronic renal failure.

Chronic renal failure is defined as irreversible destruction of nephrons with resultant loss of renal function; the condition is stable on a short-term basis but ultimately progressive (see Chapter 40). Usually the cause of chronic renal failure is not known; therefore, specific therapy cannot be implemented to reverse the condition.

5. What are the goals of dietary treatment for chronic renal failure?

Reduced renal function results in excesses or deficiencies related to nutritional status, electrolyte concentrations, acid–base balance, hydration status, retention of waste products, inadequate metabolism or excretion of exogenous substances, and neuroendocrine balance. The goal of treatment is to minimize these excesses and deficiencies. Furthermore, chronic renal failure is a dynamic process; therefore, routine monitoring and adjustment are necessary. The mnemonic **NEPHRONS** is based on these goals:

Approximate Nutrient Profiles from Selected Diets Formulated for Treatment of Urinary Tract Diseases in Cats[1]

DIET	KCAL[2]/SERVING[3]	AS FED					DRY MATTER				AMOUNT/100 KCAL			
		WATER (%)	CRUDE PROTEIN (%)	CRUDE FAT (%)	CRUDE FIBER (%)	NFE (%)	CRUDE PROTEIN (%)	CRUDE FAT (%)	CRUDE FIBER (%)	NFE (%)	CRUDE PROTEIN (GM)	CRUDE FAT (GM)	CRUDE FIBER (GM)	NFE (GM)
C/d[4]	285/cup	7.8	31.8	15.0	0.7	39.3	34.5	16.3	0.8	42.6	8.6	4.0	0.2	10.6
	423/14.25 oz can	76.1	10.4	5.2	0.8	6.0	43.4	21.7	3.3	25.1	10.0	5.0	0.8	5.7
C/d oxl[4]	286/cup	8.1	31.5	15.4	1.0	38.9	34.3	16.8	1.1	42.3	8.5	4.1	0.3	10.4
	162/5.5 oz can	76.3	9.9	4.7	0.4	7.4	41.8	19.8	1.9	31.2	9.6	4.5	0.4	7.1
Control Formula[5]	411/cup	10.0	31.0	21.0	1.3	32.3	34.4	23.3	1.4	35.9	7.9	5.3	0.3	8.2
	93/3 oz can	78.0	10.7	7.0	0.2	4.0	48.6	31.8	0.9	18.2	9.8	6.4	0.2	3.7
Control pHormula[6]	410/cup	12.0	32.0	14.0	3.0	32.4	36.4	15.9	3.4	36.8	7.8	3.4	0.7	7.8
	175/6 oz can	85.0	6.0	7.0	0.1	1.1	40.0	46.7	0.7	7.3	5.8	6.8	0.1	1.1
CV[7]	223/5.5 oz can	70.7	12.5	7.9	0.3	6.8	42.5	26.8	1.0	23.1	8.7	5.5	0.2	4.7
H/d[4]	506/14.25 oz can	70.8	12.7	7.8	0.1	6.8	43.4	26.7	0.3	23.3	10.2	6.2	0.1	6.2
K/d[4]	519/cup	7.5	26.1	25.7	0.6	35.9	28.2	27.8	0.7	38.8	6.1	6.1	0.1	8.4
	584/14.25 oz can	70.1	8.2	11.4	0.8	6.8	28.2	39.2	2.8	23.4	5.7	7.9	0.6	4.7
Low pH/S[8]	441/cup	10.0	33.4	16.7	1.7	34.3	37.1	18.6	1.9	38.2	7.9	4.0	0.4	8.1
	197/6 oz can	76.5	11.0	7.2	0.2	4.0	47.0	30.4	1.0	17.1	9.6	6.2	0.2	3.5
Low Protein[6]	385/cup	12.0	20.0	18.0	6.0	36.4	22.7	20.5	6.8	41.4	4.7	4.3	1.4	8.6
	250/6 oz can	75.0	8.0	11.0	1.0	3.1	32.0	44.0	4.0	12.4	5.5	7.5	0.7	2.1
Multi-Stage Renal[8]	535 kcal/cup	7.87	28.0	23.5	2.1	34.2	30.4	25.5	2.2	37.2	6.4	5.3	0.5	7.8
Mature Formula[5]	351/cup	10.0	26.7	15.0	2.2	41.5	29.7	16.7	2.4	16.1	7.4	4.2	0.6	11.5
	415/14 oz can	78.0	8.8	7.3	1.0	3.7	40.0	33.2	4.6	16.8	8.4	7.0	1.0	3.5
Moderate pH/O[8]	451/cup	10.0	32.4	16.5	1.7	34.0	36.0	18.3	1.9	37.8	7.5	3.8	0.4	7.9
	197/6 oz can	78.0	10.6	6.9	0.2	3.8	48.2	31.2	1.1	17.1	9.2	5.9	0.2	3.2
Modified Formula[5]	436/cup	12.0	25.4	21.6	1.8	36.9	28.9	24.6	2.1	41.9	6.4	5.5	0.5	9.3
	137/3 oz can	74.5	9.0	15.1	0.2	1.0	35.3	59.2	0.8	3.9	5.6	9.4	0.1	0.6

Table continued on following page

Approximate Nutrient Profiles from Selected Diets Formulated for Treatment of Urinary Tract Diseases in Cats[1] (Continued)

DIET	KCAL[2]/SERVING[3]	WATER (%)	AS FED CRUDE PROTEIN (%)	AS FED CRUDE FAT (%)	AS FED CRUDE FIBER (%)	AS FED NFE (%)	DRY MATTER CRUDE PROTEIN (%)	DRY MATTER CRUDE FAT (%)	DRY MATTER CRUDE FIBER (%)	DRY MATTER NFE (%)	AMOUNT/100 KCAL CRUDE PROTEIN (GM)	AMOUNT/100 KCAL CRUDE FAT (GM)	AMOUNT/100 KCAL CRUDE FIBER (GM)	AMOUNT/100 KCAL NFE (GM)
NF[7]	398/cup	7.4	28.5	11.9	1.1	46.9	30.8	12.9	1.2	50.6	6.5	2.7	0.3	10.7
	234/5.5 oz can	71.0	9.0	8.6	0.8	8.9	31.0	29.5	2.6	30.6	6.0	5.7	0.5	5.9
R/d[4]	224/cup	9.0	34.3	7.6	15.2	28.6	37.7	8.4	16.7	31.5	11.7	2.6	5.2	9.8
	251/14.25 oz can	75.0	8.5	1.8	7.0	7.0	34.0	7.2	28.0	28.0	13.7	2.9	11.3	11.3
S/d[4]	521/cup	7.5	32.0	24.0	0.6	30.3	34.6	26.0	0.7	32.8	7.5	5.6	0.1	7.1
	552/14.25 oz can	71.0	12.1	9.8	0.5	4.7	41.7	33.8	1.6	16.2	8.9	7.2	0.3	3.5
UR[7]	366/cup	8.7	32.4	10.6	1.4	41.6	35.4	11.6	1.5	45.6	8.0	2.6	0.3	10.3
	493/12.5 oz can	70.7	12.1	10.7	0.1	4.8	41.4	36.5	0.1	16.5	8.7	7.7	0.1	3.5
W/d[4]	246/cup	8.9	35.7	8.7	8.1	33.3	39.2	9.6	8.9	36.6	11.1	2.7	2.5	10.4
	364/14.25 oz can	74.7	10.4	4.2	3.1	6.0	41.1	16.6	12.3	23.7	11.6	4.7	3.5	6.7

[1] Based on information provided by pet food manufacturers.
[2] For conversion of kcal to KJ: 1 kcal = 4.2 KJ.
[3] Cup = one 8-ounce measuring cup.
[4] Prescription Diets, Hill's Pet Nutrition, Inc., Topeka, KS; diet information as of September 2000.
[5] Select Care Diets, Innovative Veterinary Diets, Division of Nature's Recipe Pet Foods; diet information as of September 2000.
[6] Veterinary Diets, Waltham, Leicestershire, England; diet information as of September 2000.
[7] CNM Diets, Ralston Purina, Company, St. Louis, MO; diet information as of September 2000.
[8] Eukanuba Diets, Iams Company, Dayton, OH; diet information as of September 2000.

N = **N**utrition (adequately provide)
E = **E**lectrolytes (maintain normal concentrations)
P = **p**H of blood (normalize)
H = **H**ydration (maintain adequate level)
R = **R**etention of wastes (remove or reduce)
O = **O**ther renal insults (avoid)
N = **N**euroendocrine parameters (normalize)
S = **S**erial monitoring (essential)

6. Describe the caloric requirements of cats with chronic renal failure.

Caloric requirements are presumed to be similar to those of healthy cats; however, energy intake decreases with declining renal function because of anorexia and nausea. In general, calculation of caloric requirements (maintenance energy requirements [MER]) with either of the following formulas is adequate:

$$\text{MER} = 1.5[(30\text{BW}_{kg}) + 70] \ or \ \text{MER} = 100(\text{BW}_{kg}^{0.75})$$

where BW_{kg} = body weight in kilograms. Ideally, however, energy intake should be adjusted in individual cats to maintain optimal body condition.

7. How can uremic anorexia be minimized?

Several strategies may be attempted to minimize uremic anorexia, the cause of which is multifactorial. Most cats with chronic renal failure have increased concentration of gastrin and benefit from H_2-receptor antagonist therapy (see Chapter 40). Correcting metabolic acidosis, hypokalemia, and potential B-vitamin deficiency and decreasing retention of metabolic waste products (urea nitrogen, creatinine, and organic acids) may increase appetite. Maintaining hydration status, treating anemia, and correcting systemic arterial hypertension are also beneficial. However, drug administration may result in anorexia in individual cats with chronic renal failure. Use of feeding tubes may be necessary.

Strategies That May Minimize Uremic Anorexia

1. **Correct underlying abnormalities.**
   Minimize deficits and excesses in:
   Hydration status
   Serum concentrations of nitrogenous wastes
   Serum electrolyte and mineral concentrations (sodium, potassium, phosphorus, calcium)
   Serum hydrogen ion concentration (pH)
   Serum concentrations of hormones (parathyroid hormone, erythropoietin, renin, angiotensin)
   Others
2. **Enhance palatability of diet.**
   When changing diet:
   Switch foods slowly.
   Use food with a texture to which the cat is accustomed.
   Try flavoring agents such as clam juice, tuna juice, and chicken broth.
   Attempt to add water to dry foods (this strategy usually does not work with cats).
   Try liquid enteral diets: Renal Care (Pet-Ag), Impact (Sandoz), other human liquid enteral diets.
   Warm moist food to, but not above, body temperature.
   The smell of food is important for cats; keep nasal passages open.
   Cats prefer high-protein foods
3. **Modify feeding patterns.**
   Emphasize frequent small meals.
   Offer rewards (favorite foods; maintenance foods).
   Hand feed.
   Avoid adverse associations with eating (medications, injections, others).
   Prevent food aversion. Do not offer diets for long-term management of chronic renal failure during periods of nausea and vomiting

Table continued on following page

Strategies That May Minimize Uremic Anorexia (Continued)

4. **Minimize vomiting.**
   Correct underlying abnormalities (see suggestions under 1).
   Use pharmacologic antiemetic agents:
   Cimetidine (2.5–5 mg/kg every 8–12 hr IV or PO)
   Ranitidine (2.5 mg/kg every 12 hr IV; 3.5 mg/kg every 12 hr PO)
   Metoclopramide (0.2–0.5 mg/kg every 6–8 hr IV, IM, or PO; 1–2 mg/kg every 24 hr by continuous IV infusion)
   Omeprazole (0.7 mg/kg PO every 24 hr)
   Chlorpromazine (0.25–0.5 mg/kg IM, SQ, or PO every 6–8 hr)
   Prochlorperazine (0.1–0.5 mg/kg IM or SQ every 6–8 hr)
   Use gastrointestinal coating agents and protectants:
   Antacids
   Sucralfate (0.25–1 gm/kg PO every 8–12 hr)
   Bismuth subsalicylate (2 ml/kg PO every 6–8 hr)
   Kaolin-Pectin (1–2 ml/kg PO every 4–6 hr)
5. **Implement pharmacologic appetite stimulation:**
   Diazepam (1–2 mg/cat PO, as needed, or 0.05–0.1 mg/kg IV, as needed)
   Oxazepam (0.3–0.4 mg/kg PO or 2–2.5 mg/cat PO, as needed)
   Flurazepam (0.1–0.5 mg/kg PO, as needed)
   Cyproheptadine (2 mg/cat PO every 8–12 hr)
   Androgens
6. **Use enteral feeding:**
   Hand feeding
   Nasoesophageal, esophageal, and/or gastrostomy feeding tubes.

IV = intravenously, PO = orally, SQ = subcutaneously, IM = intramuscularly.
Modified from Lulich JP, Osborne CA, O'Brien TD, Polzin DJ. Feline renal failure: Questions, answers, questions. Compen Contin Educ Pract Vet 14:127–153, 1992.

8. Is alteration of dietary lipid content or type beneficial in cats with chronic renal failure?
Studies in dogs with experimentally induced chronic renal failure have shown that a diet with 15% fat (dry matter basis) containing menhaden fish oil (high in omega-3 fatty acids) was associated with greater glomerular filtration rate and longer survival times compared with diets containing similar amounts of beef tallow or safflower oil. Similar benefits, however, have not been documented in cats.

9. Why does hypokalemia occur in cats with chronic renal failure?
Hypokalemia has been reported in approximately 20% of cats with naturally occurring chronic renal failure. Decreased dietary intake of potassium, increased urinary losses due to polyuria, increased fecal losses, and consumption of high-protein, low-potassium, acidifying diets may contribute to hypokalemia. Hypokalemia may result in metabolic acidosis, worsening renal failure, anorexia, and muscle weakness.

10. How is hypokalemia treated?
A dietary intake of 0.18 gm of potassium/100 kcal of metabolizable energy (ME) or 0.9% of the diet (dry matter basis) is recommended to maintain serum potassium concentration above 4 mEq/L. If diet alone does not maintain the desired serum concentration, supplementation with potassium gluconate should be instituted (see Chapter 40).

11. Is dietary sodium restriction beneficial in cats with chronic renal failure?
Sodium is important in fluid balance and blood pressure regulation. Although serum sodium concentrations are not usually abnormal in cats with chronic renal failure, dietary sodium restriction is important for maintaining normal extracellular fluid volume and systemic arterial blood pressure. Concomitant dietary chloride restriction also is important. Chloride may act as a direct

renal vasoconstrictor, and tubular chloride also stimulates release of renin by the juxtaglomerular cells. Renin increases renal sodium retention and stimulates angiotensin II production, promoting expansion of extracellular volume and increased systemic arterial blood pressure.

12. What are the recommended daily intakes for sodium and chloride?

Recommended daily sodium intake for cats with chronic renal failure is 10-40 mg/BWkg or 0.2-0.35% of the diet (dry matter basis). Appropriate dietary chloride requirements of cats with chronic renal failure are not known; however, a chloride level at least 1.5 times the sodium content is recommended. Because of obligatory renal sodium excretion in some animals, adaptation to a lower sodium- and chloride-containing diet should be gradual.

13. What is the most common acid–base abnormality in cats with chronic renal failure?

Metabolic acidosis occurs in at least 80% of cats with chronic renal failure. Acidosis results from dietary as well as nondietary factors. Dietary acid is derived from sulfur-containing amino acids; organic acids produced during intermediary metabolism from partial oxidation of carbohydrates, fats, protein, and nucleic acids; phosphoric acid used as a palatability enhancer; and mineral salts. In general, protein metabolism is the major source of hydrogen ions and thus acidosis. Metabolic acidosis may result in anorexia, weakness, increased muscle catabolism, hypokalemia, worsening of renal failure, and stimulation of parathyroid hormone production.

14. How is metabolic acidosis treated?

Potassium citrate is often included in diets formulated for management of renal failure as an alkalinizing agent as well as a source of potassium. The therapeutic goal is to maintain a serum total carbon dioxide concentration (or serum bicarbonate concentration) between 17 and 22 mEq/L. If diet alone does not achieve this goal, additional alkalinization using sodium bicarbonate or potassium citrate supplementation may be required (see Chapter 40). Potassium citrate may be a better choice in cats with chronic renal failure because the added potassium intake helps to offset hypokalemia, and the additional sodium load associated with sodium bicarbonate administration is avoided.

15. Describe the fluid requirements in cats with chronic renal failure.

Water balance occurs when the sum of water intake and metabolic water produced equals output. Water intake is composed of drinking water, water contained in food, and water formed during metabolism. The kidneys represent the major system involved in water output regulation. Renal failure is associated with polyuria, and the maximal urine osmolality approaches that of plasma (300 mOsm/kg or a specific gravity of 1.007–1.014). Dehydration and hypovolemia may result in worsening of renal failure; therefore, both should be prevented. Feeding a canned formulated diet provides water (most canned diets contain approximately 75% water compared with dry formulated diets, which contain approximately 10% water). If cats will not eat canned formulated diets, adding water to dry food may increase water intake (although cats are often resistant to this maneuver). Many cats require supplemental water in the form of subcutaneously administered fluids (glucose-free balanced electrolyte solutions, 100–150 ml/cat every 1–3 days). Water also may be administered through nasoesophageal or gastrostomy feeding tubes if either is used.

16. Is dietary protein restriction beneficial in chronic renal failure?

Dietary protein restriction is associated with decreased accumulation of waste products derived from protein, including urea and other nitrogenous compounds. Clinical experience confirms that dietary protein restriction is associated with amelioration of uremia. However, the influence of dietary protein restriction on progression of renal failure is controversial. In addition to decreasing nitrogenous compounds, dietary protein restriction is associated with a decreased acid load, decreased phosphorous intake, and less solute that failing kidneys must excrete. Diets formulated for management of renal failure should contain 19–23% of calories as high biologic value protein or 28–30% of the diet (dry matter basis).

Another beneficial effect of protein restriction relates to decreasing ammoniagenesis. Urinary ammonia is derived primarily from renal metabolism of glutamine. Urinary ammonia excretion increases with metabolic acidosis. Increased urinary ammonia may result in tubulointerstitial disease through activation of complement and other mechanisms. Because the majority of excreted acid is produced from metabolism of dietary protein (in particular, animal-derived protein), dietary protein restriction is associated with decreased generation of metabolic acids and, consequently, decreased urinary ammonia excretion.

17. What is the major risk of protein restriction?

Although uncommon, a potential side effect of dietary protein restriction is protein deficiency. Worsening anemia, hypoalbuminemia, loss of muscle mass, or a dry, unthrifty haircoat may be manifestations of protein deficiency. If signs of protein deficiency occur, increasing dietary protein intake may be attempted; however, care should be taken to avoid creating an imbalanced diet or worsening uremia.

18. What is renal secondary hyperparathyroidism?

Phosphorous retention and secondary hyperparathyroidism have been incriminated as causes of progressive renal failure. Phosphorous plays a critical role in energy metabolism, cell membrane integrity, acid–base balance, oxygen delivery to tissues, and carbohydrate metabolism. Secondary hyperparathyroidism is an inevitable consequence of chronic renal failure, although it is often not present until late in the course of the disease.

19. What dietary modifications may improve hyperparathyroidism?

In a study involving experimentally induced chronic renal failure in cats, a dietary phosphorous intake of 1.56% (dry matter basis) was associated with significant renal mineralization and tubulointerstitial lesions. In comparison, a dietary intake of 0.42% (dry matter basis) resulted in minimal lesions. Appropriate dietary phosphorous restriction prevents and reverses preexisting renal hyperparathyroidism. An intake of 0.4-0.6% phosphorous (dry matter basis) is recommended for cats with chronic renal failure. If dietary phosphorous restriction alone does not normalize serum phosphorous concentration, administration of phosphate binders (see Chapter 40) should be instituted.

20. What dietary treatments are helpful in managing the anemia of chronic renal failure?

Normocytic, normochromic nonregenerative anemia may occur with chronic renal failure and is believed to be due, in part, to decreased erythropoietin production by failing kidneys. Poor nutritional status and gastrointestinal blood loss secondary to uremic gastroenteropathy may further exacerbate anemia. Anemia is treated by maintaining a good nutritional plane, minimizing gastrointestinal hemorrhage, and administering erythropoietin (see Chapter 40). By providing adequate calories while minimizing uremia, a good nutritional plane can be maintained. Ameliorating metabolic acidosis decreases gastric acid secretion, thereby minimizing uremic gastroenteropathy and blood loss. If erythropoietin therapy is instituted, iron supplementation also should be provided. Iron sulfate (50–100 mg/cat/day orally initially) is the preferred therapy for iron deficiency and prevention of iron-deficient erythropoiesis in patients beginning therapy with recombinant human erythropoietin. Because iron supplementation may be associated with gastrointestinal upset and diarrhea, small divided doses may be preferable.

21. Describe the role of diet in management of systemic arterial hypertension.

Systemic arterial hypertension is common in cats with chronic renal failure (see Chapters 40 and 63). Dietary sodium restriction, dietary phosphorous restriction, and amelioration of metabolic acidosis may decrease systemic arterial blood pressure.

22. What other nutrients may be of interest in cats with chronic renal failure?

Soluble fiber may have a role in management of chronic renal failure. Soluble fiber causes bacterial proliferation in the large intestine. Bacterial growth requires a source of nitrogen that is derived primarily from blood urea, which diffuses into the large intestine. Colonic bacteria degrade urea, and the nitrogen is used for bacterial protein synthesis. Bacteria and these proteins are excreted in feces. The net effect is increased fecal urea excretion, reduced serum urea nitrogen concentration, and reduced urinary urea excretion. Although fecal excretion of urea may decrease serum urea nitrogen concentration, metabolic acids are generated from dietary protein, and if dietary protein is not reduced, the kidneys still must excrete an added acid load.

23. When should dietary modification be instituted in cats with chronic renal failure?

Dietary modification should be instituted at the time of diagnosis of chronic renal failure in cats. Dietary modification decreases the clinical signs and biochemical consequences of chronic renal failure and also is associated with a longer median survival time in cats with spontaneously occurring chronic renal failure. Dietary modification should not be attempted while animals are uremic because it may result in food aversion. Instead, a gradual dietary change should be attempted after initial management of uremia when the cat is eating voluntarily. Dietary change is easily accomplished early in chronic renal failure but becomes progressively more difficult as the disease progresses.

24. What nutrients are of concern in cats with proteinuria?

Protein-losing nephropathy is not common in cats unless it is associated with chronic renal failure or familial amyloidosis (see Chapter 43). Therefore, little information is available about its treatment in cats. Dietary modifications that may of benefit include protein restriction and other modifications appropriate for chronic renal failure.

25. Can dietary modification aid in treatment or prevention of urinary tract infections?

Bacterial urinary tract infections are uncommon in young cats but common in cats older than 10 years (see Chapters 40, 41, and 48). Induction of aciduria has been recommended in treatment of bacterial urinary tract infections; however, most cats cannot achieve a urine pH < 5.5. Most bacteria are able to propagate in urine with pH values ranging from 5.0 to 9.0; therefore, urinary acidification probably offers little benefit. Furthermore, because the incidence of bacterial urinary tract infection is greater in older cats and cats with renal failure, an acidifying diet may induce or exacerbate renal failure.

Fungal urinary tract infections are uncommon in cats; however, in cats with subclinical funguria, induction of alkaluria may clear the infection. Urinary alkalinizing agents such as sodium bicarbonate or potassium citrate or an alkalinizing diet to induce a urine pH ≥ 8.0 may be adequate for treatment of funguria if clinical signs are absent or minimal. Antifungal drugs may be necessary in symptomatic or ill cats with funguria.

26. Are there different forms of struvite uroliths?

Struvite (magnesium ammonium phosphate hexahydrate) forms in alkaline urine (see Chapter 45). Alkaluria may result from a urease-producing bacterial urinary tract infection (infection-induced struvite uroliths) or from diet (sterile struvite uroliths). Sterile struvite uroliths occur most commonly in cats; however, infection-induced struvite uroliths occur occasionally in kittens and older cats predisposed to bacterial urinary tract infections.

27. How are struvite uroliths managed?

Sterile struvite uroliths can be dissolved by inducing undersaturation of urine with magnesium, ammonium, and phosphate ions and by inducing alkaluria (see Chapter 45). These goals can be accomplished by feeding a diet that, compared with adult cat maintenance diets, is lower in protein, magnesium, and phosphorous and induces aciduria. Currently, only one feline diet is marketed to induce struvite urolith dissolution (S/D diet; see table on pages 237–238). On average, sterile struvite uroliths can be dissolved in 2–4 weeks by feeding this diet exclusively; dissolution of infection-induced struvite uroliths requires 8–10 weeks. Once sterile struvite uroliths are dissolved or removed, prevention involves dietary modification. Diets formulated to minimize recurrence of sterile struvite uroliths are lower in protein, phosphorous, and magnesium and induce aciduria. The struvite dissolution diet should be used cautiously in kittens or adult cats with chronic renal failure.

28. How are calcium oxalate uroliths managed?

Currently there are no medical protocols that induce dissolution of calcium oxalate uroliths in cats; therefore, symptomatic uroliths must be physically removed. Preventive measures include dietary modification.

29. What nutrients are of interest in the prevention of calcium oxalate uroliths?

Dietary modifications demonstrated or thought to be beneficial include moderate restriction of protein, restriction of calcium and oxalic acid, provision of adequate magnesium and phosphorous, increased moisture, and inducing neutral to alkaline urine pH. Currently three diets are formulated for management of calcium oxalate uroliths in cats (see table on pages 237–238). Consumption of these diets by healthy cats results in lowering of urine saturation to a state of undersaturation, which theoretically should be sufficient to minimize recurrence of calcium oxalate formation. Hypercalcemic cats (approximately 35% of cats with calcium oxalate uroliths) appear to respond better to higher-fiber diets supplemented with potassium citrate for alkalinization.

30. How are purine uroliths (ammonium urate and xanthine) managed?

Xanthine and uric acid are metabolic products in purine metabolism. Purines are derived primarily from protein sources, endogenous as well as dietary. They often form in acidic urine. Management of purine uroliths involves feeding a protein-restricted, alkalinizing diet similar to diets used in management of chronic renal failure. Although ammonium urate uroliths may form because of a portosystemic shunt, most purine uroliths in cats are not associated with the presence of a shunt.

31. What dietary modifications may be beneficial in managing cystine uroliths?

Cystine is a sulfur-containing amino acid composed of two cysteine molecules attached by a disulfide bond. Cystine uroliths tend to form in acidic urine because their solubility is low at low urine pH values; solubility increases exponentially in alkaline urine. Feeding a protein-restricted, alkalinizing diet is beneficial in managing cystine uroliths. These diets also are used in management of chronic renal failure.

32. Does dietary modification have a role in treating idiopathic feline lower urinary tract disease?

Idiopathic feline lower urinary tract disease refers to a complex of clinical signs due to unknown cause(s) (see Chapter 47). Cats with this syndrome have clinical signs of lower urinary tract disease (e.g., pollakiuria, stranguria, hematuria) and may have urethral obstruction due to urethral matrix-crystalline plug formation (males only), but they do not have a definable cause for the clinical signs. Male cats with matrix-crystalline urethral plugs may benefit from dietary modification to control the crystalline component of the plug. The most common mineral incorporated into urethral matrix-crystalline plugs is struvite (usually sterile struvite); however, other minerals have been reported in isolated urethral plugs.

A large proportion of affected cats (55–70%) have nonobstructive idiopathic lower urinary tract disease. The role of dietary modification in this setting is less clear. One clinical study of young adult cats with nonobstructive lower urinary tract disease reported fewer episodes of clinical signs when a struvite preventative diet was used compared with cats whose diets were not changed. A diet that induces production of a larger volume of urine may be beneficial. Canned food diets may be preferred. In addition, idiopathic lower urinary tract disease is more common in obese cats than nonobese cats; therefore, weight reduction may be beneficial.

BIBLIOGRAPHY

1. Allen TA, Polzin DJ, Adams LG: Renal disease. In Hand MS, Thatcher CD, Remillard RL, Roudebush P (eds): Small Animal Clinical Nutrition, 4th ed. Topeka, KS, Mark Morris Institute, 2000, pp 563–604.
2. Bartges JW: Calcium oxalate urolithiasis. In August J (ed): Consultations in Feline Medicine, 4th ed. Philadelphia, W.B. Saunders, 2000.
3. Lulich JP, Osborne CA, O'Brien TD, Polzin DJ: Feline renal failure: Questions, answers, questions. Comp Contin Educ Pract Vet 14:127–153, 1992.
4. Osborne CA, Lulich JP, Thumchai R, et al: Feline urolithiasis: Etiology and pathophysiology. Vet Clin North Am Small Anim Pract 26:217–232, 1996.
5. Thatcher CD, Hand MS, Remillard RL: Small animal clinical nutrition: An iterative process. In Hand MS, Thatcher CD, Remillard RL, Roudebush P (eds): Small Animal Clinical Nutrition, 4th ed. Topeka, KS, Mark Morris Institute, 2000, pp 1–19.

51. INAPPROPRIATE URINATION

Hazel C. Carney, M.S., D.V.M.

1. Define inappropriate urination.

The cat voluntarily deposits urine in one or more locations that are unacceptable to the owner.

2. Why do cats urinate inappropriately?

Cats urinate in different locations as a way of giving social information to other cats, as a way of releasing anxiety, or as a response to physiologic changes in the body.

3. How common is inappropriate urination by cats?

Inappropriate urination is the most common behavior problem in cats. Approximately 10% of all pet cats at some time in their lives are presented to a veterinarian with a complaint of inappropriate urination.

4. What steps are included in a diagnostic evaluation of feline inappropriate urination?

Complete history, physical examination, and urinalysis provide the basis for a presumptive diagnosis of the cause of the inappropriate urination and allows the clinician to begin a therapeutic regimen (see algorithm on following page).

5. What questions are important in the history of a case of inappropriate urination?

Questions about the cat's background and urination habits, characteristics of the cat's litter box, and the owner's personality and expectations for the cat are important in a thorough history of inappropriate urination.

6. If the owner is unsure which cat in a multicat household is urinating inappropriately, how do you determine the culprit?

Roll three fluorescein eye dye strips into each of two size 0 gelatin capsules. Give one cat in the family these capsules orally. Have the owner use a black light to scan the litter pan and the areas of inappropriate urination for the next 24–72 hours. The dye-containing capsules can be given to each cat sequentially until the culprit is determined.

7. What clues from the history may help to explain the cause of inappropriate urination?

- Dry stool or owner complaints of constipation may suggest early renal compromise.
- A history of difficulty in jumping up onto the couch or bed may suggest musculoskeletal pain.

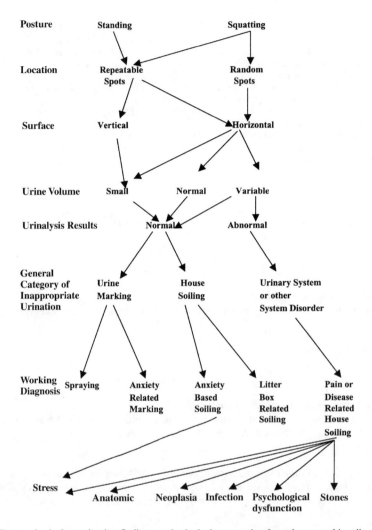

History, physical examination findings, and urinalysis are used to formulate a working diagnosis.

8. What clues from the physical examination may help to explain the cause?

- Uneven hind leg length when the hind legs are extended, a difference in the rotation of the cox-ofemoral joints, resentment of the cat to the manipulation of its hind legs, unequal hind nail lengths, or "pointing" with one leg when the cat stands may suggest musculoskeletal pain.
- Abnormal or disparate kidney size, rough or poorly compressible kidneys, or chalky white stripes on the dorsal surfaces of the cat's nails suggest declining renal function.
- If palpation of the cat's bladder (unless it is very full), causes the cat's prepuce or vulva to "wink," the cat has some bladder tenderness.
- Spines on the penis of a supposedly neutered male cat suggest occult cryptorchidism.
- Moist or chapped external genitalia or evidence of urine staining at the perineum suggests incontinence or lower urinary tract disease.
- Resentment to compression of the lumbosacral spine may suggest pain when the cat postures to urinate.
- Poor eyesight may contribute to a cat's unwillingness to use its litter box consistently.

9. What basic characteristics of feline behavior and behavioral modification do you and your client need to understand?

- The cat is a creature of habit. The more the client is a creature of habit during therapy of the cat, the greater the chance of success.
- The cat learns most quickly by constant, frequent repetition and reward but remembers the longest if trained with intermittent rewards.
- The best plan of behavior therapy establishes situations in which the cat can only succeed and blocks the chances of repeating the offending behaviors.
- All previous sites of inappropriate urination must be cleaned so that *no* residual urine smell remains.
- Modification of the environment, positive reinforcement, play therapy, aversion training, and negative reinforcement may be necessary components of the treatment plan.

10. Describe the proper technique for urine clean-up.

Urine Clean-up

---

1. Dilute white vinegar 1 to 1 with water, and saturate the soiled area. If carpet padding has urine in it, the pad also must be saturated with the vinegar water. Vinegar is cheaper than commercial odor eliminators for the initial clean-up.

2. Let set for 30 minutes.

3. Blot up all vinegar water and urine with old terry towels. Blot up any residual dampness with paper towels. Let area dry while washing the towels in X-O Odor Neutralizer (X-O Corporation, Dallas, TX) as instructed on the bottle.

4. Get close to the spot, and sniff deeply. Repeat process as many times as necessary until you can smell no urine odor. Fairly fresh spots usually take 3–4 cleanings, whereas old spots may require 8–10 cleanings. Repeat process once more, this time using plain water only. Let the area dry completely.

5. Apply one of the following urine clean-up products mixed as instructed on the label: X-O Odor Neutralizer or Nature's Miracle (Nature's Miracle, Pens 'n' People, Inc., Rolling Hills Estates, CA). If the carpet pad had any urine in it, the pad must be saturated with the odor neutralizer. Leave product in contact with surface to be cleaned as long as the label recommends.

6. Blot up odor neutralizer as you did the vinegar wash. Let dry thoroughly. For heavy, thick carpeting, you may have to put dry towels atop the carpet and weight them to help absorb absolutely all of the dampness.

---

11. What features of the cat's environment do owners need to evaluate?

The owner may need to increase the space that an individual cat has in its environment or change the environment to make a cat feel safer. An indoor cat may be less stressed if the owner builds a screened porch, deck, or patio to which the cat has access. The porch keeps the cat safe from most outdoor dangers and increases the cat's visual stimulation. The spraying cat may mark the perimeter of the porch; outside spraying "protects" the resident cat from intruders and probably is less offensive to the owners.

The owner may need to increase the vertical space available to cats by building cat trees or allowing them on top of bookcases. This strategy decreases the stress in multicat households.

12. How can the cat's carrier be used for training?

The cat's carrier can be its friend instead of an enemy. Have the owner place the open carrier in a quiet corner of the room in which the cat is most at ease and allow the cat to go in an out of the carrier whenever the cat chooses. The carrier can then be used as a haven when the cat is being trained. The cat can be confined to the carrier without feeling stressed when the owner is not home to supervise the cat's urination behavior.

13. Describe the ideal litter box.

The more the owner mimics the cat's ideal litter box, the more likely the cat is to use the litter box consistently. The ideal litter box is scrupulously clean, contains litter of a texture that the cat prefers, and is in a safe, quiet location.

14. Explain the "scrambled egg theory of litter box number."

In multicat households, the ideal number of litter boxes is 1 for each cat plus 1 for the house.

15. Give examples of positive reinforcement for cats.

- The tone of the owner's voice is important to a cat. Praise spoken in a soothing voice when the cat is seen using the litter box encourages the cat to choose the litter box again.
- Making the litter box attractive to the cat is the best positive association an owner can give for the cat. Cleanliness *is* next to godliness for cats.
- Grooming can be a positive reinforcement for some cats; so can stroking a cat gently under the chin, at the base of the left ear, or down the top of the head.

16. How should the litter box be maintained?

The owner should remove urine and stool every day and never stir wet litter into dry. A cat stepping into a litter box wants to step into a dry area. If nonclumping litter is used, the owner should empty the entire contents of the litter box once weekly. Then the box should be washed in hot, soapy water, using a soap that has no ammonia base, no pine base, and no strong odor. The box must be rinsed thoroughly; chemists say that 12 rinses with clear water are required to remove all residual odor of cleansers. The box should be dried before new litter is added. For clumping litters, this process should be repeated at least monthly. Although covered litter boxes are great for owners, cats probably equate them with an outhouse maintained by the forest service in a Southern swamp. Unless they are scooped and cleaned more often than an open box, they stink! Liners for litter boxes are convenient, but holes in liners allow urine to seep under the liner and create a source of odor that is not removed until the entire box is washed. Because of their dislike for slippery surfaces, some cats will not use a litter box with a liner.

17. Explain play therapy and give examples.

The owner should actively play with the cat each day to build its self-confidence and provide exercise. Play therapy also bonds the cat to new people. The owner can start with a few minutes at a time and then gradually increase the playtime to 15 minutes twice daily. Owners should find whatever the cat likes to do for play:

- Drag a string or a panty hose leg.
- Toss a ping-pong ball.
- Dangle a soft piece of denim tied to the end of a "fishing pole" (a good starter toy for a timid cat).
- Move a laser light pointer; mimic a scared mouse that stops, starts, and darts in several directions rather than in a straight line.
- Leave out an empty large paper grocery sack when the cat is alone; most cats cannot resist playing in them.

18. Explain aversion training and give examples.

Aversion training uses a remote-controlled device to deter a cat from urinating in an inappropriate location. It is effective only if the cat does not associate the aversion device with the owner; otherwise, the aversion device is effective only if the owner is present. Simple and effective aversion devices include the following:

- Lightweight magazines, such as *Reader's Digest,* can be tossed at a urinating cat.
- Water pistols can be squirted at a urinating cat.
- Unusual noise, such as that made by fog horns, whistles, pop cans partially filled with pennies and taped shut, a child's finger-controlled cricket noise maker, hissing noise, or clapping of hands. Owners should use these sounds when they catch the cat in the act of

inappropriate urination. The owner may have difficulty making sufficient noises without the cat seeing the owner as the source; fortunately, small devices such as a whistle or cricket toy can be carried at all times.

• Food bowls placed over areas where the cat has inappropriately urinated deter most cats because they do not like to urinate near food and water sources.

• A butter tub containing cotton balls scented with lemon or orange oil and taped shut, with small holes poked into the lid and sides, deters most cats because they do not like citrus scents.

• Slick aluminum foil, shelf paper, butcher paper, and shower curtain liners placed over areas that the owner wants the cat to avoid deter most cats because they dislike slick surfaces.

19. Should you punish a cat?

As cartoons and jokes suggest, punishment is not effective in cats unless the cat is "caught in the act." The cat perceives delayed punishment as a threat to its safety. If an owner swats a cat with his or her hand, the cat becomes afraid of the owner's hand and will resist petting also. If an owner punishes a cat near the litter box or forcibly moves the cat into the litter box, the cat may become afraid of the litter box.

20. When are drugs added to the treatment regimen?

Because almost all drugs for treatment of inappropriate urination are not approved for use in cats and because many have significant side effects, behavioral modification and changes in the cat's environment are the initial options. If inappropriate urination persists after 1–3 weeks of behavioral therapy, medication should be considered. The longer a cat urinates in any location, the more likely the cat will continue to urinate there because the presence of its own urine makes the cat feel more at home and in control. Specific drugs that have been used for treatment of inappropriate urination are discussed under each working diagnosis.

21. When can pharmacologic treatment be discontinued?

If you see no response to a particular drug after 3 weeks, the drug or starting dosage is likely ineffective and should be changed. Drugs generally require 1–5 weeks to affect the cat's neurologic and behavioral chemistry. Urination behavior should be consistently acceptable for a minimum of 3 weeks before an attempt to discontinue the drugs is made. Therefore, once drugs are started, they are given for at least 1–2 months before they are slowly tapered. At that time, the dosage usually is reduced by one half every week until a minimal effective maintenance dose is determined or no drug is needed. Sudden stoppage of the medication may cause rebound exacerbation of the undesirable behavior.

22. How do you manage suspected spraying?

1. Explain characteristics of spraying behavior to the owner.
2. Describe the characteristic posture of the spraying cat.
3. Discuss surgical treatment options.
4. Discuss behavior modification techniques.
5. Discuss possible pharmacologic therapy.

23. Why do cats spray?

The behavior communicates territoriality, possession, and sexual availability to other cats. It says, "I'm here," "It's mine," or "I'm available." The most common way that a cat marks territory is by spraying. Male cats spray more often than female cats; toms spray more often than neutered males, and queens spray more often than spayed females. In a one-cat household the chance that one cat, regardless of sex, will spray is 25%; in a household with 11 or more cats, the chance that any one cat will spray increases to 100%.

24. Describe typical spraying behaviors.

1. The cat stands with tail fully erect; there is no curve, even in the tip of the tail.
2. The cat squirts out a small amount of urine onto a vertical surface.

3. A small, anxious, intact female, especially one purchased from a large cattery, may urinate in small or normal volumes beside the litter box or near doors or windows only when she is coming into estrus; she is too timid to spray but still wants to tell male cats that she is "available."

25. What surgical options are available for spraying cats?

Gonadectomy. Within 2 months after surgery, 80–90% of cats that are spayed or castrated will no longer spray urine. The chance of spraying after gonadectomy increases if the cat had sexual experience before surgery.

Olfactory tractotomies and ischiocavernosus myectomy. Both techniques suppress spraying, but because they are technically more difficult, they are rarely used.

26. List specific behavior modification techniques for spraying cats.

1. Thoroughly clean the sprayed areas on the inside *and* outside of the house, using the technique described in question 10.

2. Actively engage the cat in play therapy at least 15 minutes daily (see question 17).

3. Increase available indoor vertical space for the cat.

4. Determine why the cat feels it must mark territory:

5. If a new adult is the cause, have the person take over feeding and other activities that the cat considers to be pleasant.

6. If the cause is new furniture or recent remodeling, limit the cat's access to times when the owner can be with the cat in the room with the new items. The owner should sit near the new items and pet or play with the cat. Let the cat rub its face on the new items, but if the cat backs up toward any item, immediately use an aversion device or pick up the cat, gently say "No," and take the cat to an area of the house where the cat is completely at ease and has not sprayed. Just before the cat is allowed into the new area, use a hormone spray (Feliway, Abbott Laboratories) daily on the new items.

7. Remove outside competitor cats if possible.

8. Block view of outside cats.

9. Cover windows with aluminum foil or vinyl view blockers for bathrooms.

10. Restrict cats to interior rooms that have no view of outside cats.

11. Decrease competition among inside cats.

12. Separate antagonistic cats.

13. Allow the spraying cat to become an indoor-outdoor cat.

14. Build a screened porch for the culprit.

15. Block sprayed areas with aluminum foil or slick shower curtain liners; the sound of sprayed urine hitting these surfaces is sometimes offensive or scary to the cat.

16. Try a "Scat Mat" type device rolled from the floor upward toward the article being sprayed. Enough of the mat should be on the floor so that the cat's hind feet contact it and trigger the alarm when the cat backs up to spray.

17. Use other invisible noise detractors whenever the cat is seen to sniff and turn its rear toward an item.

18. Use food aversion techniques.

19. If the cat sprays only one or two areas repeatedly and cannot be deterred, the owner should make an L with two litter boxes. Put one box on the floor and the second vertically inside the horizontal box. This strategy does not stop the spraying, but it contains the sprayed urine and may be acceptable to some owners.

27. What pharmacologic therapy may be used in spraying cats?

• Buspirone is a good drug to try in multicat households.

• Cyproheptadine is a safe alternative; it is the first choice if the spraying cat is cryptorchid.

• Amitriptyline, diazepam, and synthetic progestins have associated risks and should be offered only if preliminary serum chemistries and a lead II electrocardiogram (for amitriptyline) are within normal limits. The owner must be fully informed about the potential risks.

- Paroxetine may be especially useful if the spraying is territorial and motivated by aggression-dominance.
- Pheromone spray (Feliway) eliminates or decreases the frequency of spraying in 30% and 60% of treated cats, respectively.
- Flower Essences Vine and Mimulus (available at health food stores) decrease dominance- and fear-motivated spraying when given as oral drops or in drinking water and have no known adverse side effects.

28. How do you do manage suspected anxiety-based house soiling?
1. Explain to the owner the causes of anxiety in cats.
2. Describe the characteristic posture.
3. Convince the owner that cats do not urinate spitefully.
4. Discuss behavior modification plans.
5. Discuss pharmacologic therapies that help to decrease anxiety.

29. What are the common causes of anxiety in cats?
Because cats are creatures of habit, *any* change in routine may cause anxiety, especially if the cat is genetically predisposed to shyness or as a kitten did not stay with the queen long enough to be well socialized. New babies, adults, furniture, cats, puppies, walls, plants, or litter boxes can frighten a cat. Other possible causes include the following:
- Separation from its owner for different intervals
- Strained interpersonal relationships among people in the household
- Placement of the litter box in an area that is noisy or busy
- Placement of the litter box in an attic, basement, or other unpleasant setting
The act of urinating outside the litter box is also stressful to the cat because the cat is going against its own naturally fastidious nature.

30. Describe the characteristic posture associated with anxiety-related house soiling.
- The cat squats to urinate.
- The cat deposits urine on horizontal surfaces.
- The cat usually "rakes earth" before and sometimes after it urinates.
- Urine volume varies with how scared the cat may be, whether another cat or person is present, and how recently the cat previously urinated.

31. How do you convince the owner that cats do not urinate spitefully?
1. A cat deposits urine so that something or some place will smell more like itself and thus be less threatening. This principle explains why the cat may urinate on the belongings of a person that the cat dislikes.
2. A cat urinates on the owner's bed or clothes because the owner's smell is strongest there. An anxious cat urinates on these items because only there does the cat feel safe.

32. Summarize the behavior modification plan for anxiety-related house soiling.
1. Thoroughly clean all areas where the cat has urinated outside the litterbox (see question 10).
2. Attempt to determine the cause of the cat's anxiety:
   - Location of litterbox
   - Multicat household
   - Separation anxiety
   - Dislike of specific person(s)
3. Discuss pharmacologic therapies that help to decrease anxiety.

33. What specific behavior modification techniques are helpful for location anxieties?
1. Analyze both the history and the house plan to determine the locations in the house that are the quietest and most comfortable for the cat.
2. If the cat has chosen a spot that the owner does not like, the owner should camouflage the spot and place a litter box near it. When the cat is consistently using the litter box, the owner should move the box slowly by *1-inch increments* toward the preferred location.

34. What specific techniques may alleviate anxiety related to multicat thresholds?
1. Meet the "scrambled egg theory" of litter box number (see question 14).
2. Practice all aspects of litter box cleanliness.
3. Institute play therapy (see question 17).
4. Increase vertical space in the house or build screened porches to allow more separation among cats.
5. Physically separate unfriendly cats for 10–14 days, then gradually reintroduce them.

35. Describe behavior techniques for dealing with separation anxiety.
1. Have the owner stay away from the cat for gradually increasing intervals.
2. Have the owner develop a leave-taking ritual to use initially, even if just leaving the house to take out the garbage.
3. If the cat urinates on the owner's bed, lock the cat out of bedroom or cover the bed with a clear plastic shower curtain until the cat is retrained. Sometimes a litter box placed atop the shower curtain can be moved in 1-inch increments per week toward the ideal litter box location.

36. What behavior techiques are used for anxiety related to dislike of specific people?
1. Have the person assume the pleasant activities in the cat's life, such as feeding, grooming, and play.
2. Put away items belonging to the disliked person until the cat is at ease with the person. Then gradually allow the cat access to the person's belongings.

37. What drugs are available to decrease anxiety in cats?
- Buspirone may be the drug of choice for multicat households.
- Clomipramine may be better in a single cat household or when the cause of the inappropriate urination is separation anxiety.
- Pheromone spray (Feliway; see question 26) may be beneficial.
- In multicat households, consider flower essence therapies after doing personality profiles of each resident cat.

38. How do you manage suspected litter box-related house soiling?
1. Explain to the owner that the cat is house soiling because the cat dislikes something about the litter box or has a preference for the site that the cat has chosen to soil. If the cat has chosen multiple locations, the cat probably dislikes the box shape, location, or litter substrate. If the cat has chosen just one or two sites, the cat probably prefers this particular location or substrate.
2. Describe the posture that the cat uses in the inappropriate location: the cat has a normal urination posture, passes normal volumes of normal urine, and rakes earth before and after urination.
3. Look for behaviors that may suggest that the cat dislikes something about the litter box.
4. If the cat appears to dislike the litter box, try to determine why.
5. Remove or change the aspects of the litter box that the cat dislikes.
6. Thoroughly clean all areas of inappropriate urination (see question 10).
7. Try confinement therapy (see question 42).

39. List behaviors that suggest dislike of the litter box.
- The cat shakes its paws after leaving the box.
- The cat straddles the sides of the box or keeps only one or two feet in the box.
- The cat runs away from the box after using it.
- The cat does not dig in the box or cover its excrement.
- The cat starts in a squatting posture and stands up before it finishes urinating.

40. What aspects of the litter box may be displeasing to the cat?
- The cat may dislike the texture of the litter. Cats that dislike rough litter may choose soft, carpeted surfaces or fine textured material for urination.

- The cat may dislike the depth of litter in the box. Kittens and long-haired cats may prefer more shallow litter.
- The cat may dislike the smell of the litter, especially if the box is not cleaned frequently or is used by multiple cats. Cats with a smell aversion may display the Flehman response before entering the box.
- The cat may dislike the size, depth, or configuration of the box (e.g., kittens and arthritic senior cats may have difficulty with jumping into a tall box).
- The cat may dislike the location of the litter box. Cats prefer quiet, low-traffic, low-noise areas away from their food and water bowls. Some cats want two potential exits from the box so that they cannot be trapped by another animal.

41. Explain confinement therapy.

The cat is confined with its litter box in a large carrier or a small room such as a powder room. The cat is allowed out of isolation only to eat and only when owner is available to supervise the cat's activity. The goal of confinement and strict supervision is not to let the cat "make another mistake" because any mistake reenforces inappropriate behavior. One expert states that a cat must repeat a correct behavior 300 consecutive times before the new behavior replaces the old behavior in the cat's thought processes. Even without higher mathematics, one can see that the cat must urinate in the correct location for many months before it has forgotten about the old location!

42. What have you learned if the cat uses the box in confinement?

The type of litter and box size and shape are probably not the problem. The location of the box may be what the cat dislikes.

43. What if the cat does not use the litter box in confinement?

The cat probably dislikes something about the type of litter or the litter box.

44. How do you determine what the cat dislikes about the litter?

Fill separate litter boxes with a different type of litter (a substrate "smorgasbord" test). Use at least one unscented, clumping, sand type litter, one of clay, one of pellets, one lined with carpet, and one of garden soil. Put all of the boxes in the confined area with the cat and let the cat choose its favorite. Continue the test for several days. If the cat uses the same type of litter every day, the cat prefers this brand. If the cat chooses several of the boxes, the cat may need only a cleaner litter box, less litter volume, or different side height.

45. What do you do next?

If the cat uses the litter box in confinement, place the cat in confinement with the litter that the cat chose during the substrate smorgasbord test. If the cat chose carpet, use scraps of carpet initially and gradually add litter over the carpet. Some cats that rake the sides of the litter box will eliminate in a litter box with sandy litter on the bottom and carpet along the walls. Again confine the cat with the new litter until the cat has been using the box consistently for at least 2 weeks. Then gradually enlarge the area of confinement.

46. How do you prevent the cat from returning to former areas of inappropriate urination after it is let out of confinement?

1. Initially allow the cat outside the confinement area only under supervision.
2. Block access to previous sites of inappropriate urination, especially if the cat has chosen numerous places in which to urinate.
3. Divide the total meal volume among a number of food bowls equal to the number of places at which the cat inappropriately urinates. Place one food bowl over each site of inappropriate urination. Leave the food bowls in place even after they are empty each day.
4. If the cat goes one full week without inappropriately urinating, remove the food bowls one at a time. If the bowls are near a litter box, take away the innermost bowl first. Take away the

bowl for only 15 minutes or so the first day; then replace it. For each day that the cat does not urinate in the area uncovered by removing the bowl, leave the bowl away from the area for gradually increasing intervals until the cat has not inappropriately urinated in that spot for 7 days. Then take away that one bowl permanently.

5. Begin removing a second bowl, again for only 15 minutes on the first day and so on until the cat is no longer urinating inappropriately at any location.

6. If the cat used only a few areas for inappropriate urination, place litter boxes at these locations. If the cat urinates in the boxes, move them at the rate of 1 inch per week toward the preferred locations.

47. How do you manage pain- or disease-associated house soiling?

1. Explain why the cat quits using its litter box when it has cystitis or other diseases.

2. When the cat experiences pain during urination, it begins to associate the litter box with pain and leaves the box. If the pain continues at the next urination, the cat will move to a new spot again and again until the pain stops.

3. Once treatment of the primary disorder removes the pain, the cat will return to its litter box unless inappropriate urination has become a chronic habit.

4. Retrain the cat to use its litter box again after the pain is diminished with treatment of the primary condition. Consider short-term confinement (see question 42) until the cat seems to be using the litter box consistently. Gradually allow the cat unlimited access to the house.

BIBLIOGRAPHY

1. Alani MM: The Body Language and Emotion of Cats. New York, William Morrow, 1987.
2. Bateson P, Turner DC: Questions about cats. In Turner DC, Bateson P(eds): The Domestic Cat: The Biology of Its Behavior. Cambridge, MS, Cambridge University Press, 1999, pp 193–201.
3. Beaver BV: Eliminative behavior development. In Beaver BV (ed): Feline Behavior: A Guide for Veterinarians. Philadelphia, W.B. Saunders, 1992, pp 63–85.
4. Dodman NH: The writing on the wall. In Dodman NH (ed): The Cat Who Cried for Help. New York, Bantam Books, 1997, pp 101–120.
5. Graham H,Vlamis G: Bach Flower Remedies for Animals. Tallahassee, FL, Findhorn Press, 1999, pp 1–126.
6. Halip JW, McKeown DB, Luescher UA: Inappropriate elimination in cats. Part 1. Feline Pract 20:17–21, 1992.
7. Halip JW, McKeown DB, Luescher UA: Inappropriate elimination in cats. Part 2. Feline Pract 20:25–29, 1992.
8. Hunthausen W: Evaluating a feline facial pheromone analogue to control urine spraying. Vet Med 95:151–155, 2000.
9. Overall KL: Feline elimination disorders. In Overall KL (ed): Clinical Behavioral Medicine for Small Animals. St. Louis, Mosby, 1997, pp 160–194.
10. Overall KL: Diagnosing feline elimination disorders. Vet Med 93:350–382, 1998.

52. URINARY INCONTINENCE

India F. Lane, D.V.M., M.S.

1. Define urinary incontinence.

Urinary incontinence is the involuntary loss of urine. Urine leaks through the urethra, often while the cat is resting. Urinary incontinence must be differentiated from inappropriate (voluntary) urination, pollakiuria, and urine spraying in cats.

2. What mechanisms commonly lead to urinary incontinence?

Urinary incontinence results from abnormal anatomy of the ureters, urinary bladder, or urethra; poor urine storage by the urinary bladder; or weak urethral outlet tone. Functional abnormalities are caused by neurogenic and nonneurogenic disorders.

3. Is urinary incontinence common in cats compared with dogs?

Urinary incontinence is rare in cats.

4. When urinary incontinence is observed in cats, what are the common causes?

The most common causes of urinary incontinence in cats are neurologic lesions (sacral or sacrococcygeal), feline leukemia virus (FeLV)-associated urinary incontinence, and idiopathic urethral incompetence.

Causes of Urinary Incontinence in Cats

Neurologic lesions (sacral spinal cord)
Spinal malformation
Trauma
Neoplasia

Anatomic abnormalities
Congenital urethral hypoplasia
Congenital bladder hypoplasia
Ectopic ureter
Patent urachus
Ureterovaginal fistula
Perineal urethrostomy

Functional or idiopathic disorders
Idiopathic bladder hypercontractility
Feline leukemia virus-associated urinary incontinence
Acquired urethral incompetence
Urinary tract infection or inflammation
Urinary bladder neck or urethral neoplasia

Overflow urinary incontinence
Neurologic lesion (upper or lower motor neuron)
Dysautonomia
Detrusor atony (postobstructive)
Partial urethral obstruction (paradoxical incontinence)

5. What should be included in the physical examination of cats with urinary incontinence?

In addition to a general physical examination, attention to neurologic function, urinary bladder size, and expressibility of urine are important. Mental status, hindlimb proprioception, anal tone, perineal sensation, tail tone, and tail function are indicators of sacral spinal cord and higher nervous center integrity. Pupil size should be assessed. Anisocoria is often detected in cats with FeLV- associated polyganglionopathy, whereas mydriasis is a common finding in idiopathic dysautonomia.The causes of urinary incontinence are sometimes categorized by resting urinary bladder size. With a small, nondistended bladder, urinary incontinence usually is attributed to bladder hyperactivity or urethral incompetence. When incontinence occurs with a distended bladder, causes of overflow incontinence are likely. The ease of bladder expression can be used to estimate urethral outlet tone.

6. What tests are included in the initial evaluation of cats with urinary incontinence?

Urinalysis, urine culture, FeLV serum antigen testing, and abdominal radiographs are indicated in all cats with urinary incontinence. Abdominal radiographs are needed to detect uroliths or gross abnormalities of the urinary tract or spinal column. Complete blood count and serum biochemistry panel should be evaluated in cats with concurrent polyuria, urinary tract infection, or other signs of systemic illness.

7. When are additional imaging procedures indicated?

Abdominal ultrasonography may be indicated in young cats with urinary incontinence to evaluate the kidneys, ureters, and urinary bladder conformation. Excretory urography and contrast cystourethrography are indicated for further evaluation of urinary tract anatomy in cats that exhibit urinary incontinence at a young age or after surgery or trauma. Vaginourethrography also is indicated in kittens with urinary incontinence, because vaginal anomalies often accompany congenital urethral incompetence in cats.

8. What specialized diagnostic procedures are available for the evaluation of incontinent cats?

In some complex cases or cases that respond poorly to trial therapy, urodynamic or electrodiagnostic tests may be indicated to define more clearly functional and neurologic abnormalities. Urinary bladder capacity, compliance, and contractile function can be assessed with cystometry (intravesical pressure measured as the bladder is slowly distended with air, fluid, or contrast media) or specialized voiding studies. Urethral resistance can be assessed by recording urethral pressures along the length of the urethra (urethral pressure profilometry). Concurrent measurement of electromyographic activity from the perineal area adds qualitative evidence of striated urethral muscle innervation and activity during cystometric or urethral studies. Other electrodiagnostic procedures, such as spinal evoked potential and pudendal reflex recordings, may be available at teaching hospitals for more sophisticated evaluation of neurologic input to the lower urinary tract.

9. What are the distinguishing clinical features of congenital urinary incontinence in cats?

Affected kittens are female domestic short-haired cats with severe urinary incontinence, especially when resting. The urethra is anatomically hypoplastic or essentially absent. Concurrent vaginal aplasia is common; the uterine horns empty into the dorsal bladder wall. Urinary bladder hypoplasia, ectopic ureteral terminations, and renal dysplasia or aplasia also may accompany the developmental anomaly.

10. How does the presentation of ectopic ureters differ in cats and dogs?

Whereas most dogs with ectopic ureteral terminations are presented for evaluation of severe or continuous urinary incontinence, some affected kittens may exhibit minimal or no incontinence. The ectopic ureter is found during diagnostic evaluation for recurrent bacterial urinary tract infections or chronic hematuria, dysuria, or pollakiuria. At surgery, most feline ectopic ureters bypass the bladder completely, whereas most ectopic ureteral terminations in dogs tunnel through bladder or urethral mucosa. The prognosis for continence after surgical repair in cats is generally good unless overt abnormalities of the urethral and bladder are evident. Up to two-thirds of dogs with ectopic ureteral terminations continue to have some degree of urinary incontinence postoperatively.

11. What treatments are recommended for congenital urinary incontinence in cats?

Surgical correction by a specialist is recommended for congenital urinary anomalies in cats. The limited size of cat ureters necessitates command of microsurgical techniques for ureteral transplantation or neoureterostomy. Some cases of ectopic ureter with severe hydronephrosis, renal dysplasia, or pyelonephritis are managed by ureteronephrectomy as long as contralateral renal function is adequate.

Bladder neck reconstruction may be attempted in cats with urethral hypoplasia; the procedure is designed to create a longer, resistant "urethral tube." In experienced surgical hands, this procedure significantly reduces urinary incontinence. Adjunct medical treatment with phenylpropanolamine is required in some cases.

12. Summarize the mechanism of action, dosage, side effects, and contraindication of drugs used for the management of urinary incontinence in cats.

AGENT	CLASS	MECHANISM OF ACTION	RECOMMENDED DOSE	POTENTIAL SIDE EFFECTS	CONTRA-INDICATIONS
Phenylpropa-nolamine	Alpha-adrenergic agonist	Increases urethral tone	1.1–2.2 mg/kg PO every 8–12 hr	Hyperactivity Tachycardia Anorexia	Hypertension Renal failure (?) Arrhythmias
Ephedrine	Alpha-adrenergic agonist	Increases urethral tone	2–4 mg/cat PO every 8–12 hr	As above	
Oxybutynin	Anticholinergic Antispasmodic	Decreases bladder contractility	0.5 mg/cat PO every 12 hr	Ileus Vomiting Urine retention Ptyalism	
Propantheline	Anticholinergic	Decreases bladder contractility	5–7.5 mg/cat PO every 24–72 hr	As above	
Bethanechol	Cholinergic agonist	Increases bladder contractility	1.25–7.5 mg/cat PO every 8–12 hr	Ptyalism Vomiting	Urinary ob-struction

PO = orally.

13. Define dysautonomia.

Dysautonomia is a diffuse autonomic polyganglionopathy described primarily in cats in Great Britain (Key-Gaskell syndrome) but occasionally encountered in dogs or cats in the midwestern United States. The urologic disturbance is characterized by a distended urinary bladder and overflow urinary incontinence. The urinary bladder is easily expressed and contractility may improve with administration of prokinetic or parasympathomimetic agents such as bethanechol. Other clinical signs include mydriasis, prolapsed third eyelids, constipation or diarrhea, regurgitation or vomiting, and anorexia. The diagnosis is established by documenting inappropriate responses to provocative autonomic testing.

14. What treatments are recommended for FeLV-associated urinary incontinence?

FeLV-associated urinary incontinence may be caused functionally by urinary bladder overactivity or urethral incompetence. Unstable detrusor contractions at low bladder volume (also called detrusor instability) were documented in one FeLV-positive cat that responded well to administration of the anticholinergic, antispasmodic agent oxybutynin. Trial treatment with anticholinergic agents seems warranted in affected cats. If response is minimal, pharmacologic management for urethral incompetence may be considered.

15. What treatments are recommended for urethral incompetence in cats?

Although reproductive hormones are useful in the management of urethral incompetence in many dogs, they are not recommended in cats. Estrogens can induce signs of estrus or bone marrow suppression in female cats, and testosterone preparations have been minimally effective in male cats. Alpha-adrenergic agonists (phenylpropanolamine, ephedrine compounds), which stimulate urethral smooth muscle receptors, may be effective in the management of urethral incompetence in both dogs and cats.

16. When are other pharmacologic treatments indicated?
Additional pharmacologic manipulation of bladder emptying (i.e. bethanechol) may be indicated in cats with a distended urinary bladder and overflow incontinence (see also chapter 47). Manual expression or intermittent urethral catheterization may be required to maintain a small urinary bladder.

17. What is the prognosis for acquired urinary incontinence in cats?
Response to pharmacological treatments for urinary incontinence is much less reliable in cats when compared to dogs. Although some cats with feline leukemia-associated urinary incontinence may respond to anticholinergic agents, long-term prognosis is guarded. Management of lower urinary tract dysfunction associated with neurologic lesions or idiopathic urethral incompetence often is unrewarding.

BIBLIOGRAPHY

1. Baines SJ, Speakman AJ, Williams JM, et al: Genitourinary dysplasia in a cat. J Small Anim Pract 40:286–290, 1999.
2. Barsanti JA, Downey R: Urinary incontinence in cats. J Am Anim Hosp Assoc 20:979–982, 1984.
3. Holt PE: Feline urinary incontinence. In Bonagura J (ed): Kirk's Current Veterinary Therapy XII (Small Animal Practice). Philadelphia, W.B. Saunders, 1995, pp 1018–1022.
4. Holt PE: Surgical management of congenital urethral sphincter mechanism incompetence in eight female cats and a bitch. Vet Surg 22:98, 1993.
5. Lane IF, Barsanti JA: Urinary incontinence. In August JR (ed): Consultations in Feline Internal Medicine, 2nd ed. Philadelphia, W.B. Saunders, 1994, pp 373–382.
6. Lane IF: Pharmacologic management of feline lower urinary tract disorders. Vet Clin North Am Small Anim Pract 26:515–533, 1996.
7. Lappin MR, Barsanti JA: Urinary incontinence secondary to idiopathic detrusor instability: Cystometrographic diagnosis and pharmacologic management in 2 dogs and a cat. J Am Vet Med Assoc 191:1439–1442, 1987.
8. Sackman JE, Sims MH: Electromyographic evaluation of the external urethral sphincter during cystometry in male cats. Am J Vet Res 51:1237–1241, 1990.

IV. Endocrine Problems

Section Editor: Ellen N. Behrend, V.M.D., M.S., Ph.D.

53. HYPERTHYROIDISM

James K. Olson, D.V.M.

1. How common is feline hyperthyroidism?

Feline hyperthyroidism is the most common feline geriatric endocrinopathy, even though the first cases were described in the late 1970s.

2. Describe the pathophysiology of feline hyperthyroidism (thyrotoxicosis).

In 99% of cases, the cause is benign nodular adenoma(s). These nodules autonomously secrete the thyroid hormones T4 (thyroxine) and T3 (triiodothyronine) in excess, resulting in multisystemic disease. The excessive secretion has negative feedback to the pituitary, suppressing thyroid-stimulating hormone (TSH) secretion. Normal thyroid tissue atrophies because of lack of TSH from the pituitary gland and ceases secretion of T4 and T3. In the other rare 1% of cases, the cause is a mild to moderately malignant thyroid carcinoma.

3. What causes hyperthyroidism?

What initiates the hyperplasia/tumor formation is unknown, but possible risk factors have been identified and are under study. Theories of the cause of feline hyperthyroidism suggest that dietary changes (canned foods), preservatives and food additives, environmental exposures (cat litter, toxins, and pollution), increased exposure to allergens, genetic mutation (altered TSH receptor gene and G protein), and abnormal immunologic responses may be involved.

4. Describe the normal anatomy of the thyroid glands.

Most of the normal thyroid tissue is located as a single gland that is divided into two lobes located ventral to the trachea in the mid-portion of the neck between the larynx and xiphoid process. One lobe is on either side of the trachea, with no connection between them. Small amounts of ectopic thyroid tissue may be scattered throughout the ventral neck and mediastinum. The thyroid gland cannot be palpated in normal cats. Enlarged thyroid tissue in the chest cannot be palpated and can be difficult to locate at exploratory surgery.

5. What is the typical signalment of cats with hyperthyroidism?

Hyperthyroidism is a geriatric disease seen in cats aged 4–22 years, with a median age of 13 years. Hyperthyroidism is extremely rare under the age of 7 years. There is no sex or breed predilection, but Siamese and Himalayan cats have a lower incidence.

6. What historical and clinical findings are typically associated with feline hyperthyroidism?

- Weight loss or emaciation (93%)
- Enlarged thyroid lobes (80–90%)
- Behavioral changes (80%)
- Polyphagia (49%)
- Tachycardia (42%)
- Vomiting (44%)
- Polydipsia/polyuria (36%)
- Increased activity (33%)
- Diarrhea (15%)
- Gallop rhythm (15%)
- Vocalization (10%)
- Poor hair coat (10%)

Other clinical signs seen in 5–10% of cases include dyspnea, panting, large fecal volumes, and the apathetic (sick) form of hyperthyroidism characterized by decreased activity, lethargy, anorexia, depression, and weakness.

7. How does hyperthyroidism affect the body as a multisystemic disease?
A human analogy for feline thyrotoxicosis is the "stressed out speed freak" or an "adrenaline junkie."

Systemic Effects of Feline Hyperthyroidism

SYSTEM	EFFECTS
Neuromuscular	Behavioral changes, hyperactivity, muscle loss, weakness, aggression, vocalization, pacing, restlessness
Gastrointestinal	Changes in appetite, vomiting, diarrhea, maldigestion/malabsorption, large fecal volumes, vitamin and nutritional deficiencies.
Hepatic	Elevated serum enzyme activities, hepatic lipidosis
Cardiac	Systolic murmurs, tachycardia, gallop rhythm, cardiac hypertrophy, hypertension, congestive heart failure
Respiratory	Hyperventilation, dyspnea, pulmonary edema/congestive heart failure
Renal	Hypertension-induced renal damage, polydipsia/polyuria

8. Can hyperthyroid cats be diagnosed on physical examination?
Enlarged thyroid gland(s) can be palpated in 80–90% of cases. In published studies, approximately 25–30% are unilateral, 70% are bilateral, and 3–5% are ectopic.

9. What abnormalities can be detected on routine laboratory testing?
On the complete blood count, increased packed cell volume and mean corpuscular volume are seen in approximately one-third to one-half of hyperthyroid cats. Increased activities of liver enzymes are common; approximately 90% of hyperthyroid cats have increased activity of alanine transaminase (ALT), alkaline phosphatase (ALP), and/or aspartate transaminase (AST). Increased ALP activity is the most common (approximately 80% of cases), but ALT and AST increases occur in approximately 55%. Other less common biochemical abnormalities are elevated blood urea nitrogen (BUN) and creatinine (approximately 20%) and hyperglycemia (approximately 20%).

10. How is hyperthyroidism diagnosed?
Clinical signs (the first and most reliable is weight loss) give a clue to the diagnosis, and if enlarged thyroid nodules are palpated, hyperthyroidism is likely. Palpation may be the earliest and most reliable way to detect the disease, but the presence of enlarged nodules does not necessarily mean that the cat is hyperthyroid. Definitive diagnosis requires thyroid testing. The total T4 (TT4) concentration should be the first test. If the TT4 is above normal, there is a 98–100% chance that the cat is hyperthyroid. Cats with enlarged thyroid glands but normal TT4 concentrations should be considered thyroid suspects and monitored closely for hyperthyroidism.

11. Is it possible for a hyperthyroid cat to have a TT4 in the normal range?
In some hyperthyroid cats, the TT4 is in the upper half of the normal range. Total T4 concentrations fluctuate between normal and elevated levels in many mildly hyperthyroid patients. Nonthyroidal disease also may suppress TT4 into the normal range in hyperthyroid cats (i.e., euthyroid sick syndrome). If the TT4 is in the upper half of the normal range in a cat suspected of hyperthyroidism, a free T4 (fT4) level should be measured by equilibrium dialysis. Alternatively, a T3 suppression test can be done, but it is more difficult and time-consuming.

12. How is the T3 suppression test used to aid in the diagnosis of hyperthyroidism?
In borderline cases of hyperthyroidism with clinical signs but normal TT4 levels, the T3 suppression test can be used to define the condition more accurately. To perform the test, a baseline

blood sample is taken, and seven 25-mg doses of T3 are administered orally every 8 hours, starting on the morning of day 1. Two to four hours after the seventh dose is administered (day 3), a blood sample is drawn. T3 should be measured before and after T3 administration, and the concentrations should increase to ensure administration of the drug. Hyperthyroid cats have a posttest TT4 that does not suppress; the values are > 1.5 µg/dl (20 nmol/L). In normal cats or cats ill from other causes, the TT4 is suppressed below this level.

13. Does an elevated fT4 necessarily mean that the cat is hyperthyroid?

Free T4 can be elevated in up to 12% of sick, euthyroid cats. Free T4 should be measured in combination with TT4. If the fT4 is high and TT4 is in the upper half of the normal range or above, the cat is probably hyperthyroid. If the fT4 is high and TT4 is in the lower half of the normal range, the cat is probably not hyperthyroid.

14. How can a pertechnetate scan help in the diagnosis of hyperthyroidism?

In a pertechnetate or technetium scan, radiolabeled pertechnetate is injected intravenously and is concentrated by the thyroid gland. The scan can help to confirm a diagnosis of hyperthyroidism, raise the suspicion of malignant disease, and locate all abnormal tissue (even intrathoracic). For definitive diagnosis of malignancy, histopathology is required.

15. What are the three most important factors to assess in hyperthyroid patients?

Hyperthyroidism, if left untreated, eventually kills the patient. The two major organ systems most affected are the heart and kidneys. Another factor to assess, which has been underappreciated in thyrotoxicosis, is systemic hypertension.

16. How does hyperthyroidism affect the heart?

In cats with mild hyperthyroidism, the heart may be normal or have a slightly increased rate. As the disease progresses, tachycardia, gallop rhythms, myocardial hypertrophy, or, in rare cases, dilation develops. Congestive heart failure may be seen in some cats. Echocardiography cannot differentiate between hypertrophic changes due to hyperthyroidism and primary hypertrophic cardiomyopathy. Hyperthyroidism-induced hypertrophic changes revert to normal in the majority of treated patients within 6 months.

17. How does hyperthyroidism affect the kidneys?

The kidneys are a common site of geriatric disease in general, and a "normal" progressive loss of renal reserve occurs as the cat ages. Hypertension secondary to hyperthyroidism speeds the loss of nephrons. In the early stages of hyperthyroidism, increased cardiac output from hyperdynamic cardiac function increases glomerular blood flow and glomerular filtration rate (GFR). This improved function can mask low-grade renal insufficiency, and azotemia may not be detected until the cat is euthyroid. Renal disease in the aged patient can be insidious and difficult to detect accurately by laboratory testing, and hyperthyroidism can mask renal disease. Many cats with hyperthyroidism present with normal kidney laboratory values but are bordering on kidney failure. Hyperthyroidism can mask renal disease by increasing cardiac output and systemic blood pressure, thus abnormally increasing renal perfusion and GFR. If a cat treated for hyperthyroidism (medically, surgically, or with radioiodine) has "masked" kidney disease, renal failure may result when blood pressure and renal blood flow return to normal and can be life-threatening.

18. How can underlying renal disease be detected?

A methimazole challenge (administration of therapeutic doses of methimazole for 30 days) may be a reversible way to assess cats with suspected renal disease (see questions about treatment). Many cats have an increase in creatinine or BUN with correction of hyperthyroidism but show no clinical signs of renal disease; therefore, clinical status as well as blood and urine parameters must be assessed after the trial. No factors that predict whether renal failure will occur have been identified. However, some authorities believe that a urine specific gravity < 1.035 before treatment may be predictive. The hyperthyroid condition must be addressed, but kidney disease must be given equal importance in the therapeutic plan. If surgery or radioiodine therapy unmasks renal disease and failure occurs, low levels of L-thyroxine supplementation (0.1–0.2 mg/cat orally every 24 hr) can be used to increase renal perfusion and GFR to a safer, higher level. Other kidney support measures also should be part of the overall treatment.

19. How common is hypertension in hyperthyroidism?

Systemic hypertension is detected in up to 87% of hyperthyroid cats and may be one of the most significant pathophysiologic factors in hyperthyroidism. Use of new blood pressure detection systems may better define the importance of high blood pressure in cats as clinicians obtain both diastolic and systolic pressures in a more reliable and convenient manner (see Chapter 63). This manifestation appears to be caused by a combination of a hyperdynamic cardiac state, sodium retention, glomerular capillary and arteriolar scarring, low levels of renal vasodilators, loss of the autoregulation of glomerular blood pressure, and activation of the renin-angiotensin system.

20. How is hyperthyroidism treated?

Radioiodine, surgery, and medical management are options. But it is also important to practice a high level of geriatric medicine when a treatment protocol for hyperthyroidism is designed. Hyperthyroid cats are commonly over 13 years old, which makes treatment of the whole cat as a senior patient a priority.

21. How does radioiodine work? How successful is it?

Radioiodine (^{131}I) is highly selective in killing adenomatous or hyperplastic tissue wherever it is located, and response rates are high (> 95%). The abnormal tissue concentrates the radioiodine and is killed by the radioactivity, whereas normal, atrophied tissue does not take up the radioiodine and is spared. Normal thyroid function returns in most patients within 30–90 days, but up to 6 months may be required. A second treatment is needed in only about 2% of patients. Even compromised patients, when given supportive care to address concurrent disease, respond favorably to ^{131}I. Length of stays for radioiodine vary because of individual interpretation of the radiation safety policy by each state and federal regulatory agencies. The shortest stay is 2 days in Florida, and the longest stays are up to 4 weeks. The average stay is 7–10 days in most states. The cost for the procedure ranges from $750–$1,600+, depending on the length of stay and what is included in the treatment protocol.

22. Does previous medical treatment interfere with ^{131}I therapy?

Effective uptake of radioiodine by the abnormal thyroid tissue determines the efficacy of the treatment. Because hyperthyroid medication may interfere, it should be stopped 3–5 days before radioiodine treatment. Recent evidence suggests that it may be possible to continue methimazole until the time of ^{131}I administration. However, if the cat is not compromised by discontinuance of antithyroid medication, stopping for a few days before radioiodine treatment is prudent until more information is gained. After methimazole is discontinued, thyroid hormone returns to high concentrations in 24–72 hours.

23. What adverse effects and complications may be seen with ^{131}I therapy?

Side effects of treatment are few, rare, and transient; dysphagia and voice change have been documented. Clinical hypothyroidism may occur in about 2% of ^{131}I-treated cases.

24. Can surgery be used for treatment of hyperthyroidism?

If radioiodine is not available, surgery is the only other option for definitive therapy in stable patients. Success depends on the competence of the surgeon, the stability of the patient, and a proven surgical protocol. Surgery misses ectopic hyperthyroid tissue, and the only recourse is to treat either medically or with radioiodine. Because ectopic tissue is relatively uncommon, surgery leads to remission in approximately 95% of cases. The recurrence rate after surgery is approximately 5–10%, depending on the technique used.

25. What risks are associated with surgery?

Surgery and anesthesia in a compromised hyperthyroid patient have inherent risks and may cause iatrogenic injury to vital tissues (e.g. damage to the recurrent laryngeal nerve(s), leading to laryngeal paralysis, or removal of all parathyroid tissue, leading to hypocalcemia). With experienced surgeons, the rate of side effects is low (< 10%). Ideally, patients should be treated medically to resolve the hyperthyroidism before surgery to make them better anesthetic and surgical candidates. A thorough physical examination and evaluation of cardiac status are paramount. Do not use atropine in the anesthetic protocol! If the heart rate is dramatically elevated, medications such as propanolol (2.5–5 mg/cat every 8–12 hr to effect) or atenolol (6.25 mg/cat every12–24 hr to effect) may be needed to prevent arrhythmias and help contol heart rate and hypertension.

26. Does a low serum TT4 after radioiodine therapy or surgery necessarily mean that the cat is hypothyroid?

The diagnosis of clinical hypothyroidism must be made by a combination of thyroid testing and clinical signs such as lethargy, obesity, nonpruritic seborrhea sica, poor hair coat, hypothermia, and bradycardia. Only if these clinical signs are seen in combination with a low TT4 or, ideally, fT4 should thyroid supplementation (L-thyroxine, 0.1 mg orally every 24 hr) be initiated.

27. Can hyperthyroidism be treated medically?

In general, antithyroid medications are used in three scenarios:

1. As long-term therapy when ^{131}I treatment and surgery are not possible.

2. As short-term therapy preoperatively or before ^{131}I treatment to make the patient a better candidate for surgery or prolonged hospitalization. Because anesthesia can worsen hyperthyroidism-induced cardiac abnormalities, cats should be rendered euthyroid before surgery, if possible.

3. As short-term therapy to create a temporary euthyroid state in order to judge the effect of permanent correction of hyperthyroidism.

28. How effective is medical therapy?

Methimazole, which lowers circulating thyroid hormone concentrations by blocking T3 and T4 synthesis, is used most frequently. Medical therapy with methimazole is successful if the patient is stable, the client is compliant, the clinician is vigilant in performing routine blood testing (CBC, blood chemistry, and TT4 levels) to make medication adjustments, and the patient tolerates the medication. Unfortunately, if any of the above criteria are not met, treatment may not be ideal. Methimazole is effective in approximately 87% of cats. Giving pills to feline patients and lack of follow-up testing seem to be the biggest challenge to this life-long therapy. Short-term therapy is relatively inexpensive, but long-term therapy and lab tests performed for the life of the patient can be quite expensive.

29. What methimazole treatment regimen should be used?

For mild hyperthyroidism (cats that have mild clinical signs and normal or mildly elevated TT4 values), administer methimazole at 2.5–5 mg orally every 24 hr for 7–10 days. TT4 concentration, liver enzyme activities, and CBC are rechecked at that time. Timing of the post-pill TT4 determination does not matter. Ideally, the TT4 value should be in the lower half of the normal range. An increase to twice-daily dosing may be needed. During the initial 3 months, CBC, liver enzymes, and TT4 should be monitored every 2–3 weeks to assess control and monitor for serious hematologic side effects. For severe hyperthyroidism (cats with severe clinical signs and elevated TT4 usually twice the high-normal value), administer methimazole at 5 mg orally every 12 hr for 7–10 days. The first recheck should be at that time, with subsequent rechecks every 2–3 weeks as for mild disease. Increasing the dose and frequency to every 8 hr depends on the reduction of the TT4 value and clinical signs.

30. After the initial 2–3 months, how should methimazole therapy be monitored?

After the initial period, a TT4 should be measured every 3–6 months to assess control and adjust methimazole dosage as necessary. Unless clinical signs indicate the possible presence of a blood dyscrasia or hepatopathy, CBC and liver enzymes no longer need be reassessed because the likelihood of developing serious hematologic adverse effects at this point is small.

31. What clinical adverse effects are seen with methimazole? How common are they?

Clinical side effects occur in approximately 18% of cats overall and include anorexia (11%), vomiting (11%), lethargy (9%), excoriation of the face and neck (2%), bleeding (2%), and icterus (1.5%). Anorexia, vomiting, and lethargy typically occur during the first month and tend to resolve despite continuing drug administration. Treatment with methimazole should be permanently stopped in cats that develop hepatopathy or bleeding tendency or excoriate their face or neck. Myasthenia gravis has been reported after methimazole treatment in 4 cats.

32. What kind of hematologic adverse effects may be seen? How common are they?

Eosinophilia (11% of cats), lymphocytosis (7%), leukopenia (5%), thrombocytopenia (3%), and agranulocytosis (2%) may occur. The milder adverse effects—eosinophilia, lymphocytosis, and leukopenia—are usually noted within 1–2 months of initiation of treatment and are transient despite continued therapy. The more serious complications (thrombocytopenia, agranulocytosis) typically occur within the first 3 months of therapy and require discontinuation of methimazole.

33. What immunologic adverse effects may occur? How significant are they?

Immunologic effects, including positive antinuclear antibodies (ANA) and positive direct antiglobulin test (Coombs' test), have been noted. The risk of developing a positive ANA appears to increase with length of therapy and dose. Despite the presence of these abnormalities, however, no cat has shown clinical signs of a lupus-like syndrome (e.g., dermatitis, polyarthritis, glomerulonephritis, thrombocytopenia, fever) or hemolysis.

34. What other medical therapies are available?

Calcium ipodate, a radiopaque organic iodine agent, was used with some success but is no longer available. Carbimazole is metabolized to methimazole. When used at the same doses described for methimazole in question 29, carbimazole is sometimes tolerated by cats showing gastrointestinal signs when treated with methimazole. Cats that have immunologic reactions to methimazole probably will react also to carbimazole. The drug must be formulated for use. The beta-adrenergic blockers (e.g., propranolol) have no effect on thyroid hormone concentration but decrease the neuromuscular and cardiovascular effects of hyperthyroidism, such as hyperexcitability, hypertension,and cardiac hypertrophy. These agents can be used in combination with an antithyroid drug or alone if a patient cannot tolerate antithyroid medications. They can be helpful in preparing a patient for thyroidectomy or radioactive iodine by making the cat a better candidate for surgery or hospitalization.

35. What is the prognosis of treated hyperthyroidism?

With any type of treatment for hyperthyroid disease, the patient must be assessed thoroughly. Geriatric-related disease must be evaluated and treated along with hyperthyroidism. Hyperthyroidism is a killing disease and must be treated.

Medical treatment: guarded to very good, depending on medication regulation and drug side effects.

Surgical treatment: guarded to very good, depending on surgical protocol, competency of the surgeon, and follow-up care.

Radioiodine: excellent with a few exceptions. The quality of the ^{131}I protocol and hospitalized patient support is important. A 95% cure rate has been reported with one treatment.

BIBLIOGRAPHY

1. Atkins CE: Thyrotoxic heart disease. In August JR (ed): Consultations in Feline Internal Medicine, 3rd ed. Philadelphia, W.B. Saunders, 1997, pp 279–285.
2. Behrend EN: Medical therapy of feline hyperthyroidism. Comp Cont Educ Pract Vet 21:235–244, 1999.

3. Broussard JD, Peterson ME, Fox PR: Changes in clinical and laboratory findings in cats with hyperthyroidism from 1983 to 1993. J Am Vet Med Assoc 206:302–305, 1995.
4. Kass PH, Peterson ME, Levy J, et al: Evaluation of environmental, nutritional, and host factors in cats with hyperthyroidism. J Vet Intern Med 13:323–329, 1999.
5. Mooney CT, Thoday KL, Doxey DL: Carbimazole therapy of feline hyperthyroidism. J Small Anim Pract 33:228–235, 1992.
6. Peterson ME, Becker DV: Radioiodine treatment of 524 cats with hyperthyroidism. J Am Vet Med Assoc 207:1422–1428, 1995.
7. Peterson ME, Kintzer PP, Hurvitz AI: Methimazole treatment of 262 cats with hyperthyroidism. J Vet Intern Med 2:150–157, 1988.
8. Peterson ME: Hyperthyroidism. In Ettinger SJ, Feldman EC (eds): Textbook of Veterinary Internal Medicine, 5th ed., Phildelphia, W.B. Saunders, 2000, pp 1400–1419.
9. Peterson ME. Update on feline hyperthyroidism. Proceedings of the 18th Annual Veterinary Medical Forum, ACVIM, Seattle, 2000, pp 654–656.
10. Peterson ME, Graves TK, Gamble DA: Triiodothyronine (T3) suppression test: An aid in the diagnosis of mild hyperthyroidism in cats. J Vet Intern Med 4:233–238, 1990.
11. Welches CA, Scavelli TD, Matthiesen, et al: Occurrence of problems after three techniques of bilateral thyroidectomy in cats. Vet Surg 18:392–396, 1989.

54. HYPERADRENOCORTICISM

Ellen N. Behrend, V.M.D., M.S., Ph.D.

1. What is feline hyperadrenocorticism?

Classically, feline hyperadrenocorticism has been synonymous with Cushing's syndrome, which is caused by excessive secretion of cortisol from the adrenal glands. Technically, hyperadrenocorticism also applies to adrenocortical tumors that secrete any hormone. Tumors that secrete aldosterone and progesterone have been reported.

2. How common is feline hypercortisolism? Describe the pathophysiology.

Confirmed, naturally occurring hypercortisolism is rare and has been reported in approximately 88 cats since 1975. Hypercortisolism can be caused either by a pituitary tumor that excessively secretes adrenocorticotropin (ACTH), which stimulates secretion of cortisol, or an adrenal tumor that autonomously secretes cortisol. Pituitary-dependent hypercortisolism (PDH) is more common, accounting for approximately 85% of cases; the remaining 15% are due to adrenal tumors.

3. What types of pituitary and adrenal disease can be present?

Pituitary microadenomas, macroadenomas, and carcinoma (1 case) have been reported. Because clinical signs such as anorexia and disorientation, which frequently are associated with macroadenomas in dogs, are rare in cats, the majority of pituitary tumors probably are microadenomas. Approximately 50% of adrenal tumors are benign, and 50% are malignant.

4. What is the common signalment for cats with hypercortisolism?

There is no known breed or sex predisposition. Hypercortisolism is a disease of older cats; the average age is 10 years with a reported range of 4.5–15 years.

5. What historical findings are commonly associated with hypercortisolism?

Polyuria/polydipsia, polyphagia, weight loss, and lethargy are the most common historical findings. Hypercortisolemic cats without diabetes mellitus can be polyuric/polydipsic. Inappetence in hypercortisolemic dogs suggests the presence of a pituitary macroadenoma; whether the same is true in cats remains unclear.

Clinical Findings in Cats with Spontaneous Hyperadrenocortisolism*

FINDING	NUMBER OF CATS (%)
History	
Polyuria/polydipsia	52/58 (90)
Polyphagia	40/58 (69)
Weight loss	20/58 (34)
Lethargy	18/58 (31)
Weight gain	6/58 (10)
Depression	3/58 (5)
Abnormal gait	3/58 (5)
Constipation	2/58 (3)
Decreased appetite	2/58 (3)
Panting	2/58 (3)
Diarrhea	2/58 (3)
Vomiting	1/58 (2)
Physical examination	
Enlarged abdomen	41/55 (75)
Alopecia	34/58 (59)
Thin skin	25/55 (45)
Muscle atrophy	24/58 (41)
Rough or dry haircoat	17/55 (31)
Obesity	17/58 (29)
Hepatomegaly	16/55 (29)
Easily torn skin	15/58 (26)
Seborrhea	4/55 (7)
Palpable abdominal mass	3/55 (5)
Cutaneous hyperpigmentation	2/55 (4)
Folded pinnae	1/55 (2)

* This information reflects a summary of availble data from approximately 58 cats. In at least one instance, a few cats were included in two reports. Because it was not always possible to determine which data pertained to which cat in the reports, some cats may have been included twice. Because this duplication applies to 2 or 3 cats, the data should not be greatly skewed.
From Behrend EN, Kemppainen RJ: Feline adrenocortical disease. In August JR (ed): Consultations in Feline Internal Medicine, 4th edition. Philadelphia, WB Saunders, 2001.

6. What are the common physical examination findings associated with hypercortisolism?

An enlarged abdomen is the most common finding, followed by alopecia (spontaneous) and thin skin (see table above). Overall, skin changes of some form are a prominent finding. Besides spontaneous alopecia, hair may fail to regrow after clipping. Easily torn skin can be a dramatic finding, and routine hospital or grooming procedures can cause large wounds. The presence of infections or abscesses can be a historical or physical examination finding; affected sites include the upper and lower urinary tract, upper and lower respiratory tract, skin, and oral cavity. Unusual infections such as disseminated candidiasis and disseminated toxoplasmosis may occur.

7. What abnormalities of hypercortisolism are commonly noted on complete blood cell count and serum biochemical panel?

Based on experiences with dogs, a stress leukogram might be expected but is not common. Of the typical changes on stress leukogram, lymphopenia is the most consistent. Hyperglycemia is the most common biochemical change, and the majority of cats (82%) are diabetic. However, although cortisol can antagonize the actions of insulin, not all diabetic, hypercortisolemic cats are insulin-resistant. Elevations in liver enzyme activities occur in just under 50% of cases and may be seen with or without concomitant diabetes mellitus. Elevations in alkaline phosphatase activity are not as common as in dogs, because cats are believed not to have a corticosteroid-induced isoenzyme. Hypercholesterolemia is also a common finding, perhaps occurring in as many as 50%.

Clinicopathologic Results in Cats with Spontaneous Hyperadrenocortisolism

TEST	NUMBER OF CATS (%)
Complete blood count	
Lymphopenia	23/36 (64)
Eosinopenia	14/36 (39)
Neutrophilia	14/36 (39)
Monocytosis	6/36 (17)
Anemia	4/32 (13)
Leukocytosis	4/33 (12)
Neutropenia	2/36 (6)
Lymphocytosis	1/36 (3)
Biochemical profile	
Hyperglycemia	49/53 (92)
Diabetes mellitus	47/57 (82)
Elevated alanine aminotransaminase	17/34 (50)
Elevated aspartate aminotransaminase	4/9 (44)
Elevated alkaline phosphatase	12/38 (32)
Decreased total thyroxine	3/10 (30)
Elevated blood urea nitrogen	7/32 (22)
Elevated total bilirubin	3/17 (18)
Hypocalcemia	3/24 (13)
Elevated creatinine	3/25 (12)
Hypercalcemia	1/24 (4)

From Behrend EN, Kemppainen RJ: Feline adrenocortical disease. In August JR (ed): Consultations in Feline Internal Medicine, 4th edition. Philadelphia, WB Saunders, 2001.

8. How can abdominal radiography help in the diagnosis?

Hepatomegaly is a common finding, occurring in approximately 75% of hypercortisolemic cats. If an adrenal tumor is present, it may be seen. Adrenal calcification may be visualized in adrenal tumors, but since it can be seen in up to 30% of normal cats, its detection does not mean that an adrenal tumor is present.

9. What about other means of abdominal imaging?

On abdominal ultrasonography, bilaterally enlarged adrenal glands are consistent with PDH. However, feline adrenal glands can be difficult to image, and enlargement has not always been noted in cats with PDH. An adrenal tumor, if present, may be detected. Computed tomography also can be used to image the pituitary gland or the adrenal glands.

10. What tests are available for the diagnosis of hypercortisolism?

Definitive diagnosis requires adrenal testing. Screening tests used to determine whether the disease is present are the urine cortisol:creatinine ratio (UCCR), low-dose dexamethasone suppression test (LDDST), high-dose dexamethasone suppression test (HDDST), ACTH stimulation test, and the combination test. An ultra-high-dose dexamethasone suppression test, endogenous ACTH level determination, or CT scan can be used to differentiate between PDH and adrenal tumor.

11. Why are results of these tests difficult to interpret?

First, results in normal cats and cats with hypercortisolism appear to be more variable than in dogs. Second, few studies have been published examining the specificity and sensitivity of these tests in cats.

12. How accurate is UCCR in cats?

Measurement of UCCR has received little study in cats. A ratio within the normal range rules out hypercortisolism with high accuracy, possibly close to 100%. In contrast, determination of an elevated ratio is nondiagnostic because cats with hypercortisolemia or nonadrenal illness may have an elevated ratio. When an elevated ratio is found in a suspect cat, more definitive screening tests should be performed.

Screening and Differentiating Test for Hypercortisolism*

TEST	PROTOCOLS	INTERPRETATION
UCCR	Collect urine by free catch or cystocentesis. Centrifuge sample and submit super-natant.	Normal ratio (< 30) rules out hyper-cortisolism; with elevated ratio, diagnosis of hypercortisolism must be confirmed with another test.
ACTH stimula-tion test	Administer 0.125 µg of synthetic ACTH[†] IV. Draw blood samples before and 1 hr after injection.	Normal serum cortisol concentration at baseline = 10–110 nmol/L; after ACTH, normal value = 210–330 nmol/L. A post-ACTH level > 330 nmol/L is con-sistent with hypercortisolism.
LDDST	Administer dexamethasone at 0.01 mg/kg IV. Collect blood samples before and 4 and 8 hr after injection.	After dexamethasone, serum cortisol con-centration should be < 30 nmol/L. Normal suppression rules out diagnosis of hypercortisolism.
HDDST	Perform like LDDST, but administer 0.1 mg/kg dexamethasone.	Lack of suppression at 8 hr is consistent with hypercortisolism. Suppression at 4 hr with lack of suppression at 8 hr is consistent with PDH.
UHDDST	Perform like LDDST, but administer 1.0 mg/kg dexamethasone.	Suppression at 4 or 8 hr to < 30 nmol/L or to < 50% baseline is consistent with PDH.
Combination test	Take blood sample, and administer 1.0 mg/kg dexamethasone IV. Take blood sample 4 hr later, and imme-diately perform ACTH stimulation test as above.	Diagnosis of hypercortisolism is based on ACTH stimulation portion, as above. Suppression to < 30 nmol/L or < 50% baseline after dexamethasone is con-sistent with PDH. If no suppression is seen, another differentiation test must be done.
Endogenous ACTH mea-surement	Proper sample handling is critical. Collect sample in EDTA, add trasylol,[‡] and spin within 15 min. Place plasma in plastic tubes and mail cold sample overnight on ice. Sample can be stored with refrigeration for < 1 day; it should be frozen for longer storage.	Plasma ACTH concentrations should be in mid to above-normal range (> 15 pg/ml) in cats with PDH and low in cats with adrenal tumors (< 10 pg/ml).

UCCR = urinary cortisol:creatinine ratio, ACTH = adrenocorticotropin, LDDST = low-dose dexamethasone suppression test, HDDST = high-dose dexamethasone suppresssion test, UHDDST = ultra-high-dose dexam-ethasone suppression test, PDH = pituitary-dependent hypercortisolism, IV = intravenously, EDTA = ethyl-enediamine tetraacetic acid.

* The values given for interpretation are those used by the Auburn University Endocrine Diagnostic Service. Check with your own laboratory for their normal values. To convert cortisol to mg/dl, divide by 27.6.

† Cosyntropin, Organon, Inc., West Orange, NJ.

‡ A special preservative available from some endocrine diagnostic laboratories.

13. How should I use the ACTH stimulation test?

An elevated post-ACTH cortisol concentration (see table above) is consistent with a diagno-sis of hypercortisolism, but it is present in only about 81% of affected cats. Repeat testing in a previously negative cat may provide a positive result. The ACTH stimulation test has been shown to give exaggerated results in some ill cats with nonadrenal disease, and false-positive test results are possible. The ACTH stimulation test cannot be used to differentiate PDH from adrenal tumor.

14. Can a low-dose dexamethasone suppression test be used in cats?

After administration of a low dose of dexamethasone (see table in question 12), 95% of hypercortisolemic cats fail to suppress (positive result). However, some ill cats with nonadrenal disease also have inadequate suppression on an LDDST. The chance for false-positive test results limits the usefulness of LDDST in cats. However, because most hypercortisolemic cats have a positive LDDST, the negative predictive value of the test can be valuable. If the LDDST is normal, it is highly unlikely that the cat has hypercortisolism.

15. What is the diagnostic utility of the high-dose dexamethasone suppression test?

Because of the low specificity of the LDDST, the use of a higher dose of dexamethasone (see table in question 12), which causes suppression more reliably in cats with normal adrenal function, is recommended for screening purposes. When used as a screening test, a positive HDDST occurs in about 80% of hypercortisolemic cats. False-negative results may occur because a high dose of dexamethasone can cause cortisol suppression in some cats with early or mild hypercortisolism. This test appears to be more specific than the LDDST, but extensive studies have not been done.

16. How can the ultra-high-dose dexamethasone suppression test be used?

An ultra-high dose can be used to differentiate PDH and adrenal tumor (see table in question 12). This test is used once a diagnosis of hypercortisolism has been confirmed by a screening test. Suppression is consistent with the presence of PDH, but lack of suppression is consistent with either PDH or AT and another differentiation test must be used.

17. Can determination of an endogenous ACTH concentration be used to differentiate AT from PDH?

Once hypercortisolism is confirmed, plasma ACTH concentrations should be in the mid- to above-normal range in cats with PDH and low in cats with adrenal tumor. This test has been highly reliable in cats.

18. What is the combination test?

The combination of a high-dose dexamethasone suppression test and an ACTH stimulation test (see table in question 12). Each part should be interpreted as if the test were done alone, with the attendant caveats. In dogs, the combination test is hoped to be a screening test on the basis of the ACTH stimulation test and a differentiation test on the basis of the high-dose dexamethasone blood sample. Because most hypercortisolemic cats do not suppress after this dose of dexamethasone, the combination test is less likely to provide differentiation than it is in dogs. However, if both limbs of the test are positive—lack of suppression and an increased ACTH response—the diagnosis of hypercortisolism can be made with greater confidence.

19. What may be the ideal screening method for feline hypercortisolism?

Because feline hypercortisolism is an infrequent diagnosis and each test has potential for both false-positive and false-negative results, confirmation of the diagnosis is best made by demonstrating both an exaggerated cortisol response to ACTH and failure to suppress serum cortisol on an HDDST.

20. What medications are used to treat hypercortisolism?

Mitotane, ketoconazole or metyrapone may be used. Experience with all 3 is limited in cats.

21. What is the mechanism of action of mitotane? How effective is it in cats?

Mitotane (Lysodren, Bristol-Meyers Oncology, Princeton, NJ) causes selective necrosis of adrenocortical cells that secrete cortisol. Early reports suggested that mitotane was not as effective in normal cats or cats with hypercortisolism as it is in dogs. However, mitotane therapy may be successful with higher doses and/or longer induction periods than typically used for dogs.

22. Can ketoconazole therapy be used for this syndrome in cats?

Ketoconazole (Nizoral, Janssen, Titusville, NJ) decreases adrenal synthesis of cortisol through inhibition of numerous enzymes and also may antagonize glucocorticoid receptors. Ketoconazole has had mixed success in cats and commonly causes toxicity. In dogs with hypercortisolism, ketoconazole is estimated to be efficacious in < 50% of cases; successful use in cats also seems unlikely.

23. What is the mechanism of action of metyrapone? How effective is it?

Metyrapone (Metopirone, Novartis, E. Hanover, NJ) affects cortisol synthesis through inhibition of 11-β-hydroxylase, an adrenal enzyme. Its use has been highly limited and has shown mixed success, but currently it is the medical therapy of choice.

24. Can surgery be used for treatment of hypercortisolism?

Because of difficulties with medical therapy, the treatments of choice for adrenal tumor and PDH are unilateral and bilateral adrenalectomy, respectively. Surgical management appears to be highly effective overall; approximately 80% of patients survive for longer than 1 month.

25. What is the cause of postoperative mortality in cats with adrenalectomy? How can it be prevented?

Death occurred within the first month in 5 cats, 4 that underwent bilateral adrenalectomy for PDH, and 1 that underwent unilateral adrenalectomy for adrenal adenocarcinoma. Suspected causes of death included hypoadrenal crisis, renal failure, development of chylothorax secondary to extensive thrombosis of the cranial vena cava, severe pancreatitis and septic peritonitis, and sloughing of large regions of skin. Administration of metyrapone to stabilize patients preoperatively and strict adherence to postoperative medical protocols may decrease mortality rates.

26. How should cats be treated intraoperatively?

Diabetic cats should receive 50% of their usual insulin dose on the morning of surgery. With unilateral or bilateral adrenalectomy, treatment with glucocorticoids during and after surgery is required. In cats with an adrenal tumor, the contralateral adrenal gland is atrophied because constant negative feedback by the tumor to the pituitary gland decreases ACTH secretion. At the time of anesthetic induction, a continuous intravenous infusion of hydrocortisone (625 mg/kg/hr) should be initiated and continued for 24–48 hours postoperatively. At that time, prednisone (2.5 mg/cat orally every 12 hr) should be instituted.

27. Describe long-term postoperative treatment.

In cats with unilateral adrenalectomy, recovery of the unaffected gland is expected with time, and glucocorticoid therapy can be withdrawn slowly. Cats undergoing bilateral surgery should be treated as for spontaneous hypoadrenocorticism. Mineralocorticoid replacement therapy should be instituted when the hydrocortisone infusion is discontinued. Because some cats have died postoperatively from suspected hypoadrenal crisis, the importance of continuing therapy must be communicated to the owner.

28. What is the long-term prognosis for cats that survive the postoperative period?

For cats that live past the first month postoperatively, reported survival times range from 3 to > 60 months. The cause of death is varied, including suspected hypoadrenal crisis, renal failure, and expansion of a pituitary mass in cats that develop neurologic abnormalities.

29. Does diabetes mellitus resolve with treatment of hypercortisolism?

Whereas in dogs therapy for hypercortisolism alleviates insulin resistance but diabetes mellitus typically persists, the disease resolves with successful treatment of hypercortisolism in approximately 50% of cats. If the diabetes mellitus does not resolve, amelioration of the hypercortisolism should decrease insulin requirements.

30. How quickly should the clinical signs of hypercortisolism resolve once control is obtained?

Clinical signs typically resolve 2–4 months after control of hypercortisolism.

31. Can adrenal tumors secrete hormones besides cortisol?

Progesterone-secreting and aldosterone-secreting adrenal masses have been reported in 1 and 3 cats, respectively.

32. What clinical signs and physical examination findings may be seen with hyperprogesteronemia?

Clinical signs are similar to those of hypercortisolism: nonpruritic, bilaterally symmetrical alopecia; polyuria/polydipsia; and aggression. Physical examination may reveal alopecia, a greasy unkempt coat and scale, comedones at the oral commissures, thin skin with easily visible blood vessels, and bruising at venipuncture sites.

33. How can a diagnosis of hyperprogesteronemia be made?

The diagnosis is based on results of sex hormone concentration measurement before and after a standard ACTH stimulation test (see table in question 12). Progesterone will be above normal, at least in the post-ACTH sample.

34. How should a progesterone-secreting tumor be treated?

Adrenalectomy is the treatment of choice. No information is available about medical management. Postoperatively, glucocorticoid therapy may be required, at least temporarily. Progesterone can inhibit pituitary ACTH secretion, leading to atrophy of the normal gland. Glucocorticoids need to be given until the gland recovers.

35. What historical complaints, clinical signs, and physical examination findings occur with hyperaldosteronism?

Polyuria, polydipsia, nocturia, generalized weakness, collapse, anorexia, weight loss, pendulous abdomen, and blindness are reported by some owners. On physical examination, bilateral retinal detachment, hypertension, pendulous abdomen, or heart murmur may be found.

36. What abnormalities may be seen on a complete blood count and serum biochemical profile?

The complete blood cell count is generally normal. Hypokalemia is a consistent serum biochemical abnormality. Hypernatremia, increased serum bicarbonate, and elevated creatine phosphokinase (CPK) activity may be detected. Diabetes mellitus may result from the effect of hypokalemia on insulin secretion. Glycosuria despite normoglycemia also has been observed.

37. How is the diagnosis of hyperaldosteronism made?

Diagnosis of primary hyperaldosteronism is based on marked hyperaldosteronemia (at least 6 times higher than normal) in conjunction with hypertension, hypokalemia, inappropriate kaliuresis (urinary fractional excretion of potassium at least 6 times normal), normal plasma renin activity, ultrasonographic confirmation of an adrenal mass, or cytologic or histopathologic confirmation of an adrenal cortical neoplasia. Currently, a validated renin assay is not available for cats. Without such an assay, diagnosis of primary hyperaldosteronism requires that all secondary causes (e.g., states associated with peripheral edema or liver failure) be ruled out. The presence of renal failure presents a particular dilemma, because renal failure itself can lead to this constellation of abnormalities. The magnitude of aldosterone elevation may be the key to differentiation in such cats.

38. How is hyperaldosteronism treated?

Medical therapy has been only partially successful. Potassium supplementation should be provided (2–6 mEq/day) to keep the serum potassium concentration in the normal range, if possible. The best initial medication for treatment of hypertension is the aldosterone antagonist spironolactone (1–2 mg/kg orally every 12 hr), but it may not provide full control. Other antihypertensive agents may be required in combination (see Chapter 63). Unilateral adrenalectomy to remove the tumor is possible. All three cases reported have been due to carcinoma; cure may not be possible.

39. What is the prognosis?

It is difficult to make definitive statements based on results of only 3 cases, but medical therapy was not highly successful in any cat. The one cat treated by adrenalectomy survived 1 year.

BIBLIOGRAPHY

1. Ahn A: Hyperaldosteronism in cats. Semin Vet Med Surg (Small Anim) 9:153–157, 1994.
2. Behrend EN, Kemppainen RJ: Feline adrenocortical disease. In August JR (ed): Consultations in Feline Internal Medicine, 4th ed. Philadelphia, W.B. Saunders, 2001.
3. Boord M, Griffin C: Progesterone secreting adrenal mass in a cat with clinical signs of hyperadrenocorticism. J Am Vet Med Assoc 214:666–669, 1999.
4. Duesberg CA, Nelson RW, Feldman EC, et al: Adrenalectomy for treatment of hyperadrenocorticism in cats: 10 cases (1988–1992). J Am Vet Med Assoc 207:1066–1070, 1995.
5. Duesberg CA, Peterson ME: Adrenal disorders in cats. Vet Clin North Am Small Anim Pract 27:321–348, 1997.
6. Feldman EC, Nelson RW: Hyperadrenocorticism in cats. In Feldman EC, Nelson RW (eds): Canine and Feline Endocrinology and Reproduction, 2nd ed. Philadelphia, W.B. Saunders, 1996, pp. 256–261.
7. Flood SM, Randolph JR, Gelzer ARM, et al: Primary hyperaldosteronism in 2 cats. J Am Anim Hosp Assoc 35:411–416, 1999.
8. Jensen J, Henik RA, Brownfield M, et al: Plasma renin activity and angiotensin I and aldosterone concentrations in cats with hypertension associated with chronic renal disease. Am J Vet Res 58:535–540, 1997.
9. Peterson ME, Randolph JR, Mooney CT: Endocrine diseases. In Sherding RG (ed): The Cat: Diseases and Clinical Management, 2nd ed. New York, Churchill Livingstone, 1995, pp 1403–1506.
10. Schwedes CS: Mitotane (o,p'-DDD) treatment in a cat with hyperadrenocorticism. J Small Anim Pract 38:520–524, 1997.

55. HYPOADRENOCORTICISM

Ellen N. Behrend, V.M.D., M.S., Ph.D.

1. What constitutes the hypothalamic-pituitary-adrenal axis?

The hypothalamus secretes corticotropin-releasing hormone (CRH), which stimulates the anterior pituitary to release adrenocorticotropin (ACTH). ACTH, in turn, causes the adrenal glands to secrete cortisol. Cortisol then gives negative feedback to the hypothalamus and anterior pituitary, inhibiting CRH and ACTH release, respectively.

2. Define hypoadrenocorticism.

Hypoadrenocorticism is the failure of the adrenal glands to produce adequate concentrations of mineralocorticoids, glucocorticoids, or both. Spontaneous hypoadrenocorticism can be either primary or secondary. With primary hypoadrenocorticism (Addison's disease), adrenal gland dysfunction causes glucocorticoid and mineralocorticoid deficiency. Spontaneous secondary hypoadrenocorticism, due to reduced secretion of ACTH from the pituitary, has not been reported in cats. Iatrogenic secondary hypoadrenocorticism can be caused by treatment with either glucocorticoids or progestins, which lessen ACTH secretion by negative feedback. In spontaneous or iatrogenic secondary hypoadrenocorticism, reduced circulating ACTH concentrations lead to atrophy of the glucocorticoid-secreting zones of the adrenal cortex; aldosterone secretion is not affected.

3. How common is spontaneous primary hypoadrenocorticism? What causes it?

Naturally occurring hypoadrenocorticism is rare in cats, with 26 confirmed cases and 2 suspected cases reported since 1983. Most cases are idiopathic, but 2 were traumatically induced, and 2 were secondary to lymphoma. In 2 of 5 cases of idiopathic disease that went to necropsy, lymphocytic infiltration of the adrenals was noted. This finding suggests that in some cats hypoadrenocorticism results from immune-mediated destruction of adrenal tissue.

4. What signalment findings are commonly associated with spontaneous primary hypoadrenocorticism?

In 12 cats, the average age at presentation was approximately 5–6 years (range = 1.5–14 years), all were of mixed breeding, 7 were castrated males, and 5 were spayed females.

5. What historical findings are commonly associated with primary hypoadrenocorticism?

Anorexia and lethargy are the most common signs. Weight loss is also common; vomiting, a waxing and waning course, previous therapeutic response, and polyuria/polydipsia are noted less frequently. Clinical signs may be present for up to 100 days before diagnosis.

Clinical Findings in Cats with Spontaneous Hypoadrenocorticism

FINDING	NUMBER OF CATS (%)
Historical complaints	
Anorexia	14/14 (100)
Lethargy/depression	13/14 (93)
Weight loss	12/14 (86)
Vomiting	5/14 (36)
Waxing and waning course	4/14 (29)
Previous response to therapy	3/14 (21)
Polyuria/polydipsia	3/14 (21)
Sudden collapse/weakness	1/14 (7)
Physical examination findings	
Dehydration	12/13 (92)
Weakness	11/13 (85)
Hypothermia	10/13 (77)
Increased capillary refill time	5/13 (38)
Weak pulse	5/13 (38)
Inability to rise	3/13 (23)
Painful abdomen	3/13 (23)
Bradycardia	2/13 (15)
Cool extremities	1/13 (8)

From Behrend EN, Kemppainen RJ: Feline adrenocortical disease. In August JR (ed): Consultations in Feline Internal Medicine, 4th ed. Philadelphia, W.B. Saunders, 2001.

6. What physical findings are commonly associated with primary hypoadrenocorticism?

On physical examination, dehydration, weakness and hypothermia are detected in the majority of cases. Increased capillary refill time, weak pulses, inability to rise, painful abdomen, bradycardia, and cool extremities also have been observed (see table above).

7. What abnormalities of primary hypoadrenocorticism are commonly noted on complete blood cell count and serum biochemical panel?

Routine bloodwork abnormalities may suggest hypoadrenocorticism but cannot be used to make the definitive diagnosis. The most consistent abnormalities, as in dogs, are azotemia with electrolyte changes, including hyperkalemia, hyponatremia, hypochloremia, and acidosis.

Hyperkalemia is typically mild and may not be detected until days after initial presentation. The highest reported potassium value to date is 6.2 mEq/L. Hyponatremia ranges from mild to marked. Although detection of eosinophilia and lymphocytosis (i.e., lack of a stress leukogram) may be a clue to the presence of hypoadrenocorticism in a sick, stressed cat, these findings are not common. An increased red blood cell count, if seen, is most likely a result of dehydration.

Clinicopathologic Results in Cats with Spontaneous Hypoadrenocorticism*

TEST	NUMBER OF CATS (%)
Complete blood count	
Anemia	4/14 (29)
Lymphocytosis	2/13 (15)
Eosinophilia	1/13 (8)
Biochemistry profile	
Hyponatremia	15/15 (100)
Hyperkalemia	15/16 (94)
Azotemia	14/15 (93)
Hypochloremia	11/14 (79)
Decrease in total carbon dioxide	6/14 (43)
Elevated alanine aminotransferase	2/12 (17)
Elevated alkaline phosphatase	1/12 (8)
Increased total bilirubin	1/12 (8)
Increased serum calcium	1/12 (8)

* Includes two separate presentations of the same cat.
From Behrend EN, Kemppainen RJ: Feline adrenocortical disease. In August JR (ed): Consultations in Feline Internal Medicine, 4th ed. Philadelphia, W.B. Saunders, 2001.

8. Many cats with primary hypoadrenocorticism have dilute urine. What is the significance of this finding?

Of 11 cats for which urine specific gravity was determined at presentation, 7 had inappropriate urine concentration. Whether this finding represents true renal disease is unknown. Hyponatremia can cause poor urine concentrating ability by potentially leading to renal medullary washout. Urine specific gravity and renal function must be evaluated after sodium repletion to determine the true urine concentrating ability.

9. Can radiography or electrocardiography help in the diagnosis of primary hypoadrenocorticism?

As with blood work, the changes found may suggest hypoadrenocorticism but are not diagnostic. Radiography may reveal decreased lung opacity and vascular markings, suggesting hypoperfusion, and microcardia. Electrocardiographs are often normal; bradycardia and atrial premature contractions have been detected in some cats. In contrast to dogs with primary hypoadrenocorticism, tall, peaked T waves or diminished P waves due to hyperkalemia have not been detected in cats, possibly because the degree of hyperkalemia is relatively mild.

10. How is the diagnosis of hypoadrenocorticism made?

Definitive diagnosis is based on results of an ACTH stimulation test. To perform the test, administer 0.125 mg of synthetic ACTH (Cosyntropin, Organon Inc, West Orange, NJ) intravenously. Blood samples are drawn before and 1 hour after the injection. Serum cortisol concentration before and after ACTH are very low or nondetectable. Differentiation between primary and secondary hypoadrenocorticism can be made on the basis of endogenous ACTH concentrations (see Chapter 54 for sample handling). Increased endogenous ACTH confirms adrenal failure with lack of negative feedback on the pituitary; with secondary hypoadrenocorticism, endogenous ACTH is very low or non-detectable. However, differentiation is rarely necessary in cats because only iatrogenic secondary hypoadrenocorticism has been described.

11. How is hypoadrenocorticism treated?

Treatment depends on whether a hypoadrenal crisis is present or whether the patient is relatively stable.

12. What abnormalities need to be addressed therapeutically if a patient is in crisis? Which is the most important?

Therapy for a hypoadrenal crisis is directed at expanding fluid volume, supplying exogenous glucocorticoids, and correcting electrolyte abnormalities and acidosis. Fluid replacement is the most important aspect of treatment. Fluids should be given intravenously at an approximate rate of 40 ml/kg over 2–4 hours. The fluid of choice is 0.9% sodium chloride (NaCl), which provides both sodium and chloride but is potassium-deficient. However, if 0.9% NaCl is not available, Ringer's solution or lactated Ringer's solution is acceptable because potassium concentrations are low and administration dilutes serum potassium concentrations. Correction of hyponatremia should be slow to avoid neurologic sequelae.

13. What glucocorticoid should be administered to a patient with a hypoadrenal crisis?

Prednisolone sodium succinate (4–20 mg/kg IV) or dexamethasone (0.1–2.0 mg/kg IV) may be used. Prednisolone sodium succinate is the quickest-acting, followed by dexamethasone sodium phosphate and then dexamethasone. If dexamethasone sodium phosphate is used, make sure that the dose is calculated on the basis of the active ingredient. One milliliter of dexamethasone sodium phosphate usually has a total concentration of 4 mg/ml but only 3 mg/ml of dexamethasone. The 3 mg/ml figure should be used in calculations. Because prednisolone crossreacts with cortisol on most assays, an ACTH stimulation test should not be performed for 12 hours after its administration. The decision of which glucocorticoid to use depends on patient status. Because prednisolone is the most rapidly acting, it is the glucocorticoid of choice in severe crisis. Adrenal testing can be performed once the patient is stabilized.

14. What other treatments may be necessary for a hypoadrenal crisis?

Hyperkalemia may need to be addressed specifically, but this is unlikely given the mild alterations in potassium typically seen in cats with spontaneous primary hypoadrenocorticism. Intravenous administration of fluids alone causes rapid lowering of the potassium. If the potassium concentration is > 8.5 mEq/L, specific treatment options include:

- 10% calcium gluconate (0.5–1.0 mg/kg IV, given slowly over 10–20 minutes);
- Sodium bicarbonate (2–3 mEq/kg IV over 30 minutes or dose based on serum bicarbonate deficit to correct acidosis); or
- Combination of glucose and insulin (0.5 units/kg regular insulin IV followed by 1–1.5 gm dextrose per unit insulin added to the IV fluids and administered over 4–6 hours).

Calcium protects the heart from the effects of the potassium, whereas the others shift potassium from the serum into cells. Sodium bicarbonate also helps to correct acidosis but is rarely required because the acidosis is usually mild and responds well to fluid therapy.

15. Compare the response of dogs and cats to treatment.

Dogs respond rapidly whereas cats usually remain weak, lethargic and depressed for 3–5 days despite institution of appropriate therapy.

16. What long-term treatment is needed in the stable patient?

Any combination of a glucocorticoid and mineralocorticoid can be used, but complications of glucocorticoid therapy, such as diabetes mellitus, may be more likely if injectable glucocorticoids are used. Of 4 cats treated with a combination of fludrocortisone (Florinef, Apothecon, The Netherlands) at 0.1 mg/cat/day orally and prednisone at 1.25 mg/cat/day orally, one cat died suddenly of unknown causes after 47 days and the other 3 cats survived for at least 3 months. A combination of desoxycorticosterone pivalate (DOCP; Percorten-V, Novartis Animal Health, Inc, Greensboro, NC) at 10–12.5 mg/cat/month intramuscularly and methylprednisolone acetate at 10 mg/cat/month intramuscularly also has been used. Approximately 50% of dogs receiving fludrocortisone may not require further exogenous glucocorticoids, but whether this finding applies to cats is unknown. Although some dogs taking DOCP have not received glucocorticoid therapy, this practice is not recommended because DOCP has no glucocorticoid activity and the patient will always be glucocorticoid-deficient.

17. Are treatment adjustments needed during times of stress?
During times of stress, glucocorticoid requirements increase. On days of planned increased stress, the daily glucocorticoid dose should be doubled or, if the cat is not receiving glucocorticoids or is receiving an injectable form, prednisone should be administered at a dose of 0.2–0.4 mg/kg orally every 24 hr.

18. What is the prognosis for cats with hypoadrenocorticism?
For 6 cats that received long-term treatment with either DOCP or fludrocortisone for confirmed, idiopathic primary hypoadrenocorticism, the median survival was 34 months. In one cat with confirmed, traumatically induced hypoadrenocorticism, medication was eventually discontinued after adrenal recovery.

BIBLIOGRAPHY

1. Behrend EN, Kemppainen RJ: Feline adrenocortical disease. In August JR (ed): Consultations in Feline Internal Medicine, 4th edition, Philadelphia, WB Saunders, 2001.
2. Chastain CB, Graham CL, Nichols CE: Adrenocortical suppression in cats given megestrol acetate. Am J Vet Res 42:2029–2035, 1981.
3. Hypoadrenocorticism in cats. In Feldman EC, Nelson RW (eds): Canine and Feline Endocrinology and Reproduction, 2nd edition, Philadelphia, WB Saunders, 1996, pp 302–306.
4. Myers NC, Bruyette DS: Feline adrenocortical diseases: Part II – hypoadrenocorticism. Seminars Vet Med Surg (Small Animal) 9:144–147, 1994.
5. Parnell NK, Powell LL, Hohenhaus AE, et al: Hypoadrenocorticism as the primary manifestation of lymphoma in 2 cats. J Am Vet Med Assoc 214:1208–1211, 1999.
6. Peterson ME, Greco DS, Orth DN: Primary hypoadrenocorticism in ten cats. J Vet Int Med, 3:55–58, 1989.

56. DIABETES MELLITUS
Jill Lurye, D.V.M., and Ellen N. Behrend, V.M.D., M.S., Ph.D.

1. What is diabetes mellitus?
Diabetes mellitus (DM) is a metabolic disease characterized by an absolute or relative insulin deficiency that results in abnormal fuel metabolism, particularly of glucose and fat. Prolonged hyperglycemia is the most obvious consequence of insulin deficiency, but ketoacidosis and other manifestations of accelerated catabolism also occur. Because all cells require energy utilization, DM can result in abnormalities in most body systems, some of which can be fatal if untreated.

2. What are the forms of primary diabetes mellitus in humans?
Diabetes mellitus is classified as type 1 or type 2. Type 1 DM, also commonly called juvenile-onset diabetes because typically it is first evident in childhood, results from destruction of > 80–85% of pancreatic islet beta cells. It is typically immune-mediated but may be idiopathic. Type 2 DM results from three concomitant abnormalities:
1. Impaired pancreatic insulin secretion
2. Resistance of peripheral cells to insulin
3. Increased hepatic glucose production.

3. How does the human classification system apply to veterinary medicine?

Human nomenclature cannot be applied to veterinary species with complete accuracy. Evidence suggests that both type 1 and type 2 DM occur in veterinary species, but variations and overlaps in pathophysiology are likely. The presence of autoantibodies and the suggestion of autoimmune destruction of pancreatic beta cells have been occasionally reported in diabetic cats, but the presence of type 1 DM has not been established as a major pathophysiologic mechanism. It may explain the rare occurrence of DM in kittens. Most diabetic cats probably have a disease process most similar to human type 2 DM.

4. What is meant by insulin-dependent or non–insulin-dependent DM?

In the past, type 1 has been called insulin-dependent DM (IDDM) and type 2 non–insulin-dependent DM (NIDDM). This terminology is confusing when applied to veterinary patients because approximately 60–70% of diabetic cats require insulin therapy at the time of diagnosis, regardless of the underlying pathophysiology. Cats also may alternate between requiring and not requiring insulin; as many as 10–20% of insulin-dependent cats become non–insulin-dependent.

5. What is glucose toxicity?

Cats are highly sensitive to glucose toxicity. Prolonged hyperglycemia, which may be present before the diagnosis of DM, results in an additional decline in the ability of pancreatic beta cells to sense and respond to glucose concentrations. This decline further reduces insulin secretion and perpetuates the disease. Glucose toxicity also may play a role in increasing peripheral insulin resistance.

6. How can DM resolve in some cats?

Glucose toxicity may be the reason. After reduction of hyperglycemia via exogenous insulin, beta cells may regain the ability to sense glucose and secrete insulin; thus, exogenous insulin is no longer required.

7. What is secondary DM?

Secondary DM, usually called type 3, results from beta-cell dysfunction or insulin resistance caused by an unrelated disease process (e.g,. acromegaly, hyperadrenocorticism) or drug administration (e.g., progestins). If the primary problem or drug administration is eliminated, type 3 DM that has not progressed beyond initial stages will resolve.

8. How common is DM in cats?

The incidence of feline DM is estimated at 0.25–0.5% (1 in 200–400 cats). It is one of the most common endocrinopathies of cats, second only to hyperthyroidism.

9. What is the typical signalment of cats with DM?

DM can develop in cats of any breed, age, or sex; however, older (> 10 yr), obese, neutered males appear to be at increased risk.

10. What are the historical and clinical signs of DM?

In uncomplicated DM, weight loss with normal-to-increased appetite, polyuria, and polydipsia are common. Because of the insidious onset of these signs, owners may miss them until changes become severe. A poor, unkempt hair coat also may be noted. In rare instances, a gait change or plantigrade stance associated with a peripheral neuropathy may be seen. In cases of complicated DM (e.g., ketosis, hyperosmolar state, or concomitant disease, such as hepatic lipidosis), other symptoms may be seen, including anorexia, vomiting and diarrhea, lethargy, depression, and icterus.

11. How is DM diagnosed?

The diagnosis is achieved by documenting fasting hyperglycemia > 200 mg/dl and glucosuria in a cat with appropriate clinical signs. The presence of ketonuria further confirms the diagnosis.

12. Does the presence of hyperglycemia mean that a cat is diabetic?

As a result of a physiologic response to acute or chronic stress, nondiabetic cats can be hyperglycemic. Blood glucose concentration can even exceed 300 mg/dl.

13. How can DM and stress hyperglycemia be differentiated?

If the stress is acute (e.g., induced by handling or restraint), glucosuria is usually absent. If glucosuria is observed and stress is still suspected, resampling or serial sampling of blood and urine after acclimatization may be tried. Urine glucose also can be measured in a nonstressful, home environment using urine dipsticks, if needed.

14. Can measurement of glycosylated proteins aid in the differentiation?

With hyperglycemia of days to weeks in duration, certain plasma proteins (albumin and hemoglobin) become bound to glucose (glycosylated). In theory, the concentration of glycosylated protein is proportional to the blood glucose over time. The concentrations of these altered proteins can be measured in a laboratory as fructosamine or glycosylated hemoglobin, and they typically are elevated in untreated diabetic cats. However, not all diabetic cats have elevated levels; conversely, elevated levels may be seen in nondiabetics. Thus measurement of glycosylated proteins is not 100% accurate in differentiating stress from DM.

15. What other clinicopathologic changes may be seen in diabetic cats?

Other common clinicopathologic changes include hypercholesterolemia and elevations in one or more liver enzymes, ranging from mild to severe. When hyperosmolar, ketoacidotic, or concomitant disease states are present, various other laboratory findings, including evidence of hemoconcentration, hyperosmolality, acidemia, electrolyte abnormalities, and hyperbilirubinemia, may be noted.

16. How is DM treated?

Therapy consists of various combinations of weight and dietary modification, insulin therapy, and administration of oral hypoglycemic agents.

17. Why is weight correction important? How should it be done?

Correction of obesity or malnutrition diminishes insulin resistance and, in type 2 DM, improves insulin secretion. For weight loss, caloric intake should be restricted to approximately 75% of the maintenance caloric requirements of 60–70 kcal/kg/day. Underweight cats should be fed maintenance caloric requirements to achieve ideal body weight. Any attempts to alter body weight should be made gradually. Blood glucose values should be monitored closely because insulin requirements change with body condition.

18. Describe an appropriate diet for diabetic cats.

An appropriate diet and feeding schedule are important parts of diabetic control. A well-balanced diet containing adequate protein and reduced fat content is recommended most commonly, but new evidence suggests that high protein also may be beneficial. Sugars should be complex carbohydrates with minimal amounts of simple sugars. Increased dietary fiber may improve glycemic control by minimizing postprandial fluctuations in blood glucose. Diets should take into consideration any concomitant diseases.

19. Describe the ideal feeding schedule.

Consistency in amount and schedule is crucial. Insulin therapy is more successful when diet and feeding schedule are regular. Feeding schedules should minimize postprandial fluctuations in blood glucose and coordinate with the peak physiologic effects of exogenously administered insulin, if possible. The ideal schedule to minimize postprandial hyperglycemia includes multiple small meals throughout the day, but this schedule is usually impractical. Because the ideal is usually not possible, it is suggested that meals be given immediately before insulin injections, if given twice daily. If once-daily insulin is used, one meal can be given before the morning injection and one in the late afternoon or early evening.

20. What about free-choice feeding?

Free-choice feeding can be used if a cat refuses to eat scheduled meals, but the amount should be restricted to maintenance caloric requirements. The problem with this approach is that it may be difficult to tell whether the cat is eating well, and insulin may be given inappropriately.

21. What medical therapies are available?

Treatment of DM in cats can be approached by administration of either exogenous insulin or oral hypoglycemic agents, which increase insulin secretion, decrease peripheral insulin resistance, or decrease absorption of glucose from the intestinal tract.

22. When should medical therapies be used?

Insulin is the required initial therapy in ketotic patients or patients with significant systemic illness. Oral hypoglycemic agents may be used as the initial mode of therapy in relatively healthy cats with uncomplicated diabetes. Once initial glucose toxicity is resolved with insulin therapy, it may be possible to substitute oral hypoglycemic agents for insulin injections in some cats.

23. How is insulin classified?

Various insulin formulations are available. Insulin can be categorized according to source (e.g., beef, pork, or human recombinant) or type (based on onset and duration of action: short-acting, intermediate-acting, or long-acting.). Insulin is a 51-amino acid protein molecule. Several amino acid residues vary between species. Feline insulin is most similar to bovine (1-amino acid difference), followed by porcine (3-amino acid difference), and finally human (4-amino acid difference).

24. How may insulin source affect efficacy?

Variations in amino acid residues between exogenous and endogenous insulin may cause immune stimulation. Although believed to be rare, significant antibody formation against administered insulin can lead to insulin resistance. Formation of a low antibody titer, however, may actually help prolong the duration of insulin action, a desirable effect. In most situations, clinically important differences are not observed when using various sources of insulin in diabetic cats.

25. What types of insulin are available?

Characteristics of Insulin Types and Insulin Requirements for Diabetic Cats

TYPE	PRODUCTS*	SOURCE	U/ML	ROUTE	ONSET OF ACTION	AVERAGE TIME OF PEAK EFFECT	DURATION OF ACTION
Short-acting							
Regular	Humulin R	Human	100	IV, IM, SQ	10–30 min	1–5 hr	4–10 hr
	Novolin R	Human					
	Velosulin R	Human					
Intermediate-acting							
Lente	Humulin L	Human	100	SQ	< 1 hr	2–8 hr	6–14 hr
	Novolin L	Human					
NPH	Humulin N	Human	100	SQ	0.5–3 hr	2–8 hr	4–12 hr
	Novolin N	Human					
Long-acting							
PZI	PZI	Beef/pork	40	SQ	1–4 hr	3–12 hr	6–24 hr
Ultralente	Humulin U	Human	100	SQ	1–8 hr	4–16 hr	8–24 hr

IV = intravenous, IM = intramuscular, SQ = subcutaneous, NPH = neutral protamine Hagedorn, PZI = protamine zinc insulin. Humulin (Eli Lilly, Indianapolis, IN), Novolin and Velosulin (Novo Nordisk, Princeton, NJ), PZI (Blue Ridge Pharmaceuticals, Greensboro, NC).
From Feldman EC, Nelson RW (eds): Canine and Feline Endocrinology and Reproduction, 2nd ed. Philadelphia, W.B. Saunders, 1996, p 360, with permission.

26. When should short-acting insulin be used?

Short-acting insulin generally is reserved for sick diabetic cats when immediate reduction of blood glucose is desired, especially if ketoacidosis is present. Regular insulin can be adjusted frequently without significant concern for overlapping or prolonged effects of a single dose. Because intensive monitoring generally is required, its use is limited to hospitalized patients. If ketoacidosis or other complications are present at the time of diagnosis of DM, therapy with longer-acting insulin should be initiated only after resolution or stabilization of these problems.

27. When should intermediate- or long-acting insulin be used?

If no significant complications are present at diagnosis, long-term therapy with longer-acting insulins can be initiated. The choice between an intermediate- or long-acting type is based most commonly on personal preference. The classification as intermediate- or long-acting is based on humans, and both types of insulin are typically required twice daily in cats. All of these insulins have been used successfully in cats, but individual responses vary. Ultralente insulin may be associated with inconsistent absorption in approximately 33% of cats. If use of Ultralente leads to a poor response, another type of insulin may be more effective.

28. Can insulin mixtures be used to treat diabetic cats?

Occasionally insulin mixtures are used to treat human diabetics. Commercially available mixtures usually contain a combination of regular and NPH insulin in various percentages. Insulin mixtures may be useful when the onset of action of an intermediate-acting insulin alone is too slow, allowing periods of unacceptable hyperglycemia, but this requirement is rare in cats. Administration of insulin mixtures is often associated with hypoglycemia in veterinary patients.

29. How should insulin therapy be initiated?

The recommended starting dose of intermediate- and long-acting insulin ranges between 1 and 3 units (about 0.25 U/kg) subcutaneously once or twice daily (see table in question 25). In general, intermediate-acting insulins are more potent than long-acting insulins; thus the recommended starting dose of intermediate-acting insulins is lower. It is always better to err on the side of underdosing when therapy is started than to cause hypoglycemia with an overdose. If insulin therapy is to be started while the cat is in the hospital, blood glucose should be measured during the period when peak insulin effect is predicted to detect hypoglycemia if it develops. Using the lower end of the dosing range and once-daily therapy in the case of long-acting insulins may be a safer method of instituting therapy at home.

30. When does the insulin dose need to be changed?

Changes in insulin therapy are almost always needed, especially during initial management. Weight changes and resolution of glucose toxicity often play an important role during early stages of therapy. The need for changes in therapy is best determined by performing a blood glucose curve. No changes in insulin dose should be made sooner than 4–6 days after starting a given dose unless hypoglycemia occurs. This period is required for equilibration of blood glucose concentration.

31. When should a blood glucose curve be performed?

A blood glucose curve is performed after modification of insulin therapy and after an appropriate equilibration period. Glucose curves also are used as a routine monitoring tool every few months for long-term management of diabetic patients or at any time if clinical signs recur.

32. How is a blood glucose curve performed?

A blood glucose curve is made by measuring blood glucose concentration every 2 hours for a duration equal to or greater than the insulin administration interval (usually 12 or 24 hours). Blood samples may be obtained via a large-bore catheter placed at the beginning of the monitoring period or multiple venipunctures.

33. How are blood glucose curves interpreted?

The parameters that need to be assessed include the time required after injection for peak insulin effect to occur, the blood glucose nadir at the time of maximal effect, and the duration of insulin action. Blood glucose nadir values determine whether changes in insulin dosage are needed. The duration of insulin action determines the frequency of insulin administration.

34. How should insulin dose be changed with regard to blood glucose curve results?

Ideally, blood glucose values should be maintained between 100 and 200 mg/dl during any 24-hour period. This goal is rarely achieved. In most instances, it is hoped that blood glucose can be maintained under 300 mg/dl to help limit disease complications. Dosage changes should be based on blood glucose nadir values. An ideal glucose nadir is between 80 and 150 mg/dl. Nadirs above this range require increases in insulin dose. In most cases, incremental increases of 0.5–1 U per dose of insulin are appropriate. Values < 80 mg/dl require decreases in insulin dose of 10–25%. Remember that stress from hospitalization and procedures may cause blood glucose concentrations to be higher than during a cat's normal routine at home. Hypoglycemia can be life-threatening and always should be avoided.

35. How should the insulin dosing interval be determined?

Duration of insulin action is estimated by determining the period from insulin administration through the blood glucose nadir to the time when blood glucose concentration exceeds approximately 200–250 mg/dl. Once-daily insulin administration is used if the duration of insulin action is between 22 and 24 hours. If the duration of action is 10–14 hours, twice-daily insulin therapy is given, or a longer-acting insulin, if available, may be tried. For durations of action between these ranges (i.e., 15–20 hours), changes in insulin type or dose may be needed. If a long-acting insulin such as Ultralente or PZI is used, twice-daily administration of an intermediate-acting insulin, with an initial 10–25% decrease in dose, may be ideal. If a 12-hour dosing interval is not an option for owners, a small dose of regular insulin 16–18 hours after the morning dose may be tried. Caution should be used with this type of protocol because of the increased risk of hypoglycemia.

36. What is the Somogyi phenomenon?

When blood glucose levels fall below normal, counterregulatory hormones such as epinephrine and glucagon are released, quickly causing a marked hyperglycemia that can persist for hours. The hypoglycemia and subsequent physiologic response resulting in hyperglycemia are known as the Somogyi phenomenon. Prolonged hyperglycemia during a glucose curve or clinical signs of continued polyuria and polydipsia at home may be consistent with either an inadequate insulin dose or excessive insulin administration and rebound hyperglycemia. It is important to differentiate between the two before increasing insulin dosage by documentation of the blood glucose nadir. Because blood glucose values can change very quickly in response to counterregulatory hormones, excessively low blood glucose nadirs can be missed when performing a standard curve with blood glucose measurements every 2 hours. It may be necessary to perform extra glucose measurements around the time of peak insulin effect.

37. What special considerations are needed for interpreting or performing a glucose curve?

Because of the stress and associated physiologic response during hospitalized blood glucose curves, some cats are hyperglycemic throughout the testing period, falsely giving the appearance of poor diabetic control. Unnecessary increases in insulin doses may be made, putting the patient at risk for hypoglycemia. If stress-induced alterations of blood glucose curve values are suspected, hospitalization and catheter placement 24 hours before starting a glucose curve allow time for environmental adjustment and minimize handling during the glucose curve.

38. What is the best use for measurement of glycosylated proteins?

Because poorly controlled diabetic cats can have normal levels of glycosylated proteins and well-controlled diabetic animals can have elevated concentrations, they may best be used to monitor trends in an individual patient. Concentration of one of the glycosylated proteins can be measured when a cat is first diagnosed, and changes in the protein levels can be used to help assess control.

39. What period of glycemic control do glycosylated proteins reflect?

The period of glycemic control reflected by glycosylated proteins is a factor of the life span of the measured protein. In cats, glycosylated hemoglobin and fructosamine reflect glycemic control over the previous 1–2 months and 1–2 weeks, respectively.

40. What should be done for a previously well-controlled cat when therapy is no longer effective?

Insulin source, administration, and handling as well as feeding practices should be evaluated. Recent changes in insulin vials and vials more than 2 months old are suspect. Site of insulin administration also may play a role; absorption may be suboptimal in the interscapular region as compared with the lateral thorax or flank. If these factors are not a problem, a glucose curve should be performed to rule out insulin-induced hyperglycemia and to gauge insulin effectiveness. Changes in body weight, introduction of drugs such as corticosteroids or megestrol, endogenous sources of progesterone in intact females, and concomitant disease, especially urinary tract, skin, and respiratory infections, can alter diabetic control. The presence of other diseases, such as hyperthyroidism, renal disease, hyperadrenocorticism, and acromegaly, may need to be considered.

41. What is insulin resistance?

Insulin resistance is defined as the need for an insulin dose > 2.2 U/kg to maintain adequate glycemic control. Most well-controlled animals require insulin doses of < 1 U/kg. Insulin resistance should be suspected when hyperglycemia persists throughout the day despite doses > 1.5 U/kg. When insulin resistance is suspected, the same steps used to determine the cause of lack of control apply. True insulin resistance can be caused by many factors.

Causes of Insulin Resistance

Drugs: glucocorticoids, progestins
Endocrine disorders: acromegaly, hyperadrenocorticism, hyperthyroidism
Hyperlipidemia
Infection
Insulin antibodies
Ketoacidosis
Malnutrition
Neoplasia
Obesity

42. How is insulin resistance treated?

The best treatment is to remove the underlying cause. If this solution is not feasible, large doses of insulin may be necessary to maintain euglycemia, if control is possible at all.

43. What are oral hypoglycemic agents?

Oral hypoglycemic agents consist of several categories of drugs used for treatment of type 2 DM in humans. They include sulfonylureas (glipizide, glyburide, glimepiride), biguanides (metformin), thiazolidinediones (troglitazone, rosiglitazone), alpha-glucosidase inhibitors (acarbose), and transition metals (chromium, vanadium). Several of these agents have been tried in feline diabetics with variable success.

Oral Hypoglycemic Agents

PROPOSED MECHANISM OF ACTION	GENERIC DRUG (BRAND NAME)	DOSE	POTENTIAL SIDE EFFECTS	SHOWN TO BE EFFECTIVE IN SOME CATS
Sulfonylureas				
Increase insulin secretion and sensitivity Reduce hepatic glucose production	Glipizide (Glucotrol)	2.5–5.0 mg/cat PO 2–3 times/day	Hepatotoxicity Hypoglycemia Vomiting	Yes
	Glyburide (Micronase, Diabeta)	0.625 mg/cat PO every 24 hr	Same as above	No?
	Glimiperide (Amaryl)	Unknown (human dose: 1–4 mg/day)	Same as above	No
Biguanides				
Inhibit hepatic glucose production	Metformin (Gluco-phage)	Unknown (human dose: 500–750 mg/day)	Anorexia Vomiting	No
Thiazolidinediones (glitazones)				
Increase insulin receptor sensitivity	Rosiglitazone (Avandia)	Unknown (human dose: 4–8 mg/day)	Hepatotoxicity Cardiac failure	No
	Pioglitazone (Actos)	Unknown (human dose: 15–45 mg/day)	Same as above	No
Alpha-glucosidase inhibitors				
Impair glucose absorption from GI tract	Acarbose (Precose)	12.5–25 mg/cat with meals	Flatulence Soft stool, diarrhea	Yes
Transition metals				
Increase insulin receptor sensitivity	Vanadium	0.2 mg/kg/day in food or water	Anorexia Vomiting Diarrhea Renal disease	Yes
	Chromium	200 µg/cat PO every 24 hr	Unknown	No

PO = orally.
Glucotrol and Micronase: Pfizer, New York; Diabeta and Amaryl: Aventis, Bridgewater, NJ; Glucophage: Bristol-Myers Squibb, New York; Avandia: SmithKline Beecham, Philadelphia; Actos: Takeda, Lincolnshire, IL; Precose: Bayer, Pittsburgh.

44. How do oral hypoglycemics work?
Sulfonylureas increase pancreatic insulin secretion. Thiazolidinediones sensitize tissues to the effects of insulin. Biguanides are believed to act primarily by inhibiting hepatic glucose release as well as improving peripheral insulin sensitivity. How transition metals reduce blood glucose remains unclear. Possibilities include increasing insulin responsiveness at postreceptor sites, increasing insulin receptor numbers, or functioning as an insulin cofactor. Alpha-glucosidase inhibits dietary fiber digestion, decreasing postprandial glucose absorption.

45. What types of oral hypoglycemic agents have been shown to be useful in diabetic cats?
The sulfonylurea glipizide is used most commonly; it is the only oral hypoglycemic agent tested in a large number of diabetic cats. Little information is available about the efficacy and safety of other hypoglycemic agents in cats. Reports of the use of troglitazone and biguanides suggest that they may not be efficacious. The α-glucosidase inhibitor acarbose appears to have mild glucose-lowering effects and may be a useful adjunct to insulin therapy. Gastrointestinal side effects are common, however, and may outweigh the benefits. Vanadium may alleviate clinical signs of early type 2 DM.

46. Which cases are appropriate for trial therapy with glipizide?
Glipizide therapy may be most ideal in stable, nonketotic diabetic cats with mild clinical signs and normal body weight. Debilitated or ketoacidotic cats are not good candidates for glipizide. Glipizide should be tried if owners refuse to give insulin injections. Many owners who initially refuse to administer insulin subsequently agree to try insulin treatment after glipizide therapy has failed.

47. How is glipizide used in diabetic cats?

An initial dose of 2.5 mg per cat twice daily with food is recommended. Clinical signs, body weight, and medication side effects, including vomiting and icterus, should be monitored. Blood glucose, urine glucose and ketones, and liver enzyme concentrations should be checked after 1–2 weeks. If no problems have occurred, the dose may be increased to 5 mg twice daily. After 2 weeks, the cat should be reexamined and a 10–12-hour glucose curve performed. Blood glucose values < 200 mg/dl and absence of glycosuria indicate a therapeutic response. Hypoglycemia may occur in cats receiving glipizide. If response is inadequate, therapy can be continued and re-assessed every 4 weeks as long as ketoacidosis or significant weight loss and clinical signs do not develop. Response to therapy can take as long as 12 weeks. Some cats respond only when the dose is increased to 7.5 mg 2 or 3 times/day. If no response occurs after 12 weeks, glipizide administration should be discontinued and insulin therapy started. If a clinical response occurs, glipizide therapy should be stopped, and the serum glucose reevaluated in 1 week. If hyperglycemia recurs, glipizide therapy should be reinstituted, starting at half the previous dosage. If normoglycemia persists, appropriate dietary therapy should be continued and the cat routinely monitored for recurrence of clinical signs and hyperglycemia. Normoglycemia may be maintained for 12–14 months or longer.

48. What should be done if side effects occur with initiation of therapy?

Clinical signs of vomiting or icterus are usually transient. If they occur, medication should be discontinued for 5 days. If problems resolve, glipizide can be reinstituted with a gradually increasing dose. A dose of 1.25 mg twice daily can be given for 7 days. If no problems occur, the dose can be increased to 2.5 mg once daily for 7 days followed by 2.5 mg twice daily for 14 days. If problems are still absent, a dose of 5 mg twice daily can be given. If problems recur, glipizide should be stopped and insulin therapy instituted.

49. Clinical signs resolve with glipizide therapy, but blood glucose values remain consistently > 200 mg/dl. What may be the cause?

Partial responses to glipizide do occur, but stress hyperglycemia is also a possibility. Glycosylated hemoglobin or fructosamine should be measured or urine glucose assessed at home. If therapy appears to be adequate, glipizide can be continued. If control is inadequate, glipizide should be discontinued and insulin therapy started.

50. How effective is glipizide treatment?

Approximately 35–45% of cats respond to long-term therapy. Which cats will respond cannot be predicted.

51. What serious complications may occur in diabetic cats?

Diabetic ketoacidosis (DKA), hyperosmolar diabetes mellitus (HDM), and insulin overdose resulting in serious hypoglycemia can be life-threatening complications.

52. How does DKA occur?

Insulin deficiency results in an inability of peripheral tissues to utilize glucose. A relative excess of insulin counterregulatory hormones (glucagon, cortisol, catecholamines, growth hormone) occurs, perpetuating hyperglycemia. Without adequate amounts of insulin, peripheral tissues must use nonglucose energy sources, and adipose stores are mobilized. Free fatty acids undergo transformation in the liver to triglycerides or ketone bodies (including β-hydroxybutyrate, acetoacetate, and acetone). Because of the relative excess of counterregulatory hormones, particularly glucagon, ketone production predominates. Normally, peripheral tissues metabolize ketones, and their acidic nature is buffered primarily by bicarbonate. In diabetics, production can exceed utilization, and buffering systems are overwhelmed. The result is ketosis, ketonuria, and metabolic acidosis.

53. What clinical abnormalities are observed in DKA?

Vomiting, anorexia, lethargy, and depression are often reported. In previously undiagnosed diabetic patients, prior history may include clinical signs typical of DM. On physical examination, dehydration, weakness, tachypnea, and a strong acetone odor on the breath may be noted. When metabolic acidosis is severe, slow deep breathing (Kussmaul respiration) may be observed. Pathology findings usually support dehydration, metabolic acidosis, hyperglycemia, ketonemia, ketonuria, and electrolyte deficiencies, especially of sodium and potassium. Elevated liver enzymes and azotemia (usually prerenal) are also common.

54. How is DKA typically treated?

Treatment of DKA requires fluid replacement, restoration of electrolyte and acid–base balance, and reduction of hyperglycemia. Appropriate fluid and insulin therapy and identification and treatment of any underlying disease that may have precipitated the DKA are critical in achieving these goals.

55. What fluid and electrolyte therapies are used in DKA?

Adequate fluid should be administered to resolve dehydration within the first 24 hours of treatment. Normal saline is the fluid of choice. Potassium supplementation is required in patients with DKA, even if serum potassium concentration is normal to elevated on initial blood work, unless contraindicated by the presence of another disease. Because insulin therapy and correction of acidosis cause extracellular potassium to move into cells, therapy may cause severe, life-threatening hypokalemia. Typically 20–40 mEq of potassium are added to each liter of fluids, but higher levels may be needed. Potassium concentrations should be monitored as frequently as every 2–4 hours during initial therapy. Treatment of acidosis with bicarbonate therapy is not typically needed unless the acidosis is severe (arterial pH < 7.1). Replacement of circulating fluid volume and initiation of insulin therapy, which promotes metabolism of ketoacids, typically results in rapid normalization of acid–base balance. Like potassium, total body phosphorus levels also may be low despite normal levels on initial blood work; with treatment, phosphorus shifts into cells. Although development of severe hypophosphatemia is uncommon, it can be life-threatening. Phosphorus levels should be monitored regularly during initial therapy, and supplementation should be given if serum levels drop to < 2.0 mg/dl.

56. How is insulin therapy given in DKA?

Regular crystalline insulin is recommended. Because patients are dehydrated, insulin is administered intramuscularly or intravenously rather than subcutaneously to ensure absorption. If given intramuscularly, the initial starting dose is 0.2 U/kg with subsequent hourly doses of 0.1 U/kg as needed. Blood glucose levels should be monitored hourly. Because rapid reductions in blood glucose may result in cerebral edema, blood glucose levels should be maintained above 250 mg/dl for at least the first 4–6 hours. When blood glucose concentrations fall to 250 mg/dl or less, 2.5% or 5% dextrose should be added to the fluids. Insulin administration is then reduced to every 4–6 hours with dose adjustments, as needed, to control blood glucose values while avoiding hypoglycemia.

57. How is insulin administered intravenously?

Insulin can be given intravenously via continuous rate infusion (CRI) at a dose of 1.1 U/kg per 24 hours, allowing easy dose adjustments and avoiding problems with parenteral insulin absorption. A simple method of approximating this dose is to add the number of units equivalent to the body weight in kilograms to a 250-ml bag of normal saline and administer the fluid at a rate of 10 ml/hr (e.g., for a 4-kg cat, 4 units of regular insulin are added to 250 ml of fluid and administered at 10 ml/hr). When blood glucose concentration is < 250 mg/dl, the administration rate should be reduced as needed. Once clinical signs and ketonuria resolve, longer-acting insulin therapy is instituted.

58. How does HDM occur?

As in DKA, hyperglycemia results in osmotic diuresis with water and electrolyte disturbances. However, decreased renal excretion of glucose occurs in HDM, resulting in extreme hyperglycemia (usually > 600 mg/dl). Severe hyperglycemia causes an increase in serum osmolality, altering the osmotic gradient between extracellular and intracellular compartments and shifting water into the extracellular space. Severe tissue dehydration results from renal water loss as well as the shift of water out of the cells.

59. What clinical abnormalities are seen in HDM?
Neurologic abnormalities, including ataxia, disorientation, seizures, and coma, may be observed in HDM because of severe dehydration of neurologic tissue. Other historical findings similar to those noted for uncomplicated DM and DKA may be reported. Laboratory abnormalities usually include severe hyperglycemia, glycosuria (typically without ketonuria), azotemia, metabolic acidosis, and hyperosmolality (typically > 350 mOsm; normal = 285–310 mOsm). Serum osmolality can be estimated with the following formula:

$$\text{Serum osmolality} = 2(Na + K) + glucose/18 + BUN/2.8.$$

where Na = sodium, K = potassium, and BUN = blood urea nitrogen. Potassium abnormalities as seen with DKA also may occur with HDM.

60. How is HDM treated?
Treatment goals of HDM are similar to those for DKA. Treatment requires replacement of body fluids, reduction of excessive hyperglycemia, and restoration of electrolyte and acid–base balance. Appropriate fluid and insulin therapy is critical. The major difference between treating HDM and DKA is the increased risk of cerebral edema. During development of HDM, the brain accumulates idiogenic osmoles, osmotically active substances, as a mechanism to prevent dehydration of neurologic tissue. If serum osmolality decreases suddenly as a result of rapidly declining blood glucose, idiogenic osmoles do not have time to dissipate. The resultant osmotic gradient shifts water intracellularly, causing cerebral edema. Therefore, fluid deficit replacement and lowering of serum blood glucose concentration should be done slowly over a period of 24–48 hours by using smaller insulin doses than for DKA and adding dextrose to the fluids as necessary.

61. What happens with insulin overdose?
Overdosage of insulin results in hypoglycemia, which, in turn, can cause lethargy, depression, weakness, ataxia, seizures, or coma.

62. How is insulin overdose treated?
Owners should be educated about the clinical signs of hypoglycemia and instructed to apply corn syrup to oral mucous membranes if they are observed. In the hospital, an initial intravenous bolus of 50% dextrose (0.5–1 mg/kg), diluted at least 1:1 with normal saline or a balanced electrolyte solution, should be given slowly. A maintenance drip of 5% dextrose should then be started. Insulin therapy should not be reinitiated until hyperglycemia is maintained without dextrose therapy. This process may take several days, depending on the severity and duration of the hypoglycemia. Insulin therapy should be modified to prevent further episodes.

63. What is the prognosis for cats with DM?
The prognosis for cats with DM depends, in part, on owner commitment to treatment, concurrent diseases, and ease of glycemic control. In general, a guarded long-term prognosis has been suggested.

64. What important factors should owners be aware of in regard to treatment?
Owner education is critical for successful treatment. The commitment and costs required to maintain a diabetic pet should be made clear. Consistency in insulin injections or medication and feeding schedule is essential. The likelihood that dysregulation problems will be encountered during treatment should be discussed. Insulin handling and administration should be demonstrated. It is often helpful to observe the client handle and administer insulin to ensure that directions are clear and mistakes are not made. Owners should be educated about the clinical signs of hypoglycemia as well as dysregulation and be given instructions for intervention and the need for reevaluation.

65. What is acromegaly?

Acromegaly is a condition of excessive growth hormone (GH) production and secretion.

66. What causes acromegaly?

Acromegaly in cats results from a functional pituitary tumor, of which approximately 90% are macroadenomas (i.e., > 1 cm in diameter). Excessive GH has anabolic effects that may result in overgrowth of connective tissue, bone, and viscera. These effects are mediated by growth hormone-stimulated production of insulin-like growth factor-I (IGF-I) or somatomedin by the liver. Catabolic effects of GH result primarily from insulin antagonism and subsequent abnormalities in carbohydrate and fat metabolism. The net effect is promotion of hyperglycemia and ketogenesis. DM has developed in all acromegalic cats.

67. Describe the common signalment, clinical signs, and pathologic abnormalities.

Acromegaly typically occurs in older, castrated male cats. Clinical signs associated with the catabolic effects of GH tend to predominate. Typical clinical signs include polyuria, polydipsia, and polyphagia. Increases in body size with enlargement of the head, interdental spaces, and abdomen may be seen. Frequently, prognathism is present. Other abnormalities may include degenerative arthropathies; organomegaly of the heart, kidney, liver, or tongue; hypertrophic cardiomyopathy; and neurologic signs related to the presence of a pituitary mass. Hyperglycemia and glycosuria are due to DM. Hypercholesterolemia, hyperphosphatemia, elevated liver enzymes, hyperproteinemia, renal azotemia, and mild erythrocytosis also may be observed.

68. How is acromegaly diagnosed?

Feline acromegaly can be diagnosed with computed tomography or magnetic resonance imaging for visualization of a cranial mass. Documentation of increased serum GH or IGF-I levels also may be useful (Animal Health Diagnostic Laboratory, Endocrine Diagnostic Section, Michigan State University, East Lansing, MI). A commercial GH assay, however, is not currently available in the U.S. Compatible pathologic abnormalities and clinical signs also support the diagnosis.

69. How is acromegaly treated?

Radiation therapy has had short-term success in some cases. Administration of a synthetic somatostatin (octreotide) as a means of counteracting the effects of IGF-I has not been promising. Dopamine agonists have been used successfully in human acromegalics but have not been evaluated in cats.

70. What is the prognosis of acromegaly in cats?

Long-term prognosis of cats with acromegaly is poor. Because of the typically slow-growing nature of pituitary tumors in this disease, short-term prognosis may be good to guarded with reported survival times of 4–42 months. However, control of DM in cats with acromegaly is difficult; insulin doses as high as 100–200 U/day are required if the acromegaly is not controlled.

BIBLIOGRAPHY

1. Behrend EN, Greco DS: Treatment of feline diabetes mellitus: Overview and therapy. Comp Cont Educ Pract Vet 22:423–439, 2000.
2. Behrend EN, Greco DS: Treatment of feline diabetes mellitus: Evaluation of treatment. Comp Cont Educ Pract Vet 22:440–452, 2000.
3. Feldman EC, Nelson RW: Disorders of growth hormone. In Feldman EC, Nelson RW (eds): Canine and Feline Endocrinology and Reproduction, 2nd ed. Philadelphia, W.B. Saunders, 1996, pp 38–66.
4. Feldman EC, Nelson RW: Diabetes mellitus. In Feldman EC, Nelson RW (eds): Canine and Feline Endocrinology and Reproduction, 2nd ed. Philadelphia, W.B. Saunders, 1996, pp 339–391.
5. Feldman EC, Nelson RW: Diabetic ketoacidosis. In Feldman EC, Nelson RW (eds): Canine and Feline Endocrinology and Reproduction, 2nd ed. Philadelphia, W.B. Saunders, 1996, pp 392–421.
6. Feldman EC, Nelson RW, Feldman MS: Intensive 50-week evaluation of glipizide administration in 50 cats with previously untreated diabetes mellitus. J Am Vet Med Assoc 210:772–777, 1997.

7. Goossens MMC, Feldman EC, Nelson RW, et al: Cobalt 60 irradiation of pituitary gland tumors in three cats with acromegaly. J Am Vet Med Assoc 213:374–376, 1998.
8. Goossens MMC, Nelson RW Feldman EC, et al: Response to insulin treatment and survival in 104 cats with diabetes mellitus (1985–1995). J Vet Intern Med 12:1–6, 1998.
9. Lutz TA, Rand JS: Pathogenesis of feline diabetes mellitus. Vet Clin North Am Small Anim Pract 25: 527–552, 1995.
10. Peterson ME, Taylor RS, Greco DS, et al: Acromegaly in 14 cats. J Vet Intern Med 4:192–201, 1990.
11. Whitley NT, Drobatz KJ, Panciera DL: Insulin overdose in dogs and cats: 28 cases (1986–1993). J Am Vet Med Assoc 211:326–330, 1997.

57. HYPERCALCEMIA AND HYPOCALCEMIA

Rebecka S. Hess, D.V.M.

1. What are the physiologic roles of calcium?

Intracellularly, calcium mediates numerous hormonal actions and is involved in the secretion of some hormones. In addition, it is involved in muscle contraction, nerve conduction, blood coagulation, and bone formation. Because calcium has many important physiologic roles, its concentration is tightly maintained throughout the body. Ionized calcium (Ca^{2+}) is the physiologically active form.

2. Which three hormones regulate serum Ca^{2+} concentration? From what tissue are they secreted?

1. Parathyroid hormone (PTH), which is produced by chief cells in the parathyroid gland.
2. 1,25-Dihydroxycholecalciferol (calcitriol, vitamin D_3), which is produced by sequential hydroxylation of vitamin D first in the liver and then in the kidney.
3. Calcitonin, which is produced primarily by C (parafollicular) cells in the thyroid gland.

3. How do these hormones control serum Ca^{2+}?

The three major target organs of these hormones are bone, kidneys, and gastrointestinal tract. PTH increases plasma Ca^{2+} concentration mainly by stimulating bone resorption but also by increasing renal reabsorption of Ca^{2+} and stimulating production of calcitriol. Calcitriol increases plasma Ca^{2+} concentration mainly by increasing Ca^{2+} absorption from the intestine but also by stimulating bone resorption and increasing renal calcium reabsorption. Calcitonin is the only one of the three hormones that lowers Ca^{2+} concentration; it acts mainly by inhibiting osteoclast action and promoting Ca^{2+} retention in bone. Calcitonin also increases urinary excretion of calcium. The role of calcitonin in adult animals is not completely understood but appears to be minimally important.

4. How is calcium transported in blood?

Approximately 50% of calcium in blood is ionized and biologically active. Approximately 40% is protein-bound, and the remaining 10% is bound to other serum factors such as phosphate or citrate.

5. What nonhormonal factors affect serum calcium concentration?

Acid–base status and concentrations of serum phosphorus and albumin may affect serum calcium concentration. Acidosis increases plasma concentration of total and ionized calcium. As hydrogen (H^+) ions increase in acidosis, they bind plasma proteins, displacing Ca^{2+}. This process increases ionized plasma Ca^{2+} concentration. Total serum calcium also changes with acid–base status. Ionized Ca^{2+} concentration is affected by phosphorus concentration, because some Ca^{2+} is bound to phosphorus. An increase in plasma phosphorus, therefore, may result in decreased plasma ionized Ca^{2+} concentration. Total calcium concentration is affected by albumin concentration because approximately 50% of calcium is bound to albumin. Therefore, an increase in albumin concentration results in increased total calcium concentration. Conversely, hypoalbuminemia can lead to lowered total serum calcium concentration.

6. Define hypercalcemia and hypocalcemia.

In cats a total calcium concentration > 11 mg/dl is typically consistent with hypercalcemia but varies with the laboratory; a total calcium concentration < 6.5 mg/dl is consistent with significant hypocalcemia. However, ionized Ca^{2+} concentration is a more accurate and physiologically significant measure. For example, it is possible to have an abnormal total calcium measurement and normal ionized calcium concentration; if ionized calcium is normal, calcium balance overall is considered normal. Therefore, whenever possible, calcium concentration should be assessed by measurement of ionized Ca^{2+}.

7. Since serum proteins affect total calcium concentration, can total calcium concentration be corrected for serum protein concentration as in dogs?

Unlike dogs, no formula in cats can be used to correct the total serum calcium concentration for serum protein concentration.

8. How does hypercalcemia affect the kidneys?

Hypercalcemia has a profound effect on the kidneys. It may be associated with calcium deposition in any soft tissue but is particularly important in the kidneys (nephrocalcinosis). Renal tubular epithelial cells, damaged from mineralization, slough into the tubular lumen, resulting in cast formation and tubular obstruction. Renal injury is further propagated by hypercalcemia-associated vasoconstriction, which results in ischemic damage. Hypercalcemia also results in excessive secretion of calcium in urine (hypercalciuria), which predisposes animals to formation of calcium-containing uroliths.

9. Does hypercalcemia affect any other organs adversely?

Hypercalcemia usually is associated with bone resorption, which may lead to loss of normal bone architecture and pathologic fractures. Hypercalcemia also can cause polyuria with compensatory polydipsia by interfering with the response to antidiuretic hormone. Cardiac arrhythmias due to decreased intraventricular conduction may develop in some cases and are characterized by prolonged PR interval, atrioventricular block, and QRS-complex prolongation. Experimentally hypercalcemia has induced acute pancreatitis in cats by facilitating activation of pancreatic enzymes and causing pancreatic hypersecretion, but the clinical significance of these experimental findings is not known. In humans, hypercalcemia is associated with hypertension, increased platelet aggregation, thrombosis, and atherosclerosis, but whether these effects occur in cats has not been determined.

10. What clinical signs are associated with hypercalcemia in cats?

Clinical signs associated with hypercalcemia may be mild and nonspecific. The most common clinical signs in cats are gastrointestinal and include vomiting (observed most frequently) and diarrhea or constipation. Polyuria, polydipsia, neurologic signs (mainly mental dullness), anorexia, and lethargy are also common. If cystic calculi are present, clinical signs associated with the lower urinary tract (i.e., hematuria, stranguria) may be expected. If renal failure has developed, appropriate clinical signs may be present.

11. Describe the physical examination findings in cats with hypercalcemia.

Physical examination findings are usually nonspecific but may be related to the cause of hypercalcemia. For example, in one report of cats with primary hyperparathyroidism, 3 of 7 cats had a palpable parathyroid mass. A thorough physical examination should be performed in every cat with hypercalcemia to assess the parathyroid glands and kidneys, to detect palpable tumors, and to determine whether concurrent diseases are present.

12. What are the differential diagnoses for hypercalcemia?

The numerous possibilities can be remembered by the mnemonic **GOSH DARN IT**:

G = **G**ranulomatous disease, in which activated macrophages can produce calcitriol

O = **O**steolytic disease, which, if severe, can cause mild hypercalcemia.

S = **S**purious result, due to artifactual elevation of serum calcium measurement by lipemia or hemolysis (depending on laboratory technique)

H = **H**yperparathyroidism

D = Vitamin **D** toxicosis, which is seen after ingestion of cholecalciferol rodenticides

A = **A**ddison's disease, in which hypoadrenocorticism affects renal calcium excretion and gastrointestinal calcium absorption.

R = **R**enal failure

N = **N**eoplasia

I = **I**diopathic disease

T = **T**emperature; severe hypothermia may cause hypercalcemia

13. Which are the most common causes of hypercalcemia in cats?

Neoplasia, chronic renal failure, and primary hyperparathyroidism.

14. How does malignancy cause hypercalcemia?

Hypercalcemia of malignancy may result from various neoplasms, but the most common in cats are lymphosarcoma and squamous cell carcinoma. Other neoplasias associated with hypercalcemia in cats include leukemia, osteosarcoma, fibrosarcoma, undifferentiated sarcoma, and bronchogenic carcinoma. Perianal apocrine gland adenocarcinoma, multiple myeloma, thyroid adenocarcinoma, and mammary tumors are common causes of malignant hypercalcemia in dogs but not cats. Hypercalcemia of malignancy is often due to excessive secretion of parathyroid hormone-related peptide (PTHrP), a peptide that can bind to PTH receptors and mimic PTH. Alternatively, various osteoclast-activating factors may be secreted from neoplastic cells.

15. How does renal failure cause hypercalcemia?

Hypercalcemia of chronic renal failure is incompletely understood, but it may be due to lack of renal phosphorus excretion. Hyperphosphatemia results, and the phosphorus can complex with the calcium, resulting in a transient decrease in plasma Ca^{2+} concentration and compensatory secondary hyperparathyroidism. Another possible explanation for hypercalcemia of chronic renal failure is that loss of renal mass results in decreased calcitriol production. Because calcitriol inhibits PTH synthesis, decreased calcitriol concentration results in secondary hyperparathyroidism.

16. What is the underlying cause of primary hyperparathyroidism? How is it diagnosed?

Primary hyperparathyroidism in cats is usually due to a PTH-secreting parathyroid adenoma. Diagnosis is made by measurement of serum PTH concentration. With hyperparathyroidism, PTH is in the upper end of or above the normal range.

17. What other diseases have been associated with hypercalcemia?

- Nonparathyroid endocrine disorders, such as diabetes mellitus, hyperthyroidism, and, rarely, hypoadrenocorticism
- Infectious diseases, such as feline infectious peritonitis, toxoplasmosis, actinomycosis, atypical mycobacteriosis, nocardiosis, and cryptococcosis
- Lower urinary tract disease
- Liver disease
- Bone marrow disease, such as myelodysplasia and myelofibrosis

Whether some of these actually cause the hypercalcemia (e.g., liver disease) is unclear. Furthermore, urolithiasis is a common condition reported in association with hypercalcemia, but it is the result rather than the cause. In addition, mild hypercalcemia may be a normal finding in young animals.

18. How does measurement of serum phosphorus concentration aid in ranking differential diagnoses?

Primary hyperparathyroidism, vitamin D toxicosis, and neoplasia can be difficult to distinguish. With a neoplasm that secretes PTHrP or primary hyperparathyroidism, serum phosphorus is in the low-normal to below-normal range, because PTH and PTHrP increase renal phosphorus excretion. With vitamin D toxicosis, serum phosphorus is in the high-normal to above-normal range because vitamin D increases gastrointestinal phosphorus absorption.

19. How is hypercalcemia treated?

The most important component of treatment for hypercalcemia is treatment of the underlying disease. For example, if the hypercalcemia is secondary to lymphosarcoma, the most effective approach is treatment of the neoplasia. Similarly, if the cat has primary hyperparathyroidism, a parathyroidectomy is recommended. However, symptomatic treatment of hypercalcemia is warranted when clinical signs associated with hypercalcemia are severe and must be addressed before establishing the diagnosis and treating the primary cause of hypercalcemia.

20. What is the commonly used symptomatic treatment for hypercalcemia?

The most common modes of symptomatic treatment are correction of fluid deficits, saline diuresis, and furosemide administration. The sodium load that occurs with saline diuresis promotes increased renal calcium excretion. Once the cat is well hydrated, furosemide may be added. By inhibiting the sodium-potassium-chloride cotransporter in the thick ascending limb of the loop of Henle, furosemide decreases sodium reabsorption, which, in turn, causes increased calcium excretion.

21. What other options are availabcle for symptomatic therapy of hypercalcemia?

Other modes of treatment for hypercalcemia include administration of prednisone or calcitonin. Prednisone should be given only after a diagnosis has been confirmed. Prednisone may obscure a diagnosis of lymphosarcoma, potentially for weeks to months. Glucocorticoids increase urinary calcium secretion, possibly by decreasing tubular calcium reabsorption, and decrease gastrointestinal absorption. Calcitonin promotes hypocalcemia by increasing calcium retention in bone and by increasing urinary excretion of calcium.

22. Describe the pathophysiology associated with hypocalcemia.

The most important changes observed with hypocalcemia are due to increased neuromuscular excitability, which causes spontaneous skeletal muscle contraction, tetany, and possibly seizures. Effects of hypocalcemia on other organs are less dramatic and less important clinically.

23. What clinical signs are associated with hypocalcemia?

The most obvious clinical signs are neuromuscular, and the most common of these are nervousness, seizures, and tetany. Other neuromuscular signs include tense or aggressive behavior, depression, facial or foot pruritus, muscle spasms, cramping, pain, twitching, tremors, stiff gait, weakness, and disorientation. Inappetence, weight loss, vomiting, and diarrhea also may occur.

24. Describe the physical examination findings in cats with hypocalcemia.

Physical examination findings also are related mostly to neuromuscular disturbances and may include seizures or muscle fasciculations. Other nonspecific findings, such as weakness, depression, fever, hypothermia, and dehydration, may be present. Lenticular cataracts are common in humans with hypoparathyroidism and have been reported in hypoparathyroid cats.

25. What are the differential diagnoses for hypocalcemia?

Overall, the most common form of hypoparathyroidism in the cat is iatrogenic, subsequent to thyroidectomy. The most common cause of spontaneous hypocalcemia is chronic renal failure. Spontaneous hypoparathyroidism is rare. Hypocalcemia also occurs in cats with acute pancreatitis, intestinal malabsorption of vitamin D or other causes of vitamin D deficiency, eclampsia, ethylene glycol toxicity, or malnutrition and in cats that have received phosphate-containing enemas or transfusion with a large volume of citrated blood. Because calcium binds to serum proteins, hypoalbuminemia can cause a low total serum calcium measurement. However, the biologically active ionized calcium is normal and the total serum calcium measurement insignificant.

26. How is hypocalcemia treated on an emergency basis?
Emergency treatment consists of intravenous administration of calcium in the form of 10% calcium gluconate (5–15 mg/kg given slowly over 10–30 minutes). The electrocardiogram should be monitored during administration. If bradycardia, premature ventricular complexes, or prolongation of the PR interval or QRS complex is observed, calcium administration should be discontinued until the problem resolves; infusion should then be reinitiated at a slower rate. If oral supplementation with vitamin D and calcium is needed (e.g., primary hypoparathyroidism), a continuous rate intravenous infusion or subcutaneous administration of calcium is necessary to maintain adequate serum calcium concentration until oral supplementation takes effect.

27. Does hypocalcemia always need to be treated as an emergency?
Hypocalcemia should be treated if clinical signs are present, but mild hypocalcemia does not always cause clinical signs.

28. How should hypocalcemia be treated on a long-term basis?
Some causes of hypocalcemia are self-limiting (e.g., pancreatitis, eclampsia) and resolve with the underlying disease. If long-term therapy is required (e.g., spontaneous hypoparathyroidism), oral vitamin D and calcium supplementation are required initially. Vitamin D preparations include vitamin D_2 (ergocalciferol), the synthetic form of vitamin D (dihydrotachysterol [DHT]), and vitamin D_3 (calcitriol). Ergocalciferol has the longest onset of action and time required for toxicity relief, followed by DHT and calcitriol. However, calcitriol is the most expensive and requires compounding; ergocalciferol is the least costly. Oral doses of vitamin D and calcium supplementation vary with the type of preparation and must be tapered to effect in each patient. If supplementation is used, close monitoring of blood urea nitrogen, creatinine, calcium, and phosphorus is imperative—usually every 2–3 days until the dose is titrated. Hypercalcemia and hyperphosphatemia may occur with oversupplementation. Depending on the vitamin D preparation, toxicity can last for weeks. Because it is safer, calcitriol is the treatment of choice. Calcium supplementation usually can be discontinued once the effect of supplemental vitamin D is complete. Iatrogenic hypoparathyroidism secondary to thyroidectomy may be transient, lasting from days to months. If parathyroid tissue was damaged but not removed during surgery, function may be decreased only temporarily. In such cases, vitamin D therapy can be discontinued when the parathyroid recovers.

Recommended Starting Doses of Compounds Used for Treatment of Hypocalcemia[3]

COMPOUND	DOSE	COMMENTS
10% Calcium gluconate	5–15 mg/kg given slowly IV over 10–30 min if clinical signs are present	Effective immediately
Calcium carbonate	0.5–1 gm of calcium/24 hr orally	Effective within 1–3 days; may cause inappetence
Calcitriol (vitamin D_3) (0.25-μg capsule or formulate)	0.03–0.06 μg/kg/24 hr orally	Effective within 1–4 days; toxicity resolution in 1–14 days. Dose is based on therapeutic recommendations for humans; no studies of dosing in cats

BIBLIOGRAPHY

1. Cotran RS, Kumar V, Collins T: The endocrine system. In Cotran RS, Kumar V, Collins T (eds): Robbins Pathologic Basis of Disease. Philadelphia, W. B. Saunders, 1999 pp 1121–1169.

2. Feldman EC, Nelson RW: Hypercalcemia and primary hyperparathyroidism. In Feldman EC, Nelson RW (eds): Canine and Feline Endocrinology and Reproduction. Philadelphia, W.B. Saunders, 1996, pp 455–496.

3. Feldman EC, Nelson RW: Hypocalcemia and primary hypoparathyroidism. In Feldman EC, Nelson RW (eds): Canine and Feline Endocrinology and Reproduction. Philadelphia, W.B. Saunders, 1996, pp 497–516.

4. Flanders JA, Scarlett JM, Blue JT, et al: Adjustment of total serum calcium concentration for binding to albumin and protein in cats: 291 cases (1986–1987). J Am Vet Med Asoc 194:1609–1611, 1989.

5. Ganong WF: Hormonal control of calcium metabolism and the physiology of bone. In Ganong WF (ed): Review of Medical Physiology. New York, Simon & Schuster, 1999, pp 365–377.

6. Kallet AJ, Richter KP, Feldman EC, et al: Primary hyperparathyroidism in cats: Seven cases (1984–1989). J AmVet Med Assoc 199:1767–1771, 1991.

7. Kruger JM, Osborne CA: Canine and feline hypercalcemic nephropathy. Part I: Causes and consequences. Comp Cont Educ Pract Vet 16:1299–1315, 1994.

8. Kruger JM, Osborne CA: Canine and feline hypercalcemic nephropathy. Part II: Detection, cure and control. Comp Cont Educ Pract Vet 16:1445–1458, 1994.

9. Layer P, Hotz J, Schmitz-Moormann HP, et al: Effects of experimental chronic hypercalcemia on feline exocrine pancreatic secretion. Gastroenterology 82:309–316, 1982.

10. McClain HM, Barsanti JA, Bartges JW: Hypercalcemia and calcium oxalae urolithiasis in cats: A report of 5 cases. J Am Anim Hosp Assoc 35:297–301, 1999.

11. Peterson ME, James KM, Wallace M, et al: Idiopathic hypoparathyroidism in 5 cats. J Vet Intern Med 5:47–51, 1991.

12. Saul M, Genuth D: Endocrine regulation of calcium and phosphate metabolism. In Berne RM, Levy MN (eds): Physiology. St. Louis, Mosby, 1998, pp 848–871.

13. Savary KCM, Price GS, Vaden SL: Hypercalcemia in cats: a retrospective study of 71 cases (1991-1997). J Vet Intern Med 14:184–189, 2000.

14. Waters CB, Scott-Moncrieff JCR: Hypocalcemia in cats. Comp Cont Educ Pract Vet 14:497–506, 1992.

V. Reproductive Problems

Section Editor: Deb Greco, D.V.M.

58. PYOMETRA AND VAGINAL DISCHARGES

Davyd Pelsue, D.V.M.

1. What causes vaginal discharge in cats?

There are many potential causes of vaginal discharge in cats. The character of the discharge, combined with history, clinical presentation, cytology, urinalysis, other laboratory results, vaginoscopy, and diagnostic imaging, can be used to achieve a definitive diagnosis in most cats.

Differential Diagnoses for Vaginal Discharge in Cats

Serous to mucoid discharge (cornified cells on cytology)
Proestrus to estrus
Mucopurulent discharge
Primary bacterial infection
Mycoplasma spp.
Coxiella burnetii
Secondary bacterial infection
Pyometra
Endometrititis
Vaginitis/vestibulitis

Foreign body	Urinary incontinence
Neoplasia	Urinary tract infection
Stricture	

Hemorrhagic discharge
Trauma
Neoplasia
Coagulopathy

2. How do I perform vaginal cytology?

A sterile cotton swab should be introduced gently into the vestibule by directing it dorsally first, above the clitoral fossa, and then cranially. Placing a drop of sterile 0.9 sodium chloride aids in the passage of the swab. The swab then is rolled along a microscope slide several times to provide areas of varying thickness, air-dried, stained, and examined microscopically. Attention should be given to the type of epithelial cell, presence of red blood cells or neutrophils, and presence or absence of bacteria. Material draining from the vulva can be examined but does not allow accurate determination of epithelial changes.

3. What is the significance of a mucopurulent vaginal discharge?

In cats, presence of a mucopurulent vaginal discharge is usually consistent with a secondary bacterial infection. Primary infections with *Coxiella burnetii* (see Chapter 88) and *Mycoplasma* spp. are thought to be unusual. Because *C. burnetii* is a significant public health risk, care should be taken when attending to the reproductive tract of cats.

4. Define pyometra and endometritis.

Pyometra is the abnormal accumulation of purulent material in the uterus. **Endometritis** is inflammation involving only the endometrial lining of the uterus.

5. What is the difference between closed and open pyometra?

These distinctions relate to the state of the cervix. A **closed cervix** leads to greater accumulation of purulent material within the uterus. Such patients, therefore, have a greater chance of developing secondary complications such as renal dysfunction, hepatic dysfunction, anemia, cardiac arrhythmias, coagulation abnormalities, peritonitis, and septic shock. An **open cervix** allows more drainage of the purulent material from the uterus, leading to a greater degree of vaginal discharge. It is not known what specific factors lead to the development of open vs. closed pyometra.

6. How does pyometra develop in cats?

Because cats are induced ovulators, pyometra develops less frequently in cats than in dogs. In cats, ovulation is required for the formation of corpora lutea, which subsequently secrete progesterone. The influence of progesterone on the uterus can lead to cystic endometrial hyperplasia. In addition, progesterone suppresses leukocyte activity in the uterus, which may allow accumulation of mucus and inflammatory exudate to build up in the uterus. Bacterial infection is thought to ascend from the vagina while the cervix is open during proestrus and estrus.

7. Does pyometra occur only in bred cats?

Pyometra can occur in bred or unbred cats. Adequate stimulation can lead to ovulation in some unbred cats. In others, use of progesterone-containing therapeutics may be the culprit.

8. What are the clinical signs of pyometra?

Vaginal discharge occurs in just over one-half of cases. Other common signs are anorexia, lethargy, vomiting, abdominal distention, and polydipsia/polyuria. Dehydration, a palpably enlarged uterus, and fever are frequently detected on physical examination. A large proportion of cases have been in estrus within the previous 4 weeks.

9. How is pyometra diagnosed?

A presumptive diagnosis often is based on history and clinical signs. In approximately 80% of cases, the uterus is visible as a tubular fluid/soft tissue structure on survey abdominal radiographs. Ultrasound can be used to distinguish between a fluid-filled and a gravid uterus. Cytology of the vaginal discharge, if present, generally reveals the presence of large numbers of neutrophils with intracellular bacteria. Extracellular bacteria may be present as a result of contamination from the lower urinary tract.

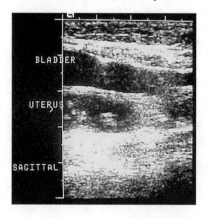

Ultrasound of an enlarged, pus-filled uterus in a cat with pyometra.

10. Are serum biochemical analysis and hematologic evaluation necessary in making the diagnosis?

Although these tests are not required, they are important in evaluating the whole patient. Common biochemical abnormalities associated with pyometra include hyperproteinemia, azotemia, and hypokalemia. Increases in liver enzyme activities also may be observed. The most common hematologic abnormality is leukocytosis with a regenerative left shift. These findings help to guide fluid and drug therapy and also act as baselines to monitor response to therapy. Cystocentesis should not be attempted in patients suspected of having pyometra.

11. What are the most common bacterial isolates associated with pyometra?

Escherichia coli, Streptococcus spp., and *Staphylococcus* spp. are isolated most commonly. However, the putrid odor and mixed flora commonly noted on cytologic exam suggest anaerobic involvement in many cats.

12. How is open pyometra treated in nonbreeding cats?

For nonbreeding cats, ovariohysterectomy (OHE) should be performed. Septic shock should be treated as indicated. A sample of the uterine discharge should be submitted for culture and antimicrobial susceptibility.

13. What alternative is available for breeding cats?

A dose of 0.1–0.25 mg/kg of natural prostaglandin $F_{2\alpha}$ ($PGF_{2\alpha}$) administered subcutaneously every 12–24 hours has proved to be effective. Before institution of therapy, a culture and antimicrobial susceptibility test of the vaginal discharge is submitted. Concurrent broad-spectrum antimicrobial therapy is instituted until antimicrobial susceptibility results return. Appropriate antimicrobial choices include beta-lactams (such as amoxicillin and cephalexin), potentiated penicillins (such as amoxicillin-clavulanic acid), and sulfonamides. Adverse reactions to $PGF_{2\alpha}$ are common, especially with the first dose. These reactions, which relate to $PGF_{2\alpha}$ actions in many tissues throughout the body, include vocalization, panting, restlessness, grooming, tenesmus, salivation, diarrhea, kneading, mydriasis, emesis, urination, and lordosis in decreasing frequency. $PGF_{2\alpha}$ is effective because it causes uterine contractions, thereby draining the pus-filled uterus. Therapy usually requires 3–5 days. Because of the common adverse reactions, hospitalization is recommended. This therapy has been shown to be 95–100% successful in returning queens to a normal estrous cycle, with 80% delivering normal litters. $PGF_{2\alpha}$ should be reserved for young, otherwise relatively healthy queens. It should not be used in sick animals because of delayed improvement of the patient.

14. How is closed pyometra treated?

OHE is the treatment of choice. Be careful to avoid the enlarged uterus when entering the peritoneal cavity to prevent rupture and spillage of uterine contents. Obtain a urine sample via cystocentesis at surgery for aerobic culture and antimicrobial susceptibility before abdominal closure. A culture of the uterine contents should be submitted for aerobic culture, anaerobic culture, and antimicrobial susceptibility. Empirical antimicrobial therapy is instituted until the results return. Appropriate choices include combination therapy with enrofloxacin and ampicillin or the use of a single-agent second-generation cephalosporin. These protocols have been used successfully in our hospital; they provide aggressive broad-spectrum coverage. Placement of drains through the cervix has been moderately successful in treating bitches with closed-cervix pyometra. This technique is more difficult in queens because of their smaller size, and results have not been reported in the veterinary literature. Therefore, their use is not recommended.

15. What are the complications of pyometra?

Death is the most serious complication, occurring in approximately 8% of cases. Causes of death include sepsis, bacterial peritonitis, renal dysfunction, and liver disease. Other complications include anorexia, lethargy, anemia, fever, vomiting, anesthetic problems, hemorrhage, dehiscence, recurrent estrus, fistulous tract formation, and urinary incontinence. Most of these complications resolve with appropriate symptomatic therapy.

16. Can cats develop "stump" pyometra?

Cats occasionally develop pyometra of the remnant of the uterus after OHE ("stump" pyometra). History, clinical signs, physical examination findings, and diagnosis are similar to those for open- or closed-cervix pyometra. The requirements for this condition are twofold: (1) remaining uterine tissue and (2) residual ovarian tissue. Treatment consists of laparotomy to remove the remaining uterine tissue and residual ovarian tissue. The incidence of stump pyometra has not been reported in the veterinary literature. At our hospital, few cases have been diagnosed. Cats can also develop "stump" granulomas, a condition that can mimic stump pyometra. In this case, the uterine stump forms a granuloma secondary to inflammatory reaction to the suture material. Treatment consists of removing suture material, if identifiable, or removal of residual uterine tissue, if needed.

BIBLIOGRAPHY

1. Davidson AP, Feldman EC, Nelson RW: Treatment of pyometra in cats, using prostaglandin $F_{2\alpha}$: 21 cases (1982–1990). J Am Vet Med Assoc 200: 825–828, 1992.
2. Hedlund CH: Surgery of the reproductive and genital systems. In Fossum (ed): Small Animal Surgery. St. Louis, Mosby, 1997, pp 544–549.
3. Kenney KJ, Matthiesen DT, Brown NO, et al: Pyometra in cats: 183 cases (1979–1984). J Am Vet Med Assoc 191:1130–1132, 1987.
4. Marretta SM, Matthiesen DT, Nichols R: Pyometra and its complications. Probl Vet Med 1:50–62, 1989.
5. Potter K, Hancock DH, Gallina AM: Clinical and pathological features of endometrial hyperplasia, pyometra, and endometritis in cats: 79 cases (1980–1985). J Am Vet Med Assoc 198:1427–1431, 1991.
6. Stone EA, Cantrell CG, Sharp NJH: Ovary and uterus. In Slatter (ed): Textbook of Small Animal Surgery. Philadelphia, W.B. Saunders, 1993, pp 1293–1307.

59. FAILURE TO CONCEIVE

Sara Stephens, D.V.M.

1. At what age do queens begin to cycle?

Female cats go through puberty, defined by onset of first estrus, at an average age of 5–10 months (range = 4–21 months). Longhaired breeds, Manx, and Persians may enter puberty later in life than shorthaired breeds. A body weight of 2.3–2.5 kg (5.0–5.5 pounds) usually must be achieved for a female cat to cycle. Cats reaching an appropriate age during the seasonal anestrus do not go though their first estrus until the breeding season begins.

2. Describe the seasonal cycle of the queen.

Cats are seasonally polyestrous, cycling for an average of 5.8 ± 3.3 days every 2–3 weeks from January through mid-October. The seasonal anestrus from mid-October through December is caused by day length: cats maintained under artificial lights for 12 continuous hours daily will cycle year round (13 ± 4.9 times/year) and may exhibit increased fertility. At least 10 hours of daylight (50 footcandles/hour) is necessary for cycling to occur. Fourteen to 16 hours of light (8–10 hours of dark) maximizes the number of cycling queens in a colony. Longhaired breeds tend to be more seasonal than shorthaired breeds.

The corpus luteum persists for about 30–40 days in the queen that ovulates and is not pregnant (pseudopregnancy). The next cycle may begin any time thereafter and usually does so within 10 days. The postpartum estrus usually occurs 2–3 weeks after weaning and is shorter in duration and less fertile. Anovulatory estrous cycles occur every 2–3 weeks during the breeding season if the queen is not bred, and it has been suggested that interestrous periods may lengthen during times of warm temperatures.

3. What hormonal factors are involved in estrus?

Gonadotropin-releasing hormone (GnRH) secreted by the hypothalamus stimulates the release of follicle-stimulating hormone (FSH) and luteinizing hormone (LH) from the pituitary gland. FSH stimulates the secretion of 17-β-estradiol from the ovarian follicle. The increasing serum concentration of estrogen triggers the follicular phases of proestrus and estrus.

4. What behavioral changes characterize proestrus and estrus?

Proestrus and estrus in the queen are not physically discernible by changes in genitalia or discharges from the reproductive tract but are recognized by behavioral changes. Proestrus is characterized by an increase in affectionate behavior and rubbing, treading with the rear feet, vocalizing, and decreasing hostility toward the male. Proestrus may not be noticed but typically lasts up to 2 days. Estrous behaviors include monotonous vocalization, increased affection, lordosis (elevation of the hindquarters with lateral deviation of the tail), and rolling. Estrus usually lasts about 6 days. Some studies suggest a shortening of estrus in bred cats, whereas others show no effect of breeding. Estrous behavior has been observed in pregnant queens, but true superfetation has not been proved.

5. How can estrus be determined?

A positive correlation has been shown between estrous behavior and cornified vaginal cytology. Cytologic studies may be useful in defining estrus in queens that exhibit no overt estrous behavior. Moistened sterile swabs should be passed quickly up to the end of the cotton, twirled, removed, and smeared. Individual cornified epithelial cells on a clear background ("clearing") indicate estrus. Cytology is also helpful in diagnosing ovarian remnant syndrome because the ovarian remnant produces estrogen.

6. What factors influence progesterone levels?

Bred cats or estrus cats that were induced to ovulate undergo a prolonged luteal phase (high serum levels of progesterone produced by the luteinized follicle). Serum progesterone concentrations rise 24–48 hours after ovulation and peak 25–30 days later.

The feline placenta either does not secrete progesterone or does so in amounts insufficient to maintain pregnancy. Apparently pregnancy-specific luteotropic hormones from the feline placenta or pituitary influence the life span of the corpus luteum. During pregnancy the corpora lutea continues to produce progesterone throughout gestation; serum concentrations gradually decline during the second half of pregnancy.

7. How does age affect reproduction in queens?

If the first pregnancy occurs after 3 years of age, litter size and neonatal survival remain poor. Reproductive performance declines after 6 years of age. Queens should be retired from breeding after 8 years of age.

8. What is the duration of pregnancy in queens? What are the reported conception rates?

The duration of pregnancy is 56–69 days (average 66 days). If pregnancy is defined as the first day on which serum progesterone concentration exceeds 2.5 ng/ml, the duration of pregnancy is 63–66 days. Reported conception rates in queens range from 68–83%.

9. When do queens ovulate?

Cats are induced ovulators; ovulation requires coital stimulation of the vagina. Lions are the only felid that are not induced ovulators. An external trigger, usually coitus, stimulates release of GnRH from the hypothalamus, which in turn stimulates release of LH from the pituitary within 2–4 hours. The LH causes ovulation in 1–3 days. The amount of LH released depends on the number of copulations and the time during the estrous cycle when copulation occurs. Queens bred only once exhibit great variability in serum LH concentrations, and fewer than 50% will ovulate. In one study, more than 4 copulations were required to ensure enough LH release to induce ovulation. More than 90% of normal domestic shorthair cats ovulate if bred 3 times daily for the first 3 days of estrus. Although cats are considered induced ovulators, several investigators have shown that 35–60% of colony cats spontaneously ovulate without coital stimulation or direct physical contact of any kind.

10. When does the tom reach puberty?
    Toms go through puberty, defined by first appearance of sperm in the ejaculate, at 8–12 months of age. Penile spines are androgen-dependent, appearing at 6–7 months of age and disappearing after castration. The testes usually are descended at birth.

11. What are the accessory sex glands in the tom?
    The prostate on the dorsolateral urethra at the neck of the urinary bladder and the bulbourethral glands, located craniolateral to the base of the penis.

12. When are mature toms capable of mating?
    Mature toms are capable of mating repeatedly over a 4–5-day period without a decrease in sperm numbers. Males maintained in 12 hours of continuous light daily show no seasonal change in breeding behavior or semen quality.

13. How is serum quality assessed?
    Retrograde ejaculation (movement of spermatozoa into the urinary bladder during ejaculation) occurs in normal toms. Collection of a urine sample by cystocentesis immediately after breeding, with centrifugation and examination of the sediment, may allow gross evaluation of semen quality.

14. Summarize the characteristics of normal feline semen.
    Semen volume varies from 0.01–0.77 ml with an average of 0.5 ml. Volume is larger with electroejaculation (EE) because of excessive stimulation of the accessory sex glands. Total number of spermatozoa in the ejaculate averages 50–60 million, with a reported range of 3–143 million, and is larger with manual collection than with EE. Motility is variable. Over 60% of the spermatozoa should have normal morphology.

15. Describe feline copulation.
    Copulation consists of mounting of the queen by the tom, positioning of the tom and erection of the penis, intromission and ejaculation by the tom, dismounting the queen, and the "after-reaction" by the queen. The "after-reaction" consists of striking out at the male (76.5%), vulvar licking (92.3%), and frantic rolling (100%). The entire copulation sequence is reported to take from 0.5–9 minutes, and the pair may copulate as many as 6 times in each of the first 2 hours. Copulation frequency then decreases. It is probably stimulation of the posterior vagina, not the cervix, that triggers ovulation.

16. Can artificial insemination be performed in cats?
    Semen collection techniques include manual collection with an artificial vagina (AV) and EE. The use of xylazine as an anesthetic in the EE process should be avoided because it may promote retrograde ejaculation of spermatozoa into the urinary bladder. Artificial insemination, either vaginal or intrauterine, is best performed 24–50 hours after medical induction of ovulation. Ovulation can be induced with GnRH administered intramuscularly at 25 µg or human chorionic gonadotropin (hCG) administered intramuscularly at 100 IU on the third day of estrus. Anesthesia of the queen before oocyte release may compromise ovulation. A pregnancy rate of 50% is reported for insemination at the time of hCG administration, with an increase to 75% if insemination is repeated 24 hours later.

17. What is infertility?
    Infertility is a broad term that refers to failure of the queen to breed, conceive, or carry a litter to term. Infertility is not a diagnosis, but a sign of one or more problems. A helpful approach to infertility in queens is to determine at which point in the breeding process the problem occurs:

1. Was estrus exhibited?
2. Was there a failure during the copulation process?
3. Did ovulation occur after copulation?
4. Was there a failure to conceive?

If the queen exhibits estrus < 18 days after being bred, no ovulation occurred. If the queen exhibits estrus at 36–40 days after breeding, she ovulated but was not fertilized. If the queen exhibits estrus after 60 days, abortion or resorption of the fetus occurred.

18. What are the three forms of anestrus in cats?
• Seasonal anestrus, related to decreasing day length (seen in most cats and considered normal)
• Primary anestrus (queens who have never exhibited estrus)
• Secondary anestrus (queens that have had at least one estrus cycle and then cease cycling)

19. What are the causes of anestrus in queens?
1. Queens housed with minimal lighting may enter a prolonged anestrus. Apparent lack of cycling may occur in queens with silent heat (normal ovarian follicular development in the absence of estrous behaviors). Silent heat may be more common in cats low in the social hierarchy. In one colony of 14 queens, 2 (14.3%) exhibited silent heat. Queens in silent heat diagnosed in estrus by weekly vaginal cytology will stand for breeding and are fertile.
2. True lack of cycling has been reported in cats with karyotypic abnormalities (38, XO), and in male pseudohermaphrodites (retained testes, female external genitalia). Cats that have errors in chromosomal sex may have gonads that are small, lack oocytes, or have both ovarian and testicular tissue (true hermaphrodites). Intersex cats may have normal karyotypes.
3. Ovarian dysfunction may result in persistent corpora lutea or luteal ovarian cysts that secrete progesterone (> 2 ng/ml). Such cats may not exhibit estrus. Luteal cysts should be confirmed with progesterone levels for several months before treating with prostaglandin $F_{2\alpha}$. Older queens may cycle less frequently.
4. Lack of cycling during false pregnancy (ovulation without conception) and nursing (lactational anestrus) is normal for cats. Lack of cycling also has been reported in cats infected with feline leukemia virus.

20. How can estrus be induced?
1. Housing a queen with other cycling queens and increasing day length to 12–14 hours may help to induce estrus.
2. FSH administered intramuscularly at 2 mg/day for 5 days should induce estrus in 4–5 days. Lower doses of FSH also may be effective: administer 2 mg on the first day, 1 mg on days 2 and 3, and 0.5 mg on days 4 and 5.
3. The GnRH analog, Decapeptyl (Organon, West Orange, NJ), may be administered subcutaneously at 1 µg/kg every 8 hours for 10 days or until signs of estrus behavior are noted.
4. Ultrapurified porcine FSH, divided into 5 daily subcutaneous doses for a total dose of 2.5 IU, followed on days 6 and 7 by 1.25 IU porcine FSH and 250 IU hCG given together intramuscularly, has resulted in supraovulation and an ovulation rate of 73%.

21. Do assays of pituitary and hypothalamic hormones help to diagnose anestrus?
The pituitary hormones, FSH and LH, and the hypothalamic hormone, GnRH, are persistently elevated in cats with ovarian/testicular aplasia or hypoplasia and after ovariohysterectomy and castration. The secretion of all three hormones is pulsatile. Because of their difficulty, assays are rarely attempted.

22. Can estradiol levels be used to diagnose anestrus?
Serum concentrations of estradiol are about a thousandfold less than those of progesterone and are often at or below the limits of detection of the assays used by many commercial endocrine laboratories. Estradiol concentrations also fluctuate widely and rapidly; thus measurement often

does not yield diagnostic results. However, estrogen levels may differentiate a queen with persistent anestrus from one with unexpressed estrus. During follicular phase (proestrus and estrus), the plasma estradiol concentrations are > 20 pg/ml. During anestrus and interestrus, the estrogen levels are < 20 pg/ml.

23. Describe the role of progesterone in the diagnosis of anestrus.

Progesterone may be assayed to differentiate pseudopregnancy from anestrus. Luteal phase serum progesterone concentration is > 2 ng/ml. If the progesterone level is < 1 ng/ml, no luteal tissue exists. The use of hormonal challenge testing may induce elevated progesterone. Blood is drawn 2–3 weeks after intramuscular administration of one 25-µg dose of progesterone. Less than 2 ng/ml indicates presence of functional luteal tissue and functional ovaries. Progesterone can be assayed to determine whether ovulation actually occurred after estrus induction with FSH- and GnRH-induced ovulation.

24. How is GnRH used to diagnose anestrus?

Intramuscular administration of a single 25-µg dose of GnRH causes a 20-fold increase in LH in anestrous queens and a 100-fold increase in estrous queens. Failure of serum LH to increase after GnRH administration indicates a possible pituitary problem. Failure of progesterone to increase after GnRH administration indicates prior ovariohysterectomy or gonadal dysfunction.

25. Discuss the role of vaginal cytology in the diagnosis of anestrus.

Vaginal cytology for detection of estrogen can be assessed every 1–2 weeks to detect queens in silent heat.

26. What causes persistent, nonovulatory estrus?

1. The queen may appear to be in constant heat because follicles form in overlapping waves. Persistent estrus may be behavioral rather than physiologic, and breeding may still lead to pregnancy.

2. Abnormally long estrus (> 16 days) and high serum estrogen levels may be due to functional cystic ovaries, functional granulosa cell tumors, or portosystemic shunts.

3. Granulosa cell tumors are the most common ovarian tumor in queens. These large unilateral tumors often are palpable; they may cause abdominal distention and produce signs of hyperestrogenism, including persistent estrus. Granulosa cell tumors are commonly malignant.

4. Ovarian remnant syndrome (ORS) is defined as the presence of functional ovarian tissue in a previously ovariohysterectomized queen. The interval between ovariohysterectomy and the first appearance of estrous behavior caused by ORS is variable, with a reported range of 2 weeks to 9 years. Individual cats may possess accessory lobes of the ovaries, but they are rare in domestic animals. All reported ovarian remnants have been found at the pedicle; in one study, 27% were bilateral.

27. Describe the diagnostic plan for cats with suspected persistent nonovulatory estrus.

1. Vaginal cytology is easily performed and is an inexpensive, accurate way to detect the presence of estrogen.

2. Ultrasound may demonstrate the presence of follicles or tumors, and serum estrogen concentrations may be elevated in queens with persistent estrus.

3. Intramuscular administration of hCG at 250 IU/day for 2–3 days or GnRH at 2.2 µg/ml/day for 3 days may luteinize follicular cysts.

4. Ovariohysterectomy is recommended if the queen does not respond quickly and ovulate.

28. What may cause copulation failure?

Because of the speed with which copulation occurs and the aggressive attitude of the cats during the process, it may be difficult to know whether copulation in fact has occurred. The queen's scream may be the only evidence that breeding has occurred. The queen should be introduced to the tom in his territory several days before estrus. Cats exhibit partner preference and may refuse to mate with one cat but mate with another. If female dominance precludes mating, the queen can be lightly sedated, a different male can be used, or 25 µg GnRH may be administered intramuscularly 1 hour before mating to increase the tom's sexual determination.

Vulvar, vaginal, and vestibular barriers, such as persistent hymenal remnants, annular strictures, hypoplasia, septal defects, and reproductive tract neoplasia, may exist in the queen. A vulvar stricture may develop in queens with a history of dystocia and preclude copulation. Contrast vaginography may be used to identify strictures and malformations.

29. What test determines whether ovulation has occurred?

Serum progesterone concentrations rise 24–48 hours after ovulation. A serum progesterone level > 2.5 ng/ml 48 hours after copulation confirms ovulation. Because progesterone is the same substance in all species, any progesterone assay may be used.

30. What causes ovulation failure?

More than 90% of normal domestic shorthair cats ovulate if bred 3 times/day for the first 3 days of estrus. Causes of ovulatory failure include breeding too late in the follicular cycle while follicles are regressing, too few breedings, and low male libido resulting in too few copulations.

The queen and tom should be allowed to breed repeatedly, and the frequency of the copulatory cry should be noted if it occurs. Ovulation may be induced physically by vaginal insertion of a metal or glass probe after breeding or medically by intramuscular administration of hCG at 250 IU on days 1 and 2 of estrus or GnRH at 25 µg on day 2 of estrus.

31. How can infertility in toms be recognized?

1. A sterile mating that induces ovulation causes the queen to enter the luteal phase (pseudopregnancy) for 45–50 days. This scenario should raise suspicion of infertility of the tom.

2. Testosterone concentrations may be nondetectable in normal intact male cats, and levels may need to be checked several times because of pulsatile secretion. Testosterone is best measured after challenge testing with either GnRH, administered intramuscularly at 25 µg with blood drawn 1 hour later (normal values = 17.3–41.6 nmol/L) or hCG at 250 IU/cat with blood drawn 4 hours later (normal values = 10.4–31.2 nmol/L). Testosterone levels should be greatest in intact toms, less in cryptorchid toms, and negligible in castrated toms.

32. How common are cryptorchidism and monorchidism in toms?

Of 1,345 cats in one study, 23 (1.7%) were cryptorchid and 2 (0.1%) were monorchid. Persian cats (29%) were overrepresented compared with other breeds (1.48%). Monorchid toms had bilateral ductus deferens, testicular arteries and veins, and cremaster muscles.

33. What are the characteristic features of cryptorchidism in toms?

- All toms with bilateral cryptorchidism have abdominally located testes.
- In toms with unilateral cryptorchidism, no predisposition for side has been noted. Of affected toms, 61% had abdominal and 39% had inguinal testes.
- A polygenic mode of inheritance for cryptochidism has been suggested, although in most species cryptorchidism has an autosomal recessive cause.

34. How should cryptorchid toms be managed?

All cryptorchid toms should be castrated bilaterally.

35. Does administration of exogenous testosterone stimulate spermatogenesis?

Testicular levels of testosterone are 50–100 times higher than serum levels. These high local levels produced by the Leydig cells stimulate spermatogenesis. Administration of testosterone does not increase spermatogenesis, however, because exogenous testosterone causes an increase in serum levels, which gives negative feedback to the pituitary to decrease LH levels. Decreased LH levels signal the Leydig cells to decrease the local production of testosterone and inhibit spermatogenesis.

36. What causes small testes in toms?

Small testes may be congenital in toms with an abnormal karyotype or acquired after fetal or neonatal panleukopenia infection. Calico and tortoiseshell male cats are often infertile. White coat is carried on an autosome. The gene for black or orange coat is carried on the X chromosome. Normal male cats with one X chromosome can exhibit either black or orange, but not both. Calico/tortoiseshell males must have two X chromosomes either as triploidy (39, XXY) or mosaicsim/chimerism (XX/XY, XXY/XY). Azoospermia is common because of seminiferous tubule dysgenesis.

37. What factors may contribute to poor libido in toms?

Age and timing may be factors in toms with low libido. Spermatogenesis begins at 5 months of age, and sexual maturity is completed by 9 months of age. Spermatogenesis and epididymal maturation take approximately 75 days. The quality of sperm decreases with age. Chronic infection can cause decreased sperm counts. Effusive feline infectious peritonitis can cause scrotal enlargement and associated testicular infection.

Diphallia, penile hypoplasia, and persistent penile frenula have been reported in cats. Adhesion of the penis to the prepuce may be a congenital lesion or result from inflammation. Hair may become impacted in rings at the base of the penis, precluding copulation after a normal mount, and can cause priapism (persistent erection). Prostate disease is uncommon in male cats.

38. How may poor libido in toms be managed?

If the tom is exhibiting poor libido, he should be housed separately from the queens. All toms should be allowed to breed within their established territories. Artifical insemination also may be used.

39. What tests are appropriate in all infertile toms and queens?

Serum biochemical panel, urinalysis, feline leukemia virus antigen test, feline immunodeficiency virus antibody test, and total T4 concentration. In appropriate situations, karyotyping may be informative.

40. How is early embryonic death differentiated from failure to conceive?

Pregnancy loss in the first 3 weeks of gestation is also called early embryonic death and cannot be distinguished from failure to conceive. Until an early pregnancy test becomes available for cats, early embryonic death is unlikely to be diagnosed or treated effectively.

41. What causes conception failure in the queen?

- Insufficient luteal phase due to premature luteolysis may cause a decline in progesterone < 1 ng/ml at 2–4 weeks after breeding. Serum progesterone concentrations < 2 ng/ml indicate lack of the luteal tissue necessary to continue pregnancy.
- Conception failure after copulation and ovulation may be due to cystic endometrial hyperplasia (CEH), subclinical uterine infection, lack of patency of the reproductive tract in the queen, or poor semen quality in the tom.
- Pyometra (CEH with overlying infection and subsequent development of purulent intrauterine fluid) occurs most commonly during the luteal phase of increased progesterone secretion in nonpregnant cats that were induced to ovulate. Bacteria ascend from the vagina more easily during this time. The organisms are usually from the normal vaginal flora; *Escherichia coli* is the most common isolate, but other organisms have been cultured.

42. Define CEH. What causes it?

CEH is a progressive, irreversible, proliferative change of the uterine lining. It is common in cats older than 5 years. CEH results from repeated exposure of the endometrium to estrogen and progesterone, and it cannot be induced experimentally with either hormone alone. Repeated ovulatory cycles that do not result in pregnancy can increase the risk of pyometra in older queens. Cats with CEH may be asymptomatic or infertile. Hyperactivity and pacing have been associated with infertility and CEH in 1 cat.

43. Describe the signs and symptoms of CEH and pyometra.

In one study of 25 cats with CEH or pyometra, 20 had corpora lutea on the ovaries at the time of ovariohysterectomy, despite no recent history of breeding or exposure to male cats.

Cats with pyometra present with variable signs, depending on the degree of cervical patency. Clinical signs reported in 183 cats with CEH/pyometra included vaginal discharge (59%), anorexia (40%), lethargy (32%), abdominal distention (17%), vomiting (16%), and polyuria/polydispia (9%). Leukocytosis and a left shift occur less commonly than in dogs; one study reported an incidence of 66% and 45%, respectively. See Chapter 58 for a discussion of treatment issues.

44. How should infertile queens be evaluated?

- In addition to the tests listed in question 39, infertile queens should be tested for toxoplasmosis.
- Ultrasound does not detect the normal uterus or ovaries, but fetal resorption with thickening of the uterine horns, endometritis, follicular cysts, and neoplasia may be detected.
- Infusion of saline into the uterine horns with a small-gauge needle can determine patency of uterine horns and oviducts. Both horns should fill uniformly, and saline should leak through the oviducts. The uterotubular junction is tight (closed) in proestrus.

45. Any final comments about infertility in cats?

The cause of most breeding disorders is inappropriate breeding management. Proper housing, nutrition, and preventative care, including vaccinations, and parasite and disease control, need to be discussed with the breeder. Timing of mating is also crucial and requires careful observation. It is important to work with the breeder through one or more estrous cycles. The highest fertility rate is seen in 1–6-year-old queens. Diagnostic evaluation of older females may not be warranted.

BIBLIOGRAPHY

1. Baldwin CJ, Peter AT: Use of ELISA test kit for estimation of serum progesterone concentrations in cats. Feline Pract 24:27–31, 1996.
2. Brockus CW: Endogenous estrogen myelotoxicosis associated with functional cystic ovaries in a dog. Vet Clin Pathol 27: 55–56, 1998.
3. Cain JL: Disorders of feline reproduction. In Morgan R (ed): Handbook of Small Animal Practice, 3rd ed. Philadelphia, W.B. Saunders, 1997, pp 645–648.
4. Feldman EC, Nelson RW: Feline reproduction. In Feldman EC, Nelson RW (eds): Canine and Feline Endocrinology and Reproduction. Philadelphia, W.B.Saunders, 1996, pp 741–768.
5. Grooters AM: Diseases of the ovaries and uterus. In Birchard SJ, Sherding RG (eds): Saunders Manual of Small Animal Practice, 2nd ed. Philadelphia, W.B. Saunders, 2000, pp 1016–1028.
6. Johnson CA: Disorders of the estrus cycle. In Nelson RW, Couto CG (eds): Small Animal Internal Medicine. Mosby, St. Louis, 1998, pp 842–844, 846–892.
7. Johnston SD, Root MV: Managing infertility in purebred catteries. In August JR (ed): Consultations in Feline Internal Medicine, 3rd ed. Philadelphia, W.B. Saunders, 1997, pp 581–586.
8. Millis DL, Hauptman JG, Johnson CA: Cryptorchidism and monorchism in cats: 25 cases (1980–1989). J Am Vet Med Assoc 200:1128–1130, 1992.
9. Purswell BJ: Diseases of pregnancy and puerperium. In Leib MS, Monroe WE (eds): Practical Small Animal Internal Medicine. Philadelphia, W.B. Saunders, 1997, pp 463–464.
10. Root M, Johnston S, Olson P: Estrous length, pregnancy rate, gestation and parturition lengths, litter size, and juvenile mortality in the domestic cat. J Am Anim Hosp Assoc 31:429–432, 1995.
11. Root Kustritz MV: Reproductive abnormalities of the queen, infertility in the queen and tom cat, and anatomy and normal reproductive physiology of the queen and tom cat. A series of lectures presented at the American Association of Feline Practitioners' Winter Meeting in Park City, Utah, February 6 and 7, 2000.
12. Schwartz S: Stereotypic pacing associated with ovarian and uterine anomalies in a Siamese cat. Feline Pract 24:29–32, 1996.
13. Soderberg SF: Infertility and disorders of breeding. In Birchard SJ, Sherding RG (eds): Saunders Manual of Small Animal Practice, 2nd ed. Philadelphia, W.B. Saunders, 2000, pp 1050–1059.
14. Von Reitzenstein M, Archbald LF: Theriogenology question of the month. J Am Vet Med Assoc 216:1221–1223, 2000.

60. PREGNANCY LOSS

Sara Stephens, D.V.M.

1. What is the length of gestation in queens?
The duration of pregnancy in queens is 56–69 days. In one cat colony, the average gestation was 66 days. The onset of pregnancy is defined as the first day on which plasma progesterone is > 2.5 ng/ml. If progesterone rise is used as a starting point, the length of gestation in the queen is 63–66 days.

2. How is pregnancy diagnosed in queens?
After ovulation, the egg is in the oviduct for 5–6 days. Fertilization is presumed to occur within the oviducts. The blastocysts become localized and recognized as spherical enlargements within the uterus by day 13–14 of gestation. Trophoblastic attachment occurs near day 15 after coitus. The fetal stage occurs when the thoracic cavity of the embryo closes at about 4 weeks when the fetuses have a crown-to-rump length of 2.4 cm. Progesterone concentrations during the first 20 days of pregnancy are similar to those in pseudopregnant cats. After day 20, the plasma progesterone is increased in pregnant cats. The placenta begins to synthesize and secrete progesterone after day 30 of gestation.

In one study, a serum progesterone concentration > 5 ng/ml at 6 or more days after breeding was indicative of pregnancy with 81% accuracy. Pregnancy diagnosis in the cat is easily accomplished by ultrasonography 16–30 days after breeding, by abdominal palpation 21 days after breeding, and by radiography 37 days after breeding. If a single radiograph is not definitive for pregnancy, a second radiograph taken 5 days later should show progressive mineralization from proximal to distal. Fetal viability is best accessed by ultrasonography, which may demonstrate the fetal heart as early as day 16. Fetal numbers and gestational age are best assessed by radiography.

3. In what ways can pregnancy loss occur?
- Embryonic death
- Resorption of the fetus
- Abortion of the fetus
- Retention of mummified or macerated fetuses
- Stillbirths

4. What causes pregnancy loss in queens?
There are maternal, fetal, and environmental causes of pregnancy loss in the queen. Often the outcome depends on the stage of gestation when the queen is affected; gestational age of the fetus determines whether a nonviable fetus will be resorbed or aborted. Pregnancy resorption with no vulvar discharge occurs before day 30 of gestation. Abortion occurs in the second half of pregnancy. Any fetus delivered before 60 days of gestation will be stillborn.

5. Define abortion.
Abortion results in fetal loss and occurs after mid-gestation in cats. Abortion usually is accompanied by discharge of fluid or fetal tissue. Any hemorrhagic vaginal discharge is abnormal during the second-to-eighth week of pregnancy. The queen may remain clinically healthy despite resorbing fetuses or aborting a litter. Queens may abort part of litter and carry the rest to term. Sometimes it is difficult to tell an aborting cat from one with an open cervix pyometra.

6. What maternal factors may cause abortion?
Any serious systemic disease can result in resorption or abortion of fetuses. Uterine diseases that can cause abortion include chronic endometritis, cystic endometrial hyperplasia, and uterine adhesions.

7. How is abortion diagnosed?

Definitive diagnosis of abortion is hard to make unless a fetus is expelled. Habitually aborting queens with multifocal placental necrosis and subsequent fetal autolysis during the third or fourth week of gestation have been reported.

8. What are some environmental causes of pregnancy loss in queens?

Poor nutrition, trauma, and stress, such as shipping or bringing the cat to a new home, can cause pregnancy loss in a queen. Taurine deficiency causes a postimplantation defect that is associated with a decline in progesterone.

9. How is early embryonic death differentiated from failure to conceive?

Pregnancy loss in the first 3 weeks of gestation is also called early embryonic death and cannot be distinguished from failure to conceive. Until an early pregnancy test becomes available for cats, early embryonic death is unlikely to be diagnosed or treated effectively.

10. Can low plasma progesterone cause pregnancy loss?

Yes. Low progesterone makes the endometrium a poor substrate for implantation of the blastocyst. This clinical scenario appears as an infertile cycle. Resorption or abortion can also occur when the plasma progesterone is < 1 ng/ml; serum progesterone concentrations must be > 2 ng/ml to support pregnancy.

11. What is the source of gestational progesterone in cats?

The source of gestational progesterone in cats is debated. Studies have shown that cats have a normal pregnancy despite ovariectomy at 45–50 days' gestation, indicating a placental source of progesterone in late gestation. However, other recent studies have indicated that cats ovariectomized at day 45 of gestation abort; thus, the maintenance of the corpus luteum may be crucial for a normal pregnancy in the queen. To diagnose hypoluteoidism, both progesterone drop and early pregnancy have to be confirmed with ultrasound. Hypoluteoidism is probably an uncommon cause of pregnancy loss in the queen.

12. How is progesterone measured in cats?

Progesterone is measured by radioimmunoassay (RIA) and enzyme-linked immunosorbent assay (ELISA). The structure of progesterone does not vary among species; any progesterone assay may be used to determine progesterone levels in queens. Hemolysis and lipemia may affect results.

13. What may cause early embryonic death?

Possible causes of early embryonic death include taurine deficiency, abnormalities of follicular or luteal function, abnormalities of the genital tract, cystic endometrial hyperplasia, genetic fetal defects, and subclinical uterine infection.

14. What is the most common infectious cause of abortion in queens?

Viral agents are the most commonly reported infectious cause of abortion in queens. Examples include feline herpes virus 1 (FHV-1, rhinotracheitis), panleukopenia, feline infectious peritonitis (FIP), feline immunodeficiency virus (FIV), feline calicivirus, and feline leukemia virus (FeLV).

15. When does abortion due to FHV-1 occur?

Abortion secondary to FHV-1 usually occurs at 5–6 weeks of gestation and is probably secondary to upper respiratory infection in the queen. FHV-1 infection can result in abortion, mummification, and stillborns.

16. How does panleukopenia affect pregnancy in queens?

Panleukopenia virus attacks tissue with a high mitotic rate. The queen may have adequate neutralizing antibodies for self-protection but insufficient immunity for the developing fetuses.

Panleukopenia can cause early embryonic loss, abortion of mummified or macerated fetuses, and stillbirths. Kittens also may be born blind, with hydrancephaly, and/or ataxia due to retinal, cerebral, and/or cerebellar degeneration. Prenatally infected kittens may have retinal dysplasia. Antemortem definitive diagnosis can be difficult, because many cats have antibodies against panleukopenia but titers only rise during acute viremia.

17. Discuss the role of feline coronaviruses in pregnancy loss.
Feline coronaviruses have been suggested as a cause of failure to conceive, abortion, stillbirth, and congenital defects as well as the fading kitten syndrome (kitten mortality complex). Abortion due to infection with FIP is thought to occur late in gestation and is associated with prolonged vaginal bleeding. However, an epidemiologic study failed to link feline coronavirus with reproductive failure or neonatal kitten mortality; thus its causative role in abortion is controversial.

18. How does FIV affect pregnancy in queens?
In utero transmission of FIV leads to several pathogenic consequences, including arrested fetal development, abortion, stillbirth, subnormal birth weights, and birth of viable, virus-infected, and asymptomatic but T-cell–deficient kittens.

19. Discuss the role of FeLV in pregnany loss.
FeLV has been reported to cause abortion from 3 weeks to term. FeLV can result in infertility, early embryonic death, resorption of fetuses, and abortion of normal-appearing fetuses. In late pregnancy, fetuses may acquire lymphocyte-associated virus transplacentally, or the neonate may be infected from the queen's milk or saliva. Such kittens may fail to thrive. The queen also may develop pyometra and endometritis due to immunosuppression and then become infertile. Seronegative healthy carriers have been identified. Positive cats should be removed from the cattery with retesting at 90-day intervals until no positive cats are identified on two consecutive tests. FeLV is a fragile virus. Routine cleanliness interrupts spread of disease in the environment. Vaccination of negative cats is also helpful.

20. What is the risk of abortion due to calicivirus?
To date, only 2 cats have had calicivirus isolated from the genital tract after abortion. Thus the true risk is unknown.

21. What are the bacterial causes of abortion in queens?
Bacterial infection of the uterus and subsequent pregnancy loss is uncommon in healthy cats housed in a clean environment. Cats aborting due to *Escherichia coli*, staphylococcal, or streptococcal uterine infection usually present with anorexia, depression, fever, straining, and a fetid, yellow-brown vaginal discharge. The discharge should be cultured, and amoxicillin therapy (22 mg/kg orally every 12 hr) should be instituted pending culture results. Bacterial abortion may occur in cats infected with FeLV secondary to virus-induced immunosuppression. The bacterial pathogens causing abortion are usually present in normal vaginal flora.

22. What are the rickettsial causes of abortion in queens?
Coxiella burnetii is a rickettsial agent that can cause abortion. Cats may acquire the infection by tick bites or ingestion or inhalation of organisms while feeding on infected body tissues or milk. Although the true incidence of this infection in cats in unknown, *C. burnetii* has been grown from the vagina of normal cats in Japan. There have been frequent reports of people becoming infected with Q fever after exposure to aerosols from a contaminated environment or fomites from feline parturient or aborted tissues (see Chapter 88).

23. Can protozoal agents cause abortion?
Toxoplasmosis is a common tissue protozoan that occasionally causes abortion. Most queens infected with toxoplasmosis are asymptomatic carriers, but systemically ill queens may abort because of placentitis. Toxoplasmic abortion usually occurs if the first exposure occurs early in gestation.

24. What drugs are associated with abortion or birth defects in cats?

Drugs associated with abortion include hormones (androgens, bromocriptine, estrogens, glucocorticoids), anticancer drugs, anesthetics (barbiturates, halothane, methoxyflurane), and chloramphenicol. Misoprostol causes abortions due to the effect of prostaglandin on the reproductive tract. Teratogenic drugs include primidone, griseofulvin, ketoconazole, amphotericin-B, ciprofloxacin, and enrofloxacin, nonsteroidal anti-inflammatory drugs, tetracycline, aminoglycosides, metronidazole, aspirin, propranolol, dimethylsulfoxide (DMSO), glucocorticoids, diethylstilbestrol (DES), estradiol cypionate (ECP), testosterone, mibolerone, progesterone, diazepam, midazolam, vitamin A, and vitamin D. Teratogens present during the first 26 days often cause cephalic, ocular, otic, and/or cardiac abnormalities, whereas those present in the next 26 days are more likely to cause palate, cerebellar, and/or urogenital defects.

25. What other factors may cause abortion?

Fetal causes of abortions include genetic fetal defects, such as X-monosomy, autosomal trisomy, and mosaicism. Uterine torsion, ectopic pregnancy and, possibly, hypocalcemia are rare causes of abortion. Females older than 7–8 years tend to cycle irregularly, to have smaller litters, and to have more problems with abortions and kittens with congenital defects.

26. Are all causes of stillbirths known?

The average rate of stillbirths is 12.9% with a range of 4.7–22.1%. Anatomic abnormalities are found in 20% of kittens that are stillborn or die within the first 3 days of life, and most congenital abnormalities have no identifiable cause. Most birth defects have no identifiable cause, and subsequent breedings are often uneventful.

27. What can be done to determine the cause of pregnancy loss?

Pregnancy can be confirmed by day 20 of gestation with ultrasound, and fetal viability can be monitored. Ultrasound also may be used to confirm pregnancy loss before day 20. Breeding records should be scrutinized to identify inherited problems. After an observed abortion, the queen should receive a thorough physical examination and ophthalmic examination. Routine tests in most cases include complete blood cell count, serum biochemical panel, FeLV antigen test, FIV antibody test, panleukopenia antibody test, *T. gondii* antibody test, urinalysis, and progesterone concentration. Hysterotomy can be done to obtain tissue for histology, microbial isolation, and karyotyping of fetal tissue. Necropsy and histopathology should be performed on aborted or stillborn fetuses.

28. What can be done to decrease pregnancy losses?

Vaccinations should be up to date, and queens should be given antihelmintics before breeding. All cats should be housed indoors in a clean environment. If the cats are gang-housed, multiple litter boxes should be provided and kept clean to lessen coronavirus exposure. The food should be of high quality; raw meat should not be fed during gestation to lessen the risk for toxoplasmosis. All breeding females should test negative for FeLV and FIV. No drugs causing abortion or birth defects should be given during pregnancy. Vaccines should not be given during pregnancy.

29. What contraceptives are available for cats?

Progestogens can prevent pregnancy in cats. Megestrol acetate (Ovaban; Schering-Plough, Kenilworth, NJ) is given at 2.5 mg orally every 24 hr for up to 2 months or 5 mg/day for 3 days, followed by 2.5 mg/week for up to 18 months. Side effects of progestogens in cats may be severe and include mammary carcinoma, mammary hypertrophy/fibroadenoma complex, uterine disease, diabetes mellitus, and suppression of the adrenal cortex. Progestogens are not approved for use as contraceptives in cats in the U.S. Preliminary studies in cats have shown that the slow-release subdermal implant levonorgestral (Norplant) is effective in suppressing estrus for 12 months with no adverse effects except the development of cystic endometrial hyperplasia.

Mibolerone (Checque; Pharmacia & Upjohn, Kalamazoo, MI), an androgen approved for use as a contraceptive in dogs, cannot be used safely in cats because the side effects include thyroid dysfunction, hepatocellular lesions with increased systemic arterial pressure and cholesterol, thickening of the cervical dermis, and clitoral hypertrophy. The mortality rate is significant with doses as low as twice the estrus suppression dose. Contraceptive vaccines that immunize against the zona pellucida surrounding the feline ova also may be used for contraception, but this method is not currently available.

30. How should an unwanted pregnancy be terminated?

No drugs are approved for feline pregnancy termination in the United States, but several protocols have been used. Mating should be confirmed with a vaginal smear to look for clearing (absence of noncellular debris) and sperm. Estrogen is not recommended immediately after mating, but megestrol acetate in a single oral dose of 2.0 mg during estrus has been reported to prevent implantation. Pregnancy termination in cats can be effected surgically (ovariohysterectomy) or medically. Medical methods include prostaglandin $F_{2\alpha}$ ($PGF_{2\alpha}$; Lutalyse, Pharmacia & Upjohn) at 500–1000 µg/kg for 2 days at mid-gestation; cloprostenol (Estrumate; Bayer, Shawnee Mission, KS) at 5 µg/kg subcutaneously for 2 days; and the prolactin inhibitor/dopamine agonist, cabergoline (Dostinex; Pharmacia & Upjohn), at 5 µg/kg orally for 10–12 days at mid-gestation. A combination of daily oral administration of cabergoline (5 µg/kg) and cloprostenol injections (5 µg/kg subcutaneously) every 2 days appears to be a reliable, safe, and practical method for terminating pregnancy at day 30 of pregnancy, when a diagnosis of pregnancy by palpation or ultrasonography can easily be made. All five queens treated in one study aborted in 9 ± 1 day without side effects except a mild hemorrhagic vulvar discharge. Progesterone concentrations were < 1 ng ml by day 38.

A $PGF_{2\alpha}$ abortifacient protocol, administered near day 45 of gestation, was effective in 3 of 4 cats in one study. On the first day, 0.2 mg/kg/day was given, followed by 0.5 mg/kg/day. The cats were treated subcutaneously twice daily until abortion occurred or for up to 5 days. All cats receiving $PGF_{2\alpha}$ had decreasing concentrations of progesterone during treatment. Cats that aborted had < 1 ng/ml, whereas cats that did not abort had > 1 ng/ml of progesterone. Cats should be hospitalized during the administration of prostaglandins. Nesting behavior may be observed 1–2 days before the abortion, and a temperature drop similar to the one observed with normal parturition may be seen within 24 hours of abortion.

BIBLIOGRAPHY

1. Baldwin C, Evans LE: Evaluation of natural prostaglandin therapy for pregnancy termination in the domestic cat. Feline Pract 28:16–21, 2000.
2. Baldwin CJ, Peter AT: Use of ELISA test kit for estimation of serum progesterone concentrations in cats. Feline Pract 24:27–31, 1996.
3. Cain JL: Disorders of feline reproduction. In Morgan R (ed): Handbook of Small Animal Practice, 3rd ed. Philadelphia, W.B. Saunders, 1997, pp 645–647.
4. Fascetti AJ: Preparturient hypocalcemia in four cats. J Am Vet Med Assoc 215:1127–1129, 1999.
5. Grooters AM: Diseases of the ovaries and uterus. In Birchard SJ, Sherding RG (eds): Saunders Manual of Small Animal Practice, 2nd ed. Philadelphia, W.B. Saunders, 2000, pp 1022–1026.
6. Johnson CA: False pregnancy, disorders of pregnancy, parturition, and the postpartum period. In Nelson RW, Couto CG (eds): Small Animal Internal Medicine. St. Louis, Mosby, 1998, pp 889–892.
7. Johnston SD, Root MV: Managing infertility in purebred catteries. In August JR (ed): Consultations in Feline Internal Medicine, 3rd ed. Philadelphia, W.B. Saunders, 1997, pp 581–586.
8. Nagaoka H, Sugieda M, Akiyama M, et al: Isolation of *Coxiella burnetii* from the vagina of feline clients at veterinary clinics. J Vet Med Sci 60:251–252, 1998.
9. Onclin K, Verstegen J: Termination of pregnancy in cats using a combination of cabergoline, a new dopamine agonist, and a synthetic PGF2 alpha, cloprostenol. J Reprod Fertil Suppl 51:259–263, 1997.
10. Purswell BJ: Diseases of pregnancy and puerperium. In Leib MS, Monroe WE (eds): Practical Small Animal Internal Medicine. Philadelphia, W.B. Saunders, 1997, pp 465–466.
11. Root Kustritz MV: Reproductive abnormalities of the queen, and anatomy and normal reproductive physiology of the queen and tom cat. A series of lectures presented at the American Association of Feline Practitioners' Winter Meeting in Park City, Utah, February 6 and 7, 2000.
12. Smith KC: Herpesviral abortion in domestic animals. Vet J 153:239–244, 253–268, 1997.
13. Van Vuuren M, Geissler K, Gerber D, et al: Characterization of a potentially abortigenic strain of feline calicivirus isolated from a domestic cat. Vet Rec 144:636–638, 1999.

VI. Polysystemic Problems

Section Editor: Michael R. Lappin, D.V.M., Ph.D.

61. OBESITY AND POLYPHAGIA

Heather E. Connally, D.V.M., M.S.

1. Define obesity.
Obesity is defined as a body weight 20% above the ideal weight for breed, sex, and species. Obesity is the most common nutritional disorder in cats (prevalence between 20% and 40%).

2. What are the primary differential diagnoses for an apparently obese cat?
Before a definitive diagnosis of obesity is made, a thorough physical examination should be performed to rule out other conditions resulting in a large patient, such as pregnancy, peripheral edema, subcutaneous emphysema, intraabdominal organomegaly (especially hepatic or splenic enlargement), abdominal masses, or ascites (see Chapter 37).

3. How do you determine whether a patient is obese?
Body condition scoring scales range from 1 to 5 or 1 to 9. In both scales, 1 is an emaciated animal. Depending on the scale used, 3 or 5 is an ideal weight and 5 or 9 is grossly obese. The assessment is based in part on ability to palpate the outline of the ribs. Ribs obscured by subcutaneous fat suggest obesity, whereas ribs that are readily visible without palpation indicate emaciation.

4. What are the risk factors for obesity in cats?
Risk factors associated with obesity in cats include apartment dwelling, inactivity, middle age, male gender, neutering, type of food, and mixed breeding. Overweight cats are more likely to be fed prescription diets rather than grocery store brands. In addition, purebred cats, such as Siamese and Abyssinians, are generally leaner than cats of mixed breed.

5. Can neutering lead to obesity?
Studies have demonstrated that ovariohysterectomy and castration result in a decrease in maintenance energy requirements in adult cats. Castrated males gain more weight as fat than intact males. In other studies, cats that were neutered at 7 weeks or 7 months of age had an increase in falciform ligament fat and body weight compared with intact controls. In addition, food intake increases significantly after neutering.

6. Which metabolic conditions are associated with weight gain and obesity?
Metabolic conditions that lead to obesity, such as hypothyroidism in dogs, are rare in cats. However, they may include hyperadrenocorticism (see Chapter 54), acromegaly (see Chapter 56), and hypothyroidism. In most instances, hypothyroidism and hyperadrenocorticism are iatrogenic, caused by treating hyperthyroidism (see Chapter 53) and overuse of glucocorticoids, respectively. Only one case of spontaneous adult-onset hypothyroidism has been documented in cats. Congenital hypothyroidism generally causes failure to thrive rather than obesity in affected kittens. If the abdomen of a kitten with congenital hypothyroidism appears distended, it is most likely secondary to constipation or obstipation, which can be confirmed radiographically. In cats with hyperadrenocorticism and acromegaly, it must be determined whether the enlarged abdomen is due to organomegaly or true obesity.

7. What are the potential negative sequelae of obesity?

Risks that have been associated with obesity in the cat include a higher likelihood for the development of hepatic lipidosis (see Chapter 30), diabetes mellitus (see Chapter 56), lower urinary tract disease, constipation (see Chapter 27), lameness (secondary to osteoarthritis and soft tissue injuries), nonallergic skin conditions, and possibly cardiac disease and exacerbation of chronic respiratory conditions. Risks associated with anesthesia and surgery also are increased in obese patients. Hepatic lipidosis generally is associated with a recent history of anorexia. Diabetes mellitus may be associated with a history of polyuria, polydipsia, polyphagia, and weight loss. Lower urinary tract disease generally accompanies a history of straining to urinate, frequent urination, or inappropriate urination. Constipated cats generally spend an excessive amount of time in the litter box, vocalize, strain to defecate, and may produce small amounts of watery feces. The most common skin problems associated with obesity include dry, flaky skin and feline acne. These abnormalities may reflect difficulties in grooming.

8. What are the most important historical findings in cats with obesity?

It is important to question the owner carefully about the eating habits of the obese cat, including diet type (both meals and snacks), amount, and frequency of feedings. This information allows calculation of daily caloric intake, which helps to determine whether caloric overconsumption contributes to obesity. In addition, it is important to gain insight into the energy expenditure of the cat. Factors to consider include whether the cat is housed primarily indoors or allowed indoors and outdoors, whether other animals live in the home, lifestyle and body appearance of the owner, and age-associated decrease in activity. Other historical habits of the cat, such as polyuria and polydipsia (see Chapter 39), can aid in the diagnosis of concurrent disease. Determine whether prescription drugs are administered; glucocorticoids, phenobarbital, cyproheptadine, benzodiazepines, and megestrol acetate increase appetite.

9. What must be done before implementing a weight-loss program?

First and foremost, it is essential that the owner recognizes the need for weight reduction in the cat and is willing to participate vigilantly in a weight-reduction program. During the initial examination, it is important to completely screen the patient's medical record and history for medical conditions that may be exacerbated by a change in diet (e.g., lower urinary tract disease, constipation, food sensitivity). In addition, a thorough physical examination should be performed as well as a minimal database of screening tests, including complete blood count (CBC), serum biochemical profile, and urinalysis. These laboratory data can be assessed for alterations in blood glucose, liver enzymes, and evidence of urinary tract disease. In addition, if problems arise during the program, the baseline laboratory data are available for reference.

10. What is the best diet to use for weight reduction?

Maintenance diets should not be used for a weight-loss program because the time taken to achieve the optimal weight is prolonged (over months) and owner frustration caused by the cat's constant attempts to obtain extra food may bring a premature end to the program. In addition, nutritional deficiencies may develop as important essential nutrients and micronutrients are underfed with restriction of maintenance-type diets. At this point the best diet for weight reduction is unknown. Published studies have demonstrated the efficacy of a high-fiber, low-fat diet in safely promoting weight loss in obese cats. High-fiber, low-fat diets also significantly improve insulin sensitivity in cats with subclinical or clinical carbohydrate intolerance. Low-fiber, low-fat diets also may be effective for weight loss as well as more palatable to cats. In addition, a recent study demonstrated that a high-fat diet in cats, unlike in people and dogs, may promote increased fat oxidation. This finding may mean that a high-fat, high-protein diet in cats can promote weight loss. At this time, however, no studies have been completed to determine the long-term efficacy and safety of either diet type.

11. How is a weight-loss program developed for an obese cat?

The diet must be palatable to the patient, and acclimation to the new diet must occur over 7 days. This approach helps to ensure that the new diet is tolerated. If it is not, a new diet must be chosen until an acceptable formulation is found. The amount of the specified diet that the cat should receive daily can be calculated from the formula and table below.

Divide the total daily food quantity into 2 or 3 meals per day. On recheck visits for weight determination every 2 weeks, be sure to use a single calibrated pediatric scale. The goal is to lose 1.0–2.0% of initial body weight per week over at least 16–18 weeks. This rate is safe and does not induce hepatic lipidosis. If the cat is not losing weight or if the body weight stabilizes before the goal weight is achieved, restrict caloric intake by 10%. If the weight loss is > 2.5% per week, increase caloric intake by 15%. Once the goal weight is achieved, the food dose can be recalculated based on maintenance energy requirement using a maintenance diet.

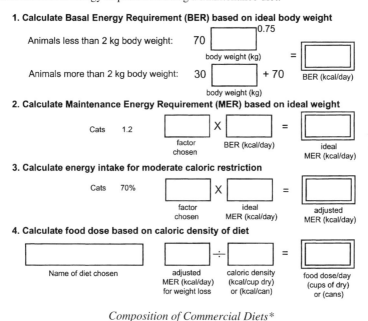

Composition of Commercial Diets*

PRODUCT	CALORIC CONTENT (AS FED BASIS)			FAT CONTENT (GM/100 GM DM)		PROTEIN CONTENT (GM/100 GM DM)	
	KCAL/GM[†]	KCAL/CUP–DRY[‡]	KCAL/CAN[§]	CAN	DRY	CAN	DRY
Hill's feline products							
Maintenance	4.1	503	447	25.5	23.0	45.3	33.8
Maint light	3.2	243	346	12.1	9.0	45.0	40.8
Growth	4.6	555	661	34.0	26.8	49.0	37.1
W/d	**3.2**	**244**	**377**	**16.8**	**9.3**	**41.5**	**38.8**
R/d	**3.0**	**226**	**296**	**9.1**	**9.1**	**36.0**	**37.1**
Purina feline products							
CNM UR	3.9	366	493	36.5	11.6	41.4	35.4
CNM NF	3.9	398	—	—	12.9	—	30.8
CNM OM	**2.8**	**283**	—	—	**7.7**	—	**37.0**
Iams feline products							
Lamb and rice	4.5	461	248	29.6	23.3	45.5	35.6
Less active[#]	**3.9**	**348**	**205**	**15.9**	**15.6**	**45.5**	**31.1**
Rest'd cal	**3.9**	**298**	—	—	**8.9**	—	**35.6**

* Weight reduction diets in boldface.
[†] Dry form only as example; can form differs slightly.
[‡] Volume reference: 8-oz. measuring cup.
[§] Hill's products: 14.25 oz per can; Purina products: 12.5 oz per can; Iams products: 6.0 oz per can
[#] Canned chicken and rice formula.
Hills Nutrition, Inc., Topeka, KS; Ralston Purina Company, St. Louis, MO; Iams Company, Dayton, OH.

12. Define polyphagia.

Polyphagia is food consumption in excess of caloric need. Because regions within the central nervous system (CNS) control hunger, satiety, and eating behaviors, polyphagia is classified as either primary (CNS problem), or secondary (systemic problem affecting the CNS).

13. What are the primary differential diagnoses for polyphagia?

Primary causes of polyphagia include psychogenic factors (e.g., stress, introduction of more palatable diet); destructive lesions of the satiety center, such as trauma and space-occupying lesions (neoplasia, abscess); and infection. Drugs such as glucocorticoids, anticonvulsants, antihistamines, progestins, benzodiazepines, and amitraz can induce polyphagia. The many potential causes of secondary polyphagia include increased metabolic rate (physiologic or pathologic), decreased energy supply, and disease states for which the mechanism is unknown. A physiologic increase in metabolic rate induced by cold temperature, lactation, pregnancy, growth, and increased exercise can cause an increase in feed consumption. Hyperthyroidism (see Chapter 53) and acromegaly (see Chapter 56) can cause pathologic increases in metabolic rate. Diabetes mellitus (see Chapter 56), hypoglycemia, decreased intake because of a low-calorie diet, and malassimilation syndromes (e.g., pancreatic exocrine insufficiency, infiltrative bowel disease, parasites [see Chapter 19], lymphangiectasia) can cause a decrease in energy supply that may lead to an increase in consumption. Diseases for which the cause of polyphagia is unknown include hyperadrenocorticism (see Chapter 54) and portosystemic shunt (see Chapter 35). In addition, diseases not commonly associated with polyphagia but for which it has been documented include feline infectious peritonitis (see Chapter 38), lymphocytic cholangitis (see Chapter 29), and spongiform encephalopathy.

14. How can the history aid in diagnosis of polyphagia?

The most important initial diagnostic tool is the history. On the basis of a thorough history many conditions can be ruled out, and possibly a diagnosis can be made. First, one must determine whether the increase in food consumption is accompanied by maintained weight, weight loss or weight gain. There may be no weight change early in the disease process. However, if the cat has gained weight, the cause is most likely primary or drug-induced. Physiologic polyphagia can lead to weight gain (e.g., pregnancy or growth) or maintenance of weight (e.g., lactation, living in a cold environment, increased exercise). Polyphagia secondary to pathologic conditions generally results in weight loss because the nutrient demand is not met. Exceptions include acromegaly and hyperadrenocorticism, which usually are associated with weight gain. History can reveal trauma, signs of CNS disease, new stress in the household (e.g., introduction of a new animal), current diet (more palatable or low-calorie), drug administration, pregnancy, lactation, exposure to a cold environment, or increased exercise. Many metabolic diseases are accompanied by a history of polyuria and polydipsia. There may be a recent behavior change or an increase in activity, as with hyperthyroidism. Abnormal feces characterized as soft, voluminous, and malodorous can be seen with malassimilation diseases. Neurologic signs such as depression, weakness, ataxia, disorientation, and seizures can be seen with hypoglycemia or portosystemic shunt.

15. How should one approach the polyphagic cat diagnostically?

The physical examination is the next diagnostic step. A careful neurologic examination, good abdominal palpation, and palpation of the neck for a thyroid "slip" may aid in ranking CNS disease, pregnancy, infiltrative bowel disease, hyperadrenocorticism, and hyperthyroidism on the differential list. Distinct changes in conformation may suggest acromegaly or hyperadrenocorticism. A minimal database including CBC, serum chemistry profile, and urinalysis should be performed. Results of these screening tests, in addition to the history, may suggest the need for further diagnostic work-up, such as thyroid function tests, liver function tests, or adrenal function tests. Fecal examination for parasites and evaluation for other causes of malabsorption or maldigestion may be warranted in some cats. Radiography or ultrasonography also may be considered, especially if pregnancy is suspected. Endoscopy or exploratory surgery and biopsy of the gastrointestinal system may be required to rule out other malassimilation syndromes.

Analysis of cerebrospinal fluid or more advanced diagnostic imaging such as computed tomography or magnetic resonance imaging may be necessary to rule out CNS disease.

BIBLIOGRAPHY

1. Behrend EN: Polyphagia. In Ettinger SM (ed): Textbook of Veterinary Internal Medicine, 5th ed. Philadelphia, W.B. Saunders, 2000, pp 104–107.
2. Bouchard GO, Sunvold GD: Dietary modification of feline obesity with a low fat, low fiber diet. In Reinhart GA, Carey DP (eds): Recent Advances in Canine and Feline Nutrition, vol II. Wilmington, DE, Orange Frazer Press, 1998, pp 183–192.
3. Burkholder WJ, Toll PW: Obesity. In Hand MS, Thatcher CD, Remillard RL, Roudebush P (eds): Small Animal Clinical Nutrition, 4th ed. Marceline, MO, Walsworth Publishing, 2000, pp 401–430.
4. Center S: Safe weight loss in cats. In Reinhart GA, Carey DP (eds): Recent Advances in Canine and Feline Nutrition, vol II, Wilmington, DE, Orange Frazer Press, 1998, pp 165–181.
5. Fettman MJ, Stanton CA, Banks LL, et al: Effects of neutering on body weight, metabolic rate and glucose tolerance of domestic cats. Res Vet Sci 62:131–136, 1997.
6. Fettman MJ, Stanton CA, Banks LL, et al: Effects of weight gain and loss on metabolic rate, glucose tolerance, and serum lipids in domestic cats. Res Vet Sci 64:11–16, 1998.
7. Lester T, Czarnecki-Maulden G, Lewis D: Cats increase fatty acid oxidation when isocalorically fed meat-based diets with increasing fat content. Am J Physiol 277:R878–R886, 1999.
8. Scarlett, JM, Donoghue S: Associations between body condition and disease in cats. J Am Vet Med Assoc 212:1725–1731, 1998.
9. Wolfsheimer KJ: Obesity. In Ettinger SM (ed): Textbook of Veterinary Internal Medicine, 5th ed. Philadelphia, W.B. Saunders, 2000, pp 70–72.

62. ANOREXIA AND WEIGHT LOSS

Cynthia L. Bowlin, D.V.M.

1. Define anorexia.

Anorexia is defined as the lack or loss of appetite for food. Food intake less than daily caloric requirement over time results in weight loss.

2. What causes anorexia?

Anorexia is a clinical sign of an underlying problem. Some authorities classify anorexia into primary causes, secondary causes, and pseudoanorexia. **Primary anorexia** is caused by diseases that affect the areas of the brain housing the appetite and satiety centers. **Secondary anorexia** has many pathologic and nonpathologic causes. Pathologic causes of secondary anorexia include pain, loss of smell, inflammation, fever, infection, toxins, neoplasia, and gastrointestinal, metabolic, or neurologic disorders. Nonpathologic conditions that may cause secondary anorexia include lack of diet palatability, strong dietary preferences, and environmental stress. Cats with **pseudoanorexia** have diseases that affect the mechanics of prehension and swallowing or painful diseases of the mouth or pharynx. An example is lymphocytic plasmocytic stomatitis; affected cats have an appetite but often do not eat.

3. What causes weight loss?

Weight loss results from decreased caloric intake or increased caloric requirement. Decreased caloric intake results from decreased consumption, absorption, or utilization. Examples of decreased consumption include decreased desire for food caused by disease, inability, or reluctance to eat and insufficient availability of food. Examples of decreased absorption include diseases of the gastrointestinal tract, liver, biliary system, and pancreas that cause maldigestion or malabsorption. Diabetes mellitus is an example of the lack of utilization of ingested food. Weight loss as a result of increased caloric requirement occurs with increased metabolism and utilization. Examples include pathologic conditions such as hyperthyroidism, neoplasia, or fever and non-pathologic conditions such as lactation or exercise.

Causes of Anorexia and Weight Loss

DECREASED CALORIC INTAKE	INCREASED CALORIC REQUIREMENT
Appetite with reduced food intake	Increased nutrient loss
Starvation	Vomiting/diarrhea
Food preference	Burns/wounds
Pain	Increased nutrient need
Inability to prehend, chew, or swallow	Surgery/trauma
Environmental factors	Infection
Appetite with adequate food intake	Fever
Malabsorption/maldigestion	Burns
Poor food caloric density/digestibility	Growth
Anorexia or inappetance	Lactation
Neurologic disease	Increased exercise
Pain	Decreased nutrient utilization
Loss of smell	Diabetes mellitus
Fever	Portosystemic shunt
Inflammation/infection	
Toxins	
Neoplasia	
Metabolic disorders	
Systemic disease	
Gastrointestinal disorders	

4. What are the pathophysiologic consequences of anorexia and weight loss in cats?

Cats are obligate carnivores that require a regular intake of certain nutrients to maintain health. During periods of reduced caloric intake, malabsorption/maldigestion, or increased caloric utilization, cats mobilize stores to meet metabolic needs. However, cats do not have the ability to store and/or synthesize certain amino acids and soon show signs of nutritional deficiencies. For example, cats are unable to synthesize the amino acid arginine, an important part of the urea cycle. During periods of reduced protein intake, the highly active protein catabolic hepatic enzymes of cats produce ammonia from the deamination of protein for energy. But without arginine to complete the conversion of ammonia to urea, hyperammonemia and its toxic affects quickly result. Cats require 8 times more vitamin B than dogs. Deficiency in B vitamins alone can precipitate or perpetuate an anorexic episode. Idiopathic hepatic lipidosis occurs most frequently in previously obese cats when calorie intake is restricted for any reason (see Chapter 30).

5. How long can cats survive without eating?

Inadequate food intake may be more detrimental to the patient than the underlying disorder. Even short-term fasting of a few days has been shown to have a negative effect on the immune system, gastrointestinal system, heart muscle, kidneys, liver, and endocrine systems. Healing is significantly hampered by lack of adequate nutrition. Early resumption of eating after an anesthetic, dental, or surgical procedure greatly enhances recovery, especially in debilitated, very young, and aged patients. Unless there is a medical indication for fasting (e.g., preoperative fasting, vomiting, acute gastritis, pancreatitis), adequate nutritional support should begin immediately. If inappetence or anorexia is predictable, as after surgery or dental work, provision for nutritional support should be part of the original treatment plan.

6. How can the history aid in determining the cause of anorexia and weight loss?

Identifying the cause of anorexia and/or weight loss starts with a complete and thorough history:

- Does the cat show an interest in foods that are offered?
- Is the cat attempting but failing to prehend the food? (The cat has an appetite but is unable or unwilling to eat.)
- What and how much is the cat eating? More or less than usual? Often in multi-cat households it is difficult to access how much an individual cat is consuming, but this crucial information affects the diagnostic plan. Recommend that the affected cat be isolated to measure food intake and appetite.
- Has there been a diet change? Cats are relatively insensitive to the caloric content of food and ingest relatively constant volumes of dry matter volumes. Changing to a lower calorie food usually results in weight loss.
- Has there been a change in the environment (e.g., move or new baby)?
- Where is the cat fed? Is food always accessible?
- Is there something or someone that would make the cat reluctant to approach the food or eat (e.g., dog, dominant cat, children)?
- Have other foods been offered? To what effect?

This information will help to differentiate pathologic from nonpathologic causes of anorexia and weight loss. If acceptable (to the cat) and adequate food is provided and polyphagia accompanies weight loss, the cat most likely has a disease that causes malabsorption/maldigestion, increased requirement of calories (e.g, hyperthyroidism), or decreased utilization of calories (e.g., diabetes mellitus). All of these diseases and the metabolic derangements that accompany their progression can result in a state of true anorexia.

7. How does the physical examination aid in the assessment of anorexia and weight loss?

If anorexia or inappetence is suggested by the history, the physical examination should provide additional direction in identifying the cause. If possible, weight loss should be verified objectively by serial weight comparisons. Significant weight loss can occur in an obese cat before it becomes subjectively apparent. Conversely, loss of a few ounces can be significant in a small or geriatric cat. A thorough examination of the oral cavity is necessary to rule out acute or chronic dental disease, neoplasia, stomatitis, or diseases that affect prehension, swallowing, or smell. A CNS evaluation should be done to rule out diseases that may cause primary anorexia. Fever in cats commonly suppresses the appetite; for the classical diagnostic plan, see Chapter 64. The chest should be auscultated thoroughly for cardiac murmurs, gallops, or arrhythmias to rule out cardiac disease. Visual observation of respiration, percussion, and auscultation should be done to evaluate the patient for upper or lower airway disease. Most animals that cannot breathe do not eat, and in cats respiratory disease can be subtle until well advanced. Complete digital palpation of the abdomen often identifies masses, organomegaly, pain, abnormal kidney size or shape, constipation, intestinal abnormalities, or urogenital disease. Examination of the eyes, including the fundus, may suggest infectious disease (feline infectious peritonitis, toxoplasmosis) or CNS disease. The ears should be evaluated for disease or polyps that may cause pain or affect smell and/or swallowing. Thorough examination of the coat and skin completes the physical evaluation and may suggest parasites, dehydration, toxins, or chronicity evident by poor coat quality or lack of self-grooming.

8. Describe the initial diagnostic plan.

If the cause of anorexia and/or weight loss is not found after evaluation of the signalment, history, and physical examination, then a complete blood count, serum biochemical profile, urinalysis, feline leukemia virus antigen test, feline immunodeficiency virus antibody test, and total T4 concentration (in cats > 5 years of age) usually are performed. Radiographs, ultrasound examination, or more advanced imaging such as magnetic resonance or computed tomography is warranted if a cause is not confirmed with the initial data.

9. What is the best diet for the cat?

The one the cat will eat! It is far more important that the cat eats than that the cat eats a specific diet. Although many nutrient-controlled diet formulations have been developed over the past

20 years for nutritional treatment and support of specific diseases, the diet will do no good and may actually do more harm if the cat refuses or is reluctant to eat it. Cats have such strong taste preferences and such a propensity to develop malnutritional disease quickly that, whenever the diet is changed, every cat should be monitored closely, even on a daily basis, to ensure consumption of an adequate volume of food. If consumption is not adequate, the diet must be changed to one that is acceptable to the cat. When cats with chronic renal failure are forced to eat renal diets, many succumb more to inadequate nutrition than to renal disease. Even novel protein diets used in diagnosis and treatment of food allergy need to be monitored closely for intake volume. I have seen cats lose 50% of body weight because they were offered only a specific diet that they did not accept. Foods should be measured and serial body weights checked regularly until stable. A cat will die before it will eat something that it does not like.

10. What are the treatments for anorexia?

No method of nutritional support substitutes for proper identification and treatment of the underlying cause of anorexia, which should be the primary goal. In the interim, various methods of nutritional support and appetite stimulation should be provided.

11. What dietary manipulation can I try?

Taste, odor, and texture of food play a large role in acceptability. Cats may develop a learned aversion to foods previously associated with nausea, vomiting, or cramping and subsequently reject them, even if previously preferred. Trying various types of foods (moist vs. dry kibble), strained baby formula meats, semimoist textures, fruits, vegetables, or others may entice the anorexic cat to resume eating. Feeding of liquefied or strained meat diets by hand or syringe often stimulates the cat to begin eating. Any medication given orally to a cat can cause gastrointestinal upsets, even if no vomiting or diarrhea is apparent. Always be sure that the cat has resumed eating before starting oral medications, and if a cat that has been eating reduces its food intake, loses weight, or stops eating, consider that oral medication may be at fault.

12. Should I try appetite stimulants?

Appetite stimulating drugs can be used in the short term to encourage food intake in recovering cats or cats for which a cause has been identified but cannot be eliminated. Too often these drugs are used instead of exhausting the search for a cause of the anorexia and weight loss. That temptation must be avoided. Measurement of food intake and serial weight monitoring must be done to assess the effectiveness of the drugs and the success of meeting caloric needs. If the response to drugs is inadequate or if long-term nutritional support is expected, other means of parenteral or enteral nutritional support should be instituted as soon as possible.

Appetite-stimulating Drugs

DRUG	DOSE	POTENTIAL SIDE EFFECTS
Cyproheptadine (Periactin) Merial Limited, Iselin NJ	1–2 mg PO every 8–24 hr	Extreme excitability and aggression
Megestrol acetate (Ovaban) Schering-Plough, Madison, NJ	0.5 mg/kg/24 hr PO for 3–5 days, then once every 5 days	Diabetes, mammary hyperplasia/neoplasia, pyometra
Prednisolone	0.25–0.5 mg/kg/24hr PO	Immune suppression, hyperglycemia
Stanozolol (Winstrol) Sanofi, New York	1–2 mg/cat PO every 12 hr	Hepatotoxicity (rare)
Vitamin B complex	2 ml/L fluids in IV	
Diazepam (Valium) Roche, Basel	0.2 mg/kg IV every 2 hr	Sedation, short effectiveness
Oxazepam (Serax) Wyeth-Ayerst, Philadelphia	1.25–2.5 mg/cat PO every 18–24 hr	Sedation potentially less than diazepam

13. Should enteral or parenteral nutritional support be used in anorexic cats?

Compared with the parenteral route, enteral nutrition has fewer complications and is more physiologic, less expensive, and technically easier. Hyperalimentation is the administration of adequate nutrients to malnourished patients or patients at risk. Enteral hyperalimentation provides nutrients to a functional gastrointestinal tract—for example, through a nasoesophageal, esophagostomy, gastrostomy, or enterostomy tube. Parenteral hyperalimentation provides nutrients intravenously. Enteral nutritional support also maintains gastrointestinal integrity: "If the gut works, use it." The parenteral route may be used when the gastrointestinal tract cannot adequately maintain and absorb nutrients (vomiting, severe diarrhea, intestinal resection or obstruction), when stimulation of the pancreas is to be avoided because of pancreatitis, or when additional support is indicated in severely malnourished cats. Factors that make total parenteral nutrition (TPN) more difficult include catheter placement and management (maintaining sterility and avoiding sepsis from formula or catheter site), need for specialized equipment (infusion pump), constant patient monitoring, and diet preparation and storage.

14. What methods are used for enteral feeding of cats?

Generally oral administration of food is most efficient, easier, and safer; it also stimulates hormonal and neural centers to enhance digestion and absorption of nutrients. The further aboral the materials are placed, the more complicated delivery and composition of the formulas become. Other available techniques include nasoesophageal, nasogastric, pharyngostomy, esophagostomy, gastrostomy, and jejunostomy tubes.

15. Are nasoesophageal and nasogastric tubes effective?

Although nasoesophageal and nasogastric tubes are quick and easy to place in cats, the type of nutritional support that can be provided is limited because of their small size. Soft polyvinyl and red rubber feeding tubes from 3–5 French (Jorvet Specialty Products, Loveland, CO; Sherwood Medical, St. Louis, MO) are easy to insert with little or no local anesthesia or sedation. Nutritionally complete, commercially available liquid diet preparations are available for use with tubes of this size:

- Jevity (Abbott Labs, Columbus, OH: 1.06 kcal/ml; 4.20 gm/100 kcal of protein, 3.48 gm/100 kcal of fat; 310 mOsm/kg)
- Osmolite HN (Abbott Labs, Columbus, OH: 1.06 kcal/ml; 4.44 gm/100 kcal of protein, 3.68 gm/100 kcal of fat; 310 mOsm/kg)
- Clinicare Feline (Abbott Labs, North Chicago, IL: 0.92 kcal/ml; 4.60 gm/100 kcal of protein, 3.68 gm/100 kcal of fat; 310 mOsm/kg)

An Elizabethan collar is usually required to prevent the patient from rubbing or dislodging the tube, although many cats resent the presence of the collar. To provide adequate quantities of nutrients, a feeding pump and constant infusion are necessary, thus restricting the use of this feeding method to hospitalized cats requiring minimal, short-term nutritional support.

16. Why have esophagostomy tubes become increasingly popular?

Esophagostomy tubes have become increasingly popular in recent years because of ease of placement and lack of required special instrumentation. This technique has largely replaced the pharyngostomy tube.

17. How are esophagostomy tubes placed?

The cat is anesthetized and intubated, and a mouth gag is applied to keep the mouth open. With the cat in right lateral recumbency, the area on the left side of the neck from the wing of the atlas to the scapula is clipped and surgically prepared. With the curved tip pointed upward toward the skin, a 6–8-inch curved Carmalt forcep is inserted into the throat and down the esophagus to the mid-neck area. Upward pressure is applied, and a scalpel blade is used to incise through the skin, subcutaneous tissues, and esophagus just over the tip of the forcep. The end of the tube is cut just above the side fenestration to allow better flow of formula. The tube is laid along the outside of the cat, measured from the tenth rib to the forcep tip, and marked. The mark places the distal end of the tube in the preferred lower esophagus, not into the stomach. The forcep tip is opened, and the distal end of the tube is grasped and withdrawn from the mouth with the forcep. The distal end of the tube is then turned back on itself and directed down the esophagus. The forcep can aid in directing and advancing the tube into the esophagus. Light traction on the tube at its exit point from the neck as the tip passes helps to relieve the bend in the tube and assists further advancement down the esophagus to the point previously marked. The tube is secured to the skin of the neck with a Chinese finger-trap suture or by gluing the tube to an adhesive tape wing and suturing to the skin of the neck. The tube is laid up over the neck and secured again dorsally, with one skin suture, to keep the tube accessible. A gauze pad with antibiotic ointment is applied over the incision, and the neck is wrapped lightly with a gauze bandage and secured. Systemic antibiotics are required for 5–7 days until the stoma forms and the incision heals. The bandage should be changed every other day until healing is complete. A light neck wrap after healing helps to keep the cat from dislodging the tube.

18. How is the esophagostomy tube used for feeding?

The esophagostomy tube is well tolerated by cats and can be as large as 10–16 French, allowing adequate size for feeding of blenderized canned food. Feedings should begin with frequent (every 2–3 hours) small servings (5–15 ml). If vomiting is not a problem, feeding volume can be increased and frequency decreased until the total daily caloric requirement is met. Most cats tolerate 50–60 ml per feeding. The tube should be kept plugged. Clogged tubes often can be relieved by pressure or injection of cola to dissolve the clog. Cats can and will eat with the esophagostomy tube in place. Once the cat is eating sufficiently on its own, the tube can be removed without sedation.

19. When should gastrostomy tubes be used?

Gastrostomy tube placement frequently is used if other diagnostic procedures are performed, such as exploratory laparotomy or endoscopy for procurement of biopsies. Another indication for gastrostomy tube placement is disease above the stomach that precludes use of the oral or esophageal route; for example, a cat that has undergone mandibulectomy for neoplasia and/or is no longer able to prehend, chew, or swallow food properly.

Various methods of gastrostomy tube placement have been described. Gastrostomy tubes are well tolerated in cats and can be used for months or years. Once the stoma has formed, the gastrostomy tube can be removed and cleaned or replaced with mild or little sedation. Gastrostomy tubes are indicated if longer-term nutritional support is anticipated (months or years) because their larger diameter allows more variety in diet and tube formula selection. The new "button" gastrostomy tubes lie close to the body wall, thus decreasing the chance of dislodgement.

20. When are jejunostomy tubes used?

The jejunostomy feeding tube is indicated in any cat that is undergoing oral, esophageal, gastric, pancreatic, duodenal, or biliary tract surgery in which the intestinal tract distal to the surgical site is functional. Patients with preexisting protein-calorie malnutrition that must undergo major abdominal surgery are candidates for early feeding via a jejunostomy tube. Celiotomy is required for placement, but the cat can begin a liquid diet into the jejunostomy tube immediately after surgery. Complications include premature removal, tube-induced jejunal perforation, and subcutaneous leakage; however, proper technique minimizes these complications. Frequently, gastrostomy tubes are placed at the same time for use when jejunostomy feedings are no longer required.

21. What unique facts about cats should be kept in mind?

- A cat will die before it will eat something that it does not like. Cats never get "hungry enough" to eat whatever is available.
- Weigh feline patients regularly. An 8-ounce weight loss can be far more significant than a 5-pound weight gain.
- Oral medications can cause anorexia.
- Cats develop learned aversions to foods previously associated with a negative experience, such as pain, nausea, vomiting, cramping, bad flavor, or hidden medications. Try something different.

• Start at an early age to feed the cat a variety of foods with different textures and smells. Diet variety should be the rule for the cat.
• Treat the cat, not the lab test. If lab values improve but the patient deteriorates, think of food intake.
• We do not know the nutritional requirements of cats.

BIBLIOGRAPHY

1. Crisp MS: Nutritional management of the critical patient. In Birchard SJ, Sherding RG (eds): Saunders Manual of Small Animal Practice. Philadelphia, W.B. Saunders, 1994, pp 29–37.
2. Hill, R: Feline enteral and parenteral nutrition. In Gumbs MW, Sokolowski JH (eds): Proceedings of the Waltham Feline Medicine Symposium in Association with The North American Veterinary Conference. Waltham, MA, 1999, pp 42–50.
3. Macy, DW, Ralston, SL: Cause and control of decreased appetite. In Kirk RW (ed): Current Veterinary Therapy X. Philadelphia, W.B. Saunders, 1989, pp 30–36.
4. Norsworthy GD: Tube feeding anorexic cats. From Instructions for Tube Feeding Anorexic Cats. Bloomington, IN, Cook Veterinary Products, 1998.
5. Seim HB, Willard M: Postoperative care of the surgical patient. In Fossum TW (ed): Small Animal Surgery. St Louis, Mosby, 1997, pp 65–85.
6. Seim, HB: Feeding tube placement. In Gumbs MW, Sokolowski JH (eds): Proceedings of the Waltham Feline Medicine Symposium in Association with The North American Veterinary Conference. Waltham, MA, 1999, pp 6–14.

63. SYSTEMIC HYPERTENSION

Drew Weigner, D.V.M.

1. Define systemic hypertension.

Systemic hypertension is a consistently elevated systolic or diastolic arterial blood pressure (BP). **Systolic pressure** is generated by contraction of the ventricles. Normal systolic pressure varies greatly from 118 to 170 mmHg. One report suggests normal systolic pressure may be somewhat higher in cats older than 11 years. Many clinicians use a value of 150 mmHg for normal systolic pressure in a clinical setting (i.e., by indirect methods). **Diastolic pressure** is the arterial BP during relaxation of the ventricles. Diastolic pressure is clinically difficult to measure but should be approximately 100 mmHg. Variations in reported data probably are due to differences in technique and equipment as well as method of restraint or anesthesia. Accordingly, each practice should establish its own normal parameters.

2. What are the other types of hypertension?

1. **Pulmonary arterial hypertension** describes elevation of BP in the pulmonary arteries. It is associated most commonly with chronic obstructive pulmonary diseases and dirofilariasis.
2. **Pulmonary venous hypertension** denotes increased BP in the pulmonary veins and occurs most frequently with congestive heart failure.
3. **Portal hypertension** is elevation of BP in the portal system of the liver. It can result from systemic hypertension but is more relevant clinically as a component of portosystemic shunts or chronic endstage liver diseases.

3. What are the major causes of systemic hypertension?

Systemic hypertension in cats is most commonly due to underlying diseases. Approximately 50% of cats with chronic renal failure have systemic hypertension. The incidence may be higher with hyperthyroidism. Occasionally, diabetes mellitus is associated with systemic hypertension. Uncommon causes include pheochromocytoma, hyperaldosteronism, and kidney transplantation.

Hypertension also may be a rare sequela of erythropoietin administration. Although suspected, hypertension from primary vascular disease (known as essential hypertension) has not been documented in cats. Furthermore, although hypertension can lead to secondary cardiac hypertrophy and resultant heart failure, no evidence suggests that heart disease causes hypertension.

4. What methods are available to determine arterial BP?

The gold standard for blood pressure measurement is direct arterial cannulation, usually of the carotid or femoral artery. Because special equipment and often anesthesia are required, indirect measurement is more common. However, indirect measurement typically understates blood pressure obtained by direct methods. Accordingly, a "correction factor" is sometimes added to indirect blood pressure readings.

5. How is indirect BP determined?

As in humans, a cuff is used to occlude a peripheral artery. The cuff pressure is decreased gradually until blood flow resumes. The cuff pressure at that point is the systolic pressure. The pressure remaining when blood flow temporarily ceases between heartbeats is the diastolic pressure. Accurate determination of diastolic pressure may not be possible via indirect measurement.

6. What is the preferred method for measuring systolic BP in cats?

Doppler ultrasonography is used most commonly to detect arterial blood flow. Doppler flow detection is less expensive and generally more accurate than other methods, particularly at higher pressures. Unfortunately, diastolic pressure cannot be measured with this technique. A correction factor of 14 mmHg has been suggested when systolic pressure is measured via Doppler: actual BP = Doppler BP + 14 mmHg, where actual BP is the value obtained by direct measurement.

7. Where is BP usually measured in cats?

Blood flow usually is measured at the plantar or palmar common digital arteries (proximal to the metatarsal or metacarpal pads, respectively) or the coccygeal artery with the cuff placed proximally. Ideally, pressures are determined with the patient in lateral recumbency so that the limb is at the same level as the heart, although it is not known how much this position affects blood pressure results.

8. What cuff size is appropriate for use in cats?

Use of an appropriate cuff size is important to obtain accurate determinations. Ideally, the width of the cuff should be 40% of the limb circumference. For most patients, a 2.5-cm cuff is appropriate. Cats that weigh over 7 kg or are obese or heavily muscled may require a 3.0-cm cuff. For practical purposes, it is easier to use a sphygmomanometer with an integral bulb/dial and a single tube that can be operated with one hand (Propper Manufacturing, Long Island City, NY).

9. What other indirect techniques of BP measurement are used in cats?

1. **Oscillometric methods** detect oscillations in cuff pressure to determine systolic, diastolic, and mean blood pressure. Although reasonably accurate at normal or low pressures, accuracy decreases markedly as the pressure increases.

2. **Plethysmography**, a newer method, uses infrared radiation to determine blood pressure. Although one report equates its accuracy with that of the Doppler technique, its use has yet to be critically evaluated in cats.

10. What is the "white coat effect"?

The "white coat effect" described in human medicine is a spurious elevation of blood pressure from stress during measurement in a clinical setting. It has been described in cats as increasing systolic pressure by 18 mmHg. Allowing patients 15 minutes to acclimate to the clinical environment before measurement of BP minimizes this effect. To increase accuracy and reproducibility, multiple determinations are recommended. One method is to obtain five readings, discard the highest and lowest, and average the remaining three.

11. What are the common signalment findings of systemic hypertension?

Systemic hypertension is more common in geriatric cats but may occur in patients of any age with predisposing conditions. Although systemic hypertension has no breed or sex predilection, it should be suspected in all cats with renal disease, such as Abyssinian cats with amyloidosis (see Chapter 40).

12. What are the common historical findings of systemic hypertension?

Systemic hypertension is called "the silent killer" because signs of early-to-moderate hypertension are vague or absent. Most cats do not exhibit overt clinical signs of systemic hypertension until systolic pressure exceeds 200 mmHg. Most cats with systemic hypertension have a history of weight loss, including obese diabetics. Appetite increases frequently in cats with hyperthyroidism and occasionally in cats with diabetes mellitus but may be normal or decreased in cats with renal disease. Astute owners may observe increased thirst or urination. Overt clinical signs are often acute and severe, including blindness from detached retinas, dyspnea from heart failure, and seizures or other neurologic signs of cerebral vascular hemorrhage. Anecdotally, excessive nocturnal vocalization has been reported in many hypertensive patients.

13. Describe the common physical examination findings of systemic hypertension.

Physical examination abnormalities are usually those of the primary disease process. Examples include small, irregularly marginated kidneys in cats with chronic renal failure and enlarged thyroid glands in cats with hyperthyroidism. Other findings relate to the effects of hypertension. Bounding pulses, increased intensity of heart sounds, and/or a gallop rhythm may be noted, usually in relation to secondary ventricular hypertrophy. Retinal artery tortuosity, retinal hemorrhage, and retinal detachment may be detected on ophthalmic examination. Seizures or other neurologic signs of cerebral vascular hemorrhage also may be present.

14. What is the initial diagnostic plan for systemic hypertension?

Indirect measurement of systolic blood pressure is essential to diagnose systemic hypertension. Because systemic hypertension is usually secondary to underlying diseases, complete blood count, serum biochemical profile, total T4 concentration, and urinalysis also should be performed.

15. What other tests are useful in determining the cause of systemic hypertension?

Direct or indirect ophthalmoscopy detects hyphema, retinal hemorrhage, or retinal detachment. Chest radiographs are useful for evaluating dyspnea associated with pleural effusion or pulmonary edema. Ultrasound techniques can be used to assess the degree of cardiac changes and primary causes of renal disease. Magnetic resonance imaging or computerized tomography with angiography to detect intracranial hemorrhage is ideal when neurologic symptoms are present.

16. Why are cats with systemic hypertension sometimes presented as emergencies?

Dyspnea from pleural effusion or pulmonary edema is the most common cause of emergency presentation of systemic hypertension. Although rare, intractable seizures or unilateral neurologic signs from intracranial hemorrhage also present as emergencies. Blindness is an uncommon emergency presentation. Indeed, some owners are unaware that the cat is blind until it is diagnosed during a thorough physical examination.

17. What is the initial treatment for systemic hypertension?

Although it is appropriate to decrease BP in patients with systemic hypertension, initial management may be directed toward treatment of acute symptoms such as dyspnea or seizures. Nitroglycerine may be particularly useful in fulminant cardiac failure secondary to systemic hypertension. Amlodipine, a calcium channel blocker, is reported to decrease blood pressure within 8–9 hours of oral administration in humans, but feline pharmacokinetics have not been determined.

Products Commonly Used for the Control of Feline Systemic Hypertension*

Sodium-restricted diets (several renal diets are commercially available)

Angiotensin-converting enzyme inhibitors
Enalapril   0.25–0.5 mg/kg orally every 12–24 hr
Lisinopril   0.5 mg/kg orally every 24 hr

Beta blockers
Propranolol   2.5–5.0 mg orally every 8–12 hr
Atenolol   2 mg/kg or 6.25–12.5 mg/cat orally every 24 hr

Calcium channel blockers
Amlodipine   0.18 mg/kg or 0.625–1.25 mg/cat orally every 24 hr
Diltiazem   0.5–2.5 mg/kg orally every 8hr

Emergency vasodilators
Nitroglycerine ointment 2%   ¼ inch cutaneously every 6–8 hr

Diruretics
Furosemide   1–2 mg/kg orally every 12 hr
Spironolactone   1–2 mg/kg orally every 12 hr

* When drugs are used for the treatment of systemic hypertension, start at the low end of the dose range and monitor arterial blood pressure and renal function parameters every 3–4 days until they are stabilized.

18. What should I use for long-term control of systemic hypertension?

In otherwise clinically normal cats with moderate hypertension, BP control may be attempted initially with low-salt diets (Dry Hills Prescription Diet and canned Waltham Low Protein are palatable to most cats). Symptomatic patients or patients with systolic pressures > 200 mmHg before or 170 mmHg after sodium restriction also should be medicated. The most effective medications for systemic hypertension are amlodipine and atenolol. Amlodipine is more reliably effective, but atenolol is the treatment of choice for patients with severe tachycardia, particularly with suspected hyperthyroidism. Angiotensin-converting enzyme inhibitors (enalapril, captopril, lisinopril), and diuretics (furosemide, spironolactone) are less effective in most cats and should be used with caution if concurrent renal failure is present. (See figure.)

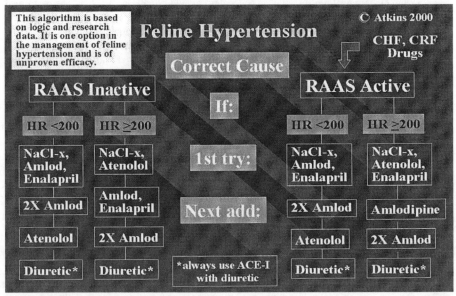

Medical management of feline hypertension. RAAS = renin-angiotensin-aldosterone system. NaCl-x = sodium restriction. (Courtesy of Clarke Atkins, D.V.M., with permission.)

19. What is the long-term prognosis for cats with systemic hypertension?
The prognosis for cats with manageable systemic hypertension depends on the underlying disease. Early detection and control of hypertension may slow the progression of renal disease and improve prognosis. Hyperthyroidism generally has a good prognosis when diagnosed before the onset of heart failure. Control of hyperthyroidism may resolve systemic hypertension in some cases. The prognosis of diabetic patients depends on the degree of glycemic control, but most patients do well on diet and insulin therapy. Acute blindness, if detected and treated within hours, may reverse if the retinas reattach. Uncontrollable systemic hypertension has a poor prognosis, regardless of the underlying cause.

BIBLIOGRAPHY

1. Belew AM, Bartlett T, Brown SA: Evaluation of the white-coat effect in cats. J Vet Intern Med 13:134–142, 1999.
2. Binn SH, Sisson DD, Buoscio DA, et al: Doppler ultrasonographic, oscillometric sphygmomanometric, and photoplethysmographic techniques for noninvasive blood pressure measurement in anesthetized cats. J Vet Intern Med 9:405–414, 1995.
3. Bodey AR, Sansom J: Epidemiological study of blood pressure in domestic cats. J Small Anim Pract 39:567–573, 1998.
4. Bonagura J, Stepien RL: Vascular diseases. In Birchard SJ and Sherding RG (eds): Small Animal Practice. Philadelphia, W.B. Saunders, 1994, pp 496–497.
5. Caulkett NA, Cantwell SL, Houston DM: A comparison of indirect blood pressure monitoring techniques in the anesthetized cat. Vet Surg 27:370–377, 1998.
6. Goodwin J-K: Systemic hypertension. In Norsworthy GD, Crystal MA, Fooshee SK, Tilley LP (eds): The Feline Patient. Baltimore, Williams & Wilkins, 1998, pp 413–416.
7. Grandy JL, Dunlop CI, Hodgson DS, et al: Evaluation of the Doppler ultrasonic method of measuring systolic arterial blood pressure in cats. Am J Vet Res 53:1166–1169, 1992.
8. Grosenbaugh DA, Muir WW: Blood pressure monitoring. Vet Med 93:48–59, 1998.
9. Henik RE, Snyder PS, Volk LM: Efficacy of amlodipine in the treatment of systemic hypertension in cats with chronic renal failure. J Am Anim Hosp Assoc 33:226–234, 1997.
10. Plotnick AN, Greco DS: Endocrine hypertension. In August JR (ed): Consultations in Feline Internal Medicine, 3rd ed. Philadelphia, W.B. Saunders, 1997, pp 163–168.
11. Polzin DJ, Osborne CA, James KM: Medical management of chronic renal failure in cats. In August JR (ed): Consultations in Feline Internal Medicine, 3rd ed. Philadelphia, W.B. Saunders, 1997, pp 331–332.
12. Snyder PS: Amlodipine: A randomized blinded clinical trial in cats with systemic hypertension. J Vet Intern Med 12:157–162, 1998.
13. Sparkes AH, Caney SM, King MC, et al: Inter- and intraindividual variation in Doppler ultrasonic indirect blood pressure measurements in healthy cats. J Vet Intern Med 13:314–318, 1999.
14. Thornhill JA: Hypertension, systemic. In Tilley LP, Smith FWK (eds): The Five Minute Veterinary Consult. Baltimore, Williams & Wilkins, 1997, pp 706–707.

64. ELEVATED BODY TEMPERATURE

Kristy L. Dowers, D.V.M.

1. What is considered an elevated temperature in cats?

A rectal temperature > 39.2° C (102.5° F) in cats should be investigated. Rectal temperature is the most accurate reflection of core body temperature. Human ear thermometers may be useful to estimate core body temperature in cats that are stressed and/or difficult to handle but are less accurate because of the shape of a cat's ear canal. When ear thermometers are used, the rectal setting should be used, and 1° F should be added to the temperature reading.

2. Does an elevated temperature mean that the cat has a fever?

The two main rule-outs for elevated temperature are true fever and hyperthermia. Hyperthermia can be caused by stress, excitement, exercise, elevated ambient temperature, or heat stress/stroke. If a cat appears normal except for the elevated temperature, the rectal temperature should be confirmed a second time after the cat has been allowed to remain calm with the owner in a quiet area for 15–20 minutes.

3. Describe the mechanism for elevated temperature due to hyperthermia.

Body temperature regulation occurs in the hypothalamus, which attempts to maintain core temperature at 38.3–38.8° C (101–102.0° F). This normal range is known as the thermoregulatory set point. With hyperthermia, the thermoregulatory set point remains unchanged, but increased muscle activity, metabolic activity, or ambient temperature causes an increase in core body temperature. The body responds by attempting to return the body temperature to the set point range, primarily by panting. Sweating is not as important because cats have few sweat glands and their skin is fur-covered.

4. Describe the mechanism for elevated body temperature due to fever.

In contrast to hyperthermia, the thermoregulatory set point is adjusted upward with fever. Exogenous pyrogens (e.g., bacteria, viruses, fungal agents, parasites, tissue necrosis, immune-mediated disease) activate mononuclear cells and neutrophils. These activated leukocytes release endogenous pyrogens such as interleukin-1, tumor necrosis factor, and interferons. Endogenous pyrogens, unlike exogenous pyrogens, can cross the blood-brain barrier and directly alter the thermoregulatory set point. Alternatively, endogenous pyrogens can stimulate the production of prostaglandins or cyclic adenosine monophosphate (cAMP) and therefore indirectly affect the set point. The body then attempts to raise the core temperature to the new set point by conserving (vasoconstriction) or generating heat (shivering).

5. What is the advantage of fever for the body?

1. Fever enhances the body's immune response:
   - Leukocyte mobility, phagocytic activity, and lymphocyte transformation increase.
   - Lysosomes break down more easily, releasing more proteolytic enzymes.
   - Interferon production rises.
   - Leukocytes have enhanced bactericidal capabilities.

2. Fever is thought to be detrimental to microorganisms by inhibiting their growth, reducing the availability of iron nutrients for bacteria, and interfering with bacterial iron chelation.

6. At what point is fever detrimental?

Fevers > 41.1° C (106.0° F) may be harmful to cellular metabolism. Permanent brain and organ damage can occur with fevers > 41.4° C (106.5° F). Cats with core body temperatures in these ranges should be treated immediately.

7. What physical examination findings accompany fever?

Most of the clinical signs of fever are nonspecific. Examples include anorexia, depression, reluctance to move, hyperpnea, and muscle or joint pain. Specific clinical signs are attributable to the inciting cause and organ system involved. For example, a cat with hemobartonellosis also may have anemia and icterus in addition to the nonspecific signs of fever.

8. What are the primary causes of fever in cats?

There are five major groups of differentials to consider in the febrile cat: (1) infectious (bacterial, rickettsial, viral, fungal, parasitic), (2) inflammatory (e.g., pancreatitis), (3) primary immune-mediated, (4) neoplasia, and (5) drug-induced. A fever that has lasted for 2 weeks and does not have an apparent cause is defined as a **fever of unknown origin**.

9. What are the most common causes of infectious fever in cats?

ORGANISM	CLINICAL DESCRIPTION	DIAGNOSTIC TESTS	TREATMENT
Viral			
Feline leukemia virus (FeLV)	Any age; intermittent fever; chronic infections; weight loss; anemia; thrombocytopenia	FeLV antigen test	Supportive therapy; treat infections; manage weight loss/anorexia
Feline immuno-deficiency virus (FIV)	Older cats; intermittent fever; chronic infections, weight loss; gingivitis/stomatitis	FIV antibody test	Supportive therapy; treat infections; manage weight loss/anorexia
Feline infectious peritonitis (FIP)	Cats < 2 yr or > 10 yr old. Effusive form; peritoneal/pleural effusion. Noneffusive form: neurologic/ocular signs; signs of specific organ involvement; persistent fever	Tissue diagnosis (biopsy)	No known therapy; fatal disease
Panleukopenia	Young, unvaccinated cats; vomiting, diarrhea, dehydration, fever, leuko-penia	Parvoviral antigen test of feces; electron micros-copy	Supportive therapy: fluids, nutrition, anti-biotics (broad spec-trum)
Feline herpes-virus 1	Any age; sneezing; oculonasal dis-charge; conjunctivitis; ocular ulce-rations; variable fever	Clinical signs; IFA, virus isolation, or PCR of nasal/con-junctival scrapings	Supportive therapy: anti-biotics with secondary bacterial infection
Feline calcivirus	Any age; serous oculonasal discharge; mild conjunctivitis; oral ulceration; biphasic fever	Clinical signs; viral isolation	Supportive therapy: anti-biotics with secondary bacterial infection
Bacterial			
Bite wound abscesses	Outdoor cats; pain, heat, swelling at abscess site; anorexia; fever	Aspirate; hetero-genous population of bacteria	Drain abscess; antibiotics (penicillin)
Feline plaque (*Yersinia pestis*)	Any age; history of hunting in endemic areas; flea exposure; fever; anorexia; submandibular lymphadenopathy	Cytology; bipolar staining for cocco-bacilli; IFA	Zoonosis! Isolation; anti-biotics (doxycycline or enrofloxacin)
Tularemia (*Francisella tularensis*)	Younger cats; exposure to rabbits; fever; icterus; lethargy; depression; oral ulcers, septicemia	IFA or culture from lymph nodes, blood, urine, bone marrow	Zoonosis! Isolation; anti-biotics (doxycycline or enrofloxacin)
Ehrlichiosis (*Ehrlichia risticii/canis*)	Any age; intermittent fever; hyper-esthesia; joint pain; lymphadenop-athy; variable appetite	*E. canis* and *E. risticii* serum antibody titers; PCR	Supportive therapy; anti-rickettsial drugs (doxycycline)
Songbird fever (*Salmonella* spp.)	Any age; indoor/outdoor with history of hunting birds; vomiting; diarrhea; fever; septicemia	Blood and fecal cultures	Antibiotics if septicemic (broad spectrum)

Table continued on following page

ORGANISM	CLINICAL DESCRIPTION	DIAGNOSTIC TESTS	TREATMENT
Bacterial *(continued)*			
Haemobartonellosis *(Haemobartonella felis)*	Any age; pale mucous membranes; icterus; anorexia; depression; severe regenerative hemolytic anemia	Marginated blood smear; PCR	Supportive therapy (transfusions); antibiotics (doxycycline, enrofloxacin)
Chlamydiosis *(Chlamydia psittaci)*	Any age; purulent oculonasal discharge; conjunctivitis; fever	Conjunctival scraping cytology: inclusion bodies in epithelial cells	Supportive therapy; antibiotics (doxycycline or chloramphenicol topically)
Protozoal			
Toxoplasmosis *(Toxoplasma gondii)*	Any age; fever; dyspnea; icterus; abdominal pain; uveitis; chorioretinitis; neurologic signs; intermittent fever; lethargy; depression	Tissue diagnosis (biopsy); IgM and IgG serum aqueous humor or CSF titers	Supportive therapy; antibiotics (clindamycin)
Cytauxzoonosis *(Cytauxzoon felis)*	Any age; high fever; dyspnea; anemia; thrombocytopenia; splenomegaly	Blood cytology: "signet ring" organisms within erythrocytes	Supportive therapy; antiprotozoals (imidocarb or diminazene)
Fungal			
Histoplasmosis *(Histoplasma capsulatum)*	Younger cats (< 4 yr); peripheral and visceral lymphadenopathy; dyspnea; fever; weight loss	Cytology: intracellular (macrophages) thin capsule; serology inaccurate	Itraconazole; fluconazole; amphotericin B
Blastomycosis *(Blastomyces dermatitidis)*	Any age (more common in dogs); respiratory signs; ocular signs; fever; weight loss	Cytology: extracellular, broad-based budding yeast; serology: antibody tests	Itraconazole; fluconazole; amphotericin B
Coccidioidomycosis *(Coccidioides immitis)*	Any age (rare in cats); skin lesions; fever	Ctyology: extracellular double-walled; serology: antibody tests	Itraconazole; fluconazole; amphotericin B
Cryptococcosis *(Cryptococcus neoformans)*	Any age; sneezing; stertorous breathing; chronic nasal discharge; skin lesions; low-grade fever	Cytology: extracellular, thick capsule; serology: antigen tests	Itraconazole; fluconazole; amphotericin B

IFA = immunofluorescent assay, PCR = polymerase chain reaction, IgM = immunoglobulin M, IgG = immunoglobulin G, CSF = cerebrospinal fluid.

10. What are the common causes of inflammatory fever in cats?

DISEASE	CLINICAL DESCRIPTION	DIAGNOSTIC TESTS	TREATMENT
Pancreatitis	Any age; chronic, intermittent form; anorexia; lethargy; variable abdominal pain; icterus	Serum TLI; ultrasound; biopsy; lipase activity of peritoneal effusion	Supportive therapy: fluids, nutrition; antibiotics; ± glucocorticoids
Cholangiohepatitis	Any age; icterus; vomiting; anorexia; fever in suppurative form	Abdominal ultrasound; liver biopsy with culture and sensitivity testing	Antibiotics if suppurative; glucocorticoids if nonsuppurative
Meningoencephalitis	Any age; recurrent seizures; multifocal neurologic signs; vomiting; diarrhea; fever	None. CSF analysis to rule out other causes of seizures	No known therapy; possible viral etiology

Table continued on following page

DISEASE	CLINICAL DESCRIPTION	DIAGNOSTIC TESTS	TREATMENT
Myocarditis/ diaphragmitis	Any age; biphasic fever at 10 days and 3–4 weeks; hyperesthesia; lymphadenopathy; cardiac signs	None. Rule out other causes of fever, cardiac disease	No known therapy; multifactorial etiology

CSF = cerebrospinal fluid.

11. What are the most common causes of immune-mediated fever in cats?

DISEASE	CLINICAL DESCRIPTION	DIAGNOSTIC TESTS	TREATMENT
Systemic lupus erythematosus	Rare in cats; multiple systemic signs; fever; weight loss; cutaneous lesions	ANA titers; skin biopsies	Immunosuppression
Primary hemolytic anemia	Anemia; icterus; fever, anorexia	Work-up for *Haemobartonella felis*; FeLV/FIV tests	Treat underlying cause; immunosuppression
Idiopathic thrombocytopenia	Rare in cats; fever; lethargy; petechiae	FeLV/FIV tests	Treat underlying cause; immunosuppression
Idiopathic polyarthritis	Uncommon in cats; stiff, painful joints; fever; lethargy	Arthrocentesis	Treat underlying cause; immunosuppression

ANA = antinuclear antibody, FeLV = feline leukemia virus, FIV = feline immunodeficiency virus.

12. What neoplasms most commonly cause fever in cats? What are the clinical signs and symptoms?

Any neoplasm may cause fever, but the most common is lymphoma. Cats of any age may be affected. Signs and symptoms are attributable to the organs involved; fever may be persistent or intermittent.

13. How is fever related to neoplasms diagnosed and treated?

Diagnosis depends on blood work, imaging, titers of feline leukemia virus and feline immunodeficiency virus, bone marrow aspirates, and biopsies. Treatment depends on the specific tumor.

14. What drugs may induce fever in cats?

The most common examples are tetracycline and amphotericin B. Cats of any age may be affected. The fever is disproportionate to clinical signs in an otherwise healthy cat. Treatment is discontinuance of the drug.

15. How do the history and signalment help rank the differential diagnoses?

Young cats, especially those with outdoor access, are more likely to have infectious causes of fever. Examples include abscessed bite wounds, feline leukemia virus (FeLV), feline plague, tularemia, and salmonellosis (song-bird fever). Fever of unknown origin in older cats is more likely to be due to neoplasia or chronic infections such as FeLV and feline immunodeficiency virus (FIV). Purebred cats may have a genetic predisposition for feline infectious peritonitis (FIP). Travel history to fungal-endemic areas, current medications, and exposure to ticks and fleas are important historical findings that help to prioritize the differential list.

16. What specific physical examination findings are helpful?

A good physical examination can direct your approach to febrile cats. An oral examination may reveal dental disease, pale mucous membranes, petechiae, or icterus. Heart murmurs and decreased lung sounds are identified with auscultation of the chest. Muscles, joints, and bones should be palpated for evidence of pain. Abdominal palpation allows you to assess pain, organomegaly, peritoneal effusion, and irregular kidneys. A fundic examination should be performed in every cat because infectious diseases such as *Cryptococcus neoformans*, *Toxoplasma gondii*, and FIP can cause ocular lesions. In some cats, however, the only presenting sign is fever.

17. What is the recommended diagnostic work-up for fever of unknown origin?
- Complete blood count
- Serum biochemistry panel
- Urinalysis with or without urine culture
- Fecal examination
- FeLV antigen test
- FIV antibody test
- Serum T4 concentration (> 5 years old)

Chest and abdominal radiographs are also recommended, especially if the physical examination and/or blood work do not reveal the cause of the fever. Abdominal ultrasound may be necessary to evaluate organomegaly, suspected pancreatitis, mass effects, or peritoneal effusion. Blood cultures, both aerobic and anaerobic, are indicated in many cats with fever because a cause may not be apparent in the preliminary work-up.

18. What is the optimal technique for performing blood cultures?
Three separate blood cultures should be obtained over 2 hours, preferably during a period of fever. Fresh venipuncture samples are preferred. At least 3–5 ml of blood should be collected for each sample; care should be taken not to oversample cats with concurrent anemia. The skin over the jugular vein should be shaved and prepared as for a surgical procedure. Sterile gloves should be worn. After the sample is collected aseptically, a new needle should be used to introduce the blood into the culture medium. Do not refrigerate the culture. It should be kept at room temperature if incubation at 37° C is not immediately available.

19. How should hyperthermia be treated?
As mentioned above, all cats with core body temperature > 41.1° C (106.0° F) should be treated immediately. The goal in cats with hyperthermia or heat stroke is rapid cooling of the core body temperature to 39.4°C (103.0° F) within 30–60 minutes. Cooling can be accomplished by soaking the cat's fur with cool water, using fans to promote evaporative cooling, and applying ice packs to the inguinal, axillary, and jugular vein areas. Intravenous fluid therapy should be used carefully; excessive fluids during initial cooling can lead to pulmonary edema. Once the target temperature of 39.4° C is achieved, cooling measures should be stopped. Shivering and heat production are induced at temperatures below this level. The cat should be monitored carefully after initial cooling for complications of heat stroke, including renal failure, hepatic failure, cerebral edema, and disseminated intravascular coagulation.

20. How should fever of unknown origin be treated?
Intravenous therapy with room temperature fluids can reduce a high fever and improve the cat's sense of well-being. The underlying cause should be identified and treated primarily. Examples include antibiotic therapy for infectious causes, glucocorticoids for immune-mediated and inflammatory causes, and surgery or chemotherapy for neoplasia. As with hyperthermia, fevers > 41.1° C (106.0° F) should be treated using the techniques described above. Most true fevers, however, do not exceed 41.1° C (106.0° F).

21. Should drugs such as dipyrone or aspirin be used?
Dipyrone and other nonsteroidal anti-inflammatories such as aspirin and flunixin meglumine are contraindicated for treatment of heat stroke. These drugs decrease the hypothalamic set point (which is normal with heat stroke) and may exacerbate the gastrointestinal ulceration and renal damage that can occur with heat stroke. For treatment of true fever, aspirin can be administered at 5 mg/kg orally every 24 hr. Use of dipyrone is discouraged because dosages for cats are not well established, and the side effects include bone marrow suppression and clotting abnormalities, especially with long-term use.

BIBLIOGRAPHY

1. Dunn JK, Green CE: Fever. In Green CE (ed): Infectious Diseases of the Dog and Cat, 2nd ed. Philadelphia, W.B. Saunders, 1990, pp 64–71.
2. Johnson KE: Pathophysiology of heatstroke. Comp Cont Educ Pract Vet 4:141–144, 1982.
3. Lappin MR: Fever, sepsis, and principles of antimicrobial therapy. In Leib MS, Monroe WE (eds): Practical Small Animal Internal Medicine. Philadelphia, W.B. Saunders, 1997, pp 829–836.
4. Larson RL, Carithers RW: A review of heat stroke and its complications in the canine. N Z Vet J 33:202–206, 1985.
5. Lorenz MD: Pyrexia (fever). In Lorenz MD, Cornelius LM (eds): Small Animal Medical Diagnosis, 2nd ed. Philadelphia, J.B. Lippincott, 1993, pp 15–22.
6. Lorenz MD: General (polysystemic) problems: Pyrexia, anorexia, weight loss, and obesity. In Lorenz MD, Cornelius LM, Ferguson DC (eds): Small Animal Medical Therapeutics. Philadelphia, J.B. Lippincott, 1993, pp 25–26.

65. JOINT DISEASE

Catriona M. MacPhail, D.V.M.

1. How is joint disease typically classified?

Joint disease is initially categorized as either inflammatory or noninflammatory. Inflammatory arthritis may have an infectious or immune-mediated etiology. Immune-mediated arthropathies can be further classified as erosive or nonerosive. The classic noninflammatory joint disease is osteoarthritis, a low-grade inflammatory condition that results in destruction of articular cartilage, typically secondary to injury or chronic abnormal wear.

Classification of Feline Joint Diseases

Noninflammatory
  Degenerative: osteoarthritis
  Congenital: Scottish fold arthropathy

Inflammatory

Infectious	*Noninfectious*
Erosive	Erosive
Sepsis	Feline chronic progressive polyarthritis
L-forms	Rheumatoid arthritis
Nonerosive	Nonerosive
Mycoplasmal	Systemic lupus erythematosus
Viral	Drug-induced
Calcivirus	Vaccine-associated
Feline infectious peritonitis	Chronic inflammatory response
	Idiopathic

2. Define polyarthritis.

Polyarthritis is an inflammatory joint disease involving two or more joints, usually with a specific etiology. It is less common in cats than in dogs. Typically systemic illness accompanies inflammatory joint changes. Systemic signs include pyrexia, anorexia, malaise, and occasionally lymphadenopathy.

3. What is the initial diagnostic plan for cats with suspected joint disease?

Thorough physical, orthopedic, and neurologic examinations help to differentiate among bone, joint, muscle, or neurologic sources of pain and lameness. Multiple joint involvement also may be identified. Radiographs and synovial fluid analysis are the hallmark diagnostic tests for joint disease. Other diagnostic tests vary based on the suspected disease. Radiographs help to confirm suspicions of osteoarthritis, identify possible septic arthritis, and determine whether a polyarthritis is erosive or nonerosive. Multiple distal joints should be radiographed if immune-mediated polyarthritis is suspected. Nonerosive inflammatory joint disease typically causes radiographic abnormalities other than soft tissue swelling and joint capsule distention. The overall cell count and predominant cell type in the synovial fluid can help differentiate among the multiple causes of arthritis. Synovial fluid analysis also can be used to monitor response to therapy.

4. How are joint taps performed and analyzed?

Mild-to-heavy sedation is often required to perform arthrocentesis. Select the joints with obvious effusion for initial sampling. However, if polyarthritis is suspected, multiple joints should be sampled, particularly the carpi and tarsi. Often only a small amount of synovial fluid is obtained. Therefore, tests on the fluid should be prioritized. If only a drop or two of fluid is retrieved, cytologic assessment helps to estimate differential cell counts, thus distinguishing between inflammatory and noninflammatory joint disease. Viscosity can be subjectively assessed as joint fluid drips from the needle onto a slide or culturette. Other tests that can be performed on synovial fluid include determination of total nucleated cell count and total protein concentration, mucin clot test, and aerobic bacterial, anaerobic bacterial, and mycoplasmal cultures.

5. What are the characteristics of normal joint fluid?

Normal joint fluid is clear, colorless, and highly viscous. Normal protein count is < 2.5 gm/dl with a total nucleated cell count < 3000 cells/μl (primarily mononuclear cells).

6. Why is osteoarthritis often not recognized in cats?

Osteoarthritis is a chronic, slowly progressive disorder that may be insidious in onset. Because of a cat's small size and ability to redistribute weight to other limbs, subtle gait abnormalities often go unrecognized by owners. Other clinical signs associated with osteoarthritis in cats include behavior or temperament changes, anorexia, dull hair coat, decreased jumping ability, and decreased activity level.

7. Where does osteoarthritis most often occur in cats?

Osteoarthritis is thought to occur most commonly in the shoulders and elbows of older cats. Hip dysplasia is a common cause of coxofemoral osteoarthritis in dogs but has received relatively little attention in cats. A recent feline population study found a 6.6% breed-dependent radiographic incidence of hip dysplasia. Purebred cats, predominantly Maine coons and Himalayans, are particularly overrepresented.

8. How can osteoarthritis be managed in cats?

As with canine osteoarthritis, areas to address for the management of osteoarthritis include:
- Nutrition and weight management
- Exercise modification
- Drugs
- Surgery

9. Discuss pain control in cats with osteoarthritis.

Pain control is difficult because many available drugs are not safe to use in cats. Newer nonsteroidal anti-inflammatory drugs can be used in cats but only for short-term relief. Potential choices for chronic administration include aspirin, piroxicam, butorphanol, or corticosteroids; however, owners must be educated about potential side effects. Glucosamine/chondroitin sulfate supplement administration has been described with anecdotal reports of improved quality of life.

10. List the drugs used to treat feline joint disease, their indications, and appropriate doses.

Drugs Used to Treat Feline Joint Disease

NAME	INDICATION	DOSE	COMMENTS
Aspirin	Analgesic, anti-inflammatory	10–25 mg/kg PO every 24–48 hr	
Auranofin	Immunosuppressive	0.05–2 mg PO every 12 hr	Not to exceed 9 mg/24 hr
Aurothioglucose	Immunosuppressive	1 mg/cat IM every 7 days, then 1 mg/kg IM every 7 days	Can be tapered after 2–4 wk to every 30 days
Azathioprine	Immunosuppressive	1.1 mg/kg PO every 48 hr	Use with caution
Butorphanol	Analgesic	1 mg/cat PO every 12 hr	
Carprofen	Analgesic, anti-inflammatory	4 mg/kg PO oncer	Use with caution
Chlorambucil	Immunosuppressive	0.25–0.5 mg/kg PO every 48–72 hr	
Chloramphenicol	Antimicrobial	25–50 mg/kg PO every 12 hr	
Cosequin	Disease-modifying	1 capsule PO every 24 hr	Sprinkle on food
Cyclophospha-mide	Immunosuppressive	2.5 mg/kg PO every 48 hr up to 3 wk 7 mg/kg IV every 7 days	Use with caution
	In conjunction with prednisone/prednisolone	2.5 mg/kgd PO every 24 hr for 4 days, then off 3 days	
Doxycycline	Antimicrobial	5–10 mg/kg PO every 12 hr	
Ketoprofen	Analgesic, anti-inflammatory	1 mg/kg PO every 24 hr	Limit 5 days
		2 mg/kg SC every 24 hr	Limit 3 days
Prednisone/prednisolone	Immunosuppressive	2–4 mg/kg PO every 24 hr divided	
Piroxicam	Anlagesic/anti-inflammatory	0.3 mg/kg PO every 48–72 hr	Use with caution

PO = orally, IM = intramuscularly, IV = intravenously.

11. What environmental changes may benefit cats with osteoarthritis?
Easier accessibility to food, toys, and bedding allows the cat to avoid large leaps up and down, thereby decreasing stress on affected joints. Weight loss for obese cats or improved nutrition for thin cats also may be of some benefit.

12. What surgical options are available for treatment of cats with osteoarthritis?
Surgical options are limited to femoral head and neck excision for coxofemoral arthritis and amputation. Arthrodesis can be performed in distal joints, such as the carpus or tarsus, but these joints are affected more commonly by inflammatory arthritides.

13. Why are cats less likely to develop infectious arthritis than dogs?
Systemic infections commonly localize in joints because of the abundant blood supply of the synovial tissue. Monoarticular disease is more likely than polyarticular disease, and previously damaged joints are more likely to be infected. Typical infections include urinary tract or prostatic infections, pyoderma, and bacterial endocarditis. These conditions are relatively rare in cats compared with dogs. More commonly, bacterial arthritis occurs in neonates with omphalophlebitis or neonates that nurse from queens with postparturient uterine or mammary gland infections.

14. Infection by what cell wall-deficient bacteria may cause erosive polyarthritis?

L-forms are mutant, wall-deficient bacteria derived from many different species. Infection is characterized by distal asymmetric polyarthritis that causes articular cartilage destruction, metaphyseal lysis, and periosteal proliferation. Cats may become nonambulatory with elevated body temperature. Distal joints are markedly swollen with occasional development of fistulating tracts erupting from the distended joint capsule. Subcutaneous draining abscesses are another manifestation of the infection. The thick brown exudate is pyogranulomatous inflammation.

15. How is L-form bacterial infection diagnosed?

Diagnosis is based on consistent clinical signs, cytologic and radiographic findings, elimination of other possible causes of erosive polyarthritis, and response to treatment. The L-form bacterium is difficult to isolate and identify. However, affected cats respond quickly to oral tetracycline. Joint changes are irreversible; if marked instability is present, arthrodesis may be a consideration.

16. Infection by what cell wall-deficient bacteria may cause nonerosive polyarthritis?

Mycoplasma spp. are normal flora in certain organ systems in the body. However, they are opportunistic secondary pathogens that may cause problems in immunocompromised animals or animals receiving penicillins or cephalosporins. Several cases of mycoplasmal arthritis in cats have been reported. Clinical signs are similar to those of other nonerosive arthritides. Mycoplasmal organisms can be isolated from the joint fluid by culture. Recently, *M. felis* was isolated from the joints of a cat with polyarthritis, and DNA was detected in joint fluid by polymerase chain reaction. Mycoplasmal infections are generally responsive to tetracyclines, chloramphenicol, fluoroquinolones, and aminoglycosides.

17. What are the other infectious causes of polyarthritis in cats?

- Feline calicivirus (FCV) infection causes a short-lived limping syndrome in kittens infected naturally or experimentally. Other clinical signs include elevated temperature, hyperesthesia, and ulceration of the tongue or palate. This syndrome also may occur after immunization of kittens with vaccines containing live FCV. Signs typically last 48–72 hours.
- Mild-to-severe synovitis has been reported in cats with the effusive form of feline infectious peritonitis (see Chapter 38). Affected cats typically show no signs of lameness or discomfort.
- An epidemiologic association between polyarthritis in cats and the presence of *Ehrlichia* spp. antibodies (see Chapter 78) was recently reported.
- Although cats develop *Borrelia burgdorferi* antibodies, polyarthritis due to infection by this bacterium has not been well documented.

18. Aside from septic arthritis and bacterial L-form polyarthritis, what other differential diagnoses must you consider in cats with erosive polyarthritis?

Several cats have been reported to have positive rheumatoid factor titers concurrent with erosive polyarthritis. However, rheumatoid arthritis is not well characterized in cats. A criterion for diagnosis has not been established for cats, as it has for humans and dogs. Feline chronic progressive polyarthritis (FCPP) is a rare condition that occurs in male cats. Although the etiology is probably immune-mediated, an association with feline leukemia virus (FeLV) and feline syncytia-forming virus (FeSFV) is suspected.

19. What are the two forms of FCPP?

The **periosteal proliferative form** occurs only in young male cats. Typical clinical signs include elevated temperature, marked joint pain, distal limb stiffness and lameness, and regional lymphadenopathy. The carpi and tarsi are the most commonly affected joints, and usually the disease is symmetrical. Radiographic changes lag behind clinical signs; however, typical abnormalities include periosteal proliferation, osteophytosis, subchondral bone lysis, and joint space collapse. Fibrous ankylosis may be present in advanced cases. Diagnosis of FFCP is usually by exclusion of infectious causes of erosive arthritis. Immunosuppressive drug therapy is the treatment of choice; corticosteroids alone lessen the severity of clinical signs but do not slow the progression of the disease. Combination therapy with corticosteroids and cyclophosphamide or azathioprine has been more successful, achieving remission in approximately 50% of treated cats.

The **erosive or deforming form** of FFCP is less common and occurs mostly in older cats. The disease is slowly progressive, and clinical signs develop gradually. Joint deformities occur in the carpal, metacarpophalangeal, metatarsophalangeal, and interphalangeal joints. Radiographic changes include severe subchondral bone erosion, relatively mild periosteal proliferation, and joint subluxation or luxations. Information about treatment and prognosis of this form of FFCP is limited, although immunosuppressive therapy probably is indicated.

20. Describe the association between FFCP and FeSFV.

FeSFV is a retrovirus of the subfamily Spumarininae. The incidence of FeSFV infection is high among both normal and diseased cats. The prevalence in a cat population varies between 4% and 50%. Vertical transmission is possible: at least 50% of kittens born to infected queens are infected at birth. FeSFV has not been associated with any disease, although in one study the virus was present in 100% of cats affected with FFCP. However, polyarthritis cannot be reproduced with FeSFV isolated from diseased cats. Concurrent FeLV infection was found in 70% of these cats, and concurrent infection with feline immunodeficiency virus (FIV) is also common. It is postulated that FeLV and FIV alter the host immune system to potentiate the ability of FeSFV to produce disease, manifesting primarily as an arthropathy through immune complex deposition in the synovium. However, this theory has yet to be verified.

21. Discuss specific causes of immune-mediated nonerosive polyarthritis.

Systemic lupus erythematosus (SLE) is a chronic, immune-mediated polysystemic disease that is not as well characterized in cats as in dogs. Polyarthritis is only one manifestation of the disease. Other clinical signs include dermatitis, lymphadenopathy, conjunctivitis, glomerulonephritis, and fever. Lameness and joint pain are often overlooked, and polyarthritis is typically diagnosed from arthrocentesis that shows an increased cell count primarily consisting of nondegenerate neutrophils. The presence of antinuclear antibodies (ANA) in the blood is a potentially diagnostic feature of SLE. However, a positive ANA titer alone does not diagnose SLE. If other causes of nonerosive polyarthritis have been ruled out, a cat with consistent clinical signs and a positive ANA titer is likely to have SLE.

A **chronic inflammatory process or antigenic source** can cause secondary polyarthritis. Immune complexes become trapped in the synovial membrane, initiating a marked inflammatory response. Sources of immune complexes include chronic bacterial or parasitic infection, neoplasia, and recent drug or vaccine administration. When the cause of immune-mediated nonerosive joint disease is undetermined, it is referred to as **idiopathic polyarthritis**.

22. How are immune-mediated nonerosive polyarthritides diagnosed and differentiated?

The clinical history of immune-mediated polyarthritides is fairly similar. Often the disease is cyclic and associated with periods of fever, malaise, and anorexia. The joints can be grossly swollen and are painful on manipulation. The smaller distal joints are more often affected, and radiographic changes are minimal to nonexistent.

Synovial fluid analysis retrieves a nontoxic neutrophilic inflammation and cultures are negative. Serologic tests include ANA titer, LE-cell preparation, and rheumatoid titer. Results of these tests must be considered in relation to history, clinical signs, and results of other diagnostic tests to distinguish among various etiologies.

23. What drugs are used to treat immune-mediated polyarthritis?

Immunosuppressive doses of corticosteroids are the cornerstone of therapy for immune-mediated disease. However, some patients may require combination therapy with cyclophosphamide, chlorambucil, or gold salts. Supportive care such as rest, dietary management, and exercise modification, should not be overlooked.

24. What type of arthropathy is associated with Scottish fold cats?

The folded ears of Scottish fold cats are due to an abnormality in the ear cartilage caused by a simple autosomal dominant gene. Cats that are homozygous for the gene develop generalized cartilage abnormalities. This condition is manifested by a shortening and thickening of axial and appendicular bones, resulting in a short, crouched appearance. Clinical signs include progressive lameness and stiffness as joint involvement advances. The joints of the distal hindlimbs are usually affected most severely. Medical management of pain and lameness is the only available therapy.

BIBLIOGRAPHY

1. Bennet D: Treatment of the immune-based inflammatory arthropathies of the dog and cat. In Kirk RW (ed): Kirk's Current Veterinary Therapy XII. Philadelphia, W.B. Saunders, 1995, pp 1188–1204.
2. Bennet D, Nash AS: Feline immune-based polyarthritis: A study of thirty-one cases. J Small Anim Pract 29:501–523, 1988.
3. Carro T: Polyarthritis in cats. Compend Cont Educ Pract Vet 16:57–67, 1994.
4. Carro T: L-Forms and mycoplasmal infections. In August JR (ed): Consultations in Feline Internal Medicine, 2nd ed. Philadelphia, W.B. Saunders, 1994, pp 13–20.
5. Hardie EM: Management of osteoarthritis in cats. Vet Clin North Am 27:945–953, 1997.
6. Keller GG, Reed AL, Lattimer JC, et al: Hip dysplasia: A feline population study. Vet Radiol Ultrasound 40:460–464, 1999.
7. Pederson NC, Morgan JP, Vassuer PB: Joint diseases of dogs and cats. In Ettinger SJ (ed): Textbook of Veterinary Internal Medicine. 5th ed. Philadelphia, W.B. Saunders, 2000, pp 1862–1885.
8. Stubbs CJ, Holland CJ, Reif JS, et al: Feline ehrlichiosis: Literature review and serologic survey. Comp Cont Educ Pract Vet 22:307–317, 2000.

66. MUSCLE DISEASES

Catriona M. MacPhail, D.V.M.

1. What are the most common muscle diseases (myopathies) of cats? How are they classified?

Although most are rare, there are multiple causes of myopathy in cats. Some myopathies can be diagnosed indirectly using history and routine blood tests (hypokalemic myopathy). Others are classified by histologic appearance of tissue collected by biopsy. Myopathies can be inflammatory or degenerative, depending on the cause. Inflammatory myopathies are further classified into immune-mediated or infectious causes. Degenerative myopathies are congenital or acquired.

Feline Myopathies

Degenerative	**Endocrine**
Congenital	Hyperthyroidism
Muscular dystrophy	Hyperadrenocorticism
Myotonia	**Inflammatory**
Nemaline rod myopathy	Immune-mediated (idiopathic)
Myasthenia gravis	Infectious
Acquired	Bacterial
Myasthenia gravis	Protozoal
Myositis ossificans	Parasitic
Metabolic	**Vascular**
Hypokalemia	Ischemic neuromyopathy

2. What are the most common clinical signs associated with myopathies?

Generalized weakness is the predominant sign associated with skeletal muscle disorders. Other clinical signs include tremors, stilted gait, abnormal posturing, muscle pain, palmigrade or plantigrade stance, and variable lameness. Muscle atrophy, fibrosis, and contracture may be apparent in advanced myopathies. Cats with generalized weakness are more likely to present with cervical ventroflexion than dogs because cats lack the nuchal ligament that helps to maintain normal neck posture.

3. What are the other possible differential diagnoses for generalized weakness in cats?

Toxicities, neuropathies, nutritional deficiencies, cardiopulmonary disease (including anemia), and hypoglycemia can present with generalized weakness. The most common toxins associated with weakness include pyrethroid insecticides and organophosphates. Thiamine deficiency has been reported to cause a responsive generalized weakness, because thiamine is essential for aerobic metabolism. Cats with mild-to-moderate hypoglycemia, most commonly associated with insulin overdose, may present with acute generalized weakness before showing any neurologic abnormalities. Cats with polyneuropathy associated with diabetes mellitus typically present with hindlimb weakness and plantigrade stance.

4. What is the initial diagnostic plan for cats with suspected myopathy?

A thorough history, physical examination, and neurologic examination should help to differentiate between musculoskeletal, neurologic, and cardiopulmonary causes of generalized weakness. Complete blood cell count, serum biochemical panel, and urinalysis may further characterize metabolic and endocrine causes. Complete blood count helps to rule out anemia as a cause of weakness, and leukocyte counts may reflect a systemic inflammatory response. Hypokalemia is one of the most common causes of myopathy in cats. Serum potassium concentrations usually must be < 3.0 mEq/L to produce clinical signs. Renal azotemia may or may not be detected concurrently. Activities of creatine kinase (CK) and aspartate aminotransferase (AST) may be elevated, although some muscular diseases may cause few enzymatic changes. Therefore, normal CK and AST activities should not be used to rule out muscle disease. Urinalysis is crucial to identify renal disease, urinary tract infections, or glucosuria. Serum total T4 concentration should be measured in cats with suspected myopathy that are > 5 years of age.

5. What are the most important clinical aspects of hypokalemic myopathy?

Hypokalemia caused by decreased intake or increased excretion is frequently recognized in cats, especially those with chronic renal disease (see Chapter 40). Generalized weakness and cervical ventroflexion are common clinical abnormalities. A heritable form of hypokalemic myopathy has been detected in Burmese kittens that demonstrate intermittent muscle weakness and cervical ventroflexion, beginning at 2–6 months of age. Hypokalemia causes muscle weakness by increasing resting membrane potential, which makes skeletal muscle more refractory to stimuli. Clinical signs usually resolve after potassium supplementation.

6. How is potassium supplementation achieved?

Mildly affected cats are given potassium gluconate at 2 mEq per 4.5 kg body weight orally every 12 hr (Tumil-K; Daniels, St. Petersburg, FL). Periodic evaluation of potassium levels dictates the need for chronic administration.

Severely affected cats (< 2.5 mEq/L) require parenteral administration of potassium-supplemented fluids. Potassium should be administered cautiously via the intravenous route (0.5–1.0 mEq/kg/hr), diluted in a balanced electrolyte solution. Serum potassium concentrations should be monitored periodically during the infusion, and treatment should be discontinued once serum levels have reached 3.5 mEq/L. Electrocardiographic monitoring is also critical to observe for dysrrhythmias associated with hyperkalemia. Rapid administration of intravenous fluids may worsen hypokalemia by expanding venous vascular volume, which dilutes serum potassium concentrations. Critically low serum potassium values (< 2.0 mEq/L) may lead to respiratory arrest due to profound muscle weakness. Dopamine administration (0.5 mcg/kg/min, IV) is an alternative; dopamine causes translocation of potassium from the intracellular to extracellular fluid.

7. What is the diagnostic plan for cats with suspected myopathy when routine testing is inconclusive?

Electromyography (EMG) and muscle biopsy are commonly used. EMG helps to differentiate among neuropathies, neuromuscular junction disorders, and myopathies. EMG changes are fairly similar, regardless of the etiology of the myopathy. Muscle biopsy is used for definitive diagnosis. However, EMG findings help to characterize the distribution of the disease. EMG abnormalities consistent with muscle disease include polyphasic decreased motor unit action potentials, single sharp wave or trains of positive sharp waves, bizarre high-frequency waves, and myotonic discharges. Fibrillation potentials classically indicate denervation but can be seen in polymyositis and muscular dystrophy. Nerve conduction velocity studies should be normal.

8. How is the site for muscle biopsy chosen?

The pathologist should be consulted for preferred methods of sample acquisition and handling to obtain reliable results. The biopsy site should be based on history and clinical findings, although ideally multiple muscles should be sampled. EMG may be used to identify affected muscles, but needle insertion sites should be avoided during sample collection. For diffuse diseases, easily accessible superficial muscles such as the biceps femoris (distal third), long head of triceps (distal third), forelimb superficial digital flexor (proximal third), and lateral gastrocnemius (proximal third) usually are chosen.

9. How is the muscle biopsy collected?

Biopsies usually are collected under general anesthesia, but heavy sedation and local analgesia may be used as an alternative. Muscle samples should be handled as atraumatically as possible. Stay sutures can be used to help manipulate the tissue. A muscle sample is obtained (without any overlying fascia) by using a scalpel blade or fine, sharp scissors and incising parallel to the long direction of the muscle fibers. Take care to avoid significant neurovascular structures. A typical biopsy sample measures $1 \times 2 \times 1$ cm. After sampling, the biopsy is wrapped in saline-damped sponge, placed in a watertight container, and forwarded to the pathology laboratory as soon as possible. Processing can be delayed up to 30 hours as long as the sample is kept moist and cool (0–4°C). If a preservative is to be used, glutaraldehyde is preferred, because formalin fixation causes marked contraction artifacts. Electron microscopy evaluation requires the muscle to be stretched without excessive tension to prevent contraction or damage to the myofibers. Ideally special biopsy clamps are used to keep the muscle slightly stretched. Alternatively, stay sutures or small pins can keep a muscle slightly stretched across a tongue depressor.

10. What is idiopathic polymyositis? How is it managed?

Feline idiopathic polymyositis is an acquired inflammatory myopathy. Affected cats have an acute onset of weakness with marked cervical ventroflexion. Diagnosis is made by exclusion of other causes of myopathy with supportive EMG and muscle biopsy abnormalities. Histopathologic findings include severe myofiber necrosis and phagocytosis, lymphocytic inflammation, and fibrosis. Spontaneous recovery occurs in 30% of cats. Prednisone therapy may alleviate signs, but recurrence is common.

11. What are the common infectious causes of polymyositis? How are they managed?

Bacterial polymyositis is uncommon in companion animals, but when it occurs in cats, it typically is associated with *Pasteurella multocida*, although anaerobic infections must be considered. Localized myositis results from external trauma, such as bite wounds, whereas polymyositis typically is a manifestation of an overall disease process in which infection is spread hematogenously from a distant site. Clinical signs include muscle pain and swelling, pyrexia, and occasionally fistulation. Empirical antimicrobial therapy is based on the most likely contaminant. In general, an antibiotic with a broad gram-positive and anaerobic spectrum is a good first choice.

Toxoplasma gondii is associated more commonly with respiratory, ocular, or gastrointestinal signs in cats, although the organism may be found in the musculoskeletal and nervous systems. Typical musculoskeletal signs include abnormal gait, shifting leg lameness, mild-to-moderate hyperesthesia on muscle palpation, and muscle atrophy. Diagnosis is based on serologic evidence of active infection (high IgM and IgG titers), exclusion of other causes of muscle disease, and clinical response to treatment. The drug of choice is clindamycin, 10–12 mg/kg orally every 12 hr (Antirobe; Upjohn, Kalamazoo, MI). Systemic signs usually begin to subside within 24–48 hours of initiation of treatment, but muscle atrophy may take several weeks to resolve.

Trichinella spiralis seldom causes musculoskeletal signs, although cats are thought to be more susceptible to infection than dogs. Sarcocystis cysts have been found in the muscle of cats, but they are thought to be incidental and nonpathogenic.

12. What endocrine disorders are commonly associated with myopathy?

Muscle tremors and generalized weakness have been reported in cats with hyperthyroidism. Thyroid hormone excess is thought to affect mitochondrial oxidative phosphorylation. Total body water loss and hypokalemia associated with hyperthyroidism also may contribute to generalized weakness (see Chapter 53). Although rare in cats, hyperadrenocorticism has been associated with muscle weakness. Glucocorticoid excess increases muscle protein catabolism and inhibits synthesis of myofibrillar proteins, resulting in progressive loss of skeletal muscle mass (see Chapter 54).

13. Define muscular dystrophy.

Muscular dystrophy refers to a group of inherited muscle disorders characterized by progressive degeneration of skeletal muscles. X-linked disorders have been described in both dogs and cats. The disease in cats is characterized by generalized skeletal muscle hypertrophy, whereas in dogs marked muscle atrophy is typically present. Other clinical signs in cats include generalized muscle stiffness and decreased agility. Because of muscle stiffness, affected cats characteristically have to fall to one side in order to lie down. Dysphagia, vomiting, and regurgitation result from tongue protrusion, megaesophagus, and diaphragmatic hypertrophy, which frequently lead to fatal complications. Serum activity of CK is dramatically increased. Muscle biopsies reveal myofiber degeneration, necrosis, and multifocal mineralization. Immunohistochemical staining definitively diagnoses muscular dystrophy by demonstrating lack of the gene dystrophin in skeletal and cardiac muscle.

14. What other causes of feline myopathies may be diagnosed by muscle biopsy?

Nemaline myopathy has been described in a small number of cats and is characterized by a generalized weakness that progresses to tremors, hypermetric gait, and muscle atrophy. Muscle biopsy reveals marked fiber size variation with severe atrophy of type IIa fibers and scant type I fibers. Nemaline rods, which arise from the Z bands of myofibers, are seen throughout.

Myositis ossificans has been reported in isolated dogs and cats in both localized and generalized forms. Clinical signs include weakness, muscle pain and swelling, and firm, palpable enlargements in affected muscles. Muscle biopsy demonstrates excessive connective tissue between muscle fibers with inflammation that can progress to replacement of muscle by fibrous tissue and heterotropic bone in severe cases.

A **rare inherited myopathy** has been reported in Devon Rex kittens between 1 and 6 months of age. Neurologic examination is normal as well as CK activities. Muscle biopsy demonstrates marked dystrophic changes, although the mechanism responsible is unknown at this time.

15. What are myotonic myopathies?

Myotonia is a condition in which active muscle contraction continues after voluntary effort or stimulation has ceased. Congenital myotonia has been reported in several kittens. Typical clinical signs include stiff, stilted gait that improves with activity and nonpainful hypertrophy of appendicular muscles. Myotonia is best diagnosed by EMG, which reveals classic myotonic discharges. Muscle biopsies demonstrate mild nonspecific changes but are helpful in ruling out other causes of myopathies.

16. What are the muscular manifestations of feline aortic thromboembolism/ischemic neuromyopathy?

Thrombolic occlusion of the caudal aorta secondary to underlying cardiomyopathy results in acute motor dysfunction in the hindlimbs (see Chapter 17). Physical examination reveals weak-to-absent femoral pulses, cool hindpaws, and hard, swollen, painful muscles. Concurrent multisystemic signs may result from embolization of renal, gastrointestinal, and pulmonary vasculature. Histologically, affected muscles have areas of focal necrosis, marked architectural change, and hypertrophic fibers. If vital organ systems are not affected, most cats show slow clinical improvement over time with the reestablishment of collateral circulation.

17. Describe the clinical aspects of myasthenia gravis.

Myasthenia gravis is suspected in cats with progressive generalized weakness that is exacerbated by exercise. Additional clinical signs may include megaesophagus, dysphagia, and the presence of a cranial mediastinal mass (thymoma). The disease can be either congenital or acquired. The acquired form is an immune-mediated disease with antibodies directed at the acetylcholine receptors. Acquired immune-mediated myasthenia gravis is confirmed by demonstration of increased serum acetylcholine receptor autoantibodies. The congenital form of myasthenia gravis is rare in cats, and the diagnosis can be difficult, because affected cats do not have receptor autoantibodies. The diagnosis is based on characteristic clinical signs, EMG, and response to therapy. EMG demonstrates a decremental response of evoked action potentials with repetitive nerve stimulation. Intravenous administration of edrophonium chloride transiently improves clinical signs and EMG results. Edrophonium should be administered to cats with caution because a potentially life-threatening cholinergic crisis may develop. This risk can be minimized by pretreatment with atropine or immediate intravenous administration of atropine if problems develop. Successful treatment of feline myasthenia gravis has been reported with pyridostigmine bromide.

BIBLIOGRAPHY

1. Amann JF: Techniques of skeletal muscle biopsy. In Bojrab MJ (ed): Current Techniques in Small Animal Surgery, 4th ed. Baltimore, Williams & Wilkins, 1998, pp 91–94.
2. Blot S: Disorders of skeletal muscles. In Ettinger SJ (ed): Textbook of Veterinary Internal Medicine, 4th ed. Philadelphia, W.B. Saunders, 1999, pp 684–690.
3. Braund KG: Skeletal muscle biopsy. Semin Vet Med Surg 4:108–115, 1989.
4. Cuddon P: Feline neuromuscular disease. In Kirk RW (ed): Current Veterinary Therapy XI. Philadelphia, W.B. Saunders, 1992, pp 1024–1030.
5. Dow SW, LeCouteur RA, Fettman MJ, et al: Potassium depletion in cats: Hypokalemia polymyopathy. J Am Vet Med Assoc 191:1563–1567, 1987.
6. Ducoté JM, Dewey CW, Coates JR, et al: Clinical forms of acquired myasthenia gravis in cats. Comp Cont Educ Pract Vet 21:440–447, 1999.
7. Hickford FH, Jones BR: Congenital myotonia in the cat. In Kirk RW (ed): Current Veterinary Therapy XIII. Philadelphia, W.B. Saunders, 2000, pp 987–989.
8. Jones BR: Hypokalemic myopathy in cats. In Kirk RW (ed): Current Veterinary Therapy XIII. Philadelphia, W.B. Saunders, 2000, pp 985–987.
9. Kornegay JN: Lower motor neuron tetraparesis: neuromuscular disease. Probl Vet Med 3:378–390, 1991.
10. Shelton GD: Diseases of the muscle and the neuromuscular junction. In Sherding RG (ed): The Cat: Diseases and Clinical Management, 2nd ed. New York, Churchill Livingstone, 1994, pp 1569–1576.
11. Taylor SM: Selected disorders of muscle and the neuromuscular junction. Vet Clin North Amr 20:59–75, 2000.

67. UVEITIS

Tammy L. Miller, D.V.M., M.S., and Cynthia C. Powell, D.V.M., M.S.

1. What is uveitis?

Uveitis is any condition that involves inflammation of the uveal tract. It is one of the most important ocular diseases in cats.

2. Describe the structure of the uvea.

The uvea constitutes the vascular portion of the eye and consists of three main components:

1. The **iris** forms the most anterior portion and is the boundary between anterior and posterior chambers. Inflammation of the iris is termed *iritis*.

2. The **ciliary body** is the middle portion of the uvea that is responsible for formation of aqueous humor and accommodation. Inflammation of the ciliary body is termed *cyclitis*. Together the iris and ciliary body are considered the anterior uvea.

3. The **choroid**, located between the sclera and retina, supplies oxygen and nutrients to the outer layer of the retina and the optic nerve. It is considered the posterior uvea. Inflammation of the choroid is termed *choroiditis*. Inflammation of the choroid typically also affects the retina, in which case it is termed *chorioretinitis*.

3. Define endophthalmitis and panophthalmitis.

Inflammation of the entire uveal tract is termed *endophthalmitis*. When endophthalmitis is coupled with scleral and corneal inflammatory changes, it is termed *panophthalmitis*.

4. How is uveitis classified?

• Location (anterior, posterior)
• Duration (acute, chronic, recurrent)
• Pathology (e.g., granulomatous, suppurative)
• Cause (trauma, infection, neoplasia, immune-mediated)

5. What determines the clinical manifestations of uveitis?

The clinical appearance of uveitis depends on location, duration, and severity. Clinical signs of uveitis in cats are generally subtle and divided into those that affect either the anterior (iris and ciliary body) or posterior (choroid) segment.

6. Describe the clinical signs of anterior uveitis.

1. Photophobia, blepharospasm, enophthalmos, elevation of the third eyelid, and epiphora manifest as ocular pain. Pain is common with acute uveitis but may be absent with mild or chronic cases.

2. Injection of conjunctival and episcleral vessels results in a "red eye."

3. Low intraocular pressure (IOP) occurs when aqueous humor formation is impaired by inflammation of the ciliary body. A difference > 5 mmHg between eyes is considered significant. If uveitis is complicated by secondary glaucoma, IOP can be elevated or in the normal range if the decrease in IOP caused by uveitis is counterbalanced by the impairment of aqueous humor outflow associated with secondary glaucoma.

3. Aqueous flare is cloudy aqueous humor that results from influx of cells and protein when the blood-ocular barrier is disrupted as a result of uveal inflammation.

4. Corneal edema can result from effects of inflammation on the corneal endothelium and ranges from perilimbal to generalized.

5. Keratic precipitates are inflammatory cells in the aqueous humor that are deposited on the corneal endothelium. Normal convection currents of the aqueous humor cause the precipitates to be located primarily on the ventral half of the cornea.

6. Miosis results from direct effects on the iris sphincter of inflammatory mediators such as prostaglandins. Its absence does not rule out uveitis because mild miosis is difficult to detect.

7. Iritis is manifested by vasodilatation and increased vessel permeability that can produce a subtle-to-pronounced change in iris color. The iris may appear swollen and have a thin coat of fibrin and cells, giving it a velvety appearance. Rubeosis iridis is the proliferation of small vessels on the iris surface.

8. Hyphema.

9. Hypopyon.

7. What clinical signs indicate chronic or previous inflammation in the anterior segment?

1. Posterior synechia are adhesions to the anterior lens capsule that may cause the pupil to be irregularly shaped and impair its ability to respond to light or dilating agents.

2. Iris bombé forms when posterior synechia involve the entire pupil margin and prevent aqueous humor from moving from the posterior chamber to the anterior chamber and exiting through the filtration angle. The accumulation of aqueous humor behind the iris causes it to billow forward and is associated with increasing IOP and glaucoma.

3. Peripheral anterior synechia are adhesions of the peripheral iris to the corneal endothelium secondary to iris swelling or iris bombé.

4. Glaucoma.

8. Describe the clinical manifestations of posterior uveitis.

Clinical signs of posterior uveitis are often difficult to observe. Focal or diffuse hyporeflectivity of the retina indicates active fluid accumulation. This inflammatory subretinal transudation or exudation may result in retinal hemorrhage and retinal detachment. Chronic inflammation may result in loss of the normal tapetal color and loss of retinal pigment epithelial cells and choroidal pigmentation. Posterior uveitis almost always extends to involve the retina. Chronic chorioretinitis results in degeneration of the involved retina. Inactive chorioretinitis lesions appear hyperreflective.

9. What are the differential diagnoses of uveitis in cats?

Causes of uveitis in cats can be endogenous or exogenous and are listed in the tables below. In contrast to dogs, systemic infectious disease is more commonly found to be the cause of uveitis in cats. Appropriate treatment of uveitis, therefore, requires proper diagnosis, because the uveitis may be the first indication of a serious or life-threatening illness. Clinical or serologic evidence of systemic disease is detected in 25–90% of cats with uveitis.

Primary Endogenous Differential Diagnoses for Uveitis in Cats

Infectious	Infectious *(continued)*
Bacterial	Viral
Bartonella henselae	Feline immunodeficiency virus (FIV)
Ehrlichia spp.	Feline leukemia virus (FeLV)
Mycobacterium spp.	Feline infectious peritonitis (FIP)
Mycotic	**Neoplastic**
Blastomyces dermatitidis	Metastatic
Candida albicans	Lymphosarcoma
Coccidioides immitis	Others
Cryptococcus neoformans	Primary
Histoplasma capsulatum	Ciliary body adenoma
Parasitic	Ciliary body adenocarcinoma
Cuterebra spp.	Diffuse iris melanoma
Metastrongylidae	**Immune-mediated**
Protozoal	Lens-induced
Toxoplasma gondii	**Idiopathic**

Primary Exogenous Differential Diagnoses for Uveitis in Cats

Trauma	Keratitis
Secondary bacterial infection	Ulcer
Sterile inflammation	Infection
Ocular surgery	**Drug or toxin**
Secondary bacterial infection	Pilocarpine
Sterile inflammation	Latanoprost

10. How do you determine the cause of uveitis in cats?

A good history, physical examination, and a minimal database of complete blood chemistry, serum biochemical profile, and urinalysis are essential. Thoracic and abdominal radiographs as well as abdominal ultrasonography may be indicated if a neoplastic or infectious process is suspected. Outdoor cats should be routinely tested for *Toxoplasma gondii*, feline leukemia virus (FeLV) and feline immunodeficiency virus (FIV). Cats raised in a cattery or < 2 years of age should be routinely screened for coronaviruses. Ocular fluids can be used for cytology, culture and sensitivity, polymerase chain reaction (PCR), and determination of antibody content.

11. What are the four most common causes of systemic endogenous uveitis in cats?

1. *T. gondii*
2. Feline infectious peritonitis (FIP)
3. FIV
4. Lymphoma with or without serologic evidence of FeLV

12. What are the ocular signs of *T. gondii* infection?

Ocular toxoplasmosis can result in anterior or posterior uveitis and may be unilateral or bilateral.

13. Do all field strains of *T. gondii* induce ophthalmic disease?

The disease-inducing potential of *T. gondii* probably varies, because relatively few of the many seropositive cats have ophthalmic disease. The actual prevalence of ocular toxoplasmosis in naturally exposed cats is unknown because it is difficult to confirm the diagnosis. Recent work suggests that ocular toxoplasmosis may occur in kittens infected transplacentally or in the postnatal period.

14. How do you diagnose ocular toxoplasmosis?

Serologic evaluation for *T. gondii* infection should include assays that detect IgG and IgM. *T. gondii*-specific IgM is detected for days to weeks in subclinically infected cats but may be of high magnitude in cats with clinical toxoplasmosis. Serum IgG antibodies develop approximately 2 weeks after infection and remain elevated in cats for years after exposure. A 4-fold increase in IgG titer over 2–3 weeks or an IgM titer > 1:256 indicates recent or active infection. Cats with ocular toxoplasmosis may be seropositive for IgM and seronegative for IgG, particularly if they are FIV-seropositive. Detection of local antibody production or *T. gondii* DNA in aqueous humor may aid in the diagnosis of ocular toxoplasmosis (Veterinary Diagnostic Laboratory, College of Veterinary Medicine and Biomedical Sciences, Colorado State University, Fort Collins, CO).

15. What are the ocular signs of FIP?

Bilateral granulomatous anterior uveitis may be present. Clinical findings range from iritis, large keratic precipitates, clots of fibrin and blood in the anterior chamber, pyogranulomatous cuffing of the retinal vasculature, and chorioretinitis to retinal hemorrhage and retinal detachment.

16. Are ocular lesions most often seen with the effusive or noneffusive form of FIP?

Ocular lesions are most often seen with the noneffusive, or dry form of FIP.

17. How do you diagnose FIP?

Diagnosis of FIP-associated ocular disease is difficult because of the nonspecific nature of available coronavirus serum antibody tests. Positive coronavirus serum antibodies document only exposure to coronavirus and do not correlate with FIP. In addition, results of blood reverse transcriptase polymerase chain reaction (RT-PCR) do not correlate with FIP. Characteristic ocular lesions in the presence of rising serum antibody titers suggest the diagnosis particularly, if the appropriate signalment and history are also present (see Chapter 38). If effusions are present, characteristic findings aid in the diagnosis of FIP (see Chapter 38).

18. What are the ocular signs of FIV?

Anterior uveitis and pars planitis are the most common ocular findings in cats with FIV. The uveitis is typically chronic and mild. A higher incidence of glaucoma has been associated with or without uveitis in FIV-positive cats.

19. In what two ways can FIV produce uveitis?

Directly: through the local production of FIV antibodies and antigens.

Indirectly: immunodeficiency associated with FIV can result in opportunistic infections such as *T. gondii* and *C. neoformans*.

20. How is ocular disease due to FIV diagnosed?

It is difficult to prove that ocular inflammation is due to FIV. Presence of serum antibodies against FIV usually correlates with current infection but cannot be used to prove illness due to infection. Currently, the only way to document FIV-associated uveitis is to exclude all other known causes in a seropositive cat.

21. Can feline herpesvirus 1 (FHV-1) cause intraocular disease?

FHV-1 DNA and local FHV-1 antibody production were detected in the aqueous humor of cats with suspected idiopathic uveitis. These results show that FHV-1 can enter the eyes of cats and, in addition to keratoconjunctivitis, may be associated with uveitis. Serum antibody detection is of no benefit in the diagnosis of FHV-1 uveitis because most cats are vaccinated or previously exposed to FHV-1. Aqueous humor can be tested for FHV-1 by PCR commercially (Veterinary Diagnostic Laboratory, College of Veterinary Medicine and Biomedical Sciences, Colorado State University, Fort Collins, CO).

22. Is *Bartonella henselae* associated with uveitis in cats?

Cats are the apparent reservoir host for *B. henselae*. Although clinical disease is rare, 55-81% of cats are seropositive. *B. henselae* is one of the causes of cat-scratch disease in humans, and uveal tract inflammation has been reported in association with infection. *Bartonella* spp. was suggested as a likely cause of anterior uveitis in one cat based on the presence of antibody production in aqueous humor and response to doxycycline. *Bartonella* spp., therefore, may be able to invade the eyes of cats and result in uveitis.

23. How does FeLV cause ocular disease?

FeLV has not been shown to cause primary ocular disease. Ocular disease associated with FeLV is manifested in two ways:
- Metastatic lymphosarcoma of the anterior uvea and neurologic tissue
- Opportunistic infections secondary to immunosuppression

24. How is FeLV-associated ocular disease diagnosed?

The clinical presentation of neoplastic infiltration of the uveal tract and resultant uveitis may vary widely. Nodular or diffuse infiltration of the posterior or anterior uveal tract is possible. Although isolated ocular lymphosarcoma is rare, many cats present primarily for ocular signs. A search for neoplastic involvement of other organs should be made. Cats with lymphosarcoma should be staged (I–V) and FeLV status should be determined because both are related to treatment response and prognosis (see Chapter 68). Ocular involvement is by definition stage V lymphosarcoma. Aqueous humor cytology may be diagnostic in cases in which obvious lymphosarcoma cannot be identified in other organs. Testing for FeLV is always indicated in cats with uveitis whether or not lymphosarcoma is suspected, because opportunistic infection may be present. The enzyme-linked immunosorbent assay (ELISA) for detection of the p27 antigen in the blood (serum) is a useful screening tool for FeLV, but a positive immunofluorescent assay (IFA) correlates better with persistent viremia (see Chapter 76). A positive FeLV test does not prove ocular disease due to the virus, nor does a negative test rule out lymphosarcoma. Most FeLV-positive cats do not have lymphosarcoma, and 20–70% of cats with confirmed lymphosarcoma are FeLV-negative.

25. What is idiopathic uveitis? How is it diagnosed?

Idiopathic uveitis is any uveitis in which a cause cannot be identified. Unfortunately, a cause is not identified in 10–70% of cats with uveitis. The lymphocytic-plasmocytic infiltration of the anterior uvea found on histopathology in eyes lacking an etiologic diagnosis suggests that it may be immune-mediated. Whether this immune-mediated reaction is a true autoimmune disease or triggered by other antigenic stimulation remains to be determined in cats.

26. What are the goals of treating uveitis in cats?

Nonspecific
1. Stop or decrease the inflammation.
2. Prevent or control the complications caused by inflammation.
3. Relieve pain

Specific
1. Address etiologic agents (e.g., virus, bacteria, fungi).
2. Address specific causes of inflammation (e.g., foreign body, corneal ulcer, luxated lens).

27. How should you treat uveitis in cats?

Specific therapies for treating infectious agents are addressed in other chapters. In general, clindamycin hydrochloride is used for toxoplasmosis (see Chapter 11), doxycycline is used for *B. henselae* (see Chapter 85) and feline ehrlichiosis (see Chapter 78), and itraconazole or fluconazole is used for *C. neoformans* (see Chapter 4). Nonspecific therapies are listed in the table below.

Drugs Commonly Used to Treat Uveitis in Cats

Glucocorticoids
Topical (every 1–12 hr)
  Dexamethasone sodium phosphate 0.1% (solution), 0.5% (ointment)
  Prednisolone acetate 1% (suspension)
Oral (0.5–2.2 mg/kg every 12–24 hr)
  Prednisolone (5-mg tablet)
  Prednisone (5- or 20-mg tablet)

Subconjunctival agents
Betamethasone (0.75 mg/eye)
Methylprednisolone acetate (4 mg/eye)
Triamcinolone (4 mg/eye)

Nonsteroidal anti-inflammatory drugs (NSAIDs)
Topical (every 6–12 hr)
  Diclofenac 0.1% (solution)
  Flurbiprofen 0.03% (solution)
  Ketorolac 0.5% (solution)
  Suprofen 1% (solution)
Oral
  Acetylsalisylic acid (80-mg tablet every 48–72 h)r
  Ketoprofen (12.5 mg tablet; 2mg/kg initially; 1mg/kg/day maintenance)

Table continued on following page

Drugs Commonly Used to Treat Uveitis in Cats (Continued)

Mydriatic/cycloplegic (parasympatholytic) agents
Topical
Atropine sulfate (0.5% and 1% solution and ointment every 8–24 hr)
Tropicamide (0.5% and 1% [solution] every 6–12 hr)

---

28. What is the main difference in treatment of anterior and posterior uveitis?

Systemic therapy is the treatment of choice for posterior uveitis. Systemic glucocorticoid administration must be used with caution if an infectious process is suspected.

Topical therapy is the treatment of choice for anterior uveitis. If inflammation is not well controlled, addition of subconjunctival or systemic medication may be necessary.

29. For what two reasons are topical and subconjunctival glucocorticoids contraindicated in the treatment of uveitis in the presence of corneal ulceration?

1. Inhibition of wound healing
2. Augmentation of collagenase activity in the cornea

30. When should you use subconjunctival glucocorticoids?

This form of treatment should be used only in cases of severe intraocular inflammation as an adjunct to topical or systemic steroids or in cases in which frequent topical therapy is not possible. A serious disadvantage to this method is inability to withdraw the medication if complications arise.

31. When should topical and systemic NSAIDs be used in cats?

There is little information about their use in cats. NSAIDs should be considered only when glucocorticoids are contraindicated. Topical NSAIDs may complicate bacterial corneal infections and are not recommended. Systemic NSAIDs should be used with caution in cats because they have been associated with potentially severe side effects, such as vomiting, diarrhea, gastrointestinal ulceration and hemorrhage, and bone marrow suppression.

32. How do you relieve the ocular pain associated with uveitis?

Mydriatics/cycloplegics relieve pain by relaxation of ciliary body and iris spasm. The duration and frequency of use depend on the severity of the inflammation.

33. What are the potential sight-threatening complications of failure to control intraocular inflammation?

- Posterior synechiae
- Glaucoma
- Cataracts
- Lens luxation
- Retinal degeneration
- Retinal detachment

BIBLIOGRAPHY

1. Brightman AH, Ogilvie GK, Tompkins M: Ocular disease in FeLV-positive cats: 11 cases (1981–1986). J Am Vet Med Assoc 198:1049–1051, 1991.
2. Chavkin MJ, Lappin MR, Powell CC, et al: Seroepidemiologic and clinical observations of 93 cases of uveitis in cats. Prog Vet Comp Ophthalmol 2:29–36, 1992.
3. Chavkin MJ, Lappin MR, Powell CC, et al: *Toxoplasma gondii*-specific antibodies in the aqueous humor of cats with toxoplasmosis. Am J Vet Res 55:1244–1249, 1994.
4. Davidson MG, Nasisse MP, English RV, et al: Feline anterior uveitis: A study of 53 cases. J Am Anim Hosp Assoc 27:77–83, 1991.
5. English RV, Davidson MG, Nasisse MP, et al: Intraocular disease associated with feline immunodeficiency virus infection in cats. J Am Vet Med Assoc 196:1116–1119, 1990.
6. Lappin MR: Opportunistic infections associated with retroviral infections in cats. Semin Vet Med Surg (Small Anim) 104:244–250, 1995.

7. Lappin MR, Black JC: *Bartonella* spp. infection as a possible cause of uveitis in a cat. J Am Vet Med Assoc 214:1205–1207, 1999.
8. Lappin MR, Kordick DL, Breitschwerdt EB: *Bartonella* spp. antibodies and DNA in aqueous humor of cats. J Fel Med Surg 2:61–68, 2000.
9. Lappin MR, Marks A, Greene CE, et al: Serologic prevalence of selected infectious diseases in cats with uveitis. J Am Vet Med Assoc 201:1005–1009, 1992.
10. Maggs DJ, Lappin MR, Reif JS, et al: Evaluation of feline herpes-specific antibodies and DNA in aqueous humor from cats with or without uveitis. Am J Vet Res 60:932–936, 1999.
11. Martin CL, Stiles J: Ocular infections. In Greene CE (ed): Infectious Diseases of the Dog and Cat, 2nd ed. Philadelphia, W.B. Saunders, 1998, pp 658–672.
12. Peiffer RL Jr, Wilcock BP: Histopathologic study of uveitis in cats: 139 cases (1978–1988). J Am Vet Med Assoc 198:135–138, 1991.
13. Powell CC, Lappin MR: Uveitis in cats. Part 1: Definitions and causes. Comp Cont Educ Pract Vet [in press].
14. Powell CC, Lappin MR: Uveitis in cats. Part 2: Diagnostic and treatment plans. Comp Cont Educ Pract Vet [in press].
15. Stiles J: The cat. In Gelatt KN (ed): Veterinary Ophthalmology. Philadelphia, Lippincott Williams & Wilkins, 1999, pp 1448–1473.

VII. Hemolymphatic Problems

Section Editor: Christine S. Olver, D.V.M., Ph.D.

68. LYMPHADENOPATHY AND LYMPHOMA

Elizabeth A. McNiel, D.V.M., M.S., Ph.D.

1. How is lymphadenopathy recognized?

On physical examination, determination of lymphadenopathy may be quite subjective. "Normal" lymph node size varies among individuals and as a function of lymph node location, age of the animal, body condition, and conformation. Variation in lymph node size can even be based on environmental factors such as geographical location. Although pronounced lymphadenopathy is usually obvious to both the pet owner and the veterinarian, mild lymph node enlargement may be difficult to appreciate and may go unrecognized. The potential difficulty in identifying this problem underscores the importance of a thorough physical examination, including palpation of peripheral lymph nodes and regular reassessment of lymph nodes. As a disease progresses, the lymphadenopathy may become more evident.

2. What causes lymphadenopathy in cats?

The primary differential diagnoses for generalized lymphadenopathy in cats are infectious diseases; immune-mediated, inflammatory. and neoplastic diseases are less common. The reverse may well be true for dogs, depending on geographical location. Generalized lymphadenopathy in dogs is commonly caused by multicentric lymphoma. In cats, multicentric lymphoma is diagnosed relatively infrequently.

Causes of Lymphadenopathy in Cats

Infections	Inflammatory/immune-mediated disorders
Bacterial	Hypereosinophilic syndrome (cause is unknown
Bartonella henselae	but may be a neoplastic process)
Mycobacterium spp	Polyarthritis
Yersinia pestis	Polymyositis
Norcardia spp.	
Actinomyces spp.	**Neoplastic processes**
Ehrlichia spp.	Lymphoma
Viral	Leukemia
Feline leukemia virus (FeLV)	Metastatic neoplasia
Feline immunodeficiency virus	
Panleukopenia	**Benign lymphadenopathy**
Parasitic	Benign hyperplasia resembling lymphoma—
Toxoplasma gondii	with or without FeLV infection
Fungal	Plexiform vascularization
Blastomyces dermatitidis	
Coccidioides immitis	
Cryptococcus neoformans	
Histoplasma capsulatum	

3. How should lymphadenopathy be approached diagnostically?

If lymphadenopathy is clearly secondary to some other process, specific diagnostic tests may be unnecessary. Unexplained lymphadenopathy should be approached systematically, regardless of species and underlying etiology (see algorithm below).

In cases of chronic lymphadenopathy without obvious cause, advanced diagnostics should be considered. Flow cytometry is now available at a number of veterinary institutions for evaluation of peripheral blood, bone marrow, and single cell suspensions of lymphoid tissue to detect cell surface antigens and measure relative DNA content. Flow cytometric detection of cell surface antigens is helpful in differentiating a homogenous, clonal population of lymphoid cells consistent with lymphoid neoplasia from a mixed population consistent with an immunologic process. Altered DNA content also can be evaluated when neoplasia is suspected, as many tumors are not diploid.

Recently, polymerase chain reaction (PCR) of lymphoid tissue, blood, or bone marrow, detecting clonal expansions of lymphoid cells with unique antigen receptor gene rearrangements, has been added to the armamentarium of diagnostic tests for lymphoma in dogs. The test is under evaluation for use in cats. PCR is used to detect a clonal population of lymphocytes in blood or tissue sample and also the immunophenotype (B or T cell) of that population. This information provides support for a diagnosis of lymphoma and potentially provides prognostic insight. PCR may be useful for cases of unexplained lymphadenopathy, lymphocytosis, and hypercalcemia. For information on the status of PCR, contact the Colorado State University Diagnostic Laboratory at (970) 491-1281.

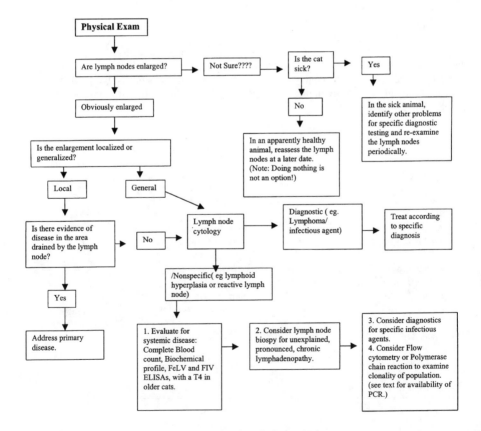

Diagnostic approach to lymphadenopathy in cats.

4. Describe the clinical presentation of feline lymphoma.

Cats with lymphoma are usually "sick." The clinical signs depend on the organ system affected. For example, spinal lymphoma may be associated with hind limb paralysis, alimentary lymphoma is often characterized by vomiting, and nasal lymphoma results in signs of upper respiratory disease. Generalized lymphadenopathy is a relatively uncommon presentation for cats with lymphoma and, like mediastinal lymphoma, may become increasingly infrequent. The changing prevalence of FeLV antigenemia in cats with lymphoma may account for this decrease. Cats with multicentric and mediastinal lymphoma are frequently FeLV-positive. Over the past 15 years, the number of cats with lymphoma that test positive for FeLV has decreased from about 70% to 20–30%. The change in FeLV prevalence accompanies a shift in the anatomic site of lymphomas (alimentary lymphoma seems to be most common) and in the age of cats affected (cats with lymphoma that are FeLV-negative are older than cats that are FeLV-positive).

5. What laboratory abnormalities are associated with lymphoma?

Laboratory findings are usually nonspecific. Anemia is common and may result from any combination of chronic illness, bone barrow infiltration by neoplastic cells, or immune-mediated or infectious disease (e.g., FeLV). Lymphocytosis is probable with lymphoid leukemia. Hypercalcemia of malignancy has been reported but is much less common than in dogs. Azotemia may result from hypercalcemia or nephric lymphoma. Hyperglobulinemia occurs in some cats and may be polyclonal or monoclonal.

6. How is lymphoma diagnosed?

Histologic evaluation of tissue is the most definitive diagnostic technique for lymphoma, particularly with the use of immunohistochemical stains for B- and T-cell surface markers. Cytology also may be diagnostic. A diagnosis of lymphoma based on lymph node cytology should be viewed cautiously, however, because benign lymphoid hyperplasia has been described in cats. Cytology in such cases may be difficult to distinguish from lymphoma. If other lymph nodes are enlarged, mandibular lymph nodes should be avoided when samples are collected for cytologic evaluation because hyperplasia is particularly common at this site. As mentioned for the work-up of lymphadenopathy, flow cytometry and PCR can be valuable diagnostic tools.

7. Why do cats get lymphoma?

FeLV is known to cause lymphoma in cats (see Chapter 76). The prevalence of FeLV-positive lymphomas appears to have declined in recent years. It is not known whether this decrease is a result of management changes, such as testing and vaccination, or a change in the typical virus. Feline immunodeficiency virus may indirectly result in lymphoma (see Chapter 77). Many lymphomas do not have an obvious retroviral etiology; their cause is unknown. Because cancer is a genetic disease, it is assumed that induced and inherited mutations in cancer-associated genes play a role in lymphoma development in cats.

8. What treatments are available for cats with lymphoma?

Chemotherapy and radiation therapy are the most effective modalities for treating lymphoma in any species. Chemotherapy is indicated in most cases because of the disseminated, systemic nature of many feline lymphomas and may be used as the sole treatment modality for alimentary, renal, and multicentric disease. Prednisone used as a single agent results in a short remission and improvement in clinical signs in about one-half of treated cats. Multiagent chemotherapy regimens are the mainstay of therapy. The addition of doxorubicin to the standard combination therapy with cyclophosphamide, vincristine, and prednisone appears to improve prognosis. Unfortunately, few prospective studies compare various chemotherapeutic combinations for efficacy and toxicity in cats with a single type of lymphoma. The available information is insufficient to select the "optimal" protocol for all situations (see table on following page).

Appealing attributes of radiation therapy in the treatment of lymphoma include the exquisite sensitivity of lymphoid cells to radiation and the ability to localize the dose. Radiation therapy

Chemotherapy for Feline Lymphoma

	COP	COP + IDARUBICIN/DOXORUBICIN	VCM	UWM
Week 1	Vincristine, 0.75 mg/m² Cyclophosphamide, 300 mg/m² PO Prednisone, 40 mg/m³/day PO	Vincristine, 0.75 mg/m² Cyclosphosphamide, 250 mg/m² PO Prednisone, 40 mg/m³/day PO	Vincristine, 0.025 mg/kg IV, + L-asparaginase, 400 IU/kg IP	Vincristine, 0.7 mg/m² IV, + L-asparaginase, 400 IU/kg IM Prednisone, 2 mg/kg/day PO
Week 2	Vincristine, 0.75 mg/m² Prednisone, 40 mg/m³/day PO	Vincristine, 0.75 mg/m² Prednisone, 40 mg/m³/day PO	Cyclophosphamide, 10 mg/kg IV	Cyclophosphamide, 250 mg/m² IV Prednisone, 2 mg/kg/day PO
Week 3	Vincristine, 0.75 mg/m² Prednisone, 40 mg/m³/day PO	Vincristine, 0.75 mg/m² Prednisone, 40 mg/m³/day PO	Vincristine, 0.025 mg/kg IV	Vincristine, 0.7 mg/m² IV Prednisone, 1 mg/kg/day PO
Week 4	Vincristine, 0.75 mg/m² Cyclophosphamide, 300 mg/m² PO Prednisone, 40 mg/m³/day PO	Idarubicin, 2 mg/kg PO for 3 days *or* Doxorubicin, 25 mg/m² every 3 wk	Methotrexate, 0.8 mg/kg IV or PO	Doxorubicin, 20 mg/m² IV Prednisone, 1 mg/kg/day PO
Week 6				Vincristine, 0.7 mg/m² IV
Week 7				Cyclophosphamide, 250 mg/m² IV *or* Chlorambucil, 1.4 mg/kg PO *or* Cytosine arabinoside, 600 mg/m² SQ divided twice daily for 2 days (renal lymphoma)
Week 8				Vincristine, 0.7 mg/m² IV
Week 9				Doxorubicin, 20 mg/m² IV
Week 11				Vincristine, 0.7 mg/m² IV
Week 13				Cyclophosphamide, 250 mg/m² IV *or* Chlorambucil, 1.4 mg/kg PO *or* Cytosine arabinoside, 600 mg/m² SQ divided twice daily for 2 days (renal lymphoma)

Week 15	Vincristine, 0.7 mg/m² IV		
Week 17	Methotrexate, 0.8 mg/kg IV		
Week 19	Vincristine, 0.7 mg/m² IV		
Week 21	Cyclophosphamide, 250 mg/m² IV, *or* Chlorambucil, 1.4 mg/kg PO *or* Cytosine arabinoside, 600 mg/m² SQ divided twice daily for 2 days (renal lymphoma)		
Week 23	Vincristine, 0.7 mg/m² IV		
Week 25	Doxorubicin, 20 mg/m² IV		
Maintenance	Continue vincristine/cyclophosphamide every 3 wk for 1 yr	Repeat (1) idarubicin every 3 wk until recurrence or 11 mo *or* (2) doxorubicin, 25 mg/m² every 3 wk for 6 mo or until relapse	Repeat weeks 1–4 Prednisone, 5 mg/day PO	Continue prednisone 1 mg/kg every other day after week 5; repeat weeks 11–25 at 2-week intervals for 1 yr (week 52); repeat at 3–4 week intervals for second year

COP = cylophosphamide, vincristine, and prednisone; VCM = vincristine, cyclophosphamide, and methotrexate; UWM = University of Wisconsin–Madison; PO = orally, IV = intravenously, IP = intraperitoneally, SQ = subcutaneously.

should be considered for localized lymphomas, drug-resistant lymphomas, and cases in which a primary mass results in severe dysfunction. Excellent results are reported for irradiation of cats with nasal lymphoma. As radiation therapy becomes increasingly available to veterinarians, its role in the treatment of lymphoma is likely to expand.

9. How much toxicity is expected with treatment?

Quality of life is a primary concern in the treatment of any veterinary problem, including cancer. The most commonly used chemotherapeutic protocols are designed to cause minimal toxicity. Gastrointestinal (GI) toxicity (anorexia, vomiting, and diarrhea) is the most common side effect, but it is dose-dependent and usually self-limiting. It is possible to achieve acceptable levels of GI toxicity in most cases through the use of supportive measures and individually designed dose and administration schedules. Bone marrow suppression and most drug-specific toxicities are uncommon in cats. Cats on long-term chemotherapy lose their whiskers!

Toxicity due to radiation is classified as acute (concurrent with or shortly after treatment) or late (> 6 months after treatment). Late effects are extremely unlikely in the treatment of lymphoma with standard-dose protocols. Acute effects depend on the site. In nasal irradiation, mucositis of the nasal and oral cavity is probable. For superficial treatments, there is the possibility of moist or dry skin desquamation. These effects can be minimized with appropriate treatment planning and are of limited duration (a few weeks).

10. What is the prognosis for feline lymphoma?

Without treatment, cats with lymphoma do not live very long (see questions 11 and 12), particularly because most cats are sick at the time of diagnosis. For treated cats, the prognosis is quite variable and usually unpredictable in individual patients. Site, clinical stage, and FeLV status have an effect on outcome.

11. How does FeLV status influence outcome?

Cats that are FeLV-positive may respond well to chemotherapy initially but have median survival periods of just a few months. Mediastinal and multicentric lymphoma is commonly associated with FeLV infection.

12. How do anatomic site and clinical stage affect outcome?

The table below provides the staging scheme recommended by the World Health Organization for feline lymphoma. For the various anatomic sites and clinical stages, the response of individual cats may vary a lot. Overall, 50–70% of cats treated for lymphoma achieve complete remission with median remission times of 2–4 months and median survival times of about 4–6 months. Cats surviving for years after treatment are frequently reported, particularly with solitary nasal lymphoma (and perhaps other stage I lymphomas) and with some alimentary lymphomas. Cats that achieve complete remission initially respond better than those cats that do not. The heterogeneity in the response of feline lymphomas probably reflects diversity in the disease. Subclassifications based on immunologic markers, genetic mutations, and chromosome rearrangements may be of considerable value as prognostic factors. Research in these areas is ongoing.

Clinical Stages of Feline Lymphoma

Stage I	Single node or solitary extranodal site, including mediastinum
Stage II	Regional lymph node involvement; resectable gastrointestinal mass
Stage III	Generalized lymph node involvement; unresectable abdominal disease; epidural tumor
Stage IV	Stages I–III with liver or spleen involvement
Stage V	Stages I–IV with bone marrow involvement
Substage A	No systemic signs
Substage B	Systemic signs

BIBLIOGRAPHY

1. Elmslie RE, Ogilvie GK, Gillette EL, et al: Radiotherapy with and without chemotherapy for localized lymphoma in 10 cats. Vet Radiol 32:277–280, 1991.
2. Jeglum KA, Whereat A, Young K: Chemotherapy of lymphoma in 75 cats. J Am Vet Med Assoc 190:174–178, 1987.
3. Meleo KA: The role of radiotherapy in the treatment of lymphoma and thymoma. Vet Clin North Am Small Anim Pract 27:115–129, 1997.
4. Mooney SC, Hayes AA, MacEwen EG, et al: Treatment and prognostic factors in lymphoma in cats: 103 cases (1977–1981). J Am Vet Med Assoc 194:696–702, 1989.
5. Moore AS, Cotter SM, Frimberger AE, et al: A comparison of doxorubicin and COP for maintenance of remission in cats with lymphoma. J Vet Intern Med 10:372–375, 1996.
6. Moore AS, Ruslander D, Cotter SM, et al: Efficacy of, and toxicoses associated with, oral idarubicin administration in cats with neoplasia. J Am Vet Med Assoc 206:1550–1554, 1995.
7. Moore FM, Emerson WE, Cotter SM, et al: Distinctive peripheral lymph node hyperplasia of young cats. Vet Pathol 23:386–391, 1986.
8. Rassnick KM, Mauldin GN, Moroff SD, et al: Prognostic value of argyrophilic nucleolar organizer region (AgNOR) staining in feline intestinal lymphoma. J Vet Intern Med 13:187–190, 1999.
9. Vail DM, Moore AS, Ogilvie GK, et al: Feline lymphoma (145 cases): Proliferation indices, cluster of differentiation 3 immunoreactivity, and their association with prognosis in 90 cats. J Vet Intern Med 12:349–354, 1998.
10. Zwahlen CH, Lucroy MD, Kraegel SA, et al: Results of chemotherapy for cats with alimentary malignant lymphoma: 21 cases (1993–1997) [see comments]. J Am Vet Med Assoc 213:1144–1149, 1998.

69. NEUTROPHILIA AND NEUTROPENIA

Armando R. Irizarry-Rovira, D.V.M.

1. Define neutrophilia and neutropenia.

Neutrophilia is an absolute increase in the number of neutrophils circulating in the peripheral blood (circulating neutrophil pool). **Neutropenia** is an absolute decrease in the number of neutrophils circulating in the peripheral blood. The number of circulating neutrophils, as measured in a complete blood count (CBC), is a one-time snapshot, the result of the balance among production, distribution, utilization, and destruction of neutrophils.

2. What causes neutrophilia?

In general, neutrophilia can be caused by four main conditions, acting singly or in combination:

1. Epinephrine release/administration. Epinephrine is released during excitement, fear, and/or exercise. The leukogram changes associated with epinephrine are also referred to as **physiologic leukocytosis**.

2. Corticosteroid release/administration. Endogenous corticosteroids are released during injury, pain, prolonged emotional stress, abnormal body temperature, and hyperadrenocorticism. The leukogram picture of neutrophilia and accompanying lymphopenia associated with corticosteroids is commonly referred to as **stress leukogram**. Epinephrine- and corticosteroid-mediated neutrophilias are commonly seen in veterinary patients.

3. Inflammation. This important cause of neutrophilia is elicited by both infectious and noninfectious causes.

4. Myeloproliferative disease (MPD). Although rarely seen, feline patients with acute myelogenous leukemia with differentiation (AML-M2) and chronic myelogenous leukemia (CML) may present with neutrophilia.

Primary Differential Diagnoses for Neutrophilia in Cats

Epinephrine release/administration
  Fear
  Excitement
  Exercise
Corticosteroid release/administration
  Trauma or injury
  Pain
  Prolonged emotional stress
  Abnormal body temperature
  Hyperadrenocorticism
  Exogenous administration (length of effect depends on short- vs. long-acting formulation)
  Metabolic imbalance (diabetic ketoacidosis, hyperthyroidism, ethylene glycol toxicosis)
Inflammation
  Infectious
    Bacterial infections (various)
    Systemic fungal infections
    Viral infections (feline infectious peritonitis virus, feline herpesvirus 1)
    Rickettsial infections (*Haemobartonella felis*, ehrlichiosis)
  Immune-mediated
    Autoimmune hemolytic anemia
    Immune-mediated arthritis
  Necrosis
    Infarctions, gangrene
    Tumor necrosis
  Trauma
    Surgery
    Gunshots
    Other trauma
  Foreign bodies (intestinal, oropharyngeal, migrating grass awns, iatrogenic)
Neoplasms
  Myeloproliferative disease
  Lymphosarcoma
  Adenocarcinoma
  Tumor necrosis
  Neoplasms in general may cause inflammation, pain, and "stress" (neutrophilia is common in small
    animals with neoplastic diseases)
  Paraneoplastic syndrome (production of cytokines by neoplastic cells)

---

3. By what mechanisms do the causes listed above lead to neutrophilia?

Neutrophilia is elicited by three general mechanisms, acting singly or in combination with each other: (1) neutrophil redistribution, (2) increased bone marrow production, and (3) decreased egress from the peripheral blood to the tissues.

4. Explain the mechanism of neutrophil redistribution.

Neutrophils may be redistributed from the marginal neutrophil pool (MNP) to the circulating neutrophil pool (CNP). The MNP is not sampled during routine blood collection; it consists of neutrophils that are found rolling along arteriolar and venular endothelial surfaces or have transiently ceased moving within capillaries. Redistribution of neutrophils from the MNP to CNP can be caused by corticosteroids (endogenous or exogenous) and/or epinephrine (endogenous or exogenous). Generally, in cats the MNP-to-CNP ratio is 3:1; therefore, dramatic increases in circulating neutrophils may result from redistribution into the CNP. Neutrophils also may be redistributed from the bone marrow mature neutrophil storage pool to the total blood neutrophil pool by corticosteroids and inflammation.

5. When does bone marrow increase production of neutrophil precursors?

Increased bone marrow production of neutrophil precursors occurs when there is demand for neutrophils in the peripheral tissues. Trauma, infections, immune-mediated cell injury, and certain neoplasms cause neutrophilia by eliciting the release of chemical mediators (cytokines, growth factors) that stimulate neutrophil precursors to proliferate and differentiate. Certain tumors (carcinomas) may be the direct source of these chemical mediators. Increased neutrophil production also occurs in certain rare types of MPD (e.g. AML-M2, CML). In 80% of human cases of CML, a reciprocal translocation between chromosomes 9 and 22 in the leukemic cells results in the formation of the Philadelphia chromosome. The protein product of this oncogene has tyrosine kinase activity that results in the marked proliferation of granulocytic precursors. Although chromosomal abnormalities are seen in feline leukemia virus (FeLV)-positive cats in general and FeLV-positive cats with leukemia, characteristic chromosomal abnormalities specifically associated with the development of MPD in cats are not documented.

6. What causes decreased egress of neutrophils from peripheral blood into tissues?

Decreased egress of neutrophils from peripheral blood into tissues occurs in combination with the other mechanisms mentioned above but is due primarily to the effects of corticosteroids. Although not currently recognized in cats, neutrophilia also may result from congenital defects in leukocyte adhesion, such as leukocyte adhesion molecule (β2 integrin) deficiency in dogs and cattle.

7. How can the signalment help in ranking the differential list for neutrophilia?

Neutrophilia due to endogenous epinephrine release (physiologic leukocytosis) is frequently seen in young cats; however, it may be seen in cats of any age. Neutrophilia due to endogenous corticosteroid release or inflammatory diseases may be seen in cats of any age. Neutrophilia due to MPD is seen in FeLV-infected cats. Cats with MPD are generally younger (< 5.5 years old).

8. How can the history help in ranking the differential list?

Neutrophilia due to endogenous epinephrine release (physiologic leukocytosis) is frequently seen in healthy cats that are excited or frightened during the visit to the veterinarian. It is also seen in cats that vigorously struggle during restraint or blood collection. Neutrophilia due to endogenous corticosteroid release is seen in cats affected by stressful conditions such as severe, painful injuries or, less commonly, diseases that cause endogenous corticosteroid release, such as primary or secondary hyperadrenocorticism (polyuria/polydipsia associated with diabetes mellitus, poor haircoat, skin infections, skin bruising). Patients with neutrophilia due to inflammatory diseases present with a variety of clinical histories. For example, the patient may have a history of lethargy, anorexia, being hit by a car (trauma), recent surgery (sterile foreign body, dehiscence), or diabetes (diabetic ketoacidosis). Inflammation in diabetic ketoacidotic patients may develop from the combined effects of immunosuppression and hyperglycemia (which predispose to bacterial infections) or in association with pancreatitis. Patients affected with MPD may have a history supportive of FeLV (multiple cat household, outdoor cat, previous positive FeLV test), hemorrhages (thrombocytopenia, coagulation factor deficiency due to liver involvement), lethargy, anorexia, or masses (lymphadenomegaly).

9. How can the physical examination help in ranking the differential list?

Neutrophilia due to endogenous epinephrine release in healthy cats may be characterized by increases in heart and respiratory rate, blood pressure, and muscular activity. Neutrophilia due to endogenous corticosteroid release in cats with primary or secondary hyperadrenocorticism may be associated with potbelly appearance, rough hair coat, and thin fragile skin. Patients with neutrophilia due to inflammatory diseases may present with a multitude of physical examination abnormalities, including fever, depression, elevated heart and respiratory rates, distended and/or painful abdomen (pyometra, peritonitis, hemoabdomen, surgical dehiscence, foreign bodies), dyspnea (pyothorax, pneumonia), nasal discharge (feline viral rhinotracheitis, foreign bodies, neoplasia), space-occupying masses (neoplasia, abscesses), pale mucus membranes (anemia due to *H. felis*), and splenomegaly and/or hepatomegaly (neoplasia, diffuse fungal or bacterial infection). Cats affected with MPD may present with organomegaly, elevated heart and respiratory rates, fever, hemorrhages, pallor, icterus, and lymphadenopathy.

10. What are the typical CBC findings in cats with epinephrine-induced neutrophilia?
Epinephrine-induced neutrophilia is mild-to-moderate (12,500–25,000 cells/µl) and transient (usually 20–30 minutes in duration). It may be accompanied by lymphocytosis or a normal lymphocyte count. An elevated packed cell volume (PCV) may be seen due to splenic contraction secondary to the effects of epinephrine. A second blood sample collected a few hours later when the cat is calmer helps to confirm the diagnosis (i.e., the leukogram will be within reference ranges).

11. Describe the typical CBC findings in cats with corticosteroid-induced neutrophilia.
Corticosteroid-induced neutrophilia is mild-to-moderate (12,500–25,000 cells/µl), not associated with a left shift, and frequently accompanied by lymphopenia and eosinopenia. Monocytosis secondary to corticosteroids is an inconsistent finding in cats. Corticosteroid-induced leukogram changes, specifically lymphopenia, also may be seen with inflammatory disease.

12. What are the typical CBC findings in cats with neutrophilia of mild inflammatory disease?
Neutrophilia may be the only leukocyte abnormality associated with mild inflammatory changes. Neutrophil counts of 12,500–25,000 cells/µl with no other significant leukogram change may be difficult to differentiate from neutrophil counts seen with corticosteroids and epinephrine. Although not specifically studied in cats, fibrinogen levels may increase with inflammation and help to differentiate neutrophilia of inflammation from neutrophilia induced by epinephrine or corticosteroids. Fibrinogen levels should be within normal reference values in patients with corticosteroid or epinephrine-induced neutrophilia that do not have inflammatory, neoplastic or hemostatic abnormalities. Hyperfibrinogenemia also is seen in neoplastic conditions (due to inflammation, increased synthesis from tumor cells or secondary to cytokine production by the tumor cells) and in certain species with compensated intravascular coagulation.

13. Describe the CBC findings that suggest more severe inflammatory disease.
Neutrophil toxicity (cytoplasmic basophilia, foaminess, increased numbers of Döhle bodies) and circulating immature neutrophils (bands, metamyelocytes, and myelocytes) indicate inflammation of increased severity. Circulating immature neutrophils are referred to as a left shift and indicate that the bone marrow is not able to meet the demand for mature neutrophils. The more pronounced the left shift and the toxic change, the more severe the inflammatory insult. Moderate to severe neutrophilia (>30,000 cells/µl) is seen with localized, long-standing infections such as pyothorax, pyometra, and peritonitis. Severely elevated neutrophil counts (50,000–75,000 cells/µl) with a prominent left shift are also referred to as a leukemoid reaction and can be difficult to differentiate from certain forms of MPD (e.g., AML-M2, CML). The neutrophilia associated with MPD may be mild-to-severe and accompanied by significant numbers of immature neutrophils (e.g., AML-M2 and CML with blast crisis [not described in cats]). Select cytopenias (e.g., nonregenerative anemia) may accompany the leukemic changes. Caution is warranted in cats suspected of feline panleukopenia virus (FPLV) infection because dramatic left shifts during the recovery phase may be reminiscent of myelogenous leukemia. Repeating the CBC on subsequent days should help to clarify this distinction. Neutrophilic series mature in cats recovering from FPLV but not in cats with leukemia.

14. What is the diagnostic plan for cats with neutrophilia after an epinephrine or corticosteroid response is ruled out?
The plan usually includes a serum biochemical panel and urinalysis. Patients with epinephrine-induced neutrophilia may exhibit mild-to-marked, transient hyperglycemia with resulting glucosuria. Patients with corticosteroid-induced neutrophilia may exhibit mild and potentially persistent hyperglycemia. The hyperglycemia induced by corticosteroids should not exceed the renal threshold for glucose.

Serum FeLV antigen test and feline immunodeficiency virus antibody test should be performed. Other diagnostic procedures (e.g., diagnostic imaging, cytology, histopathology, microbiology) may be necessary to characterize the process eliciting neutrophilia (see questions 15 and 16). Bone marrow evaluation should be pursued in unexplained, persistent neutrophilia or when leukocyte morphology or the magnitude of neutrophilia raises suspicion of leukemia. Bone marrow aspirates are useful for detecting the presence of morphologically bizarre neoplastic/dysplastic hematopoietic precursors or abnormal distribution of hematopoietic precursors in the marrow (i.e., too many immature cells).

15. How do imaging techniques aid in the ranking of differential diagnoses?

Radiographs, ultrasound, computed tomography scan, or magnetic resonance imaging may be used in some cases to aid in detecting organomegaly, effusion, space-occupying masses, and localizing lesions. Abnormalities are expected in patients with some inflammatory conditions and some patients with leukemic disease.

16. When are aspirates or biopsies indicated?

Aspirates or biopsies are indicated when space-occupying lesions, effusions, organomegaly, or abnormal organ shape and appearance are present. Exploratory surgery may be required to obtain diagnostic samples. Aspirates are generally easier to perform and less expensive and can be examined almost immediately. Tissue biopsies are necessary to examine tissue architecture and determine the extent of involvement of a particular organ or location. Bone marrow aspirates and biopsies are indicated in suspected cases of leukemia. A coagulation profile should be performed before sampling procedures are done in bleeding patients and patients suspected of having liver disease or coagulation abnormalities.

17. What are the predominant causes of neutropenia?

In general, neutropenia can be caused by five main conditions, acting singly or in combination: (1) severe, sudden tissue demand; (2) neutrophil redistribution; (3) abnormalities in bone marrow neutrophil production; (4) ineffective granulopoiesis; and (5) peripheral neutrophil destruction.

Primary Differential Diagnoses for Neutropenia in Cats

Severe, sudden tissue demand for neutrophils
Infection (various bacteria causing diseases such as peritonitis, pyothorax, and pneumonia)
Redistribution of neutrophils from CNP to MNP
Infection (gram-negative endotoxemia)
Abnormalities in bone marrow neutrophil production
Drugs
Azathioprine
Griseofulvin
Chloramphenicol
Sulfa-trimethoprim combinations
Human G-CSF (cats initially respond with neutrophilia but later develop antihuman G-CSF
antibodies that cross-react with feline G-CSF)
Radiation therapy
Neoplastic disease

Myeloproliferative disease	Metastatic neoplasia
Myelodysplastic syndrome	Systemic mast cell tumor
Lymphoproliferative disease	

Infections
Feline leuekmia virus (FeLV)
Feline immunodeficiency virus
Feline infectious peritonitis virus (particularly in cats coinfected with FeLV)
Feline panleukopenia virus
Histoplasmosis
Idiopathic abnormalities

Ineffective granulopoiesis
  Drug-related (anticancer drugs, griseofulvin, chloramphenicol, azathioprine, others)
Peripheral neutrophil destruction
  Corticosteroid-responsive (suggests an immune-mediated mechanism), "hypersplenism"
  Paraneoplastic syndrome (immune-mediated mechanism may be involved): dermal squamous cell
    carcinoma

G-CSF = granulocyte colony-stimulating factor, CNP = circulating neutrophil pool, MNP = marginal neutrophil pool.

18. What is the most common cause of a severe, sudden tissue demand for neutrophils?

Severe, sudden tissue demand, which is probably the most common cause of neutropenia in cats, is due primarily to inflammation (infectious or noninfectious) and results from the release of potent chemical signals that attract neutrophils to the inflammatory site.

19. When does neutrophil redistribution occur?

During endotoxemia due to gram-negative infections, neutrophils shift from the CNP to the MNP as a result of the release of various cytokines that increase neutrophil adhesion to endothelial surfaces.

20. What may cause abnormalities in bone marrow neutrophil production?

Various infectious agents (FeLV, feline immunodeficiency virus [FIV], feline panleukopenia virus [FPLV], histoplasmosis), chemicals (anticancer drugs, griseofulvin, chloramphenicol), toxins (mycotoxins), neoplastic diseases (lymphoproliferative disease, myeloproliferative disease, metastatic neoplasm), myelodysplastic syndromes, and idiopathic disease can lead to a decrease in the proliferating pool of neutrophil precursors.

21. Explain ineffective granulopoiesis.

In cats with ineffective granulopoiesis, neutropenia is present concurrently with bone marrow hyperplasia or normal bone marrow cellularity. This condition may be due to an immune-mediated destructive process directed at a single type or multiple types of neutrophil precursors. Many causes of abnormalities in bone marrow neutrophil production also may cause ineffective granulopoiesis. Ineffective granulopoiesis is seen in cats with FeLV and/or FIV infection and cats with myelodysplastic syndromes. It may be seen after administration of certain drugs (sulfa-trimethoprim, anticancer drugs, griseofulvin, chloramphenicol). FeLV-associated neutropenia is more common than FeLV-associated myeloproliferative disease. The marrow is frequently hypercellular in FeLV-associated neutropenic patients.

22. What causes peripheral neutrophil destruction?

Immune-mediated destruction, "hypersplenism" (sequestration in the spleen or removal of neutrophils by splenic macrophages), administration of certain drugs, and paraneoplastic syndrome associated with cutaneous squamous cell carcinoma (an immune-mediated mechanism may be involved).

23. How can the signalment help in ranking the differential list?

The specific signalment can vary with the particular cause of the neutropenia. Some diseases affect cats of any age (endotoxemia, toxins, intestinal foreign bodies), whereas others affect specific age groups:
  • FIV is more commonly seen in older (> 5 years of age), outdoor, male cats.
  • FeLV-affected cats are generally younger (< 5 years of age).
  • Cats < 1 year of age are at increased risk for disseminated histoplasmosis.
  • Cats infected with FPLV are generally < 1 year of age.

- Cats most susceptible to FIPV tend to be young (6 months to 2 years of age) or geriatric (14–15 years of age).
- The mean age of cats with MPD is 3–5.5 years old.

24. How can the history help in ranking the differential list?

The history varies with the specific cause and may not be suggestive of neutropenia. For instance, fever, anorexia, and lethargy may be reported by the owner but are clearly not specific for neutropenia. The history is important in determining whether the cat is at increased risk for viral disease (e.g., outdoor cats and cats that live in multiple-cat households are at increased risk for FIV and FeLV). Cats affected with FIPV have histories reflecting multisystemic disease. Neutropenic patients often present with a clinical history of specific organ system involvement. For example, diarrhea may be seen with FPLV and FeLV and intestinal foreign bodies with perforation, neoplasia involving the intestines, or septicemia. Dyspnea may be seen in patients with acute pneumonia. Patients with abnormalities in bone marrow neutrophil production may have a history of administration of marrow-suppressive drugs, FeLV-positive status, or multiple "lumps" (lymphadenomegaly associated with systemic neoplasia). Patients with peripheral neutrophil destruction or ineffective granulopoiesis may have a history of recent drug administration.

25. How can physical examination findings help in ranking the differential list?

Physical examination findings may be nonspecific or vary with the specific cause of neutropenia. Patients with neutropenia due to severe, sudden demand for neutrophils may present with a multitude of abnormalities, including fever, depression, elevated heart and respiratory rates, distended and/or painful abdomen (pyometra, peritonitis, ruptured intestine), or dyspnea (pyothorax). Cats with abnormalities in bone marrow neutrophil production may have evidence of systemic neoplasia or infection (organomegaly, space-occupying masses, icterus) and pancytopenia (pale mucous membranes due to anemia, petechiae due to thrombocytopenia).

26. How can the CBC help to determine the cause of neutropenia?

Cats with inflammatory disease, endotoxemia, or septicemia have inflammatory leukograms (left shift, neutrophil toxicity). Leukemic patients may have atypical cells in the circulation. Pancytopenias may be present in patients with abnormalities in bone marrow neutrophil production and ineffective granulopoiesis. Patients with peripheral neutrophil destruction may have neutropenia as the only hematologic abnormality (immune-mediated neutropenia, cyclic neutropenia). Leukoerythroblastic (immature white and red blood cells) reactions may be seen in patients with bone marrow infiltration by massive numbers of neoplastic or inflammatory cells.

27. Describe the initial diagnostic plan for cats with neutropenia.

If the neutropenia is an incidental finding (i.e., the cat is not ill), a repeat CBC may be used to confirm neutropenia. CBC, peripheral blood smear evaluation, serum biochemical analysis, FeLV and FIV testing, and bone marrow aspirate and biopsy should be obtained in persistently or ill neutropenic cats. CBC and peripheral blood smear evaluation are necessary to identify other hematologic and bone marrow production abnormalities (pancytopenia, leukemia). Additional diagnostic tests may be necessary, including imaging examinations (radiography, ultrasonography), microscopic examination of cytologic preparations, tissue biopsies and effusions, microbiologic culture, and serology. Patients must be examined carefully for the presence of an inflammatory focus (abscess), systemic neoplasia, or systemic infection.

28. Can routine biochemical testing aid in the ranking of differential diagnoses?

Biochemical testing and urinalysis may be helpful in localizing a particular disease process or documenting the extent of the disease. Coagulation profiles are recommended in patients with hemorrhage or liver involvement and patients suspected of having coagulation abnormalities. Cats affected with FIPV often have hyperglobulinemia (polyclonal or monoclonal gammopathy). Serum protein electrophoresis is recommended to characterize the hyperglobulinemia.

29. How do imaging techniques aid in the ranking of differential diagnoses?

Imaging techniques (radiography, ultrasonography) help to detect organomegaly, fluid in body cavities, and space-occupying masses; to localize lesions; and to direct biopsies (ultrasonography). Abnormalities are expected in patients with some inflammatory conditions and some patients with leukemic and neoplastic disease.

30. When are aspirates or biopsies indicated?

Aspirates or biopsies are indicated in patients with space-occupying lesions, effusions, organomegaly, or abnormal organ shape and appearance. Exploratory surgery may be required to obtain diagnostic samples. Bone marrow aspirates and biopsies are indicated in suspected cases of MPD and pancytopenia. In cases of bone marrow hypoplasia, aspirates may produce low numbers of cells. Bone marrow core biopsies may help to differentiate a poor aspirate sample from true hypoplastic bone marrow and hypoplasia associated with myelofibrosis from hypoplasia seen with other conditions (e.g., FPLV). Tissue biopsies are necessary to examine tissue architecture and determine the extent of involvement of a particular organ or location. A coagulation profile should be performed before sampling procedures in bleeding patients and patients suspected of having liver disease or coagulation abnormalities.

31. Describe the initial treatment plan for cats with neutrophilia and neutropenia.

Intravenous fluids are indicated in most sick patients, particularly those that are dehydrated. Patients with infectious diseases (bacterial, fungal) should be treated with appropriate antimicrobial therapy. Patients with immune-mediated diseases frequently benefit from immunosuppressive therapy. Patients with neoplastic disease, depending on the stage of the disease, may benefit from anticancer chemotherapy or surgery. Other treatments depend on the primary disease process.

BIBLIOGRAPHY

1. Baldwin CJ, Ledet AE: Pancytopenia. In August JR (ed): Consultations in Feline Internal Medicine, 2nd ed. Philadelphia, W.B. Saunders, 1994, pp 495–502.
2. Bjoersdorff A, Svendenius L, Owens JH, et al: Feline granulocytic ehrlichiosis: A report of a new clinical entity and characterization of the infectious agent. J Small Anim Pract 40:20–24, 1999.
3. Duncan JR, Prasse KW, Mahaffey EA: Leukocytes. In Veterinary Laboratory Medicine: Clinical Pathology. Ames, IA, Iowa State University Press, 1994, pp 37–62.
4. Hall RL: Interpreting the leukogram. In August JR (ed): Consultations in Feline Internal Medicine, 2nd ed. Philadelphia, W.B. Saunders, 1994, pp 489–494.
5. Hawkins EC: Investigation and management of neutropenia. In August JR (ed): Consultations in Feline Internal Medicine. Philadelphia, W.B. Saunders, 1990, pp 343–348.
6. Kidd R: Interpreting neutrophil numbers. Vet Med 86:975–978, 1991.
7. Linenberger ML, Shelton GH, Persik MT, Abkowitz JL: Hematopoiesis in asymptomatic cats infected with feline immunodeficiency virus. Blood 78:1963–1968, 1991.
8. Meyer DJ, Harvey JW: Evaluation of leukocytic disorders. In Veterinary Laboratory Medicine: Interpretation and Diagnosis. Philadelphia, W.B. Saunders, 1998, pp 83–109.
9. Raskin RE: Myelopoiesis and myeloproliferative disorders. Vet Clin North Am 26:1023–1042, 1996.
10. Rojko JL, Hardy WD Jr: Feline leukemia virus and other retroviruses. In Sherding RG (ed): The Cat: Diseases and Clinical Management. New York, Churchill Livingstone, 1994, pp 263–432.
11. Thoday KL, Mooney CT: Historical and laboratory features of 126 hyperthyroid cats. Vet Rec 131:257–264, 1992.
12. Thrall MA, Grauer GF, Mero KN: Clinicopathologic findings in cats with ethylene glycol intoxication. J Am Vet Med Assoc 184:37–41, 1984.
13. Tyler RD, Cowell RL, Meador V: Bone marrow evaluation. In August JR (ed): Consultations in Feline Internal Medicine, 2nd ed. Philadelphia, W.B. Saunders, 1994, pp 515–523.
14. Ward H, Couto CG: Myeloid leukemias. In August JR (ed): Consultations in Feline Internal Medicine, 3rd ed. Philadelphia, W.B. Saunders, 1997, pp 509–513.
15. Wellman ML, Hammer AS, DiBartola SP, et al: Lymphoma involving large granular lymphocytes in cats: 11 cases (1982–1991). J Am Vet Med Assoc 201:1265–1269, 1992.

70. EOSINOPHILIA AND EOSINOPENIA

Robin W. Allison, D.V.M.

1. Define eosinophilia and eosinopenia.

Eosinophilia refers to increased numbers of circulating eosinophils (depending on the laboratory reference range, usually > 1,200–1,500 cells/μl). **Eosinopenia** is rarely recognized because the low normal value for eosinophils in cats is zero.

2. In what tissues are eosinophils most abundant?

After production in the bone marrow and release into peripheral blood, eosinophils migrate after only a few hours in circulation into various tissues, where they can survive for several days. Eosinophils generally are most abundant in submucosal and mucocutaneous areas (skin, respiratory tract, gastrointestinal tract, and genitourinary tract).

3. What are the normal functions of eosinophils?

The characteristic pinkish-red cytoplasmic granules of eosinophils (rod-shaped in cats) contain a wide variety of chemical constituents with different functional roles. In general, eosinophils are important in controlling tissue parasites and regulating allergic and acute inflammatory responses. Specifically, eosinophils migrate into tissues in response to local chemoattractants, including antigen–antibody complexes involving IgE, mast cell products such as histamine, activated complement components, and cytokines such as interleukin-2 and eotaxin. Once in tissues, eosinophils interact through surface receptors, eventually releasing potent granule contents (e.g., major basic protein, histaminase, phospholipase D) and lipid mediators (e.g., leukotrienes, platelet-activating factor). These reactive substances have a diverse array of local effects, including antibody-mediated parasite killing, inhibition and inactivation of mast cell products such as histamine and serotonin, amplification of the inflammatory cascade via cytokine release, tissue injury through collagen degradation, and alterations in vascular permeability.

4. How does eosinophilia occur?

Blood eosinophilia may result from:
- Increased production
- Increased release from bone marrow
- Redistribution from the marginal pool
- Prolonged intravascular survival

The first two mechanisms are probably responsible for most instances of eosinophilia and occur in response to cytokines produced by activated T lymphocytes (primarily interleukin 5). Redistribution may occur in association with neutrophilia and lymphocytosis during the epinephrine-induced excitement response. Prolonged survival may be important in some hypereosinophilic syndromes.

5. What causes eosinopenia?

Although of limited significance, eosinopenia may result from stress associated with illness and exogenous corticosteroid administration. Concurrent lymphopenia supports a diagnosis of true eosinopenia due to stress.

6. What are the primary causes of eosinophilia?

Inflammatory disorders, frequently parasitic or allergic in origin, involving the skin, respiratory tract, or gastrointestinal tract (GI) are common causes of eosinophilia. Flea allergy, bronchial asthma, eosinophilic granuloma complex, and eosinophilic gastroenteritis are the most common underlying diseases in cats. Less frequent causes include neoplasia (e.g., mast cell tumor, lymphoma, eosinophilic leukemia), fungal, viral, or bacterial infections, and hypereosinophilic syndrome (HES). HES is characterized by blood eosinophilia, bone marrow hyperplasia of eosinophil precursors, and multiple organ infiltration by eosinophils; it may be difficult to distinguish from eosinophilic leukemia.

Diseases Associated with Eosinophilia in Cats

Gastrointestinal diseases	**Respiratory disease**
Coccidiosis	*Aleurostrongylus abstrusus*
Eosinophilic enteritis*	*Dirofilaria immitis*
Giardia spp.	Feline bronchial asthma*
Hookworms*	*Paragonimus kellikotti*
Inflammatory bowel disease (chronic)	Pneumonia (bacterial, viral)
Roundworms*	Pneumothorax
Tapeworms*	Rhinitis/sinusitis (chronic)
Toxoplasma gondii	Upper respiratory infection (chronic)
Infectious diseases	**Skin diseases**
Feline infectious peritonitis	Atopy
Feline leukemia virus	*Ctenocephalides felis**
Feline panleukopenia	Eosinophilic granuloma complex*
Viral upper respiratory disease	Flea allergy dermatitis*
Neoplasia	Food hypersensitivity
Lymphoma	*Notoedres cati*
Mast cell disease (systemic, cutaneous)	*Otodectes cyanosis*
Myeoloproliferative disorders	Pemphigus foliaceous
Solid tumors (uncommon)	Miscellaneous
Myxosarcoma	Cardiomyopathy
Basal cell tumor	Feline urologic syndrome
Squamous cell carcinoma	Focal inflammatory disorders
Salivary adenocarcinoma	Hyperthyroidism
Sweat gland adenocarcinoma	Renal failure
Transitional cell carcinoma	Soft tissue trauma
	Suppurative processes

* Most common causes.

7. Describe the initial diagnostic plan for cats with eosinophilia.

Initial evaluation should be aimed at excluding parasitic and allergic disorders and can be directed by the clinical signs.

8. What tests are appropriate for cats with respiratory signs?

For cats exhibiting respiratory signs such as dyspnea, tachypnea, or wheezing, appropriate diagnostic tests include thoracic radiographs, *Dirofiliaria immitis* antibody and antigen testing, fecal flotation, and Baermann examination (see Chapter 8). If bronchial or alveolar lung disease are present, eosinophilic inflammation may be evident in a tracheal wash, indicating a hypersensitivity reaction that could be allergic or parasitic. Occasionally parasite larvae or ova also may be present in the wash, but often multiple fecal examinations are necessary to identify parasites that have been coughed up and swallowed.

9. What tests are useful in cats with skin disease?

Cats with skin disease should be examined for fleas, have skin scrapings or cultures to identify ectoparasites or other microorganisms, and may require skin biopsies, food trials, or allergy testing. Fine-needle aspiration or surgical biopsy can be used to evaluate masses.

10. Describe the elements of GI tract evaluation.

GI evaluation should include an oral examination for eosinophilic granuloma, fecal flotation, fecal wet mount examination, and abdominal radiographs (see Chapter 18). Endoscopy or exploratory laparotomy may be indicated with cytology or biopsy of any identified lesions used to prove eosinophilic inflammation. Hypoadrenocorticism is another cause of eosinophilia and GI signs (see Chapter 55).

11. What additional diagnostic tests may be needed?

Once the more common parasitic and allergic disorders have been ruled out, other causes such as hematopoietic or nonhematopoietic neoplasia and various infectious and inflammatory diseases should be pursued. Bone marrow aspirates; ultrasound-guided aspirates of enlarged abdominal organs such as liver, spleen, or lymph nodes; and cytologic evaluation of any thoracic or abdominal effusion may be helpful.

12. How is eosinophilia treated?

The underlying disease must be identified and treated to resolve the eosinophilia. HES and eosinophilic leukemia in cats have been treated with corticosteroids with some short-term improvement, but long-term results have been poor.

BIBLIOGRAPHY

1. Center SA, Randolph JF, Erb HN, et al: Eosinophilia in the cat: A retrospective study of 312 cases (1975 to 1986). J Am Anim Hosp Assoc 26:349–358, 1990.
2. Center SA, Randolph JF: Eosinophilia. In August JR (ed): Consultations in Feline Internal Medicine. Philadelphia, W.B. Saunders, 1991, pp 349–358.
3. Corcoran BM, Foster DJ, Fuentes VL: Feline asthma syndrome: A retrospective study of the clinical presentation in cats. J Small Anim Pract. 36:481, 1995.
4. Couto CG, Wellman M: Disorders of leukocytes and leukopoiesis. In Sherding RG (ed): The Cat: Diseases and Clinical Management. New York, Churchill Livingstone, 1994, pp 721–737.
5. Huibregtse BA, Turner JL: Hypereosinophilic syndrome and eosinophilic leukemia: A comparison of 22 hypereosinophilic cats. J Am Anim Hosp Assoc 30:591–599, 1994.
6. Jain NC: The eosinophils. In Essentials of Veterinary Hematology. Philadelphia, Lea & Febiger, 1993, pp 247–257.
7. Power HT, Ihrke PJ: Selected feline eosinophilic skin diseases. Vet Clin North Am Small Anim Pract 25:833–850, 1995.

71. BLEEDING PROBLEMS

Michael R. Lappin, D.V.M., Ph.D., and Christine Olver, D.V.M., Ph.D.

1. What are the primary differential diagnoses for cats with evidence of bleeding?

Cats presented for evaluation of clinical findings consistent with hemorrhage usually have one of the four following conditions:

1. Local vascular disease
2. Disorders of hemostasis
3. Hypertension
4. Generalized vascular disease (vasculitis)

Local diseases of blood vessels (e.g., trauma, tumors, chronic inflammation) are the most common conditions resulting in bleeding in cats. Widespread vasculitis is rare in cats. Hypertension usually results only in retinal hemorrhage, but epistaxis and bleeding into the central nervous system occur in some cats (see Chapter 63). Although apparently less common than in dogs, disorders of hemostasis do occur in cats. One study found abnormalities in 38 of 85 clinically ill cats assessed for coagulopathies.

2. How can disorders of hemostasis be classified?

Primary hemostasis is basically the primary platelet plug that develops at the site of a defect in a vessel wall. As the primary platelet plug is forming, fibrin is deposited in the diseased area (**secondary hemostasis**) via activation of soluble and cell-associated coagulation pathways.

3. Describe the mechanisms of primary hemostasis.

Platelets bind to adhesive glycoproteins in the exposed subendothelium of damaged blood vessels, forming the primary platelet plug that continues to grow as platelets aggregate. Primary hemostasis helps to control local hemorrhage for seconds to minutes. Primary hemostasis disorders can be divided into disorders resulting in platelet function deficits or disorders resulting in thrombocytopenia. Platelet function deficits in cats are apparently rare; von Willebrand's disease has been reported in several cats. Mechanisms leading to thrombocytopenia include decreased production, increased destruction, or increased consumption of platelets.

4. Describe the disorders associated with secondary hemostasis.

Defects in secondary hemostasis can be grouped into disorders leading to factor decrease or absence or factor inhibition. Examples of factor decrease or absence include decreased production due to hepatic insufficiency; congenital lack; failure to convert procoagulants to coagulants (factors II, VII, IX, and X) due to vitamin K absence (cholestatic liver disease or malabsorption syndromes) or vitamin K antagonism (some rodenticides); and consumption due to disseminated intravascular coagulation (DIC).

5. Where are clotting factors produced?

With the exception of von Willebrand's factor and factor VIII, circulating polypetide clotting factors are produced exclusively by the liver.

6. Which clotting factors are vitamin K–dependent?

Factors II, VII, IX, and X.

7. Which factor is the most significant component measured by the one-stage prothrombin time (OSPT)?

Factor VII.

8. How is a balance maintained between clot formation and clot dissolution?

- When secondary hemostasis is activated, fibrinolysis also occurs.
- Tissue activators of plasminogen include urokinase and tissue plasminogen activator.
- Activation of plasminogen generates plasmin, which degrades fibrinogen and fibrin to fibrinogen degradation products (FDPs).
- Physiologic anticoagulants include antithrombin III (ATIII), which inhibits thrombin (factor II), activated factors X, IX, XI, and XII, and kallikrein, and the vitamin K-dependent proteins S and C, which inhibit factors V and VIII. ATIII is produced by the liver and potentiated by heparin.

9. Describe the clinical findings of hemostatic disorders.

Petechiae and ecchymoses are most common with primary hemostatic disorders. Mucous membranes and the retina are the areas with the highest sensitivity for detection of petechiae. Cats with secondary hemostatic disorders can be clinically normal. Factor abnormalities often result in deep-tissue and body-cavity bleeding. Bleeding tendencies may not be evident until vessels are traumatized (e.g., at surgery). Other clinical findings depend on the primary disease and the site of hemorrhage. For example, cats with warfarin toxicity resulting in hemothorax usually present with lethargy, dyspnea, and restrictive breathing pattern.

10. What tests are used to help classify hemostatic disorders?

The tests used most commonly include platelet count, activated clotting time (ACT), and bleeding time (BT) because each can be performed easily in the feline hospital in an emergency situation without expensive equipment. Machines (SC2000 Coagulation Analyzer; Synbiotics, San Diego, CA) available for in-clinic use can perform the OSPT and activated partial thromboplastin time (APTT). These tests also can be performed accurately in commercial laboratories if the samples are handled appropriately. Fibrinogen degradation products (FDP), thrombin time (TT), proteins induced by vitamin K absence or antagonism (PIVKAs), von Willebrand's factor, ATIII, and other specific factor assessments are sometimes needed. With the exception of FDP, platelet count, and ACT, coagulation tests are performed on citrated plasma. After collection, citrated blood should be centrifuged immediately and the plasma frozen until assayed. When collecting samples for assessment of hemostasis, make a clean venipuncture to avoid liberating procoagulant tissue factors.

11. Summarize the test results associated with hemostatic disorders in cats.

DISEASE	PLATELET COUNT	ACTIVATED CLOTTING TIME	BLEEDING TIME	DIAGNOSIS
Primary hemostasis				
Thrombocytopenia	Decreased	Slight prolongation	Prolonged	Varies with primary disease
von Willebrand's disease and other platelet dysfunction diseases	Normal	Normal or prolonged with concurrent factor VIII hemophilia	Prolonged	Measurement of von Willebrand's antigen
Secondary hemostasis				
Hemophilia	Normal	Prolonged unless factor VII deficiency	Normal	Specific factor assessment
Hepatic insufficiency	Normal	Prolonged	Normal	Serum biochemical panel, bile acids, imaging, biopsy
Cholestatic liver disease or malabsorption syndromes	Normal	Prolonged	Normal	Serum biochemical panel, imaging, biopsy
Vitamin K antagonist rodenticides	Normal	Prolonged	Normal	Measurement of PIVKA or warfarin byproducts

12. How are platelet count and morphology assessed?

Platelets can be counted or estimated by microscopic examination of a stained thin blood smear. Under oil immersion, each platelet per field is equivalent to 15,000/µl; normal cats have 11–19 platelets per field. Whenever thrombocytopenia is detected, evaluate for evidence of platelet clumps, which may signify falsely lowered numbers. Giant platelets may indicate the release of immature platelets from an appropriately active bone marrow, making decreased production of platelets less likely. Spontaneous hemorrhage from thrombocytopenia usually does not occur unless the count is < 50,000/µl. The platelet count of normal cats should be > 200,000/µl.

13. How is ACT assessed?

Assessment of ACT requires only a special tube (Becton Dickinson Microbiology Systems, Rutherford, NJ) and a 37°C incubator. The test estimates decreases in factors in the intrinsic and common pathways and thus is similar to the APTT. However, platelet phospholipid affects the ACT but not the APTT. Thus, extreme thrombocytopenia (< 50,000/µl) may result in a slight prolongation of the ACT (10–15 seconds). ACT does not detect decreases in factor VII (extrinsic pathway). However, factor VII hemophilia is either nonexistent or extremely rare in cats. Cats with ACT < 165 seconds should be considered normal.

14. Describe the assessment of bleeding time.
Bleeding time evaluates platelet function and thus is not indicated in cats with thrombocytopenia. Platelet function abnormalities are rare in cats since von Willebrand's disease is uncommon. If bleeding time is assessed, the lip should be gently rolled back and held in place lightly with gauze under light sedation. A Simplate device (Organon Teknika Corp., Durham, NC) is applied gently to the mucosa, and the trigger is released to make a measured incision. Filter paper or gauze is used to wick away excessive blood but should not touch the incision or risk dislodging the platelet plug. A normal mucosal bleeding time is < 2.5 minutes.

15. When are other tests indicated?
Results of the initial screening tests determine which other tests are needed:
• OSPT detects abnormalities in the extrinsic and common pathways; APTT detects abnormalities in the intrinsic and common pathways.
• Von Willebrand's factor can be measured to assess for von Willebrand's disease.
• PIVKAs are procoagulants of the vitamin K-dependent factors II, VII, IX, and X and increase in plasma if vitamin K is absent or antagonized (see questions 19–23).
• FDPs are products of fibrinolysis and are increased in cats with DIC.
• ATIII is consumed in DIC, resulting in decreased activity; thus, ATII activity can be used to aid in the diagnosis (see questions 26–28).

16. What causes decreased production of platelets in cats?
Decreased production of platelets can be caused by a number of different syndromes. Thrombocytopenia is often extreme, and other cell lines (neutrophils and erythrocytes) are decreased with some diseases. Bone marrow aspiration or biopsy may be needed to diagnose the specific syndrome. Diseases likely to be encountered include:
• Myelophthisis due to infiltrative lymphoma, leukemias, or multiple myeloma
• Feline leukemia virus-associated myelosuppression (see Chapter 76)
• Immune–mediated disease directed at megakaryocytes
• Drug induced bone marrow suppression
In a study of 41 cats with thrombocytopenia, FeLV and myeloproliferative neoplasia accounted for 44% of the cases. Primary immune-mediated thrombocytopenia was suspected in only 1 cat.

17. What causes increased platelet utilization, consumption, or destruction in cats?
Increased platelet utilization, consumption, or destruction occurs rarely in cats. The degree of thrombocytopenia is mild to moderate. Diseases that may be encountered include:
• Idiopathic immune-mediated thrombocytopenia (rare compared with dogs)
• Systemic lupus erythematosus (extremely rare compared with dogs).
• Disseminated intravascular coagulation (see questions 26–28).
• Modified live vaccines, which may cause transient thrombocytopenia that usually is inapparent clinically (see Chapter 82).
• Platelet utilization at sites of hemorrhage due to trauma or secondary hemostatic problems (e.g., rodenticide toxicity), which may cause mild thrombocytopenia
• Feline ehrlichiosis (see Chapter 78).
• Any disease resulting in vasculitis (e.g., sepsis) can result in thrombocytopenia due to local consumption of platelets.

18. Summarize the approach to management of platelet problems.
The primary disease should be identified and treated. Whole blood transfusion may be indicated if extreme anemia is occurring. Fresh whole blood transfusion does not provide many

platelets but may be indicated if active bleeding is occurring. Suspected primary immune-mediated thrombocytopenia is managed like immune-mediated hemolytic anemia (see Chapter 72).

19. Does von Willebrand's disease occur in cats?

Compared with dogs, this disease is extremely rare in cats. Expected findings include a prolonged bleeding time due to platelet dysfunction (decreased von Willebrand's antigen) and a normal platelet count, with or without a prolongation in ACT or APTT (depending on the presence of concurrent factor VIII deficiency) (see question 9).

20. What are other inherited coagulation abnormalities?

Factor XII deficiency is an autosomal recessive trait that appears to be the most common inherited secondary hemostatic disorder in cats. Most cats are subclinically affected, but increased hemorrhage may be noted after surgical procedures. Factor VIII deficiency, factor IX deficiency, combined factor VIII and XII deficiency, combined factor IX and XII deficiency, and vitamin K-dependent multifactor coagulopathy of Devon Rex cats are reported sporadically.

21. With what disorders is vitamin K absence associated?

- Hepatic lipidosis and cholangiohepatitis. Bile salts are required for the absorption of vitamin K because it is a fat-soluble vitamin.
- Malabsorption syndromes. Fats and vitamin K must be absorbed from the gastrointestinal (GI) tract.
- Anorexia and administration of antimicrobials that decrease anaerobic bacterial flora in the GI tract. Vitamin K comes from the diet as well as GI bacterial flora.

22. With what disorder is vitamin K antagonism usually associated?

Anticoagulant rodenticides.

23. What test results are associated with vitamin K absence or antagonism?

- ACT, OSPT, and APTT are usually increased by the time active hemorrhage occurs.
- Because factor VII has the shortest half-life, OSPT is the most sensitive test for detection of toxicity in cats that are not bleeding.
- PIVKAs increase. In one study, the PIVKA test was more sensitive than other coagulation tests.
- Mild thrombocytopenia may occur, probably from utilization of platelets at sites of hemorrhage.

24. How do cats become intoxicated with rodenticides?

Cat are thought to be intoxicated by rodenticides from direct ingestion of the bait or ingesting rodents that have ingested the rodenticide.

25. Describe the management of cats with suspected vitamin K absence or antagonism.

1. Collect samples needed for further diagnostic tests.
2. Administer vitamin K_1 subcutaneously at a loading dose of 2.5–5.0 mg/kg; it should not be given intravenously because of the risk of an anaphylactoid reaction.
3. Give vitamin K_1 orally at 1.0–5.0 mg/kg every 12 hours, depending on the form of rodenticide ingested. Lower doses given for 7–10 days are usually effective for first-generation drugs such as warfarin. Diphacinonone, chlorphacinone, brodifacoum, and bromadiolone (second-generation drugs) usually require the high end of the dose for up to 6 weeks.
4. When given orally, vitamin K_1 should be given with a fatty meal to increase absorption.
5. Give whole blood transfusion if needed for anemia or uncontrollable hemorrhage.
6. Coagulation tests generally start improving within 12 hours because procoagulants are rapidly converted to active coagulants in the presence of vitamin K.

7. Treat with oral vitamin K for a minimum of 2 weeks

8. Stop treatment and assess ACT or OSPT 2 days later. If the results are normal, further treatment is not needed. If the results are prolonged, repeat the treatment cycle.

26. Describe the signs and symptoms of hemostatic abnormalities associated with liver insufficiency.

Because most coagulation factors are produced at least in part by the liver, hepatic insufficiency can ultimately result in factor deficiencies. Factor deficiencies typically occur only in late-stage liver disease when other clinical abnormalities are usually present, including cachexia, GI signs, ascites, and low concentrations of blood urea nitrogen, albumin, cholesterol, and glucose (see hepatic disease chapters). ACT, OSPT, and APTT are expected to be prolonged as hepatic function worsens. Thrombocytopenia may be present in cats with concurrent DIC or severe inflammation. Because clotting factors are not produced, there is no dramatic response to vitamin K as seen with cholestasis.

27. Describe the management of hemostatic abnormalities associated with liver insufficiency.

There is no specific treatment except to attempt to remove the primary disease process so that hepatic function improves.

28. What is DIC?

DIC is the result of a primary disease process that activates widespread intravascular coagulation as a result of endothelial damage, massive platelet activation, or release of tissue procoagulants. One example is feline infectious peritonitis; in one study, all 6 experimentally inoculated cats developed coagulation test results consistent with DIC. After a brief period of hypercoagulability that is difficult to document, platelets and factors are consumed, ultimately resulting in bleeding.

29. How common is DIC in cats?

Although DIC in cats is thought to be rare, 21% of cats at the Ohio State University with hemostatic screening procedures had findings consistent with DIC. The authors considered cats to have evidence of DIC if four of the following were present.

- Thrombocytopenia   • Low ATIII concentration
- Prolonged APTT   • Positive FDPs
- Prolonged OSPT   • Schistocytes
- Low fibrinogen concentration

In another study of thrombocytopenic cats, 5 of 41 were considered to have DIC.

30. How is DIC treated?

Treatment of DIC in cats has not been objectively assessed. General recommendations based on treatment of people and dogs include:

1. Remove the primary cause if possible.

2. Give low-dose heparin in an attempt to lessen disseminated coagulation (90–200 U/kg-subcutaneously every 8 hours).

3. Give blood components to replenish ATIII and clotting factors.

BIBLIOGRAPHY

1. Bay JD, Scott MA, Hans JE: Reference values for activated coagulation time in cats. Am J Vet Res 61:750–753, 2000.
2. Boudreaux MK, Weiss RC, Cox N, et al: Evaluation of antithrombin-III activity as a coindicator of disseminated intravascular coagulation in cats with induced feline infectious peritonitis virus infection. Am J Vet Res 50:1910–1913, 1989.
3. Center SA, Warner K, Corbett J et al: Proteins invoked by vitamin K absence and clotting times in clinically ill cats. J Vet Intern Med 14:292–297, 2000.
4. Couto CG, Hammer AS: Disorders of hemostasis. In Scherding RG (ed): The Cat: Diseases and Clinical Management, 2nd ed. New York, Churchill Livingstone, 1994, pp 739–753.

5. Hart SW, Nolte I: Hemostatic disorders in feline immunodeficiency virus-seropositive cats. J Vet Intern Med 8:355–362, 1994.
6. Jordan HL, Grindem CB, Breitschwerdt EB: Thrombocytopenia in cats: A retrospective study of 41 cases. J Vet Intern Med 7:261–265, 1993.
7. Maddison JE, Watson AD, Eade IG, et al: Vitamin K-dependent multifactor coagulopathy in Devon Rex cats. J Am Vet Med Assoc 197:1495–1497, 1990.
8. Randolph JF, DeMarco J, Center SA, et al: Prothrombin, activated partial thromboplastin, and proteins induced by vitamin K absence or antagonists clotting times in 20 hyperthyroid cats before and after methimazole treatment. J Vet Intern Med 14:56–59, 2000.
9. Rivera-Ramirez PA, Deniz A, Wirth W, et al: Antithrombin III activity in healthy cats and its changes in selected diseases. Berliner-und-Munchener-Tierarztliche-Wochenschrift 110:440–444, 1997.
10. Thomas JS, Green RA: Clotting times and antithrombin III activity in cats with naturally developing diseases: 85 cases (1984–1994). J Am Vet Med Assoc 213:1290–1295, 1998.
11. Weiss DJ: Uniform evaluation and semiquantitative reporting of hematologic data in veterinary laboratories. Vet Clin Pathol 13:27, 1988.

72. IMMUNE-MEDIATED HEMOLYTIC ANEMIA

Michael R. Lappin, D.V.M., Ph.D.

1. What are the primary differential diagnoses for pale mucous membranes in cats?

Pale mucous membranes are usually the result of **anemia** or **hypoperfusion** (shock). These two problems are differentiated by packed cell volume (PCV). In cats, anemia is defined as PCV < 27.

2. Describe the two types of anemia.

Anemia is classified as **regenerative** or **nonregenerative**. By definition, regenerative anemia is characterized by reticulocyte counts > 50,000/μl; nonregenerative anemia has < 50,000/μl (see Chapter 79). Because it takes 3–5 days after acute development of anemia for maximal reticulocytosis to appear, acute anemia initially may appear as nonregenerative.

3. How are regenerative anemias initially classified?

The two primary differential diagnoses for regenerative anemia are **hemolysis** and **blood loss**. Hemolytic regenerative anemia can be **intravascular** or **extravascular**. Intravascular hemolysis can lead to hemoglobinuria and pink plasma. Extravascular hemolysis usually has icteric serum or plasma. Blood can be lost into body spaces (e.g., hemothorax, hemoabdomen) or out of the body (e.g., epistaxis, gastrointestinal hemorrhage). If blood is lost out of the body, total protein concentrations are usually decreased, whereas total protein concentrations usually are normal with blood loss into a body cavity and hemolytic anemias.

4. What forms of hemolytic anemia occur in the cat?

- Immune-mediated
- Infectious
- Microangiopathic
- Drug- or toxin-related
- Metabolic
- Congenital

5. Describe the two basic types of immune-mediated hemolytic anemia.

Immune reactions can result in destruction of erythrocytes. With **primary** immune-mediated hemolytic anemia, the immune reaction is directed specifically against erythrocyte antigens. Sytemic lupus erythematosus (SLE) can be associated with primary immune-mediated hemolytic anemia. Primary immune-mediated hemolytic anemia appears to be more common in dogs than in cats. With **secondary** immune-mediated hemolytic anemia, the immune reaction is induced by other causes; erythrocyte damage occurs secondarily. In cats, most immune-mediated hemolytic anemias are secondary to drugs or infectious agents.

6. Describe the basic mechanism of infectious hemolytic anemia.

In cats, the most common causes of hemolytic anemia are infectious. The primary infection starts a specific immune response that damages erythrocytes secondarily. In dogs, secondary immune-mediated hemolytic anemia is thought to be associated with modified live vaccines. This mechanism is suspected in cats as well but has not been well documented.

7. How is infectious hemolytic anemia diagnosed and treated?

Diagnosis is based on cytologic demonstration of the organism (e.g., *Haemobartonella* spp., *Cytauxzoon felis*), serologic testing (e.g., feline leukemia virus [FeLV], feline infectious peritonitis [FIP] virus), or polymerase chain reaction (e.g., *Haemobartonella* spp.). Treatment is based primarily on removal of the primary agent. Occasionally, glucocorticoids are required to lessen the secondary immune reaction as the primary cause is removed. For example, doxycycline and glucocorticoids are commonly given concurrently to cats with severe agglutination due to hemobartonellosis (see Chapter 74).

8. Describe the mechanism of microangiopathic hemolytic anemia.

Erythrocytes can be damaged when passing through abnormal vessels, resulting in schistocytes or fragments. Disseminated intravascular coagulation (fibrin strands), dirofilariasis, and splenic tumors or hematomas can damage red blood cells.

9. How do drugs and toxins cause hemolytic anemia?

Some drugs or toxins (e.g., acetaminophen, benzocaines) result in Heinz body anemia, which is usually regenerative (see Chapter 73). Other drugs and toxins induce nonregenerative anemia (see Chapter 79). Secondary immune-mediated hemolytic anemia can be induced by propothiouracil, a drug previously used to treat hyperthyroidism. Secondary immune-mediated hemolytic anemia is thought to occur in some dogs with repeated exposure to beta-lactam antibiotics. This mechanism is suspected in cats as well but has not been documented.

10. What is the most common metabolic cause of hemolytic anemia in cats?

Extreme hypophosphatemia during treatment of ketoacidotic cats results in increased red blood cell fragility and resultant lysis.

11. What are the congenital causes of hemolytic anemia in cats?

Congenital defects can result in erythrocyte fragility and hemolytic anemia. Pyruvate kinase deficiency in Abyssinian cats is one example. Neonatal isoerythrolysis also occurs in some cats (see questions 20 and 21).

12. Why does primary immune-mediated hemolytic anemia occur?

The initiating cause is unknown. Antibodies are developed that attach to erythrocytes, and the cells are removed by the reticuloendothelial system (extravascular hemolysis) or lysed after complement fixation (intravascular hemolysis). IgM or IgG antibodies can be involved. IgM is commonly associated with agglutination. Cold agglutinin disease is a rare manifestation of primary immune-mediated hemolytic anemia in cats. IgM antibodies interact with the surface of the erythrocyte only at temperatures < 37°C. Agglutination in peripheral vessels results in ischemic necrosis of the ear tips, tail tip, and, rarely, distal extremities. The immune reaction can be directed at erythrocyte precursors (pure red cell aplasia). In this syndrome, the anemia is nonregenerative (see question 16). Disease sometimes occurs in littermates, suggesting a genetic predisposition.

13. Describe the signalment of immune-mediated hemolytic anemia in cats.

The signalment varies with the primary disease. Examples include:
- Neonatal isoerythrolysis occurs in 1–2-day-old kittens.
- FeLV infection is most common in young cats.
- Drug reactions can occur at any age.
- Because of the small number of reported cases of primary immune-mediated hemolytic anemia in cats, it is impossible to specify an association with age or sex.

14. What are the historical clues to immune-mediated hemolytic anemia in cats?

Cats with secondary immune-mediated hemolytic anemia often have historical evidence of the primary cause. Examples include:
- Cats with haemobartonellosis may be infested with *Ctenocephalides felis*.
- Cats with cytauxzoonosis come from specific regions of the United States and may have history of exposure to *Dermacenter variabilis*.
- The mating of a blood type A tom with a blood type B queen predicts neonatal isoerythrolysis.
- The cat may be from an FeLV-infected cattery.
- Drugs or vaccines may have been given recently.

15. Describe the clinical presentation of cats with immune-mediated hemolytic anemia.

Nonspecific presenting complaints usually include weakness or lethargy, depression, inappetence, elevated respiratory rate, polyuria, and polydipsia. On rare occasions, the owner notices pale mucous membranes, icterus, or necrosis of ear or tail tips (cold-agglutinin disease). Nonspecific physical examination abnormalities may include pale mucous membranes, elevated heart and respiratory rates, heart murmur, icterus, splenomegaly, low-grade fever, lymphadenopathy, depression, necrosis of ear or tail tips, and weakness.

16. What is pure red cell aplasia?

Pure red cell aplasia develops when erythrocyte precursors are damaged by a primary immune-mediated reaction. The anemia is usually severe and poorly regenerative, or reticulocytes are absent but platelet and neutrophil numbers are normal. Cytologic examination of bone marrow cells reveals a decrease in erythroblasts and an increase in small lymphocytes. In a report of 9 cases, cats were between 8 months and 3 years of age and were seronegative for FeLV antigen. Pale mucous membranes, heart murmur, lethargy, and anorexia were the most common clinical findings. Each cat responded to immunsuppressive therapy with glucocorticoids and cyclophosphamide or cyclosporine (see question 23).

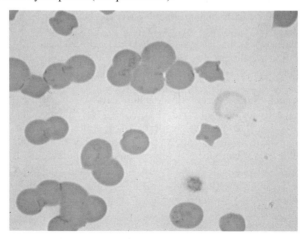

Microscopic agglutination in a cat with *H. felis* infection. Note the clumps of red blood cells.

17. What is the diagnostic plan for cats with suspected hemolytic anemia?

Complete blood cell count, reticulocyte count, platelet count, and total serum protein concentration are the minimal diagnostic tests for evaluation of anemia. If a regenerative anemia is present, the total serum protein concentration is normal; if there is no evidence of body cavity hemorrhage, hemolytic anemia is most likely. Careful examination of the blood smear is imperative for evaluation for hemoparasites, spherocytes, schistocytes, microscopic agglutination, or Heinz bodies, which further direct the diagnostic plan. It is difficult to detect spherocytes cytologically in cats because normal erythrocytes are small and dense. If agglutination is present, rule out massive rouleaux formation by mixing 1 drop of EDTA blood with 1 drop of saline and repeating the cytologic examination. Agglutination is not dispersed by saline.

18. What is the only way to prove primary immune-mediated hemolytic anemia?

Exclude all known secondary causes. Use the history to exclude drug- or vaccine-associated disease. FeLV antigen testing and cytologic evaluation for *H. felis* are imperative. If *H. felis* is not detected cytologically in EDTA blood smears or fresh blood smears, polymerase chain reaction should be performed (HESKA Diagnostic Laboratory, Fort Collins, CO). Direct Coombs' testing can detect antibodies on the surface of erythrocytes in cats with no evidence of microscopic agglutination or spherocytes. However, positive results occur with most secondary causes of immune-mediated hemolytic anemia and have been detected in normal cats. If hyperbilirubinemia is present, hemolysis is probably extravascular. If the plasma is pink, intravascular hemolysis is likely.

19. How is pure red blood cell aplasia diagnosed?

The anemia is usually nonregenerative, but platelet and neutrophil numbers are normal. Bone marrow aspiration for cytologic evaluation is required to provide evidence of disease. Erythroblasts are absent or reduced in number, and increased proportions of small lymphocytes are noted.

20. Why does neonatal isoerythrolysis occur in some kittens?

Toms with blood type A always produce kittens with blood type A, regardless of the blood type of the queen. Blood type A kittens born to blood type B queens can develop neonatal isoerythrolysis. Passive transfer of anti-A antibodies from the queen to the kittens in milk results in hemolytic anemia.

21. How is neonatal isoerythrolysis diagnosed and treated?

Weakness, depression, pale mucous membranes, and pigmenturia are the most common findings. Diagnosis can be confirmed by blood-typing the tom and queen. Kittens should be removed from the queen when clinical signs are noted and hand-reared. After 2–3 days, they can be returned to the queen because at that time passive transfer of antibodies no longer occurs. Treatment is supportive.

22. Is SLE a common cause of hemolytic anemia in cats?

SLE has rarely been documented in cats. It is primarily an immune complex disease, but cytophilic antibodies directed at circulating erythrocytes or erythrocyte precursors occur in some cases, resulting in immune-mediated hemolytic anemia. Other common clinical findings include leukocytosis, leukopenia, neutropenia, lymphopenia, fever, neurologic abnormalities, lymphadenopathy, polyarthritis, myopathy, dermatitis, oral ulceration, and progessive renal failure. In Pedersen's study, the cats were positive for antinuclear antibodies in serum, and most responded to immune suppressive therapy.

23. How is primary immune-mediated hemolytic anemia treated?

There is no consensus for the most appropriate protocol because the disease is so rare in cats. The following table lists the dosages of drugs that may be considered for treatment.

Drugs Used in the Management of Primary immune-mediated Hemolytic Anemia

DRUG	DOSE
Dexamethasone	0.25–1 mg/kg IV once acutely 0.2–0.4 mg/kg PO every 24–48 hr for maintenance
Chlorambucil (Leukoran)	2 mg/cat PO every 24–48 hr for maintenance
Cyclophosphamide (Cytoxan)	50 mg/m^2 PO 4 days weekly or every 48 hr acutely
Cyclosporine (Sandimmune)	5–10 mg/kg PO every 12–24 hr acutely or for maintenance in resistant cases
Methylprednisolone acetate (Depo-Medrol)	2–4 mg/kg IM every 3–4 wk for maintenance
Prednisolone	2–4 mg/kg PO every 12–24 hr for induction acutely 0.5–2 mg/kg PO every 24–48 hr for maintenance

IV = intravenously, PO = orally, IM = intramuscularly.

24. How is dexamethasone used?

Many clinicians give rapid-acting dexamethasone intravenously when the diagnosis is made in an attempt to suppress as quickly as possible macrophage removal of antibody-coated erythrocytes. Oral dexamethasone typically is used only if the cat fails to respond to prednisolone or becomes resistant.

25. Discuss the role of prednisone or prednisolone.

On day 2 of therapy, one of these drugs is usually started orally as long-term maintenance therapy. Some clinicians believe that cats respond more consistently to prednisolone. Once anemia is resolved, the dose is generally decreased by no more than 25% every 2 weeks. Complete blood count should be performed at each recheck examination. Cats are relatively resistant to the adverse effects of glucocorticoids. However, a reasonable dose for long-term prednisone or prednisolone is 0.5 mg/kg orally every 24–48 hours. Most cats do not have evidence of glucocorticoid-induced illness with this protocol. In cats that are difficult to treat with oral medications, methylprednisolone acetate (DepoMedrol) may be given intermittently by intramuscular injection in an attempt to control the disease.

26. When is cyclophosphamide used?

Cyclophosphamide (Cytoxan) is an alkylating agent used with prednisone or prednisolone for acute management of primary immune-mediated hemolytic anemia and SLE. It should be considered for use in cats with severe autoagglutination or intravascular hemolysis. Because vomiting, diarrhea, and bone marrow suppression may occur in cats, cyclophosphamide is not used for chronic management.

27. Describe the role of chlorambucil.

If an alkylating agent is needed chronically, chlorambucil (Leucoran) should be used. It should be considered in cats with refractory hemolytic anemia or severe side effects associated with glucocorticoids.

28. When is cyclosporine used?

Cyclosporine (Sandimmune) typically is used in conjunction with glucocorticoids for acute management of primary immune diseases, as a rescue drug when other drugs fail, or when the syndrome is resistant to other treatments.

29. What other agents may be considered?

Danazol and human gammaglobulin have been used to treat immune-mediated hemolytic anemia in dogs, but little is known about their use in cats. Blood transfusion or hemoglobin replacement products should be administered if clinically indicated. Oxyglobin administration in cats has been associated with pulmonary edema.

30. What is the prognosis for primary immune-mediated hemolytic anemia?
Generally guarded, particularly if intravascular hemolysis, autoagglutination, or pulmonary thromboembolic disease is present. In one study of 9 cats with pure red cell aplasia, all responded to therapy, but most required chronic administration of immunosuppressive drugs. Pulmonary thromboembolic disease is a common cause of death in dogs with primary immune-mediated hemolytic anemia; whether this complication is common in cats is unknown.

31. What is the prognosis for secondary immune-mediated hemolytic anemia?
Some causes have a good prognosis. For example, *H. felis*, vaccines, and drug induction of secondary immune-mediated hemolytic anemia theoretically should resolve when the inciting cause is removed and appropriate treatment administered. The prognosis of FeLV-associated hemolytic anemia is more guarded.

BIBLIOGRAPHY

1. Adams LG, Hardy RM, Weiss DJ, et al: Hypophosphatemia and hemolytic anemia associated with diabetes mellitus and hepatic lipidosis in cats. J Vet Intern Med 7:266–271, 1993.
2. Bridle KH, Littlewood JD: Tail tip necrosis in two litters of Birman kittens. J Small Anim Pract 39:88–89, 1998.
3. Dunn JK, Searcy GP, Hirsch VM: The diagnostic significance of a positive direct agglutination test in anemic cats. Can J Comp Med 48:349–353, 1984.
4. Faircloth JC, Montgomery JK: Systemic lupus erythematosus in a cat presenting with autoimmune hemolytic anemia. Fel Pract 11:24–26, 1981.
5. Ford S, Giger U, Duesberg C, et al: Inherited erythrocyte pyruvate kinase (PK) deficiency causing hemolytic anemia in an Abyssinian cat. J Vet Intern Med 6:123, 1992.
6. Gunn Moore DA, Day MJ, Graham MEA, et al: Immune-mediated haemolytic anaemia in two sibling cats associated with multicentric lymphoblastic infiltration. J Fel Med Surg 1:209–214, 1999.
7. Heise SC, Smith RS, Schalm OW: Lupus erythematosus with hemolytic anemia in a cat. Feline Pract 3:14–19, 1973.
8. Hitt ME, McCaw DL: FeLV infection, hemolytic anemia and hypocellular bone marrow in a cat: Treatment with protein A and prednisone. Can Vet J 29:737–739, 1988.
9. Lusson D, Billiemaz B, Chabanne JL: Circulating lupus anticoagulant and probable systemic lupus erythematosus in a cat. J Fel Med Surg 1:193–196, 1999.
10. Pedersen NC, Barlough JE: Systemic lupus erythematosus in the cat. Feline Pract 19:5–13, 1991.
11. Person JM, Sicard M, Pellerin JL: Autoimmune haemolytic anaemia in the cat: A clinical and immunopathological study of five cases. Rev Med Veterin 148:107–114, 1997.
12. Scott DW, Schultz RD, Post JE, et al: Autoimmune hemolytic anemia in the cat. J Am Anim Hosp Assoc 9:530–539, 1973.
13. Stokol T, Blue JT: Pure red cell aplasia in cats: 9 cases (1989–1997). J Am Vet Med Assoc 214:75–79, 1999.
14. Utroska B: Autoimmune hemolytic anemia in sibling cats. Vet Med Small Anim Clin 75:1699–1701, 1980.

73. HEINZ BODIES

Stacy B. Smith, D.V.M., Rick L. Cowell, D.V.M., M.S.,
and Karen E. Dorsey, D.V.M.

1. What is a Heinz body?

A Heinz body, also known as a Schumach body or erythrocyte refractile body, is a precipitate or clump of denatured hemoglobin.

2. How are Heinz bodies formed?

Heinz bodies are formed during oxidative injury to erythrocytes. Any chemical, endogenous or exogenous, that inhibits glutathione reduction within the erythrocyte can lead to denaturation of hemoglobin.

3. Can Heinz bodies be detected on a routine blood smear?

Heinz bodies sometimes can be seen on blood smears, but generally they do not stain well with routine hematologic stains. On blood smears they appear as faint or unstained areas near the edge of, or protruding from, the surface of the red blood cell (RBC).

4. If Heinz bodies are suspected from a blood smear, how can their presence be confimed?

New methylene blue stain can be used to stain another blood smear. Heinz bodies are easily recognized as dark staining structures near the periphery of the erythrocytes.

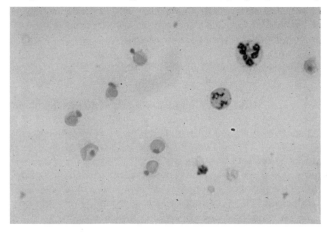

Scattered RBCs containing dark-staining Heinz bodies, one aggregate reticulocyte, and one neutrophil (new methylene blue stain; original magnification 250 ×).

5. What makes cats more susceptible to Heinz body formation than other species?

The feline hemoglobin molecule contains 8–10 sulfhydryl groups that are readily oxidized, whereas the hemoglobin of most other species contains 4 or fewer sulfhydryl groups.

6. When Heinz bodies are formed, why do higher numbers continue to circulate in the peripheral blood of cats compared with other domestic species?

Most species have a sinusoidal spleen, which is efficient at removing RBCs that contain Heinz bodies. Cats have a nonsinusoidal spleen, which is ineffective at removing such RBCs.

7. When Heinz bodies are seen on a feline blood smear, are they diagnostic of disease?

Heinz bodies can be seen in apparently healthy and nonanemic cats. In normal cats they tend to be small (0.5–1 mm).

8. How do Heinz bodies contribute to clinical disease?

Heinz bodies are formed during oxidative injury to the erythrocyte. Some cells with Heinz bodies lyse, whereas others remain in the circulation. Cells that remain in the circulation have a shortened life span and fragile cell membrane. These characteristics can lead to mild-to-severe anemias.

9. What are the most common pharmacologic agents known to cause Heinz body formation in cats?

Although numerous agents can lead to Heinz body formation, the most commonly administered are acetaminophen, DL-methionine, methylene blue, and benzocaine-containing products. Consecutive-day use of propofol also may induce increased Heinz body formation in cats.

10. Besides drugs, what other mechanisms cause increased Heinz body formation?

Increased numbers of Heinz bodies can occur in association with certain systemic diseases, including diabetes mellitus, hyperthyroidism, and lymphoma. Specific food additives, including onion products and propylene glycol, also induce formation of Heinz bodies.

11. What clinical signs are seen with Heinz body-associated problems?

Signs associated with anemia such as pale mucous membranes, weakness, tachycardia, tachypnea, lethargy, and icterus may occur with Heinz body-associated anemia. The severity of these signs depends on the acuteness of the developing anemia.

12. How should Heinz body anemias be treated?

The inciting cause needs to be identified. In the case of toxic causes, the involved agent needs to be discontinued. In systemic illness, the underlying process needs to be definitively diagnosed and treated to stop Heinz body formation and associated anemia. Other supportive measures may be necessary, such as intravenous fluids and possibly blood transfusion.

13. In cats with acetaminophen toxicosis, what other process is affected by oxidative insult?

Iron is converted from the ferrous to the ferric state, thus causing methemoglobinemia.

14. What other clinical signs are seen with acetaminophen-associated methemoglobinemia?

Cyanosis, dark brown blood, dyspnea, and facial edema.

15. What additional treatments are necessary in such cases?

Induce vomiting if ingestion occurred less than 2 hours previously, and administer N-acetyl-cysteine (140 mg/kg intravenously or orally once, followed by 70 mg/kg intravenously or orally every 4 hr for 7 doses) and ascorbic acid (30 mg/kg subcutaneously or orally every 6 hr for 7 doses). Oxygen therapy may be necessary in some cases. Sometimes a single intravenous dose of methylene blue may be indicated.

BIBLIOGRAPHY

1. Andress JL, et al: The effects of consecutive day propofol anesthesia on feline red blood cells. Vet Surg 24:277–282, 1995.
2. Christopher MM: Relation of endogenous Heinz bodies to disease and anemia in cats: 120 cases (1978–1987). J Am Vet Med Assoc 194:1089–1095, 1989.
3. Christopher MM, et al: Erythrocyte pathology and mechanisms of Heinz body-mediated hemolysis in cats. Vet Pathol 27:299–310, 1990.
4. Christopher MM, et al: Heinz body formation associated with ketoacidosis in diabetic cats. J Vet Intern Med 9:24–31, 1995.
5. Ewing PJ, et al: Heinz bodies. In August JR (ed): Consultations in Feline Internal Medicine, 3rd ed. Philadelphia, W.B. Saunders, 1997, pp 469–473.
6. Maede Y, et al: Methionine toxicosis in cats. Am J Vet Res 48:289–292, 1987.
7. Robertson JE, et al: Heinz body formation in cats fed baby food containing onion powder. J Am Vet Med Assoc 212:1260–1266, 1998.

74. HEMOBARTONELLA FELIS

Séverine Tasker, B.Sc., B.V.Sc.

1. What type of organism is *Hemobartonella felis*?

Hemobartonella felis is a bacterium currently classified as a rickettsial organism. However, recent data about DNA sequences have revealed that they are more closely related to the mycoplasmal organisms, and reclassification has been recommended. In polychrome-stained blood smears, *H. felis* is pleomorphic and appears as coccoid, rod, or ring forms. The thickness of a blood smear and position of the parasite on the erythrocyte may influence the morphology of the organism, but the coccoid form is most commonly recognized. The coccoid forms range from 0.2–0.8 μm in diameter. *H. felis* appears on the surface of the erythrocyte and around the periphery of the cell; it may be found singly, in pairs, or in chains with severe infestation. Occasionally organisms may detach and lie free of the erythrocytes.

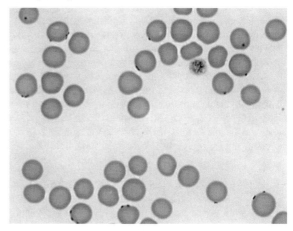

Wright-Giemsa–stained blood smear showing epicellular *H. felis* organisms attached to erythrocytes.

2. How many different strains of *H. felis* have been recognized? Discuss the differences.

Currently two strains of *H. felis* have been recognized. They vary genetically, in pathogenicity, and in morphologic appearance. The large strain (Ohio strain) is approximately twice the diameter of the small strain; experimental inoculation of cats usually results in severe anemia. With the small strains studied to date, experimental inoculation of cats results in minimal clinical signs, and anemia is not usually induced. In addition, dual infection has been documented in naturally infected cats, and experimental infection of cats with both strains results in more severe clinical disease than either strain alone.

3. What disease is associated with *H. felis* infection?

H. felis causes feline infectious anemia, a common hemolytic anemia in cats. In recent in situ hybridization studies, *H. felis* DNA sequences were physically linked to areas of known cellular pathology on feline erythrocytes. In addition, the appearance of *H. felis* DNA in blood coincides with clinical evidence of experimental infection, and the amount of DNA correlates with the number of organisms in the blood.

4. Describe the clinical findings of *H. felis* infection.

Clinical signs are often vague and nonspecific, reflecting the presence of anemia rather than *H. felis* infection per se. Anorexia, lethargy, pallor, weight loss, and depression are common.

Intermittent pyrexia is common, particularly in the acute stages of the disease. Splenomegaly and lymphadenopathy may result from extramedullary hematopoiesis and stimulation of immune responses. Icterus is rare. Organisms appear in the blood on average about 7–8 days (range = 2–20 days) after experimental inoculation of cats with *H. felis*. Cycles of parasitemia then occur. One study reported that males and cats younger than 3 years are more likely to be infected. Other risk factors include lack of vaccinations, feline leukemia virus (FeLV)-positive status, and presence of anemia. Up to 47.2% of *H. felis*-infected cats are FeLV-positive. Cats with *H. felis* infection may be more susceptible to FeLV infection, FeLV infection may activate latent *H. felis* infection, or the two organisms may be acquired under the same circumstances. An association with feline immunodeficiency virus (FIV) infection also was proposed when it was found that 40% of anemic FIV-positive cats were infected with *H. felis*. All cats infected with *H. felis* should be tested for FeLV and FIV. Cats that are retrovirus-positive may show more severe clinical disease.

5. Describe the pathogenesis of *H. felis*-associated anemia.

Hemolysis, erythrophagocytosis, and sequestration of red blood cells are the three common mechanisms. The attachment of *H. felis* to erythrocytes results in direct damage to the erythrocytic membrane, causing an increase in erythrocytic osmotic fragility and shortened erythrocyte lifespan. Erythrocyte damage also may expose hidden erythrocytic antigens or result in an alteration in erythrocytic antigens, inducing the production of antierythrocytic antibodies. Antibodies also may be directed against the organism itself, resulting in erythrocytic damage as an "innocent bystander." Positive Coombs' tests and autoagglutination have been reported in acute hemobartonellosis, indicating the presence of erythrocyte-bound antibodies. Although some intravascular hemolysis may occur by direct damage to the erythrocytes, the majority of hemolysis induced by *H. felis* is extravascular. Erythrophagocytosis occurs in the spleen, liver, lungs, and bone marrow. In addition, erythrocytes are sequestered in the spleen, where macrophages remove *H. felis* organisms from their surface ("pitting"), returning unparasitized cells into the circulation. Release of sequestered erythrocytes explains the rapid increase in packed cell volume (PCV) in some cats after clearance of *H. felis* from the circulation.

6. Is the parasitemia associated with *H. felis* infection continuous or intermittent?

After infection with *H. felis*, cycles of parasitemia occur with an average duration of 6 days between episodes, which usually last 1–2 days. PCV tends to fall in association with the appearance of *H. felis*. The clearance of parasites from the blood can be rapid, with reports of a high level of parasitemia falling to undetectable levels within hours. No relationship has been found between degree of parasitemia and severity of anemia.

7. How does splenectomy affect hemobartonellosis in cats?

In animals other than cats, splenectomy usually is required before *Hemobartonella* spp. produce clinical disease. In cats, splenectomy has little effect on incubation period or severity of disease induced by *H. felis*, although the parasitemia may last longer than in intact cats.

8. How is *H. felis* transmitted?

Experimental transmission has been demonstrated via the intravenous, intraperitoneal, and oral routes using blood from infected cats. Vertical transmission from dam to offspring has been implicated but not proven. Uninfected and infected cats housed together for several months often show no evidence of horizontal spread of infection. Many believe that infection can be spread by blood-sucking arthropods, although this theory has not yet been proved.

9. Describe the hematologic abnormalities induced by *H. felis*.

Infection by *H. felis* typically causes regenerative anemia. The severity of anemia depends on the stage of infection, but PCV usually falls to < 20%, with average values of 15–18%. Anisocytosis, macrocytosis, and polychromasia are common hemopathologic findings. Reticulocytosis occurs when anemia has been present for 3–5 days. Anemia associated with *H. felis* infection is usually categorized as a macrocytic, normochromic regenerative anemia. One study found that macrocytosis usually reflected coninfection with FeLV. In one review, 44% of *H. felis*-infected cats had nonregenerative anemia. Whether this finding was due to acute anemia or concurrent diseases is unknown. Alternatively, it is possible that *H. felis* causes anemia of chronic inflammatory disease. Platelet counts are usually normal. Changes in the white blood cell counts during hemobartonellosis are variable. Moderate neutropenia may be seen after the onset of anemia, followed by neutrophilia.

10. What are the other major differential diagnoses for regenerative anemias in cats?

Regenerative anemias result from hemorrhage and blood loss or hemolysis. The most common cause of hemorrhage in cats is trauma, but neoplasia and amyloidosis also may cause organ or blood vessel rupture. Bleeding disorders such as coagulopathies are rare in cats. Causes of hemolysis include hemobartonellosis, oxidative injury to erythrocytes (e.g., acetaminophen, methylene blue, onions), hypophosphataemia (which can develop during the treatment of diabetic ketoacidosis), and immune-mediated hemolysis secondary to infections (including *H. felis* and FeLV) or vaccinations. Hemolytic anemias in cats also result from drugs (e.g., trimethoprim-sulphonamides, methimazole), neonatal isoerythrolysis, and microangiopathies (e.g., disseminated intravascular coagulopathy).

11. How is *H. felis* infection diagnosed?

Because the organism cannot be cultured, diagnosis has been based on demonstrating the organism cytologically on blood smear or DNA in blood by polymerase chain reaction (PCR).

12. Which method best demonstrates the organism in blood films?

Romanowsky stains such as Giemsa, Wright, Wright's-Giemsa, and May-Grunwald-Giemsa and acridine orange (AO) stain can be used (see figure in question 1). AO staining is more sensitive than standard Romanowsky stains for *H. felis*, but its use is limited by the need for a fluorescent microscope. False-positive diagnoses may result from artifact generation by improper drying, improper fixation, or stain precipitation. Only fresh filtered stain solutions should be used. Stain precipitate usually is found above the plane of focus of the erythrocytes and is more dense and larger than *H. felis* organisms. Refractile artifacts, which occur when moisture adheres to the cells on the film, tend to have irregular borders and appear colorless when the erythrocytes are in focus. Other cytologic findings may be confused with *H. felis*. Because cyclical parasitemia occurs, the absence of *H. felis* organisms on blood smears does not rule out a diagnosis of hemobartonellosis. Examination of multiple fresh blood smears during the course of a day or over a few days may increase the chances of obtaining a positive diagnosis. It has been shown that ethylenediaminetetraacetic acid (EDTA) anticoagulant dislodges the organism from the erythrocyte cell surface within hours, making identification on blood smears extremely difficult. It is important, therefore, to prepare blood smears immediately after collection of nonanticoagulated blood.

Differentiation of H. felis *from Other Inclusions and Artifacts on Blood Smear*

STRUCTURE	SIZE	APPEARANCE	POSITION
H. felis	0.2–0.8 µm	Coccoid, rod- or ring-shaped	On surface of erythrocyte, often on periphery
Cytauxzoon felis (see Chapter 75)	1–4 µm	Signet ring-shaped, bipolar	Within erythrocyte, usually one organism per cell
Babesia felis	2.5–3.0 µm by 4–5 µm	Signet ring-shaped, round, pear-shaped, or Maltese cross-shaped	Usually intracellular
Stain precipitate	Variable	Round	Anywhere on blood smear
Howell-Jolly body	1–2 µm	Round	Within erythrocyte
Heinz body (see Chapter 73)	1–2 µm	Round or irregular	Within erythrocyte but at periphery; may protrude
Refractile artifact	Variable	Variable and clear	Appear to be within erythrocyte and refractile as plane of focus is changed

13. How does PCR aid in the diagnosis of hemobartonellosis?

PCR is a technique used to amplify specific fragments of *H. felis* DNA to detectable amounts. It is, therefore, an extremely sensitive test. One study claimed that as few as 52 *H. felis* organisms can be detected by PCR from blood samples.

14. How does PCR compare with cytologic examination of blood smears?

PCR has been adapted to detect both strains of *H. felis* and is more sensitive than examination of blood smears for the detection of *H. felis*. PCR has been used to identify chronically infected asymptomatic cats, indicating that a positive PCR result does not correlate with the presence of clinical disease. PCR studies have shown that anemic cats are more likely to be infected with the large strain of *H. felis* or dually infected with both strains than nonanemic cats.

15. What percentage of cats become chronically infected with *H. felis*? How can they be identified?

It is believed that all cats that recover from infection remain chronically infected with *H. felis* for an undetermined period, potentially for life. Parasitemia generally is not visible on blood smears during this period, and chronically infected cats appear clinically normal. Such cats appear to be in a balanced state in which replication of organisms is balanced by phagocytosis and removal, although reactivation of infection may occur, resulting in clinical disease. Demonstration of the presence of *H. felis* in the blood is possible by PCR.

16. Which antibiotics are routinely used for the treatment of hemobartonellosis?

Currently the tetracycline group is commonly used. The preferred tetracycline derivative is doxycycline because of fewer side effects and less frequent dosing than oxytetracycline. The recommended doxycycline dose is 5–10 mg/kg orally every 24 hours, and therapy should be continued for 14–21 days, depending on response to treatment. PCR has shown that, despite being effective for the treatment of anemia, doxycyline does not eliminate the causal organism; treated cats still become chronic carriers. Enrofloxacin also has been recommended for the treatment of hemobartonellosis (10 mg/kg/day orally for at least 14 days). Azithromycin is effective against many *Mycoplasma* spp., but a one-dose regimen (15 mg/kg orally every 12 hr) was ineffective in one group of *H. felis*-infected cats.

17. What other therapies may be of benefit in the treatment of hemobartonellosis?

Supportive care, including whole-blood transfusion, and glucocorticoid therapy for treatment of the immune-mediated component of hemolytic disease have been used in many infected cats. However, concurrent diseases (e.g., respiratory infections, toxoplasmosis) that may be exacerbated by the use of glucocorticoids should be ruled out first. Positive retroviral status does not preclude the use of glucocorticoids. Some clinicians advocate the use of glucocorticoids only if the anemia is pronounced or acute in onset and/or accompanied by autoagglutination. The recommended dose of prednisolone is 2 mg/kg/day orally, with a tapering of dosage toward the end of therapy. The value of glucocorticoids in the treatment of *H. felis* is not proven at present.

18. What is the prognosis for cats infected with *H. felis*?

The long-term prognosis for cats after recovery from uncomplicated hemobartonellosis appears to be good if a definitive diagnosis is made and therapy is instituted promptly. Recovered cats become chronic carriers and are believed to be prone to relapse of clinical disease after periods of illness or stress, although relapse is rare.

19. What is the prevalence of *H. felis* infection in the cat population?

Reports of the prevalence of *H. felis* in different cat populations vary greatly from 3.6% to 28%. This wide range may be due, in part, to the different methods of diagnosis used by different studies. The cytopathologic diagnosis of *H. felis* infection by the examination of blood smears may have both false-positive (stain precipitate, other erythrocytic inclusions) and false-negative (intermittent parasitemias, collection of blood into EDTA) diagnoses. A recent prevalence study using PCR reported that 28.0% of cats with suspected hemobartonellosis were found to be infected compared with 14.5% of control cats. The latter group of cats showed no clinical signs of hemobartonellosis, emphasizing that a positive PCR result does not equate with clinical disease.

BIBLIOGRAPHY

1. Alleman AR, Pate MG, Harvey JW, et al: Western immunoblot analysis of *Haemobartonella felis* with sera from experimentally infected cats. J Clin Microbiol 37:1474–1479, 1999.
2. Berent LM, Messick JB, Cooper SK: Detection of *Hemobartonella felis* in cats with experimentally induced acute and chronic infections, using a polymerase chain reaction assay. Am J Vet Res 59:1215–1220, 1998.
3. Berent LM, Messick JB, Cooper SK, et al: Specific in situ hybridisation of *Hemobartonella felis* with a DNA probe and tyramide signal amplification. Vet Pathol 37:47–53, 2000.
4. Bobade PA, Nash AS, Rogerson P: Feline hemobartonellosis: clinical, haematological and pathological studies in natural infections and the relationship to infection with feline leukaemia virus. Vet Rec 122:32–36, 1988.
5. Cooper SK, Berent LM, Messick JB: Competitive, quantitative PCR analysis of *Hemobartonella felis* in the blood of experimentally infected cats. J Microbiol Methods 34:235–243, 1999.
6. Cotter SM, Hardy WD Jr, Essex M: Association of feline leukemia virus with lymphosarcoma and other disorders in the cat. J Am Vet Med Assoc 166:449–454, 1975.
7. Foley JE, Harrus S, Poland A, et al: Molecular, clinical, and pathologic comparison of two distinct strains of *Hemobartonella felis* in domestic cats. Am J Vet Res 59:1581–1588, 1998.
8. Hopper CD, Sparkes AH, Gruffydd-Jones TJ, et al: Clinical and laboratory findings in cats infected with feline immunodeficiency virus. Vet Rec 125:341–346, 1989.
9. Jensen WA, Lappin MR, Kamkar S et al: Prevalence of *Hemobartonella felis* infection in cats. Am J Vet Res [in press].
10. Rikihisa Y, Kawahara M, Wen B, et al: Western immunoblot analysis of *Hemobartonella muris* and comparison of 16S rRNA gene sequences of *H. muris, H. felis,* and *Eperythrozoon suis.* J Clin Microbiol 35:823–829, 1997.
11. VanSteenhouse JL, Millard JR, Taboada J: Feline hemobartonellosis. Comp Cont Educ Pract Vet 15:535–545, 1993.
12. Westfall DS, Jensen WA, Reagan WJ, et al: Experimental infection of cats with two *Hemobartonella felis* genotypes (California and Ohio variants) and response to treatment with azithromycin. Am J Vet Res [in press].

75. CYTAUXZOON FELIS

James H. Meinkoth, D.V.M., Ph.D.

1. What type of organism is *Cytauxzoon felis*?

C. felis is a protozoan parasite somewhat similar to *Babesia* spp. Unlike *Babesia* spp., which typically are limited to erythrocytes in mammalian hosts, organisms of the genus *Cytauxzoon* have two tissue phases: piroplasms (found in red blood cells) and schizonts (found in macrophages in various organs throughout the body).

2. How do cats become infected with *C. felis*?

C. felis is a tick-transmitted parasite. *Dermacentor variabilis* is highly effective at transmitting the organism under experimental conditions and is probably the major vector for natural disease. Many wild cats, most notably bobcats, have a high prevalence of *C. felis* infection. Unlike domestic cats, infection in wild cats is typically subclinical. Tick transmission of the organism from subclinically infected bobcats to domestic cats produces fatal clinical disease in recipient domestic cats.

3. How common is cytauxzoonosis?

The incidence of cytauxzoonosis varies tremendously by geographic location and type of clientele. Cytauxzoonosis occurs in the southcentral to southeastern United States. In certain areas of Oklahoma, Missouri, and Arkansas it is not unusual for a practitioner to see 3–4 cases per week during early summer months. Conversations with practitioners indicate that the geographic distribution of *C. felis* may be expanding. As a tick-transmitted disease, cytauxzoonosis is seen in cats exposed to outdoor, particularly wooded, environments. Even in endemic areas of the country, veterinarians who work in clinics in urban environments or whose clients maintain strictly indoor cats are less likely to see the disease.

4. What clinical presentation should cause suspicion of cytauxzoonosis?

Historically, owners report an acute onset of profound depression and anorexia. Cats often are found outside after failing to return home and are reluctant to move. Prominent findings on physical examination are marked fever (commonly ≥ 106°F), dehydration, and icterus. Some cats appear to be in pain when touched and may have abnormal vocalizations. Severe mental depression and abnormal vocalizations have led some practitioners to consider rabies as the initial diagnosis. An outdoor cat from an endemic area, particularly in a rural environment, is at risk. The disease is most prevalent in the early (May–June) and late (September) summer months, when the tick host is active.

5. What causes the clinical manifestations of cytauxzoonosis?

Most clinical signs are not the result of infected red cells. Cats that are experimentally infected with only the red cell phase of the organism become parasitemic but usually do not show clinical illness, nor are they immune to subsequent challenge. The widespread infiltration of schizont-infected macrophages in various body tissues produces the profound clinical illness. Development of schizonts occurs before piroplasms are seen in peripheral blood.

6. Describe the clinicopathologic changes seen in cytauxzoonosis.

Anemia, leukopenia, and thrombocytopenia, alone or in combination, may be detected on complete blood count. Nonregenerative anemia of variable severity is the most common finding. Profound leukopenia is present in many cats and is more common later in the course of disease. Thrombocytopenia is often present, more commonly in cats that show severe clinical signs. Serum biochemical findings are variable. The most common abnormality is hyperbilirubinemia.

7. What tests are available to confirm a diagnosis?

Cytauxzoonosis is diagnosed by examining a blood smear and finding the characteristic piroplasms in red cells (see figures on following page). Serologic tests and DNA-based tests (e.g., polymerase chain reaction) have been used in research settings but are not widely available for diagnostic use, nor are they usually needed.

8. Does a lack of organisms on blood smear effectively rule out cytauxzoonosis?

Although organisms are frequently found, some cats test negative on initial evaluation of blood smears. Negative results may be due to various factors:

1. Laboratory personnel must be familiar with identifying *C. felis*.

2. The organism is easily overlooked because it is extremely small and can be present in low numbers. It is best to alert the diagnostic laboratory that cytauxzoonosis is suspected and to request specifically that the sample be examined for piroplasms. Many practitioners in endemic areas examine blood smears themselves to get a quick diagnosis.

3. Many cats simply do not have organisms in their blood at the time of initial presentation. The magnitude of parasitemia typically increases as the disease progresses, and organisms are common late in the disease course.

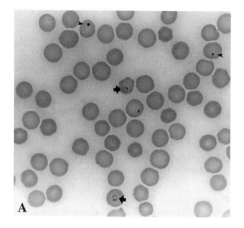

Differentiation of *C. felis* piroplasms from other red cell inclusions in feline peripheral blood. *A,* Two signet ring-shaped *C. felis* piroplasms *(arrows)* and two Howell-Jolly bodies *(arrowheads)* seen in erythrocytes. *B, Hemobartonella felis* organisms are seen as distinct chains *(arrows)* and as less distinct dots and rings *(arrow heads)*. *H. felis* is an extracellular organism, as can be seen from the position of the chains at the periphery of the cell. Organisms on the top and bottom of the cell are out of the plane of focus and appear less distinct. *C,* Stain precipitate is seen between red cells as well as on red cells. Stain precipitate superimposed on top of red cells *(arrows)* can mimic red cell parasites (Wright stain, original magnification × 330)

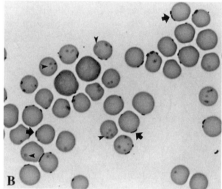

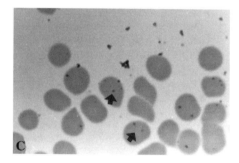

9. How can cytauxzoonosis be diagnosed when no organisms are evident on the blood smear?

The first option is to collect an additional blood sample at a later time since the magnitude of parasitemia increases as the disease progresses. It is not uncommon for animals to show significant parasitemia as few as 24 hours after having been negative on initial blood smear examination. The second option is to look for the schizont phase of the organism. They occur in macrophages in many organs of the body, but are most common in the spleen, lung and liver (bone marrow and lymph nodes are also often affected). Fine needle aspirates (or impression smears in animals that have died) of these organs often reveal numerous large schizont-laden macrophages.

Impression smear of the spleen from a cat with cytauxzoonosis. Two enlarged macrophages contain *C. felis* schizonts. The macrophagic nuclei contain large, prominent nucleoli *(arrows)*. The schizonts *(outlined by arrowheads)* are ill-defined, granular structures that completely fill and distend the cell cytoplasm (Wright stain, original magnification × 165).

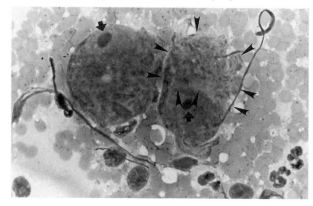

10. What is needed to look for *C. felis* on a blood smear in the clinic?

A reasonably good microscope with an oil immersion objective (100 ×) is needed because the organisms are small. They stain well with routine hematologic stains, such as Diff-Quik. The other essential ingredient is a well-made blood smear. The smears need to be thin so that a large area contains red cells that are well spread out and not crowded together. It is nearly impossible to see the organisms in thick areas of a blood smear where red cells are piled on top of each other.

The smear also must be dried well before staining. One of the biggest problems in examining for small red cell parasites is the presence of water artifact in the red cells. Water retained in red cells during the staining process appears as refractile areas that can easily be confused with parasites and also obscure identification of anything that may be within the cell. To avoid water artifact, let the smears sit for several minutes (even after they appear to have dried) before staining—or better yet, dry the smears for 15–20 seconds with a hair dryer. If you still get refractile areas, replace the fixative portion (the clear solution in Diff-Quik) of the stain set.

Besides water artifact, *C. felis* organisms must be differentiated from Howell-Jolly bodies, stain precipitate, and *Hemobartonella felis* (see figures with question 8). Howell-Jolly bodies are larger, round, dark dots that do not have the ring form typical of *C. felis*. Stain precipitate is usually abundant and seen between the cells as well as overlying the cells. *H. felis* organisms are smaller and usually form dots and chains. They can be small rings, but they do not have the nuclear area (thick "dot" on the ring) that is typical of *C. felis*.

11. How is cytauxzoonosis treated?

Recently two drugs have been advocated for treating *C. felis* infections: diminazine aceturate and imidocarb dipropionate. One recent study reported the successful treatment of 5 cats with diminazine aceturate (2.0 mg/kg/wk intramuscularly for 2 doses), a drug used to treat babesiosis and other protozoal diseases. The cats also were treated with heparin and supportive fluid therapy to prevent disseminated intravascular coagulation. Unfortunately, diminazine is not marketed in the United States.

Based on anecdotal reports and 1 case report, imidocarb dipropionate (5.0 mg/kg intramuscularly every 2 weeks for 2 doses) has been recommended as a potential therapy. Imidocarb (Imizol, Schering-Plough Animal Health, Union, NJ) is available in the United States for the treatment of canine babesiosis. Limited experience with imidocarb in Oklahoma and Arkansas has not been as promising; further studies are needed to determine efficacy.

12. Describe the prognosis for cats with cytauxzoonosis.

The prognosis for a cat infected with *C. felis* is grave. Historically, the case fatality rate has been nearly 100%, regardless of therapeutic attempts. There have been sporadic reports of cats surviving experimental or natural infection, but they are rare. Recently, some cats that had clinical signs compatible with cytauxzoonosis and *C. felis* organisms within erythrocytes at presentation recovered with supportive care in the absence of specific antiprotozoal therapy. Currently, such cases have been limited to an area of western Arkansas and eastern Oklahoma, prompting suspicion of the emergence of a less virulent strain. Infected cats are persistently parasitemic but, once recovered, have not shown recurrence of clinical signs.

13. What are the implications for other cats in the household?

It is not unusual for an owner to lose several cats to cytauxzoonosis in a short period. However, infection is not spread directly from cat to cat, even when they are housed in close contact. When multiple cats in the household are infected, it is most likely from exposure to the same population of ticks. Clinical signs in other family cats usually occur within approximately 2–3 weeks of exposure to infected ticks. The only method to determine whether other cats in the family were infected is to monitor blood smears for organisms. However, this approach has an extremely low sensitivity early in the course of infection.

14. How can cytauxzoonosis be avoided?

Limiting (or eliminating) exposure to outdoors and good external parasite control are the best methods of preventing infection with *C. felis*.

15. What public health risks are associated with *C. felis*?

The organism does not infect people. However, cats can bring ticks that may carry other zoonotic agents into the human environment.

BIBLIOGRAPHY

1. Greene CE, Latimer K, Hopper E, et al: Administration of diminazene aceturate or imidocarb dipropionate for treatment of cytauxzoonosis in cats. J Am Vet Med Assoc 215:497–500, 1999.
2. Kier AB, Greene CE: Cytauxzoonosis. In Greene CE (ed): Infectious Diseases of the Dog and Cat, 2nd ed. Philadelphia, W.B.Saunders, 1998, pp 470–473.
3. Meinkoth JH, Kocan AA, Whitworth L, et al: Cats surviving natural infection with *Cytauxzoon felis*: 18 cases (1997–1998). J Vet Intern Med 14:521–525, 2000.

76. FELINE LEUKEMIA VIRUS

Margo L. Mehl, D.V.M.

1. What is feline leukemia virus (FeLV)?

FeLV is a pancytotropic virus horizontally transmitted and capable of inducing lymphoproliferative and myeloproliferative diseases. FeLV belongs to the subfamily Oncovirinae of the family Retroviridae. Like other retroviruses, FeLV has a single-stranded RNA genome and with reverse transcriptase infects a host cell and makes a DNA copy of its genome (provirus), which is inserted into the host genome.

2. How is FeLV transmitted?

The most likely route of transmission of FeLV is continued intimate moist contact, such as mutual grooming and sharing food and water bowls. The virus can be transmitted to neonates in utero and through the milk of infected queens. Feline leukemia virus also has been transmitted via blood transfusions; therefore, FeLV-positive cats should not be used as blood donors.

3. Is FeLV stable in the environment?

FeLV is relatively fragile in the environment. It can be inactivated by ordinary hospital and household detergents, alcohol, bleach, heating, and drying.

4. Describe the typical signalment of FeLV-infected cats.

Cats with FeLV infection tend to be young (1–5 years old) at the time of diagnosis. Kittens younger than 4 months have an increased susceptibility to developing persistent viremia compared with adult cats.

5. Do all FeLV-infected cats succumb to disease?

The outcome of infection depends on many factors, including host immune response, virulence of the viral strain, dose and duration of exposure, presence of concurrent diseases, and age of the cat at time of infection. In one study, approximately 30% of virus-infected cats actually developed disease. Healthy and persistently positive cats had a median survival time of 2 years; 20% were still alive after 3 years. Disease in infected cats usually results from bone marrow or lymphoid suppression with life-threatening secondary infections or neoplastic manifestations.

6. What are the outcomes of FeLV exposure?

(1) The cat may mount an immune response, clear the virus, and become resistant to future infection; (2) some cats fail to mount an effective immune response, become persistently viremic, and succumb to FeLV-associated diseases; or (3) the virus is cleared from the plasma or serum but persists in a latent form in the bone marrow or lymphatic tissue.

7. Describe the six stages of FeLV infection.

The first stage occurs after oronasal exposure and replication of FeLV in tonsillar and pharygeal lymphoid tissues. In the second stage, the virus infects circulating small lymphocytes and monocytes. The virus is then amplified in the spleen, gastrointestinal tract, and lymph nodes which is considered the third stage of infection. The fourth stage involves bone marrow replication and infection of platelets and neutrophils. Once bone marrow cell lines are infected, peripheral viremia occurs (fifth stage). The sixth stage of infection begins with epithelial infection, which results in excretion of FeLV in saliva and urine. In the sixth stage the cat is contagious.

Stages of Feline Leukemia Virus Infection with Corresponding Test Results

STAGE	ORGANISM LOCALIZATION	TIMING	IFA RESULT	ELISA RESULT
I	Replication in local lymphoid tissues (tonsillar and pharyngeal with oronasal exposure)	2–12 days	Negative	Negative
II	Dissemination in circulating lymphocytes and monocytes	2–12 days	Negative	Positive
III	Replication in the spleen, distant lymph nodes and gut-associated lymphoid tissue	2–12 days	Negative	Positive
IV	Replication in bone marrow cells and intestinal epithelial crypts	2–6 wk	Negative	Positive
V	Peripheral viremia, dissemination via infected bone marrow derived neutrophils and platelets	4–6 wk	Positive	Positive
VI	Disseminated epithelial cell infection with virus secretion in saliva and tears	4–6 wk	Positive	Positive

IFA = immunofluorescent assay, ELISA = enzyme-linked immunosorbent assay.
Adapted from Rojko JL, Hardy WD: Feline leukemia virus and other retroviruses. In Sherding RG (ed): The Cat: Diseases and Clinical Management, 2nd ed. New York, Churchill Livingstone, 1994, pp 263–432.

8. What are the clinical findings of FeLV infection?

FeLV infection results in a wide variety of clinical findings, which result either from the virus itself or from secondary infections. Clinical manifestations of FeLV result from secondary infections due to immunosuppression, cytopenias due to retrogression of bone marrow precursor cells, or myeloid or lymphoid neoplasia. Cytopenias include nonregenerative anemia, thrombocytopenia, neutropenia, and lymphopenia. Secondary infections that appear to be worsened by concurrent FeLV infection include hemobartonellosis, toxoplasmosis, chronic stomatitis, and respiratory tract infections. Lymphosarcoma, fibrosarcoma, and myeloproliferative diseases are common FeLV-associated neoplasms.

Clinical Findings of Feline Leukemia Virus Infection

Neoplasia
  Myeloproliferative
    Megakaryocytic leukemia
    Myelomonocytic leukemia
    Erythroid leukemia
  Lymphoproliferative
    Lymphosarcoma
    Lymphocytic leukemia
Myelosuppression/myelodysplasia
  Anemia
  Neutropenia
  Thrombocytopenia

Immunosuppression and secondary syndromes
  Chronic bacterial infections
  Calicivirus
  Cryptococcus neoformans
  Dermatophytosis
  Feline infectious peritonitis
  Haemobartonella felis
  Stomatitis
  Toxoplasma gondii
Other related syndromes
  Glomerulonephritis
  Lymphadenopathy
  Osteochondromas
  Reproductive failure and abortion

9. How is FeLV infection detected?

The most commonly used tests to detect FeLV infection are enzyme-linked immunosorbent assay (ELISA) and immunofluorescent assay (IFA); both are based on the detection of viral p27 antigen (see table in question 7). ELISA is the recognized screening test for FeLV infection. Serum is the preferred media for testing individual animals because it gives fewer false-positive and false-negative results than plasma, blood, tears, or saliva. IFA detects the p27 antigen after bone marrow infection has occurred and the p27 antigen has been incorporated into leukocytes and platelets; it is used primarily as a confimatory test.

10. How are ELISA and IFA results interpreted?

There are three major reasons for negative ELISA results: (1) the cat is not infected due to lack of exposure or development of neutralizing antibodies and elimination of infection; (2) the cat is undergoing peracute infection; or (3) the cat has cleared the serum but is latently infected.

ELISA-positive cats are undergoing transient infection (stages 1–4; see table in question 8) or are persistently infected. Thirty percent of ELISA-positive cats may convert to a negative status, which is believed to be due to transient infection or development of a latent infection.

ELISA-positive cats without clinical signs of FeLV-related disease should be quarantined from other cats and immediately tested by IFA or retested by ELISA in 4–8 weeks to determine whether transient or persistent viremia is present. If results of both ELISA and IFA are positive, the cat probably will be viremic for life. If ELISA results are positive but IFA results are negative, the cat should be retested by ELISA and IFA every 4–8 weeks for up to 90 days to determine whether the ELISA becomes negative or the IFA becomes positive. If false-positive FeLV results are suspected, you should test serum from the cat with a different FeLV test.

11. What cats should be tested for FeLV infection?

All cats that go outdoors or come from unknown backgrounds should be tested for FeLV infection when first examined by the veterinarian. Cats with clinical disease consistent with FeLV infection should be tested as part of the diagnostic work-up. Cats vaccinated for FeLV infection but allowed outdoors should be tested yearly because vaccines do not give complete protection (see Chapter 81). If a cat has had a presumed exposure, it should be tested 4–8 weeks later and again 12 weeks later.

12. Can kittens be tested for FeLV infection?

Kittens can and should be tested for FeLV infection. Because ELISA is an antigen test and not affected by maternal antibodies, kittens should be tested immediately when first evaluated by the veterinarian—preferably before allowing contact with other household cats.

13. How is latent FeLV infection documented?

Latent infection occasionally is associated with clinical disease, particularly immunosuppression and cytopenias. It can be documented by IFA, virus isolation, or polymerase chain reaction on bone marrow cells.

14. What other tests are available for FeLV?

Feline oncornavirus-associated cell membrane antigen (FOCMA) and neutralizing antibodies can be detected in some laboratories but usually are not used clinically for individual cats.

15. Describe the approach to treatment of clinically ill FeLV-positive cats.

First a diagnostic work-up is performed to characterize the clinical illness and to determine whether the clinical syndrome is related directly to FeLV or to secondary invaders, for which specific treatment is administered (if available). For example, hemolytic anemia in FeLV-positive cats may be due to the virus or *H. felis*, which responds well to doxycycline. Cats with leukemia or myeloproliferative diseases generally do not respond well to available therapy and have a poor prognosis. Cats with lymphosarcoma may respond well to chemotherapy protocols, but survival times vary based on the location of lymphosarcoma and individual responses (see Chapter 68).

Bone marrow suppression from FeLV infection often results in nonregenerative anemia or pan-leukopenia syndrome, which may respond to whole-blood transfusions. Administration of human granulocytic colony-stimulating factor causes only transient increases in neutrophil count.

16. What other therapies have been used?

Many other therapies have been used in the management of FeLV-related diseases, including antivirals and immunomodulators. Immunomodulators used most frequently include interferon alpha, *Proprionibacterium acnes* (Immunoregulin), acemannan, diethylcarbamazine, and staphylococcal protein A. To date, well-designed studies assessing these therapies are not available, but beneficial effects have been suggested by some veterinarians. Use of interferon alpha (30 U orally every 24 hr) has resulted in perceived improvement in clinical well-being in some cats treated by the author. The antiviral drugs zidovudine (AZT) and 9-(2-phosphonyl-methoxyethyl) adenine (PMEA) have been assessed for the treatment of FeLV in several studies. Cats with stomatitis showed improved clinical status. AZT (5 mg/kg orally every 12 hr) may be indicated in some cats and has minimal side effects.

17. What recommendations can be made for management of FeLV-positive cats?

A single positive FeLV test in a healthy cat should be confirmed by a second test. Once a healthy cat is found to be persistently FeLV-positive, the following topics should be addressed with the owner:
- Prognosis: the median survival for an FeLV-infected healthy cat is 2 years.
- Risk to other cats: the cat should be housed indoors to lessen odds of infecting other cats.
- Secondary invaders: the cat should be housed indoors to lessen the potential for acquiring secondary infection.
- Public health risk: the risk to humans from contact with FeLV-positive cats appears to be minimal (see question 19).
- Therapeutic options
- Avoidance of stressful environments (e.g., travel, elective surgery, introduction of a new cat)
- Avoidance of glucocorticoid use, if possible
- Vaccines: if the cat is housed indoors, there is little need for vaccines. If vaccines are indicated, inactivated products should be used.

CONTROVERSIES

18. Should FeLV vaccines be used?

Vaccination for FeLV should be considered for seronegative cats with a high risk of exposure; examples include outdoor cats, indoor-outdoor cats, stray or feral cats, cats in multiple or open cat households, and cats in households of unknown FeLV status or with FeLV-positive cats (see Chapter 81). Immunity from FeLV vaccination is reported as fair-to-good and varies with different vaccines. The FeLV vaccine is considered to be a noncore vaccine by the Advisory Panel on Feline Vaccines of the American Association of Feline Practitioners. The panel recommends that cats at risk be given a series of boosters as kittens and annual boosters in the left hind-leg as distal as practical, according to the manufacturer's instructions. The vaccination site recommendations are aimed at understanding the potential causal link between vaccination and tumor development. To date, approximately 1–3 in 10,000 cats have developed vaccine-associated sarcomas after receiving adjuvanted products.

19. What public health concerns are related to FeLV?

FeLV grows in some human cell cultures. However, no study to date has shown human infection with FeLV. In separate studies, people with chronic fatigue syndrome, people with leukemia, and normal veterinarians had no evidence of FeLV infection. It is possible that a cat immunosuppressed by FeLV may shed other zoonotic agents in higher numbers than normal cats, but this theory has not been well documented. FeLV-seropositive cats with clinical signs of disease should be assessed for potentially zoonotic agents.

BIBIOGRAPHY

1. Butera ST, Brown J, Callahan ME, et al: Survey of veterinary conference attendees for evidence of zoonotic infection by feline retroviruses. J Am Vet Med Assoc 217:1475–1479, 2000.
2. Cotter SM: Management of healthy feline leukemia virus-positive cats. J Am Vet Med Assoc 199:1470–1473, 1991.
3. Cotter SM: Feline viral neoplasia. In Greene CE (ed): Infectious Diseases of the Dog and Cat, 2nd ed. Philadelphia, W.B. Saunders, 1998, pp 71–84.
4. Elston T, Rodan I, Flemming DF, et al: AAFP/AFM Vaccination Guidelines. J Am Vet Med Assoc 212:228–241, 1998.
5. Hartmann K, Donath A, Beer B, et al: Use of two virustatica (AZT, PMEA) in the treatment of FIV and FeLV seropositive cats with clinical symptoms. Vet Immunol Immunopathol 35:167–175, 1992.
6. Hartmann K, Donath A, Kraft W: AZT in the treatment of feline immunodeficiency virus infection. Part 1. Feline Pract 23:16–21, 1995.
7. Hartmann K, Donath A, Kraft W: AZT in the treatment of feline immunodeficiency virus infection. Part 2 . Feline Pract 23:13–20, 1995.
8. Rojko JL, Hardy WD: Feline leukemia virus and other retroviruses. In Sherding RG (ed): The Cat: Diseases and Clinical Management, 2nd ed. New York, Churchill Livingstone, 1994, pp 263–432.
9. Tizard I: Use of immunomodulators as an aid to clinical management of feline leukemia virus-infected cats. J Am Vet Med Assoc 199:1482–1484, 1991.
10. Weiss RC, Cummins JM, Richards AB: Low-dose orally administered alpha interferon treatment for feline leukemia virus infection. J Am Vet Med Assoc 199:1477–1481, 1991.
11. Wolf AM: CVT update: Feline leukemia virus. Bonagura J (ed): Kirk's Current Veterinary Therapy XIII. Philadelphia, W.B. Saunders, 2000, pp 280–284.

77. FELINE IMMUNODEFICIENCY VIRUS

Paul R. Avery, V.M.D.

1. What is the feline immunodeficiency virus (FIV)?

FIV, first described in 1987 in Petaluma, California, is a retrovirus of the subfamily Lentiviridae. Like all retroviruses, FIV uses the enzyme reverse transcriptase to make a DNA copy from the viral RNA once inside an infected cell. The viral DNA is then integrated into the host genome, where it persists as proviral DNA. FIV has been the focus of much research because of its importance as a feline pathogen and also because it serves as a model of human immunodeficiency virus (HIV) infection.

2. How common is FIV infection?

FIV occurs worldwide. The seroprevalence of infection within the United States is approximately 1–4% in clinically healthy cats and increases up to 14% when clinically ill cats are surveyed. These general incidence rates are relatively consistent worldwide, although higher rates of infection have been reported in regions of Japan and Australia. FIV is more prevalent in free-ranging, intact male cats. This finding is consistent with the proposed major mode of transmission: bite wounds.

3. Can FIV be transmitted by routes other than biting?

Epidemiologic evidence suggests that bite wounds are the most common means of transmission. The virus can be isolated from the saliva of infected cats and transmitted experimentally via biting. FIV also can be isolated from the semen of infected cats, and, in the laboratory setting, semen and cell culture supernatants can be used to transmit FIV. The significance of venereal transmission in the natural setting is unknown. Like HIV, FIV crosses the rectal mucosa when inoculated experimentally. In utero transmission has been demonstrated in queens chronically infected with three of the major subtypes of FIV despite the fact that peripheral blood viral loads were quite low at the time of pregnancy. Lactating queens also have been shown to transmit FIV via milk, and foster-raising kittens of FIV-infected queens can decrease the transmission rate.

The question of whether close, daily contact with an FIV-infected cat in the absence of aggression poses a significant risk of transmission has been addressed in several studies of multi-cat households. The transmission rate has ranged from 0–100%. A recent well-controlled study of a closed, 26-cat household over a 10-year period showed a 35% transmission rate of FIV despite a lack of any subjective or objective evidence of aggressive behavior.

4. Describe the progression of disease in FIV-infected cats.
Many investigators have recognized broad phases of FIV infection that are quite similar to those seen with HIV infection. The duration of each stage varies considerably in infected cats, but the general phases of progression are consistent. Some feline practitioners have combined stages 3 and 4, because the two stages are often difficult to distinguish clinically.

STAGE	CLINICAL SIGNS	HEMATOLOGY	DURATION	DETECTION	COMMENTS
1. Acute phase	With or without fever, lethargy, diarrhea Lymphadenopathy	Neutropenia	Several days to weeks Lymphade-nopathy can persist for months	May be ELISA, WB, IFA negative up to 8 or more wk Positive PCR 1–3 wk after infection	Signs mild, generally overlooked by owner Younger cats tend to have more severe signs
2. Asympto-matic carrier	Generally none	CBC generally normal CD4/CD8 T-cell ratio decreased	Quite variable; generally several yr up to 10+ yr	Generally positive on ELISA, WB, IFA, PCR	Outwardly healthy despite demonstrable immune system defects
3. Persistent generalized lymphade-nopathy	Vague signs: with or without an-orexia, weight loss, fever of unknown origin, lymphadenopathy	With or without leukopenia Anemia CD4/CD8 ratio decreased	6 months to several yr	Generally positive on ELISA, WB, IFA, PCR	Approximately one-third of infected cats present during this stage FIV may be overlooked
4. AIDS-related complex	Secondary bacte-rial infections: oral cavity, upper respiratory tract, GI tract, skin Neurologic signs and neoplasia less common	Anemia, leu-kopenia, or leukocytosis CD4/CD8 ratio decreased	6 month to 1–2 yr	Generally positive on ELISA, WB, IFA, PCR	Approximately one-half of infected cats present during this stage Opportunistic infections not present
5. AIDS	Opportunistic infections: herpes and calicivirus *Toxoplasma* spp. *Cryptosporidium* spp. *Candida* spp. *Mycobacterium* spp. *Demodex* spp. Neurologic disease (~ 5% of cats) Neoplasia	Leukopenia Anemia CD4/CD8 ratio decreased	Cats seldom survive more than a few weeks to months at this stage	Some par-ticularly debilitated cats may be negative on ELISA, WB, IFA, but most are positive Positive PCR	Only approxi-mately 10% of FIV-infected cats reach this stage

ELISA = enzyme-linked immunosorbent assay, WB = Western blot test, IFA = immunofluorescent assay, PCR = polymerase chain reaction, CBC = complete blood count.

5. How is the diagnosis of FIV infection made?

There are four major types of assays to detect FIV infection: antibody enzyme-linked immunosorbent assay (ELISA), immunofluorescent antibody assay (IFA), western blot assay (WB) and polymerase chain reaction (PCR).

6. Which test is used most commonly?

The ELISA, which detects antibodies to FIV, is the most commonly used test and the preferred screening method. Because virtually all cats that mount an antibody response to FIV become persistently infected, the presence of antibodies can be used as a surrogate marker to detect ongoing FIV infection. ELISA tests consist of microwell formats used by diagnostic laboratories and in-house kits generally marketed to the practitioner.

7. Why are WBs used for confirmation?

Western blots also detect antibodies to FIV but are more specific than the ELISA. The specificity of this assay lies in the fact that the test sera are allowed to react with particular FIV antigens that have been separated on a gel based on size. Antibodies to FIV specifically bind to antigens in the gel, producing an identifiable band pattern. Depending on which antigens are used, some FIV-specific antibodies may go undetected. Because this assay is more laborious and expensive than an ELISA, it is generally reserved as a confirmatory test for a positive ELISA.

8. How accurate are IFAs?

IFAs also detect antibodies to FIV. FIV-infected cells are fixed to a slide as the source of viral antigen, and any antibodies in the test sample are allowed to bind to these cells. Bound FIV antibodies are then detected with a fluorescent secondary antibody to feline IgG. Some laboratories report that IFA performs as well as WB and is more reliable than ELISA. Despite this fact, occasional nonspecific fluorescence has been reported, obscuring both positive and negative results and requiring interpretation by an experienced operator.

9. Discuss the role of PCR.

PCR is an extremely sensitive tool for amplifying and detecting small amounts of viral RNA or DNA, but its use thus far has generally been restricted to the research setting. The detection of viral DNA by PCR indicates that the virus has entered the cell and integrated into the host genome. Viral RNA levels indicate ongoing virus production. RNA measured with PCR has been used to monitor progression of disease in patients with HIV and FIV (experimental) infections. RNA levels also have been shown to correlate with disease stage. It is likely that laboratories performing FIV PCR will become more prevalent in the future.

10. What causes false-negative results on the ELISA?

1. Some cats may take 8 weeks or more from the time of infection to produce detectable antibodies. During this window of time, a recently infected cat can be ELISA-negative (no antibodies), yet infectious to other cats. Because of this potential, the American Association of Feline Practitioners and the Academy of Feline Medicine have issued a recommendation that animals with known or potential exposure to an FIV-infected animal be retested at least 120 days after the exposure before being declared FIV negative.

2. User error or test failure is always a potential source of a false-negative result. The test should be repeated, preferably at a reference laboratory, when the clinical index of suspicion for FIV infection is high.

3. Some FIV-positive cats can become antibody-negative late in the disease. The proposed mechanism involves severe debilitation of the immune system.

11. What causes false-positive results on the ELISA?

1. Any screening test, even one with a relatively high specificity, has the potential to produce false-positive results when used to detect a disease with a low incidence. The positive predictive value (the percent of positive results that are true positives) of a test decreases as the

incidence of the disease decreases. This point is dramatically demonstrated in the case of FIV, which may have an incidence of 1–4% in healthy cats. One study in Germany comparing the results of the PetCheck microwell ELISA (IDEXX, Portland, ME) with Western blots for screening clinically normal cats showed that more than half (59%) of the positive results were false—despite the fact that previous reports had shown that the PetCheck test had a specificity of 98.0–99.6%. This finding clearly demonstrates the importance of confirming a positive ELISA result, particularly in healthy cats.

2. A false-positive result may be seen in young kittens that received maternal antibodies in the colostrum. Maternal antibodies are transmitted to the kitten more readily than the virus itself. These passively acquired antibodies may persist for 4 months or longer and produce a positive ELISA result that may not reflect the true infection status of the kitten. For this reason, it is recommended that kittens with a positive ELISA result be retested after 6 months of age.

3. There are reports that infection with feline leukemia virus, feline infectious peritonitis, or *Toxoplasma gondii* can result in a false-positive microwell ELISA (PetChek) reading.

12. When should tests other than ELISA be used to aid in the diagnosis of FIV infection?

1. Ideally, any positive ELISA result should be confirmed with a WB, particularly in an otherwise healthy cat, because of the relatively high chance of a false-positive result.

2. In any cat with a high clinical index of suspicion for FIV and a negative ELISA test, the ELISA should be repeated at a diagnostic laboratory or PCR should be performed. In the case of user error, a repeat ELISA at a reference laboratory may result in a positive result. In the case of a severely debilitated FIV-infected cat with little or no antibody production, PCR detects the integrated provirus.

3. In kittens that may have passively received colostral antibodies, there are no advantages to a WB or IFA because they both detect antibodies. The general recommendation in such cases is to retest the kitten after 6 months of age. PCR may be helpful in young kittens because FIV DNA should be absent (PCR-negative) if the ELISA test is positive because of the passive acquisition of antibodies.

4. PCR also can shorten the retest interval in cats with an unknown recent history or known recent contact with an FIV-infected animal. A negative ELISA in this instance may misdiagnose an infected cat in which antibodies have not yet developed. The general recommendation is to retest such cats with an ELISA in 12–16 weeks. Because most cats become PCR-positive in the peripheral blood within 1–3 weeks after infection, the detection of viral DNA via PCR may allow an owner to decide whether to introduce the cat into a multicat household without having to wait 3–4 months.

13. Which parameters can be monitored over time to predict when a particular FIV-infected cat is likely to progress to AIDS?

Despite intensive monitoring of both naturally occurring and experimental infections, biochemical or hematologic prediction of impending disease progression has proved difficult. None of the routinely measured parameters in complete blood counts or biochemical panels have been shown to correlate specifically with disease stage. Cats can have intermittent cytopenias for many years before developing overt FIV-induced disease. The development of hyperglobulinemia has been documented in some FIV-infected cats, but this, too, can precede actual disease by years.

The monitoring of CD4+ T-cell counts and CD4/CD8 ratios has been quite useful in following the progression of HIV infection. Unfortunately, FIV-infected cats demonstrate a relatively early decrease in CD4+ T-cell counts that can remain low for many years before development of AIDS. Limited studies to date have not shown an apparent correlation between the CD4/CD8 ratio and clinical stage of infection.

Peripheral plasma viral RNA levels measured via PCR are routinely used to monitor HIV progression. Evidence in FIV-infected cats suggests that the magnitude of the initial virus levels can predict the rapidity with which they progress to AIDS-like illnesses. Peripheral viral loads decrease as cats move from the acute phase to the asymptomatic stage, where they remain relatively stable. Some experimentally infected cats have shown a rise in peripheral viral loads as they begin to progress to the terminal stages of infection. Further work is needed to establish the utility and practicality of monitoring viral loads over time in naturally infected cats.

14. What are the accepted treatment options for FIV-infected cats?

Clearly, general supportive care and treatment of clinical signs is as important in FIV-positive cats as in any ill animal. The judicious use of antimicrobials to treat any specific infectious agent is also critical in these often immunosuppressed animals.

Targeted treatment of the virus itself has been attempted with some of the same antiviral compounds shown to be effective against HIV. The nucleoside analogs 9-(2-phosphonomethoxyethyl) adenine (PMEA) and (S)-9-(3-fluoro-2-phosphonylmethyoxypropyl) adenine (PMPA) and 3'azido-2',3'-deoxythymidine (AZT; Retrovir, Glaxo-Wellcome, Middlesex, UK) have been shown to inhibit FIV replication. Protease inhibitors dramatically reduce HIV levels in humans with AIDS, but, despite the structural similarities between the proteases of HIV and FIV, none of the currently identified drugs is effective against FIV.

15. Discuss the use of PMEA and PMPA for the treatment of FIV infection.

In one study, 5 of 6 naturally infected cats suffering from a variety of clinical signs (diarrhea, stomatitis, gingivitis, weight loss) showed moderate-to-marked improvement when treated with PMEA at 2–20 mg/kg intramuscularly (IM) every 12 hours for 3 weeks. The improvement in oral lesions may be related to the effect of PMEA on concurrent herpes or calicivirus replication. All cats had recrudescence of clinical signs weeks to months after discontinuation of treatment, but a 3-week retreatment period induced an even longer clinical remission in some cats. Nine months after the termination of treatment, 4 of the 5 responding cats were clinically healthy. Side effects were limited to slight anemia at the highest dose (20 mg/kg IM every 12 hr). In another double-blind study, FIV-positive cats were treated with either PMEA (10 mg/kg), PMPA (25 mg/kg) or placebo IM twice weekly for 6 weeks. Both drugs caused significant improvement in stomatitis and conjunctivitis. PMEA had a greater effect on increasing CD4+ T-cell numbers and improving the cat's quality of life (based on a modified Karnofsky's score, which is used in humans with cancer) than PMPA, although PMPA had a more potent effect on decreasing the levels of circulating virus. Side effects were tolerable and consisted of mild anemia, which was more pronounced in PMEA-treated cats. Unfortunately, neither drug is readily available to the practitioner.

16. How effective and safe is AZT in FIV-infected cats?

AZT has been shown to improve general clinical status, increase CD4/CD8 ratios, and improve stomatitis in FIV-positive cats. It is equally effective when given orally or subcutaneously at a dose of 5 mg/kg twice daily. AZT is administered orally in a gelatin capsule or subcutaneously diluted in 5 ml of isotonic sodium chloride. Cats must be monitored for development of anemia, which can be associated with Heinz bodies, although the drug is generally well tolerated. Cats have been maintained on symptomatic therapy for as long as 9 months without significant side effects. AZT appears to be somewhat less efficacious in controlling FIV-induced symptoms and viral levels than PMEA and PMPA, but it is currently the only commercially available drug with demonstrated utility against FIV.

17. Is the development of resistant strains a problem in FIV-infected cats?

Strains of FIV resistant to some or all of the above drugs have been generated in experimental settings. Thus, as has proved true for HIV, long-term use in cats probably will generate viruses that are no longer susceptible to nucleoside analog drugs.

18. Discuss the connection between FIV infection and lymphoma.

Most feline lymphomas occur in cats infected with the feline leukemia virus, which, as an oncovirus, plays a direct role in causing tumors. Lentiviruses such as FIV generally are not considered direct tumor-inducing viruses, but several studies have identified an increased risk of developing lymphoma in FIV-infected cats. One epidemiologic study showed that FIV-infected cats had a five-fold increased risk for the development of lymphoid malignancies compared with FIV-negative cats

(FeLV-infected cats had a 60-fold increased risk). In addition, the lymphomas described in FIV-infected cats share many features. They tend to be high-grade immunoblastic or centroblastic B-cell tumors, the same type of lymphomas associated with HIV infection. Many theories for an indirect role of FIV in tumorigenesis have been proposed, including long-term polyclonal stimulation of B cells, which eventually may result in malignant transformation and decreased tumor surveillance due to immunodeficiency. A recent study has identified a B-cell tumor in which FIV virus was integrated at a single site, indicating that the virus had integrated prior to malignant transformation. This study raises the possibility that, in some FIV-associated lymphomas, the virus may play a more direct role in the induction of neoplastic transformation.

19. What are the prospects for the development of a commercially available FIV vaccine?

The search for a means to protect cats from FIV infection has been ongoing since the initial description of the virus in the late 1980s. Three basic approaches to vaccination have been studied: whole inactivated virus, viral subunits, and viral DNA. Despite some of the promising results shown in the experimental setting, the challenge of developing a universally effective FIV vaccine is great. Much still needs to be learned about the natural immune response to the virus, but each vaccine construct sheds more light on the subject and brings protection from FIV infection closer to reality.

20. What are the limitations of whole inactivated virus vaccines?

Whole inactivated virus preparations have induced protective immunity against the particular virus used in the vaccine but, in general, have shown little or no protection to heterologous viral isolates. Because of the high degree of variability among FIV viral strains and subtypes, this technique may not be able to afford a broad enough range of protection against natural infection. There is also concern that an inactivated whole virus preparation may have the potential to reacquire virulence once inside the cat.

21. What is the major problem with viral subunit vaccines?

Because of concerns about whole inactivated virus vaccines, subunit vaccines using portions of the viral envelope protein have been investigated. Like whole inactivated viruses, the viral subunits were capable of inducing high levels of antibodies to FIV, and some have shown partial protection against FIV infection. However, it appears that some of these subunit vaccines induced antibodies to FIV that actually enhanced subsequent infection rather than protecting cats. It is thought that the affinity of the antibodies and the identity of the particular epitopes to which they bind influences whether they result in protection or enhancement of infection. Clearly this ambiguity is a significant obstacle in the development of viral subunit vaccines.

22. What are the potential advantages of viral DNA vaccines?

The third approach that has been studied is the relatively new technique of using viral DNA as a vaccine. Molecular clones of FIV in which specific regions have been deleted to make them replication-defective have been used to vaccinate cats. There was evidence of significant protection when the cats were challenged with the same virus used as the vaccine, and in cats that were not completely protected, the severity of clinical signs was reduced. DNA vaccination holds particular promise because it can be manipulated to stimulate cellular and humoral arms of the immune system, both of which are important in controlling retrovirus replication.

BIBLIOGRAPHY

1. Addie DD, Dennis JM, Toth S, et al: Long-term impact on a closed household of pet cats of natural infection with feline coronavirus, feline leukaemia virus and feline immunodeficiency virus. Vet Rec 146:419–424, 2000.
2. Barr MC: FIV, FeLV, and FIP: Interpretation and misinterpretation of serological test results. Semin Vet Med Surg 11:144–153, 1996.
3. Beatty JA, Callanan JJ, Terry A, et al: Molecular and immunophenotypical characterization of a feline immunodeficiency virus (FIV)-associated lymphoma: A direct role for FIV in B-lymphocyte transformation? J Virol 72:767–771, 1998.

4. Egberink H, Borst M, Niphuis H, et al: Suppression of feline immunodeficiency virus infection in vivo by 9-(2-phosphonomethoxyethyl) adenine. Proc Natl Acad Sci 87:3087–3091, 1990.
5. Elder JH, Dean GA, Hoover EA, et al: Lessons form the cat: Feline immunodeficiency virus as a tool to develop intervention strategies against human immunodeficiency virus type 1. AIDS Res Human Retrovir 14:797–801, 1998.
6. Hartmann K, Kuffer M, Balzarini J, et al: Efficacy of the acyclic nucleoside phosphonates FPMPA and PMEA against feline immunodeficiency virus. J AIDS Human Retrovirol 17:120–128, 1997.
7. Hartmann K: Feline immunodeficiency virus infection: an overview. Vet J 155:123–137, 1998.
8. Hartmann K, Donath A, Kraft W: AZT in the treatmant of feline immunodeficiency virus infection. Feline Pract 23:13–21, 1995.
9. Hosie MJ, Jarrett O: Analysis of the protective immunity induced by feline immunodeficiency virus vaccination. Adv Vet Med 41:325–333, 1999.
10. Hosie MJ, Flynn JN, Rigby MA, et al: DNA vaccination affords significant protection against feline immunodeficiency virus infection without inducing detectable antiviral antibodies. J Virol 2:7310–7319, 1998.
11. Novotney C, English RV, Houseman J, et al: Lymphocyte population changes in cats naturally infected with feline immunodeficiency virus. AIDS 4:1213–1218, 1990.
12. O'Neil LL, Burkhard MJ, Diehl LJ, et al: Vertical transmission of feline immunodeficiency virus. AIDS Res Human Retrovir 1:171–182, 1995.
13. Pedersen NC, Barlough JE: Clinical overview of feline immunodeficiency virus. J Am Vet Med Assoc 199:1298–1305, 1991.
14. Shelton GH, Grant CK, Cotter SM, et al: Feline immunodeficiency virus and feline leukemia virus infections and their relationships to lymphoid malignancies in the cat: A retrospective study (1968–1988). J AIDS 3:623–630, 1990.
15. Torten M, Franchini M, Barlough JE, et al: Progressive immune dysfunction in cats experimentally infected with feline immunodeficiency virus. J Virol 65:2225–2230, 1991.

78. EHRLICHIOSIS

Cynthia J. Stubbs, D.V.M., M.S.

1. What are *Ehrlichia* spp.?

Ehrlichia spp., members of the family Rickettsiaceae, are pleomorphic, gram-negative, obligate intracellular microorganisms. Morulae, which are intracytoplasmic inclusions formed by clusters of the rickettsia, can be found transiently in mononucler cells, neutrophils, eosinophils, or platelets during acute illness. Animals known to be naturally infected by *Ehrlichia* spp. include cats, dogs, horses, ruminants, mice, and humans.

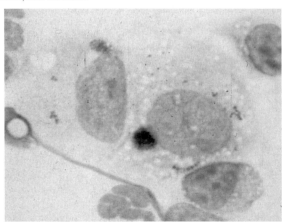

Mononuclear cell of an *Ehrlichia canis* and *E. risticii* seropositive cat containing a cluster of organisms morphologically consistent with *Ehrlichia* spp.

2. What evidence indicates that cats become infected with *Ehrlichia* spp.?

In 1986, the first naturally occurring case of feline ehrlichiosis was documented in a cat in France by Charpentier and Groulade. Intracytoplasmic inclusion bodies in neutrophils, eosinophils, and mononulcear cells that resemble *Ehrlichia* spp. morulae have been detected in naturally exposed cats in several countries, including France, Kenya, Sweden, Brazil, Thailand, and the United States. In one study, electron microscopic assessment of these *Ehrlichia*-like boides revealed organisms from 0.54–1.3 µm, intermediate in size between *E. canis* and *E. sennetsu* morulae. In other studies, morphologic descriptions of morulae were not available. To date, the only sequenced isolate from a domestic cat was genetically identical to the *Ehrlichia* spp. that causes human, canine, and equine granulocytic ehrlichiosis.

Cats have been infected experimentally with *E. risticii*, the causative agent of Potomac horse fever, and *E. equi*, which causes equine ehrlichiosis. Experimental infections of cats with *E. canis* or other ehrlichial species have not been attempted. Based on the reports of morulae in different cell types, genetic sequencing, and results of experimental infection studies, it appears that cats may be infected by more than one ehrlichial species.

3. How common is feline ehrlichiosis?

Internationally, antibodies that react with *Ehrlichia* antigens have been detected in serum of cats from Sweden, Africa, France, and the United States. In separate reports, seropositive cats were detected in Maryland, Colorado, Virgina, and California. In a national seroprevalence study of 599 cats, antibodies to E. canis and/or E. risticii were detected in 29.2%; positive cats were identified throughout the United States. Of these cats, 4.4% were seropositive for *E. canis* alone, 28.5% for *E. risticii* alone, and 3% for both species.

4. What are the most common clinical signs of feline ehrlichiosis?

A wide variety of clinical signs has been reported. The most common is fever. Other clinical signs include anorexia, weight loss, attitude changes (lethargy, depression, general malaise, irritable disposition), gastrointestinal signs (vomiting or diarrhea), pain (generalized hyperesthesia, lameness, or arthralgia), ocular discharge, pale mucous membranes, dyspnea, splenomegaly, and lymphadenopathy. Less commonly reported clinical signs include dehydration, gingivitis, polyuria, polydipsia, and tachypnea.

5. How is ehrlichiosis definitively diagnosed in cats?

- Demonstration of intracytoplasmic inclusion bodies typical of *Ehrlichia* spp. within blood leukocytes makes a definitive diagnosis of feline ehrlichiosis. However, in most ehrlichial infections of other species, morulae usually occur in detectable numbers only transiently in the acute phase of illness. In addition, detection of morulae cannot be used to determine which species of *Ehrlichia* is involved.
- Polymerase chain reaction (PCR) has been used to document ehrlichial DNA in the blood of cats. Currently PCR for Ehrlichia spp. is commercially available in at least two laboratories (HESKA Diagnostic Laboratory, Fort Collins, CO; North Carolina State University, Raleigh, NC). As more cats are assessed by PCR, it will be easier to determine which *Ehrlichia* spp. infect cats.

6. On what evidence is a presumptive diagnosis of ehrlichiosis based?

Presumptive diagnoses have been based on the combination of serum *Ehrlihcia* antibody detection (Prototek Reference Laboratory, Chandler, AZ), appropriate clinical signs, exclusion of other causes of disease, and response to treatment with antirickettsial drugs. However, because positive serologic results are seen in healthy cats as well as clinically ill cats, a diagnosis of ehrlichiosis should not be based on serologic results alone. A fourfold rise in the acute and convalescent titers also may correlate with recent or active infection. To date, no consistent pattern of titer duration has been noted in cats with ehrlichiosis. As in dogs, it appears that clearance of serum antibodies to *Ehrlichia* spp. is prolonged in some cats.

7. What laboratory abnormalities are most commonly associated with feline ehrlichiosis?
The most frequent hematologic change is nonregenerative anemia. Several cats with feline ehrlichiosis have had regenerative anemia, but they also were infected with *Hemobartonella felis*. Thrombocytopenia, neutrophilic leukocytosis, general leukocytosis, lymphocytosis, monocytosis, leukopenia, neutropenia, and lymphopenia also have been reported in some cats,
Hyperglobulinemia is a common biochemical profile abnormality in cats with feline ehrlichiosis. The increased globulin level has not been well described in the literature, but both monoclonal and polyclonal gammopathies have been reported. Other reported changes in the biochemical profile include elevated blood urea nitrogen, elevated creatinine, hyperbilirubinemia, hypoalbuminemia, hyperglycemia, hypokalemia, and elevated creatine phosphokinase activity.

8. Describe the pathogenesis of feline ehrlichiosis.
The pathogenesis is unknown, but based on clinical and laboratory findings, it is probably similar to acute *E. canis* infection in dogs.

9. How are *Ehrlichia* spp. transmitted?
The route of transmission to cats is currently unknown. Most ehrlichial species are tick-borne; cats in Kenya and the cat from Sweden were infested with *Haemaphysalis leachi* and *Ixodes ricinus*, respectively. Whether other arthropods or transport hosts are involved is not known. It is plausible that feline ehrlichiosis can be transmitted by blood transfusions, as reported in dogs. Because ehrlichial infection of cats appears to be common on the basis of serologic studies, it may be prudent to screen blood donor cats for antibodies or DNA by PCR. Further studies are needed to determine the mode of transmission to cats.

10. How is feline ehrlichiosis treated?
Antirickettsial drugs, including tetracycline, doxycycline, chloramphenicol, and imidocarb dipropionate, can be used to treat feline ehrlichiosis. Doxycycline at 5 mg/kg every 12 hours for 21 days is a commonly used protocol. Some cats require a longer course of treatment (4–6 weeks) because of recurring laboratory abnormalities. Two intramuscular doses of imidocarb dipropionate (5 mg/kg) 14 days apart appear to be safe and effective.

11. When should I do a trial of tetracycline therapy?
When a presumptive diagnosis of ehrlichiosis is based on the combination of serum antibody detection, appropriate clinical signs, and exclusion of other causes of disease, a trial of tetracycline is indicated. In dogs, clinical signs of ehrlichiosis develop before antibodies can be detected. Thus, treatment should be considered if the cat is acutely ill with appropriate clinical signs even if seronegative. It is possible that acutely infected seronegative cats are PCR-positive.

12. What public health concerns are associated with feline ehrlichiosis?
Both cats and people can be infected with a granulocytic strain of *Ehrlichia* spp. Dogs can harbor *E. chaffeensis*, the causative agent of human monocytic ehrlichiosis that cross-reacts serologically with *E. canis*. Cats are not known to be infected by *E. canis* but commonly have *E. canis* antibodies; thus, cats also may be infected with *E. chaffeensis*. Further work is required to determine whether cats are a reservoir for *Ehrlichia* spp. Cats may serve to bring infected vectors into the human environment (see Chapter 90).

BIBLIOGRAPHY

1. Almosny NRP, de Almeida LE, Moreira NS, et al: Ehrlichiose clinica em gato *(Felis canis)*. R Bras Ci Vet 5:82–83, 1998.
2. Artursson K, Malmqvist M, Olsson E, et al: Diagnosis of borreliosis and granulocytic ehrlichiosis of horses, dogs, and cats in Sweden. Svensk Veterinartidning 45:331–336, 1994.
3. Beaufils JP, Marin-Granel J, Jumelle P: *Ehrlichia* infection in cats: A review of three cases. Pratique Medicale Chirurgicate de l'Animale de Compagnie 30:397–402, 1995.

4. Bjoersdorff A, Svendenius L, Owens J, et al: Feline granulocytic ehrlichiosis: A report of a new clinical entity and characterisation of the infectious agent. J Small Anim Pract 40:20–24, 1999.
5. Bouloy RP, Lappin MR, Holland CJ, et al: Clinical ehrlichiosis in a cat. J Am Vet Med Assoc 204: 1475–1478, 1994.
6. Buoro IBJ, Atwell RB, Kipoon JC, et al: Feline anaemia associated with *Ehrlichia*-like bodies in three domestic short-haired cats. Vet Rec 125:434–436, 1989.
7. Buoro IBJ, Nyamwange SB, Kiptoon JC: Presence of *Ehrlichia*-like bodies in monocytes of an adult lioness. Feline Pract 22:36–37, 1994.
8. Charpentier F, Groulade P: Probable case of ehrlichiosis in a cat. Bull Acad Vet France 59:287–290, 1986.
9. Dawson JE, Abeygunawardena I, Holland CJ, et al: Susceptibility of cats to infection with *Ehrlichia risticii*, causative agent of equine monocytic ehrlichiosis. Am J Vet Res 49:2096–2100, 1988.
10. Jittapalapong S, Jansawan W: Preliminary surve on blood parasites of cats in Bangkhen District Area. Kasetsart J Natl Sci 27:330–335, 1993.
11. Lewis GE, Huxsoll DL, Ristic M, et al: Experimentally induced infection of dogs, cats, and nonhuman primates with *Ehrlichia equi*, etiologic agent of equine ehrlichiosis. J Am Vet Med Assoc 36:85–88, 1975.
12. Matthewman LA, Kelley PJ, Wray K, et al: Antibodies in cat sera from southern Africa react with antigens of *Ehrlichia canis*. Vet Rec 138:364–365, 1996.
13. Peavy GM, Holland CJ, Dulta SK, et al: Suspected ehrlichial infection in five cats from a household. J Am Vet Med Assoc 210:231–234, 1997.
14. Stubbs CJ, Holland CJ, Reif JS, et al: Feline ehrlichiosis. Compend Contin Educ Pract Vet 22:307–318, 2000.

79. NONREGENERATIVE ANEMIA

Dina A. Andrews, D.V.M., Ph.D.

1. Define nonregenerative anemia.

Nonregenerative anemia is defined by a decrease in red cell mass with an inadequate release of normal immature red blood cells into the peripheral circulation by the bone marrow. In recognizing nonregenerative anemia, it is important to know the duration of the anemia because the bone marrow requires approximately 5 days to respond adequately to a decrease in red cell density.

2. How is nonregenerative anemia identified on a peripheral blood smear?

Nonregenerative anemia is identified on a peripheral blood smear by a decrease in red cell density that is not accompanied by polychromasia in the monolayer portion of the smear. Polychromatophils correlate with aggregate reticulocytes, the most accurate marker of recent bone marrow regeneration in cats. Anisocytosis, nucleated red blood cells, and Howell-Jolly bodies without concurrent polychromasia are not specific indicators of regeneration.

3. What abnormal red cell morphologies provide information about the pathogenesis of nonregenerative anemia?

Nonpolychromatophilic macrocytes (large red cells) are associated with feline leukemia virus (FeLV) infection. Macrocytes also are identified in normal kittens less than 5 weeks of age. Nucleated erythroid precursors in circulation without accompanying polychromasia can be seen with myeloproliferative disease, often secondary to FeLV. Microcytes (small red cells) can indicate an early iron deficiency anemia. Poikilocytosis (cells of different shapes) are often present in iron deficiency anemia because of oxidative damage to the red cell membrane. Although not pathognomonic, dacryocytes (teardrop-shaped red cells) have been associated with myelofibrosis.

4. How is nonregenerative anemia identified by a complete blood count (CBC)?

Red cell parameters indicate a decreased hematocrit or packed cell volume. The red cell indices are most commonly normocytic and normochromic. An inflammatory leukogram can provide support for anemia due to a wide variety of infectious, noninfectious, and neoplastic conditions. Because iron sequestration and altered iron kinetics are common to these anemias, the possibility that microcytic anemia may develop in long-standing disease processes must be considered but is not a common finding.

5. Can red cell indices help to narrow the differential list?

Macrocytic/normochromic anemias are characteristic of FeLV infection. Minimal-to-mild macrocytic/normochromic anemias also may be seen in young kittens < 5 weeks old. Microcytic/ normochromic and microcytic/hypochromic anemias are characteristic of iron deficiency. Normocytic/normochromic anemias are nonspecific and can be seen with a variety of hypoproliferative anemias due to inflammation and chronic disease processes. A microcytic/normochromic anemia can be found in humans with long-standing disease processes, although this finding has not been documented in cats.

6. What laboratory tests confirm the presence of nonregenerative anemia?

A highly sensitive and cost-effective way to detect nonregenerative anemia is microscopic evaluation of the monolayer portion of a peripheral blood smear (see above). If polychromasia is questionable on the peripheral blood smear, an absolute reticulocyte count (using a vital stain, such as new methylene blue) should be performed by a laboratory familiar with the identification of feline reticulocytes. Cats have both aggregate and punctate reticulocytes. The aggregate reticulocytes mature into punctate reticulocytes within 12 hours, whereas punctate reticulocytes mature slowly over 10–14 days. Aggregate reticulocytes are the most accurate indicator of recent bone marrow response in cats, and their absolute numbers should be reported for categorizing an anemia as regenerative or nonregenerative. Although punctate reticulocyte numbers may be reported, they represent a cumulative indicator of bone marrow response because of their lengthy maturation time in the circulation and should not be used to evaluate recent bone marrow response.

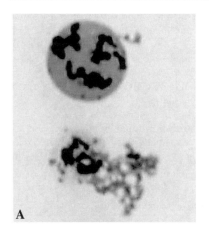 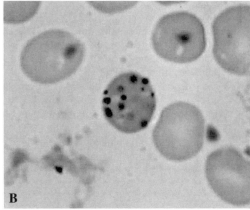

Aggregate *(A)* and punctate *(B)* reticulocytes in a cat with regenerative anemia.

7. What reticulocyte count is considered nonregenerative?

Cats do not respond as vigorously to anemias as humans and dogs, and their bone marrow reserves are small. Feline aggregate reticulocytes in health range from 0.0–0.4% of circulating erythrocytes when several reported ranges are averaged. Any increase in this percentage is considered indicative of regeneration. Caution must be used in interpreting the reticulocyte percentage as indicative of a regenerative reponse because this value does not correct for the degree of anemia. An absolute reticulocyte number is the most accurate means to evaluate regeneration. An absolute reticulocyte count of 0–50,000/μl is normal in cats, and an absolute reticulocyte count > 50,000/μl is considered indicative of regeneration. In interpreting both reticulocyte percentage and absolute reticulocyte count, the duration of the anemia and appropriateness of the regenerative response relative to the degree of anemia must be taken into consideration. For example, in an anemia of undetermined origin that has persisted for several weeks, a mild increase in aggregate reticulocyte numbers would not be considered an appropriate regenerative response. Bone marrow aspiration should be done to evaluate production of the erythroid series.

8. When can nonregenerative anemia be diagnosed confidently in a newly presenting patient?

If the underlying pathology of the disease process can support the finding of nonregenerative anemia (e.g., chronic renal failure), the diagnosis can be confidently made on initial presentation. If the patient presents with no obvious disease process on physical examination and no CBC or chemistry abnormalities that support nonregenerative anemia, the CBC should be repeated to confirm the presence of the anemia for longer than 4–5 days with no evidence of regeneration. If the nonregenerative anemia is deemed persistent, a bone marrow aspirate is warranted. Establishing a baseline aggregate reticulocyte count in patients with nonregenerative anemia is recommended so that any small increase in reticulocyte numbers due to treatment can be recognized on serial CBCs.

9. How long does nonregenerative anemia take to develop?

The time frame depends on the cause of the anemia. If the nonregenerative anemia is due to an acute inflammatory process (e.g., abscess), a decrease in red cell mass can develop within 4 days because of an increased rate of red cell destruction without an appropriate bone marrow response. Conversely, if the anemia is due to a long-standing disease process such as chronic renal failure, failure of the bone marrow to replace normally senescent red cells during their 80-day life span results in a more slowly evolving anemia.

10. What general categories of disease can cause nonregenerative anemia?

Distinguishing whether nonregenerative anemia is a singular abnormality in the CBC or accompanied by other cytopenias is extremely helpful in determining the cause of the anemia. This distinction generally differentiates anemia due to secondary or extramarrow causes from anemia due to intramarrow disease, respectively. As always, there are exceptions and overlap with the manifestations of certain disease processes, particularly FeLV and feline immunodeficiency virus (FIV) infections. Recognition of abnormal red cell morphologies, classification of the severity of anemia, and description of red cell indices are also helpful criteria.

11. What diseases result in selective nonregenerative anemia without cytopenias?

Important differential diagnoses include FeLV-induced selective red cell aplasia, iron deficiency anemia, acute inflammation, and chronic disease processes, including renal disease, endocrine disorders, immune-mediated disease, and neoplasia. If the anemia is severe, congenital or acquired pure red cell aplasia also should be considered.

Secondary Bone Marrow Failures: Nonregenerative Anemia without Cytopenias

CAUSE	SEVERITY OF ANEMIA	RED CELL INDICES	RBC MORPHOLOGY	BONE MARROW
FeLV-induced selective RBC aplasia	Mild to severe	Normocytic-normochromic or Macrocytic-normochromic	Normal: macrocytes	Variable: ineffective erythropoiesis, erythroid hypoplasia, absence of RBC precursors
Anemia of acute inflammation	Mild	Normocytic-normochromic	Normal	Erythroid hypoplasia
Anemia of chronic disease	Mild	Normocytic-normochromic	Normal	Erythroid hypoplasia

Table continued on following page

Secondary Bone Marrow Failures: Nonregenerative Anemia without Cytopenias (Continued)

CAUSE	SEVERITY OF ANEMIA	RED CELL INDICES	RBC MORPHOLOGY	BONE MARROW
Renal disease	Mild to moderate	Normocytic-normochromic	Normal; with or without Burr cells	Erythroid hypoplasia
Iron deficiency anemia	Mild (early) Mild to moderate (late)	Normocytic-normochromic (early) Microcytic-normochromic (late)	Microcytes Poikilocytosis (red cell fragmentation)	Left-shifted erythroid series, ineffective erythropoiesis
Red cell aplasia	Usually severe	Normocytic-normochromic	Normal	Absence of RBC precursors, other marrow elements normal
Acute hemorrhage (first 4 days)	Variable	Normocytic-normochromic	None	Normal

RBC = red blood cell, FeLV = feline leukemia virus.

12. What diseases cause nonregenerative anemia with leukopenia and/or thrombocytopenia?

The presence of multiple cytopenias indicates injury or destruction to the stem cell population in the bone marrow. The general category of myelophthisic disorders encompasses bone marrow failure or dysfunction due to abnormal proliferation of any or multiple cell lines, including bone marrow-occupying metastatic disease. Myeloproliferative disorders involve the clonal proliferation of one or more nonlymphoid precursors (erythroid, granulocytic, monocytic, megakaryocytic, or fibroblastic series) and are more common in cats than in dogs. An underlying FeLV infection is suspect in most cases. Circulating atypical or neoplastic cells may or may not be present. Infiltration of the marrow due to lymphosarcoma or primary lymphoid leukemias (acute or chronic) can cause similar marrow suppression. Myelofibrosis also serves as a space-occupying lesion in the bone marrow, effectively crowding out proliferating stem cells.

Myelodysplastic syndromes are characterized by multiple peripheral cytopenias in the face of a hypercellular marrow and are considered a preleukemic condition of the bone marrow, probably caused by FeLV. Abnormal morphology of the red cell, white cell, and/or megakaryocytic lineage is found in the bone marrow, and the functional result is ineffective hematopoiesis. Direct injury to the stem cell population due to administration of toxic drugs (e.g., chloramphenicol, griseofulvin, azathioprine) or idiopathic immune-mediated destruction of stem cells (aplastic anemia) also can cause primary bone marrow failure. Certain infections (e.g., cytauxzoonosis, ehrlichiosis) are also documented to cause nonregenerative anemias in addition to other cytopenias in cats.

Primary Bone Marrow Failure: Nonregenerative Anemia with Other Cytopenias

CAUSE	SEVERITY OF ANEMIA	RED CELL INDICES	RBC MORPHOLOGY	BONE MARROW
FeLV-related: stem cell damage	Moderate to severe	Normocytic-normochromic Macrocytic-normochromic	Normal macrocytes	Hypocellular
Other viral diseases (e.g., FIP, FIV)	Mild to moderate	Normocytic-normochromic	Normal	Hypocellular

Table continued on following page

Primary Bone Marrow Failure: Nonregenerative Anemia with Other Cytopenias (Continued)

CAUSE	SEVERITY OF ANEMIA	RED CELL INDICES	RBC MORPHOLOGY	BONE MARROW
Myelophthisic disorders (myelo-proliferative disease, lymphoid leukemia, lymphosarcoma)	Usually severe	Normocytic-normochromic Macrocytic-normochromic	Variable: normal, atypical/blasts, normal RBCs with no poly-chromasia	Hyperplastic mega-loblastic changes > 30% blasts in bone marrow
Myelodysplastic syndrome	Mild to severe	Normocytic-normochromic Macrocytic-normochromic	Normal	Normal to hyper-cellular Ineffective erythro-poiesis Dyserythropoiesis, dysgranulopoiesis, and/or dysthrom-bopoiesis
Myelofibrosis	Severe	Normocytic-normochromic	Normal dacryocytes	Hypocellular
Aplastic anemia	Severe	Normocytic-normochromic	Normal	Hypocellular
Feline ehrlichiosis	Mild to moderate	Normocytic-normochromic	Morulae in mono-nuclear cells	Not examined
Cytauxzoonosis	Mild to moderate	Normocytic-normochromic	Piroplasms of *C. felis* in erythrocytes, toxic neutrophils	Not examined
Drugs/chemicals	Severe	Normocytic-normochromic	Normal	Hypocellular

RBC = red blood cell, FeLV = feline leukemia virus, FIP = feline infectious peritonitis, FIV = feline immuno-deficiency virus.

13. What is the most common cause of nonregenerative anemias in cats?

There is a high incidence of nonregenerative anemias in cats with FeLV and FIV infections. Any cat with anemia should be tested for these viruses. Anemias caused by chronic disorders (e.g., inflammation, renal disease, neoplasia, immune-mediated diseases, endocrine disease, liver disease) are also common causes of nonregenerative anemia in cats.

14. Describe the classic profile of anemia due to chronic inflammation or chronic disease?

Such anemias are commonly described as mild (packed cell volume [PCV] > 20%), normocytic, and normochromic, with no evidence of regeneration (0–50,000/µl reticulocytes) and no erythrocytic morphologic abnormalities.

15. Describe the pathogenesis of anemia of chronic disease.

Anemias resulting from chronic disease are not well understood but are believed to share a common pathogenesis. Sequestration of iron in bone marrow macrophages, decreased response to erythropoietin by bone marrow, and decreased red cell life span are significant contributors. Altered iron handling is also involved based on common findings of decreased iron absorption by the gut, decreased serum iron, decreased serum iron-binding capacity, and increased tissue iron stores. Although some of these features are similar to those associated with true iron deficiency, classic hematologic features of iron deficiency anemia, such as microcytosis and hypochromasia, do not usually develop.

16. How do I treat anemia due to chronic disease?

Anemias due to chronic disease are secondary disorders. Resolution of the underlying disease process is necessary to restore normal red cell mass. Although the pathogenesis in part describes an iron-deficient state, body stores of iron are adequate, and patients do not respond to oral or injectable iron administration.

17. Describe the classic profile of anemia due to renal failure.

Anemias due to renal failure are classically mild (PCV > 20%), normocytic, normochromic, and nonregenerative. If the renal disease has been present for several months or other factors associated with renal disease have contributed to increased red cell destruction (e.g., uremia), the hematocrit may be moderately decreased (PCV = 15–19%).

18. Describe the pathogenesis of anemia due to renal failure.

The cause of the anemia is believed to be a combination of failure of the injured kidney to release adequate erythropoietin, impaired hematopoietic cell response to erythropoietin, and shortening of erythrocyte survival, probably related to metabolic injury associated with uremia.

19. Can nonregenerative anemia associated with renal failure be treated?

Although erythropoietin levels in cats with chronic renal failure are often within the normal range, a relative erythropoietin deficiency (inappropriate erythropoietin response for the degree of anemia) is believed to be present. Patients respond to recombinant human erythropoietin (rHuEpo) therapy (see Chapter 40), but its administration poses risks of anemia due to rHuEpo antibody production, seizures, systemic hypertension, and iron deficiency. The production of rHuEpo antibodies interferes with the erythropoietic effects of rHuEpo and endogenous erythropoietin. These effects are reversible on withdrawal of rHuEpo.

20. Describe the classic profile of nonregenerative anemia due to FeLV infection.

The hematologic findings are extremely varied. Anemias range from mild to severe, depending on the manifestation of the viral infection. Mild, normocytic, normochromic to macrocytic normochromic anemias (mean corpuscular volume [MCV] > 50 fl) can be present with normal leukocyte and platelet counts when viral infection results in selective depression of erythroid elements. Alternatively, infection can result in primary bone marrow disease, manifesting as pure red cell aplasia, aplastic anemia, myeloproliferative disorder, or myelodysplastic syndrome. In such instances, PCV can be dramatically decreased (< 10%) and associated with concurrent leukopenia and thrombocytopenia. Atypical erythroid (megaloblasts) or neoplastic cells may be present in the peripheral circulation and bone marrow aspirates.

21. What is the classic profile of nonregenerative anemia due to FIV infection?

The anemia is usually mild to moderate, normocytic and normochromic in subclinically infected cats. Multiple cytopenias are reported in cats with clinical evidence of disease.

22. Describe the classic profile of iron deficiency anemia.

Iron deficiency anemias are recognized infrequently in older cats as a result of chronic blood loss and malnutrition. Transient iron deficiency anemia is also recognized in kittens at approximately 5 weeks of age due to rapid growth and an all-milk diet. The classic profile for cats is a microcytic, normochromic nonregenerative anemia with prominent erythrocyte fragmentation (schistocytes, poikilocytes). However, this profile often evolves over a period of months after typically beginning as regenerative anemia. The key factor in the pathogenesis of the classic profile is insufficient hemoglobinization of red cell precursors. Normally precursor cells continue dividing until they reach a critical cytoplasmic hemoglobin concentration. At this point, cell division ceases and maturation proceeds. With iron deficiency, inadequate hemoglobinization causes precursors to undergo extra cell divisions, resulting in smaller cells. This process is first seen on the blood smear as anisocytosis due to the presence of microcytosis. Eventually, enough microcytes reach the circulation to reduce the population mean size and result in low MCV. Hypochromasia, a hallmark feature of iron deficiency in humans and dogs, is not commonly recognized in cats.

23. When is a bone marrow aspirate appropriate?
Clinical and laboratory findings often reveal the cause of nonregenerative anemia as bone marrow failure. In such cases, a bone marrow aspirate is usually not necessary. If the anemia remains unexplained or is accompanied by other cytopenias, a bone marrow aspirate is essential to determine the cause of the primary marrow failure.

24. When is it appropriate to submit a bone marrow core biopsy specimen?
A bone marrow core biopsy is most helpful when bone marrow aspirates are hypocellular. The core biopsy provides important information about cellularity of the bone marrow and recognizes fibrosis or local lesions in the bone marrow.

BIBLIOGRAPHY

1. Cook SM, Lothrop CD: Serum erythropoietin concentrations measured by radioimmunoassay in normal, polycythemic, and anemic dogs and cats. J Vet Intern Med 8:18–25, 1994.
2. Cowgill LD, James KM, Levy JK, et al: Use of recombinant human erythropoietin for management of anemia in dogs and cats with renal failure. J Am Vet Med Assoc 212:521–528, 1998.
3. Hoover JP, Walker DB, Hedges JD: Cytauxzoonosis in cats: Eight cases (1985–1992). J Am Vet Med Assoc 205:455–460, 1994.
4. Hoover EA, Mullins JI: Feline leukemia virus infection and diseases. J Am Vet Med Assoc 199:1287–1297, 1991.
5. Loar AS: Anemia: Diagnosis and treatment. In August JR (ed): Consultations in Feline Internal Medicine. Philadelphia, W.B. Saunders, 1994, pp 469–487.
6. Perkins PC, Grindem CB, Cullins LD: Flow cytometric analysis of punctate and aggregate reticulocyte responses in phlebotomized cats. Am J Vet Res 56:1564–1569, 1995.
7. Raskin RE: Myelopoiesis and myeloproliferative disorders. Vet Clin North Am 26:1023–1042, 1996.
8. Shelton GH, Linenberger ML, Abkowitz JL: Hematologic abnormalities in cats seropositive for feline immunodeficiency virus. J Am Vet Med Assoc 199:1353–1357, 1991.
9. Stokol T, Blue JT: Pure red cell aplasia in cats: 9 cases (1989–1997). J Am Vet Med Assoc 214:75–79, 1999.
10. Tvedten H, Weiss D: Erythrocyte disorders. In Willard MD, Tvedten H, Turnwald GH (eds): Small Animal Clinical Diagnosis by Laboratory Methods, 3rd ed. Philadelphia, W.B. Saunders, 1999, pp 31–37, 45–49.
11. Weiser MG: Disorders of erythrocytes and erythropoiesis. In Sherding, RG (ed): The Cat: Diseases and Clinical Management, 2nd ed. New York, Churchill Livingstone, 1994, pp 691–720.

VIII. Prevention of Diseases

Section Editor: Michael R. Lappin, D.V.M., Ph.D.

80. HOSPITAL BIOSECURITY

Michael R. Lappin, D.V.M., Ph.D.

1. Why is hospital biosecurity important?

Transmission of an infectious disease in the veterinary clinic (nosocomial infection) usually can be prevented, and it is always preferable to prevent rather than treat infections. Acquisition of an infectious disease in the hospital can be devastating for the infected cat because many hospitalized animals are extremely ill. In addition, if an infectious disease is acquired in the hospital, many clients may lose faith in their veterinary health care provider and seek veterinary care elsewhere. Some infectious agents infect cats and humans (see Chapter 83). It is extremely important to avoid zoonotic transfer of infectious agents, because many zoonotic diseases, such as plague and rabies, are life-threatening. Veterinarians should strive to understand the biology of each infectious agent so that they can counsel clients and staff about the best strategies for prevention. Vaccines available for some infectious agents can prevent infection or lessen clinical illness when infection occurs (see Chapter 81). However, vaccines are not uniformly effective and are not available for all pathogens; thus, it is paramount to develop sound biosecurity procedures to avoid exposure to infectious agents.

2. How are infectious diseases transmitted in the hospital?

Most infectious agents of cats are transmitted in fecal material, respiratory secretions, reproductive tract secretions, or urine; by bites or scratches; or by contact with vectors or reservoirs. Some infectious agents, such as *Bordetella bronchiseptica* and feline herpesvirus 1, can be transmitted by direct contact with subclinically infected cats. Thus, appropriate housing (individual cages) is extremely important. Many infectious agents are environmentally resistant and can be transmitted by contact with a contaminated environment (fomites). In addition, fleas or ticks from infested cats can contaminate the hospital and transmit infectious diseases. Thus, appropriate cleaning and disinfecting of the premises are imperative.

3. What are the common general biosecurity guidelines?

1. Recognition of risk factors associated with infectious agents is the initial step in prevention of infectious diseases.

2. Contaminated hands are the most common source of infectious disease transmission in the hospital environment.
   - Fingernails of personnel having patient contact should be cut short.
   - Personnel should not touch patients, clients, food, doorknobs, drawer or cabinet handles or contents, equipment, or medical records with soiled hands or gloves.

3. Hands should be washed before and after attending to each individual animal. Hands should be washed as follows;
   - Collect clean paper towels, and use them to turn on water faucets.
   - Wash hands for 30 seconds with antiseptic soap, taking care to clean under fingernails.
   - Rinse hands thoroughly.
   - Use paper towels to dry hands.
   - Use paper towels to turn off the water faucets.

4. All employees should wear an outer garment such as a smock or scrub suit when attending to patients. A minimum of 2 sets of outer garments should always be available, and garments should be changed immediately after contamination with feces, secretions, or exudates.

5. Footwear should be protective, clean, and cleanable.

6. Equipment such as stethoscopes, pen lights, thermometers, bandage scissors, cat carriers, percussion hammers, and clipper blades can be fomites and should be cleaned and disinfected with 0.5% chlorhexidine solution after each use if infectious disease is suspected. Disposable thermometer covers should be used.

7. To avoid zoonotic transfer of infectious diseases, food or drink should not be consumed in areas where cat care is provided.

8. All areas where cats are examined or treated should be cleaned and disinfected immediately after use, regardless of infectious disease status of the individual animal.

9. Litter boxes and dishes should be cleaned and disinfected after each use.

4. Can front-desk personnel aid in lessening transmission of infectious diseases in the clinic?

Prevention of infectious diseases starts with front-desk personnel:

1. Staff should be trained to recognize the presenting complaints for infectious agents within the geographic area of the hospital.

2. Cats with gastrointestinal or respiratory diseases are the most likely to be contagious.
   - Infectious gastrointestinal disease should be suspected in all cats with small or large bowel diarrhea, whether the syndrome is acute or chronic.
   - Infectious respiratory disease should be suspected in all cats with sneezing (especially with purulent oculonasal discharge) or coughing (especially if productive).

3. The index of suspicion for infectious diseases is increased for cats with acute disease and fever, particularly if the cat is from a crowded environment such as a breeding facility, boarding facility, or humane society.

4. Front-desk personnel should indicate clearly on the hospital record that gastrointestinal or respiratory disease is present.
   - If the presenting complaint is known before admission into the hospital, it is optimal to meet the client in the parking area to determine the risk of infectious disease before entering the hospital.
   - If infectious gastrointestinal or respiratory disease is suspected, the cat should be transported (i.e., not allowed to walk on the premises) to an examination room or isolation facility.
   - If a cat with acute gastrointestinal or respiratory disease is presented directly to the reception desk, the receptionist should contact the receiving clinician or technician immediately and coordinate placement of the animal in an examination room to minimize hospital contamination.

5. How can patient management lessen nosocomial transmission of infections?

1. Cats with suspected infectious diseases should be treated as outpatients if possible.

2. If hospitalization is required, the cat should be transported to the appropriate housing area by the shortest route possible, preferably by cat carrier to lessen hospital contamination.

3. The cat carrier and any hospital material contacted by potentially contaminated employees (including examination tables and door knobs) should be immediately cleaned and disinfected (see routine disinfection protocols).

4. If possible, all cats with suspected infectious diseases such as *Salmonella* spp., *Campylobacter jejuni*, parvovirus, feline upper respiratory disease syndrome, rabies, or plague should be housed in an isolated area of the hospital.
   - Because feline leukemia virus and feline immunodeficiency virus are not contagious if the infected cat is individually housed, seropositive cats should not be placed in the isolation area to avoid exposing them to other infectious diseases. However, they should not be allowed direct contact with other cats.

- The number of staff members entering the isolation area should be kept to a minimum. On entry into the isolation area, outerwear should be left outside and surgical booties or other disposable shoe covers should be placed over the shoes. Alternatively, a footbath filled with disinfectant should be placed by the exit and used when leaving the area (see question 6).
- When the room is entered, a disposable gown (or smock designated for the patient) and latex gloves should be put on. A surgical mask should be worn when attending cats with plague. Separate equipment and disinfectant supplies should be used in the isolation area.
- Procedures requiring general hospital facilities, such as surgery and radiology, should be postponed to the end of the day, if possible, and the contaminated areas disinfected before use with other animals.
- All biologic materials submitted to clinical pathology or diagnostic laboratories from animals with suspected or proven infectious diseases should be clearly marked as such.
- Fecal material should be placed in a plastic, screw-capped cup using a tongue depressor or wearing gloves. Place the cup in a clean area, and place the lid with a clean, gloved hand. Remove the used gloves, and place the cup in a second bag clearly marked with the name of the infectious disease suspected. The outer surface of the bag should be disinfected before leaving the isolation area.
- Disposable materials should be placed in plastic bags in the isolation area. The external surfaces of the bags should be sprayed with a disinfectant before being removed from the isolation area.
- After attending to the patient, contaminated equipment and surfaces should be cleaned and disinfected, and contaminated outer garments and shoe covers should be removed.
- Hands should be washed after discarding the contaminated outerwear. Dishes and litterpans should be cleansed thoroughly with detergent before being returned to the central supply area.
- Optimally, materials to be returned to a central supply area, such as outerwear and equipment, should be placed in plastic bags and sprayed with a disinfectant before transport.
- Cats should be discharged from the isolation area using the shortest path possible to the parking lot.

6. What basic disinfection protocols should be followed?

1. Cat beds, blankets, collar tags, and leash must go home with owner.
2. Cats should be housed individually.
3. Cats should never be moved from cage to cage.
4. Cage papers and litterpans soiled by feces, urine, blood, exudates, or respiratory secretions should be removed and placed in trash receptacles. Bulk fecal material also should be placed in trash receptacles.
5. Disinfectants do not penetrate deeply into contaminated materials such as feces; cleaning is as important or more important than disinfecting.
6. Many agents are resistant to disinfectants or require prolonged contact time to be inactivated.
7. Contaminated surfaces, including the cage or run floor, walls, ceiling, door, and door latch, should be wetted thoroughly with a disinfectant, which is then blotted with clean paper towels or mops.
8. Surfaces should be in contact with the disinfectant for 10–15 minutes if possible, particularly if known infectious agents are present.
9. Soiled paper towels should be placed in trash receptacles. If infectious diseases are suspected, the trash bags should be sealed, the surface of the bag sprayed with a disinfectant, and the trash bags discarded.
10. Contaminated surfaces in examination rooms should be cleaned to remove hair, blood, feces, and exudates.

11. Examination tables, countertops, floors, canister lids, and water taps should be saturated with disinfectant for 10 minutes, if possible.

12. Surfaces should be blotted with paper towels until dry, and the soiled towels should be placed in a trash receptacle. Urine or feces on the floor should be contained with paper towels, blotted, and placed in trash receptacles. The soiled area of the floor should be mopped with disinfectant.

13. Disinfectants are relatively effective for viral and bacterial agents but require high concentrations and long contact times to kill parasite ova, cysts, and oocysts. Cleanliness is the key to lessening hospital-borne infection with these agents, most of which are inactivated with detergent or steam cleaning. Litterpans and dishes should be cleaned thoroughly with detergent and scalding water.

BIBLIOGRAPHY

Lappin MR: Prevention of infectious diseases. In Nelson RW, Couto GC (eds): Small Animal Internal Medicine, 2nd ed. St Louis, Mosby, 1998, pp 1265–1272.

81. VACCINE RECOMMENDATIONS

Dennis W. Macy, D.V.M., and Michael R. Lappin, D.V.M., Ph.D.

1. Which vaccines should all cats receive?
The core vaccines that all cats should receive include:
- Panleukopenia (feline parvovirus)
- Rhinotracheitis (feline herpesvirus 1)
- Calicivirus
- Rabies

2. Should other vaccines be considered?
Noncore vaccines that should be administered on the basis of medical risk include:
- Feline leukemia virus (FeLV)
- Feline infectious peritonitis (FIP)
- *Chlamydia psittaci*
- *Bordetella bronchiseptica*
- *Giardia* spp.
- *Microsporum canis*

3. What types of vaccines are currently available?
Attenuated (modified-live) vaccines generally have low antigen mass and almost never induce local reactions; they can be given locally (e.g., modified-live *B. bronchiseptica* intranasal vaccine) or parenterally (e.g., modified-live panleukopenia). However, living vaccines must replicate in the host to stimulate an effective immune response.

Noninfectious vaccines include killed virus, killed bacteria (bacterins), and subunit vaccines. In general, noninfectious vaccines require higher antigen mass than modified-live vaccines to stimulate immune responses because they do not replicate in the host. Noninfectious vaccines stimulate immune responses of lesser magnitude and shorter duration than attenuated vaccines, unless adjuvants are added. Adjuvants improve immune responses by stimulating uptake of antigens by macrophages, which present the antigens to lymphocytes. Adjuvants can cause or potentiate adverse vaccine reactions; induction of vaccine-associated sarcomas in cats may be one example (see Chapter 82). Most adjuvanted vaccines studied in cats have led to pyogranulomatous reactions that may undergo malignant transformation to soft tissue sarcomas. Subunit vaccines may be superior to killed vaccines that use the entire organism because only the immunogenic parts of the organism are used; thus the potential for vaccine reactions is decreased.

Vector vaccines combine the advantages of attenuated and subunit vaccines. The DNA that codes for the immunogenic components of the infectious agent is inserted into the genome of a nonpathogenic organism (vector) that replicates in the vaccinated species. As the vector replicates in the host, it expresses the immunogenic components of the infectious agent, resulting in induction of specific immune responses. Because the vector vaccine is live and replicates in the host, adjuvants and high-antigen mass are not required, and because only DNA from the infectious agent is incorporated into the vaccine, there is no risk of reverting to the virulent parent strain, as occasionally occurs with attenuated vaccines. Only vectors that do not induce disease in the vaccinate are used.

4. Does the duration of immunity conferred by a vaccine vary?
In general, modified live virus vaccines and vector vaccines provide better cell-mediated immunity and longer duration of humoral immunity than killed or inactivated vaccines.

5. Should all adjuvanted vaccines be avoided in cats?
Because of the risk for vaccine-associated sarcomas (see Chapter 82), the nonadjuvanted product should be used when both adjuvanted and nonadjuvanted products are available. Many killed vaccines contain adjuvants, a fact that may not always be indicated on the label. Some killed feline rhinotracheitis, calcivirus, and panleukopenia (FVRCP) vaccines contain adjuvants and should not be used routinely. In addition, *Microsporum canis* and *Giardia* spp. vaccines contain adjuvants and should be avoided unless medically necessary.

6. Does the level of protection vary among vaccines for various diseases?
Some vaccines provide sterilizing immunity; infection is totally prevented if the animal is exposed (e.g., panleukopenia). Other vaccines, including those for upper respiratory disease, do not prevent infection but limit clinical signs if vaccinated cats are exposed. In general, vaccination should be expected to provide no better immunity than that conferred by recovery from the disease.

7. How often should core vaccines be given to pet cats?
• Kittens presented for vaccination between 6 and 12 weeks of age should be given an inactivated or modified live FVRCP vaccine every 3–4 weeks until 12 weeks of age.
• Kittens presented at > 12 weeks of age should be given either 2 inactivated FVRCP, 3–4 weeks apart, or 1 modified live FVRCP.
• Rabies vaccination should be based on local ordinances.
• Core vaccines should be boosted in 1 year, then every 3 years thereafter unless a rabies vaccine approved only for 1 year is used (see question 9).
• Titer and challenge studies indicate that core vaccines are effective for more than 6 years; for some antigens, such as panleukopenia, duration of immunity is probably lifelong.

8. How should the core vaccines be administered?
1. Topical (intranasal) and injectable FVRCP vaccines are available.
   • Intranasal rhinotracheitis and calicivirus vaccines induce IgA antibodies more rapidly and should be used if speed of response is important (e.g., during outbreaks).
   • Intranasal vaccines often are associated with sneezing.
   • Intranasal vaccines are not as likely as injectable vaccines to cause vaccine-associated sarcomas.
2. Injectable FVRCP vaccines should be administered subcutaneously as low as possible over the right shoulder.
3. Rabies vaccines should be given intramuscularly or subcutaneously as low as possible on the right rear limb.

9. Which rabies vaccines should be used in cats?
One nonadjuvanted rabies vaccine (Merial, Athens, GA) is currently available; at this time, it is the rabies vaccine of choice for cats. Chronic inflammation is thought to be necessary for the development of vaccine sarcomas (see Chapter 82); this product induces no chronic reaction at the injection site.

10. How often should core vaccines be given in crowded environments such as catteries or shelters?

If outbreaks occur, modified live intranasal vaccines containing feline herpesvirus 1 and calicivirus have been given to kittens as young as 2 weeks of age. In this scenario, one vaccine is usually divided among several kittens.

11. Why not use an interval longer than 3 years?

Memory T-lymphocytes probably exist for a lifetime after the administration of a modified live virus vaccine; thus vaccination intervals for some antigens probably could be longer. If recovery from the natural disease results in lifelong immunity, prolonged immunity may be expected from vaccination. Evolutionary concepts suggest that cats that are susceptible to acutely fatal diseases twice would be purged from the gene pool. For example, panleukopenia has never been reported in a cat that has received the initial set of vaccines, regardless of whether they received additional booster vaccines.

12. Can serum antibody titers be used to determine need for boosting individual cats?

Serum antibody titers are an indirect measure of protection that may be used for some diseases, but they have limitations:

1. Reproducibility from laboratory to laboratory is sometimes poor; only laboratories that have correlated titer magnitude to protection should be used (New York State Diagnostic Laboratory, Ithaca, NY; HESKA Diagnostic Laboratory, Fort Collins, CO).

2. For some diseases, mucosal and cell-mediated immunity is more important than humoral immunity for protection.

3. The presence of antibodies against panleukopenia, herpesvirus 1, and calicivirus usually predicts protection, but the absence of antibodies does not accurately predict susceptibility.

13. When should FeLV vaccination be used?

Cats that benefit the most from FeLV vaccines are young cats with a high risk of contact with FeLV carriers. For example, when exposed to an FeLV-infected cat, 12-week-old kittens and adult cats have an 85% and 15% chance, respectively, of becoming persistently infected. This age-acquired immunity limits the protection that can be attributed to the FeLV vaccine in adult cats.

- Naive cats should receive 2 vaccinations initially.
- Adjuvanted products should be administered subcutaneously or intramuscularly in the distal left rear limb because of the risk for development of soft tissue sarcomas.
- Because duration of immunity is unknown, annual boosters are currently recommended.
- The vaccine is not effective in persistently viremic cats and so is not indicated. However, administration of the vaccine to viremic or latent cats is not associated with an increased risk of vaccine reaction.
- FeLV testing should be performed before vaccination because the retrovirus serologic status of all cats should be known to maintain appropriate husbandry.

14. When should FIP vaccine be used?

The incidence of FIP is only 1 in 5000 cat households. The vaccine has been shown to be effective only in cats that do not harbor the coronavirus. Given that 20–40% of cats already harbor the coronavirus, that the maximal protection of the vaccines is 60–80%, and that the duration of protection is limited to secretory IgA, the value of the FIP vaccine in any situation is questionable. The vaccine may be indicated for seronegative cats entering a household or cattery known to be FIP-infected.

15. Should cats be vaccinated against chlamydiosis?

In the United States, *Chlamydia psittaci* infection in cats generally results only in mild conjunctivitis; therefore, whether vaccination is ever required is controversial. Use of this vaccine should be reserved for cats with a high risk of exposure to other cats and in catteries with endemic disease. Duration of immunity for chlamydial vaccines may be short-lived; thus, high-risk cats should be immunized before a potential exposure.

16. Should cats be vaccinated against bordetellosis?
Many cats have antibodies against *B. bronchiseptica*, and there are sporadic reports of severe lower respiratory disease due to bordetellosis in young kittens from crowded, stressful environments. Clinical infection in pet cats, however, is extremely rare. *B. bronchiseptica* vaccination should be considered primarily for cats at high risk for exposure. Because the disease is apparently not life-threatening in adult cats, is uncommon in pet cats, and responds to various antibiotics, routine use of the vaccine in client-owned cats seems unnecessary.

17. Should cats be vaccinated against giardiasis?
A *Giardia* spp. vaccine has been introduced for use in cats. When given twice, the vaccine lessens numbers of cysts shed and clinical disease on challenge with one heterologous strain. The vaccine is adjuvanted and given subcutaneously and ultimately may be associated with fibrosarcomas. Because the disease is usually not life-threatening and at least 90% of cases respond to therapy, routine use in client-owned cats seems unnecessary. The vaccine may have therapeutic utility in cats with recurrent or persistent infection, as was recently documented in dogs.

BIBLIOGRAPHY

1. 2000 Report of the American Association of Feline Practitioners and Academy of Feline Medicine Advisory Panel on Feline Vaccines. Nashville, TN, AAFPIAFM, 2000.
2. Burton G, Mason KV: Do postvaccinal sarcomas occur in Australian cats? Aust Vet J 75:102–106, 1997.
3. Coutts AJ, Dawson S, Binns SH, et al: Studies on the natural transmission of *Bordetella bronchiseptica* in cats. Vet Microbiol 48:19–27, 1996.
4. Lappin MR, Jensen W, Andrews J: Prediction of resistance to panleukopenia, herpesvirus 1, and calicivirus utilizing serology. J Vet Intern Med 14:364, 2000.
5. Macy DW: Are we vaccinating too much? J Am Vet Med Assoc 207:421–425, 1995.
6. Macy DW, Bergman P: Vaccine associated sarcomas in cats. Fel Pract 23:24–27, 1995.
7. Macy DW, Hendrick MW: The potential role of inflammation in the development of post-vaccinal sarcomas in cats. Vet Clin North Am 26:103–109, 1996.
8. Olson ME, Morch DW, Ceri H: The efficacy of a *Giardia lamblia* vaccine in kittens. Can J Vet Res 60:249–256, 1996.
9. Scott FW: Duration of immunity in cats vaccinated with an inactivated feline panleukopenia, herpesvirus, and calicivirus vaccine. Fel Pract 25:12–22, 1997.
10. Schultz RD: Current and future canine and feline vaccination programs. Vet Med 3:233–254, 1998.

82. VACCINE RISKS

Dennis W. Macy, D.V.M.

1. What are the most common vaccine reactions?
Vaccines are suspected to cause a number of reactions, some of which are better documented than others:

- Vaccine associated sarcomas
- Acute anaphylaxis
- Polyarthritis from modified live calicivirus vaccines
- Sneezing and nasal discharge from topical vaccines
- Fever
- Cytopenias
- Prenatal infections (modified live vaccines)
- Chronic stomatitis
- Renal disease

2. How common are vaccine-associated sarcomas?

Studies indicate an incidence of 1/1,000 to 1/10,000 in cats receiving either FeLV or rabies vaccines. Most experts believe that the incidence is 1/2,000 and 1/4,000 in cats receiving either FeLV or rabies vaccination.

3. Which vaccines are most often associated with vaccine-associated sarcomas? Why?

Adjuvanted feline vaccines, particularly FeLV and rabies vaccines, are associated most frequently with sarcoma development at injection sites. Adjuvanted vaccines produce inflammation, stimulate fibroblasts to divide, and are responsible for free radical formation, which results in oxidative damage to DNA.

4. Why do the same rabies vaccines not produce tumors in dogs?

Apparently cats are unique in terms of their susceptibility to sarcoma development. It is believed that the cat's unique species susceptibility to oxidative injury (acetominophen-associated Heinz body anemia, steatitis) is one reason for the high vaccine-associated tumor rate.

5. If granulomas and inflammation occur in all cats receiving certain adjuvanted vaccines, why do only 1–5 in 10,000 develop sarcoma?

It may depend on individual susceptibility to oxidative stress (reduced glutamine levels have been demonstrated in some cats with vaccine-associated sarcoma). Individual cats may have defects in the tumor suppressor gene, P53. Aberrations in P53 have been reported in some cats with vaccine-associated sarcomas.

6. Have sarcomas been reported after administration of products other than vaccines?

Virtually anything that results in chronic inflammation can result in sarcoma formation (e.g., sutures, polyethylene glycol tubes, parenteral antibiotics, injectable lufenuron). However, adjuvanted vaccines are the only substances that are injected repeatedly in large numbers of cats.

7. What is the time from vaccine administration to subsequent tumor formation?

Reports indicate that tumors may develop 3 months to 11 years after vaccine administration. Tumors that occur sooner than 3 months are probably due to previous vaccination or tissue injury.

8. What can be done to prevent vaccine-associated sarcomas?
1. Do not overvaccinate.
2. Limit the use of adjuvanted vaccines.
3. Avoid using any medication that produces chronic inflammation.

9. How long do postvaccinal lumps remain?

Adjuvanted vaccines produce granulomas that reach their maximal size 3 weeks after vaccination but disappear within 3 months after vaccination.

10. When should a postvaccinal lump be removed?

The Vaccine-Associated Sarcoma Task Force recommends that any lump at a vaccination site be biopsied and removed if it meets any one of the following three criteria:
1. Still present 3 months after vaccination
2. > 2 cm in size at any time after vaccination
3. Growing in size 4 weeks after vaccination.

11. What biopsy techniques should be used?

A wedge or Tru-Cut biopsy technique should be used. Fine-needle aspiration is unreliable.

12. Should granulomas be removed?

If a biopsy determines the postvaccinal lump to be a granuloma, simple marginal resection of the granuloma should be performed.

13. How should a vaccine site sarcoma be managed?

The following should be done before treatment of a vaccine-associated sarcoma:

1. Computed tomography examination should be done to determine the extent of the lesion.

2. A chest radiograph should be done to determine whether metastatic disease is present (usually 5% or less at the time of first diagnosis, but the incidence may increase to 25% in patients with prior treatment).

3. FeLV test should be performed to eliminate the possibility of a feline sarcoma virus-induced tumor. Sarcomas caused by the feline sarcoma virus do not benefit from surgery.

14. What treatment is best?

A combination of surgery, radiation therapy, and chemotherapy gives the best results.

15. Which treatment regimen should be used first?

Surgery followed by radiation therapy or radiation therapy followed by surgery have been recommended; chemotherapy usually follows radiation and surgery regimens.

16. How large a margin should be used in surgery?

Large. Margins of 2–5 cm are recommended.

17. Should I refer the surgery?

Significant improvement in disease-free interval has been shown if a referral institution does either the initial or second surgery. No difference in disease-free interval is found if multiple surgeries have been done before referral.

18. What is the prognosis?

Surgery alone: 60% recurrence rate (86% recur within 6 months); average survival is 1–1.5 years.

Radiation and surgery: 30–40% recurrence rate; average survival 700–800 days.

Some **chemotherapeutic agents** are active against vaccine-associated sarcomas but are marginally effective in increasing patient survival, perhaps adding 10% to survival time. Although a wide variety of drugs have been evaluated (including doxorubicin, carboplatin, mitoxantrone, cyclophosphamide, and vincristine), doxorubicin appears to be the most effective.

BIBLIOGRAPHY

1. Burton G, Mason KV: Do postvaccinal sarcomas occur in Australian cats? Aust Vet J 75:102–106, 1997.
2. Hendrick MJ, Brooks JJ: Postvaccinal sarcomas in the cat: Histology and immunohistochemistry. Vet Pathol 31:126–129, 1994.
3. Hendrick MJ, Goldschmidt MH: Do injection site reactions induce fibrosarcomas in cats? J Am Vet Med Assoc 199:968, 1991.
4. Hendrick MJ, Kass PH, McGill LD, et al: Commentary: Postvaccinal sarcomas in cats. J Natl Cancer Inst 86:5, 1994.
5. Hendrick MJ, Shoter FS, Goldschmidt MH, et al: Comparison of fibrosarcomas developed at vaccination sites and at nonvaccination sites in cats: 239 cases (1991–1992). J Am Vet Med Assoc 205:1425–1429, 1994.
6. Hendrick MJ, Goldschmidt MH, Shoter FS, et al: Postvaccinal sarcomas in the cats: Epidemiology and electron probe microanalytical identification of aluminum. Cancer Res 52:5391–5394, 1992.
7. Kass PH, Barnes WG, Spangler WL, et al: Epidemiologic evidence for a causal relationship between vaccination and fibrosarcoma tumorigenesis in cats. J Am Vet Med Assoc 203:396–405, 1993.
8. Macy DW, Bergman PJ: Vaccine associated sarcomas in cats. Fel Pract 23:24–27, 1995.
9. Macy DW, Hendrick MJ: The potential role of inflammation in the development of post-vaccinal sarcomas in cats. Vet Clin North Am 26:103–109, 1996.
10. Macy DW: The potential role and mechanisms of FeLV vaccine-induced neoplasms. Semin Vet Med Surg 10:234–238, 1995.
11. Macy DW, Bergman JP: Postvaccinal reactions associated with three rabies and three leukemia virus vaccines in cats. Proceedings of the 14th Annual Veterinary Cancer Society Conference, Townsend, TN, Veterinary Cancer Society, 1994, pp 90–91.
12. Smith CA: Current concepts: Are we vaccinating too much? J Am Vet Med Assoc 207:421–425, 1995.

IX. Public Health Risks

Section Editor: Michael R. Lappin, D.V.M., Ph.D.

83. ZOONOSES: OVERVIEW

Michael R. Lappin, D.V.M., Ph.D.

1. Define zoonotic disease.

Zoonotic diseases are common to, shared by, or naturally transmitted between humans and other vertebrate animals.

2. What are the most likely ways to become exposed to an infectious agent with zoonotic potential?

Transmission of zoonotic agents can occur by direct contact with the cat; indirect contact with secretions from the cat; contact with contaminated vehicles such as water, food, or fomites; or shared vectors. Some of the most common zoonoses are associated with the gastrointestinal tract (see Chapter 84) and bites and scratches (see Chapter 85). The respiratory tract (see Chapter 86), exudates (see Chapter 87), and urogenital tract (see Chapter 88) also harbor infectious agents capable of infecting humans. With some agents, infection of humans and cats occurs from a shared environment (see Chapter 89) or shared vector (see Chapter 90), but the organism is not directly transmitted from cats. Overall, the most likely ways of contracting a cat-associated infectious disease are fecal-oral contact, bites or scratches, or infected fleas or ticks in the human environment.

3. Do you have to be immunocompromised to be infected by a zoonotic agent?

Immunosuppression is common in people. The acquired immunodeficiency syndrome (AIDS) is discussed frequently, but there are many other common immunosuppressive syndromes:

• People on chemotherapy for organ transplantation, inflammatory diseases, immune mediated diseases, or neoplasia
• Older people with decrimental decreases in immune function
• Young people with poorly developed immune systems, such as the fetus
• Splenectomized people

Most zoonotic infectious agents will infect anyone regardless of immune status, but the magnitude of clinical illness is often much more severe in immunosuppressed people. For example, giardial infection of an immunocompetent person usually is associated only with transient diarrhea, whereas an immunosuppressed person may develop life-threatening disease.

4. Should immunosuppressed people own cats?

Because many agents infect both cats and human beings, it is sometimes assumed that direct contact zoonoses are common. In actuality, healthy, adult, parasite-free, indoor cats are unlikely to transmit infectious agents to people.

Families with a proven or suspected immunodeficient member are commonly told to avoid cat ownership because of potential health risks. Often these recommendations are based on inaccurate information. For example, pregnant women and immunosuppressed people are commonly told to avoid cats because of the risk of acquiring toxoplasmosis. However, it is extremely rare to acquire *Toxoplasma gondii* from touching cats; the organism is transmitted most commonly from contact with sporulated oocysts in a contaminated environment or from ingesting undercooked meats (see Chapter 84).

Cat ownership provides many health benefits; it is well recognized that pet ownership results in increased happiness and decreased depression. Thus, any decision about cat ownership should consider both potential risks and potential benefits. Veterinarians should familiarize themselves with zoonotic issues and take an active role in discussion of the health risks and benefits of pet ownership with clients so that logical decisions about ownership and management of individual animals can be made.

5. What overall recommendations can be made to an immunosuppressed person for avoidance of feline zoonoses?

As discussed previously and in Chapters 84–90, the risk of acquiring an infection from a cat is minimal. The following recommendations may further decrease the risk:

- The common enteric zoonoses occur most frequently in young cats with diarrhea from crowded environments. Thus, the cat least likely to be a zoonotic risk is a clinically normal, indoor adult from a private family.
- If possible, someone other than the immunosuppressed individual should remove fecal material produced in the home environment daily.
- The cat should be housed indoors.
- The cat should be fed only commercially processed pet food.
- The owner should not allow the cat to share utensils and should avoid licking.
- Kittens or cats with external parasites should be avoided or treated because of increased risk of *Bartonella henselae* infection and other shared vector zoonoses.
- Kittens or cats with respiratory disease, ocular disease, or skin disease should be avoided or treated.
- Physical examination and fecal examination should be performed at least once or twice yearly.
- If a new cat is desired, the immunosuppressed person should avoid direct contact while it is evaluated for zoonotic agents.
- Once the cat to be adopted is identified, a thorough physical examination should be performed.
- Fecal flotation for giardial cysts and helminth eggs, wet mount for protozoal trophozoite identification, special stains or antigen testing for *Cryptosporidium parvum*, and fecal culture for enteric bacteria can be performed to screen for enteric zoonoses.
- Blood should be collected aseptically from cats and placed in an EDTA tube for *Bartonella* culture or polymerase chain reaction; serum should be submitted at the same time for *Bartonella* antibody testing.
- Because direct contact with individual cats rarely results in toxoplasmosis, there is no indication for serologic evaluation of healthy cats.
- The cat should be routinely dewormed with a drug that kills hookworms, roundworms, and tapeworms.
- Flea and tick control should be instituted.
- Previously owned cats with clinical signs of disease associated with the gastrointestinal tract, eyes, respiratory tract, genital tract, urinary system, or skin should be evaluated for zoonotic agents by the veterinarian.

BIBLIOGRAPHY

1. Angulo FJ, Glaser CA, Juranek DD, et al: Caring for pets of immunocompromised persons. J Am Vet Med Assoc 205:1711–1718, 1994.
2. Burton B: Pets and PWAs: Claims of health risk exaggerated. AIDS Patient Care Feb:34–37, 1989.
3. Carmack B: The role of companion animals for persons with AIDS/HIV. Hol Nurs Pract 5:24–31, 1991.
4. Evans RH: Public health and important zoonoses in feline populations. In August JR (ed): Consultations in Feline Internal Medicine, 3rd ed. Philadelphia, W.B. Saunders, 1997, pp 611–629.
5. Greene CE: Immunocompromised people and pets. In, Greene CE (ed): Infectious Diseases of the Dog and Cat, 2nd ed. Philadelphia, W.B. Saunders, 1998, pp 710–717.

6. Glaser CA, Angulo FJ, Rooney JA: Animal associated opportunistic infections among persons infected with the human immunodeficiency virus. Clin Infect Dis 18:14–24, 1994.
7. Lappin MR: Feline zoonoses. In Kirk RW, Bonagura JD (eds): Current Veterinary Therapy XI Small Animal Practice. Philadelphia, W.B. Saunders, 1992, pp 284–291.
8. Olsen CW: Vaccination of cats against emerging and reemerging zoonotic pathogens. Adv Vet Med 41:333–346, 1999.
9. Patronek G: Free-roaming and feral cats: Their impact on wildlife and human beings. J Am Vet Med Assoc 212:218–226, 1998.
10. Spencer L: Study explores health risks and the human animal bond. J Am Vet Med Assoc 201:1669, 1992.
11. Tan J: Human zoonotic infections transmitted by dogs and cats. Arch Intern Med 157:1933–1943, 1997.

84. ENTERIC ZOONOSES

Michael R. Lappin, D.V.M., Ph.D.

1. What are the major classes of enteric zoonotic agents?

Bacteria, protozoans, helminths, and cestodes.

Enteric Zoonoses Associated with Contact with Cats or Their Excrement

ORGANISM	COMMENT
Bacteria	
Campylobacter spp.	Immediately infectious
Eschericia coli	Immediately infectious
Helicobacter spp.*	Immediately infectious
Salmonella spp.	Immediately infectious
Yersinia enterocolitica	Immediately infectious
Cestodes	
Echinococcus multilocularis	Ova are immediately infectious
Dipylidium caninum	Requires ingestion of flea
Protozoan–coccidians	
Cryptosporidium parvum	Oocysts are immediately infectious
Toxoplasma gondii	Oocysts are infectious after 1–5 days of incubation; exposure from environment
Protozoan–flagellate	
Giardia spp.	Cysts are immediately infectious
Helminths	
Ancylostoma braziliense	Larva infectious after > 3 days of incubation; skin penetration from larva in environment
Ancylostoma tubaeforme	Larva infectious after > 3 days of incubation; skin penetration from larva in environment
Uncinaria stenocephala	Larva infectious after > 3 days of incubation; skin penetration from larva in environment
Strongyloides stercoralis	Larva immediately infectious
Toxocara cati	Larvated ova infectious after 3–4 weeks of incubation; exposure from environment

* Zoonotic potential undetermined.

2. What are the odds of acquiring a gastrointestinal disease from my cat?

Prevalence of enteric zoonotic agents varies by region, whether cats are housed indoors or outdoors, and whether diarrhea occurs. Odds of being infected from contact with cats or cat excrement also vary with the organism (see discussions that follow). In a recent study, enteric zoonotic agents were detected in feces of 13.1% of 206 cats in north central Colorado. Although enteric zoonotic agents are common, people are unlikely to acquire infections from direct contact with cats. Most cats are fastidious and do not leave fecal material on the fur. Thus, contact with enteric zoonotic agents is probably more common from environmental contamination. Because cat fecal material is usually concentrated in one area and of small volume, extensive contamination of the home environment is probably uncommon.

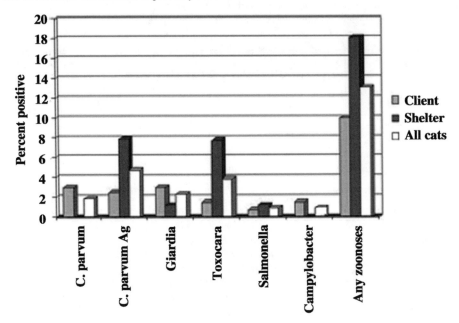

Prevalence of enteric zoonotic agents in 206 cats of north central Colorado. (Data from Hill S, Lappin MR, Cheney J, et al: Prevalence of enteric zoonotic agents in cats. J Am Vet Med Assoc 216:687–692, 2000.)

3. Which helminths are most commonly associated with infection of people?

Both cats and people can be infected with *Toxocara cati, Ancylostoma braziliense, A. tubaeforme, Uncinaria stenocephala,* and *Strongyloides stercoralis.*

4. What syndromes in humans are associated with *T. cati* infection?

Visceral larva migrans and ocular larva migrans are the two most common syndromes associated with human toxocariasis. Most cases are thought to be due to *T. canis* infection, but the same syndromes can occur after infection with *T. cati.* Infected cats pass ova into the human environment. After 3–4 weeks, the ova larvate and then are infectious. Humans are infected by ingestion of larvated ova, which release infective larvae in the gastrointestinal tract. The larvae penetrate the mucosa of the small intestine and migrate to the liver, lungs, and other organs (visceral larva migrans). The eosinophilic reaction against the larvae can result in clinical signs of disease. Manifestations include eosinophilia, abdominal pain, anorexia, nausea, vomiting fever, cough, hepatomegaly, myocarditis, and encephalitis. Asthma is more common in *Toxocara*-seropositive people than *Toxocara*-seronegative people, suggesting that toxocariasis contributes to asthma. If larvae migrate to the eye (ocular larva migrans), the eosinophilic reaction can result in severe intraocular inflammation. Adult *T. cati* worms have been detected in some infected children. Humans with toxocariasis are generally treated symptomatically with antihistamines and glucocorticoids; the use of antihelmintics is controversial.

5. Is human toxocariasis common?

Toxocara ova are environmentally resistant; when an area is contaminated, the potential for infection persists for months. In the United States, the seroprevalence of antibodies against *Toxocara* spp. is 2.8% in the general population and 4.6–7.3% in children 1–11 years of age. Thus, exposure to infective roundworms is still common. Visceral larva migrans is most common in children < 6 years of age; ocular larva migrans is most common in older children and young adults.

6. What is cutaneous larva migrans?

Cats can be the definitive host for *A. braziliense, A. tubaeforme, U. stenocephala,* and *S. stercoralis.* Ova are passed into the environment, where they larvate after several days in warm, humid conditions. Infective larva penetrate the skin of people in direct contact. Pruritic, serpiginous, erythrematous tracts occur as the larva migrate in the epidermis. *A. caninum* has been linked with eosinophilic enteritis in humans; the syndrome has not been described with hookworms that infect cats. Topical or oral administration of thiabendazole lessens symptoms in infected humans.

7. How can the potential for human infection by feline helminths be lessened?

Prevention of hookworm and roundworm infections revolves around control of animal excrement in human environments. The children's sandbox should be covered when not in use, and fecal material should be removed immediately. Geophagia and ingestion of water in the environment should be discouraged. For hookworms, direct skin contact with moist, potentially infected soil should be avoided. Anthelmintics should be routinely administered to all kittens at least twice, 14–21 days apart (see Chapter 19 for drugs and doses). In high-risk kittens, anthelmintics should be administered at 6, 8, and 10 weeks of age. Fecal flotation should be performed to assess for other parasites once or twice yearly, particularly if the cat goes outdoors, even if it is taking heartworm preventatives.

8. What human syndromes are associated with cestodes that infect cats?

Both cats and people can be infected with *Dipylidium caninum* and *Echinococcus multilocularis.* Transmission to humans occurs after ingestion of the intermediate host (flea, *D. caninum*) or by the ingestion of eggs (*E. multilocularis*). Dipylidial infection is most common in children and can lead to diarrhea and pruritus ani. Cats play a role in this infection only by bringing fleas into the human environment (see Chapter 90). Cats become infected by *E. multilocularis* when they ingest infected intermediate hosts (rodents). Cats are subclinically infected but pass infective ova into the human environment. After a human ingests ova, *E. multilocularis* onchospheres enter the portal circulation and spread throughout the liver and other tissues. Metacestodes then develop in infected tissues as hydatid cysts. The liver, lung, and brain are most commonly infected. The hydatid cysts are multilocular and grow rapidly (alveolar echinococcosis). A combination of surgical excision and drugs is used to treat the syndrome in people, but the disease has a poor prognosis. *E. multilocularis* is most common in the northern and central parts of North America but seems to be spreading with the fox population (the most common definitive host). Although the incidence of the disease is rare in humans, cats should not be allowed to hunt in endemic areas. Praziquantel has been shown to be effective for the treatment of echinococcosis (see Chapter 19).

9. Which enteric protozoans of cats also infect people?

Both cats and people can be infected with *Entamoeba histolytica, Cryptosporidium parvum, C. felis, Toxoplasma gondii,* and *Giardia* spp. *E. histolytica* has been described in cats only occasionally and is not likely to be a significant zoonosis.

10. Can the *Giardia* spp. of cats infect people?

Giardia spp. are flagellates with worldwide distribution; they cause significant gastrointestinal disease in dogs, cats, and people. The organism is believed to have a wide host range; all mammalian isolates are currently classified as *G. lamblia.* Studies of the cross-infection potential of *Giardia* spp. isolates have had varying results. In one study, *Giardia* spp. from humans were inoculated into cats; the cats were relatively resistant to infection. In another study, isoenzyme electrophoresis comparison of human and feline isolates suggested that cats may serve as a reservoir for human infections. There also appears to be a separate feline giardial genotype. Because it is impossible to determine zoonotic strains of *Giardia* spp. by microscopic examination, it seems prudent to assume that feces from all cats infected with *Giardia* spp. are a potential human health risk. *Giardia* spp. are common enteric pathogens and can be detected in feces of cats with and without diarrhea. These findings emphasize that fecal examination should be performed on all cats at least yearly, and treatment with antigiardial drugs (see Chapter 19) should be administered if indicated. Vaccination against *Giardia* spp. may be considered in cats with recurrent infection and is under evaluation as a therapeutic strategy.

11. What is cryptosporidiosis?

Cryptosporidium parvum is a coccidian that can result in severe gastrointestinal tract disease in infected people; infection of immunosuppressed people may be life-threatening. Infection is common in humans; approximately 300,000 people in Milwaukee developed cryptosporidiosis when a water purification system malfunctioned; approximately 10–20% of patients with AIDS are infected with *C. parvum* at some time during their life; and the organism commonly causes diarrhea outbreaks in daycare centers. Many infected people require hospitalization for administration of intravenous fluid therapy; people with AIDS may never be cured.

12. Do *Cryptosporidium* spp. infect cats?

C. parvum oocysts have been documented in feces of many domestic cats in the United States, Japan, Scotland, Australia, and Spain. Presence of serum antibodies can be used to estimate numbers of cats exposed to *C. parvum*. An enzyme-linked immunosorbent assay (ELISA) for detection of *C. parvum* IgG placed the seroprevalence of *C. parvum* antibodies in cats in Colorado and the United States at 15.3% and 8.3%, respectively. Oocysts or antigens of *C. parvum* were detected in feces of 5.4% of cats tested in north central Colorado.

13. Do the *Cryptosporidium* spp. that infect cats infect people?

The source of *C. parvum* infection in humans usually is undetermined; contaminated water is the most likely source. However, cryptosporidiosis has been documented in people and cats in the same environment, suggesting the potential for zoonotic transfer. Limited cross-infection studies have been performed with *C. parvum* isolates from cats. In one study, a feline isolate failed to cross-infect mice, rats, guinea pigs, or dogs. In another study, a *C. parvum* isolate from a cat cross-infected lambs. An alternative to cross-infection studies is genetic comparison of isolates. A feline genotype that varies considerably from human and cattle genotypes has been identified. The feline genotype (*C. felis*) was documented in an infected human and an infected cow, suggesting that the feline genotype can infect other mammals. A study of HIV-infected people with cryptosporidiosis found no statistical association with cat ownership, suggesting that cat contact is an uncommon way to acquire cryptosporidiosis.

14. How should cats with cryptosporidiosis be managed?

As with *Giardia* spp., it is impossible to determine zoonotic strains of *C. parvum* by microscopic examination. Thus, it seems prudent to assume that feces from all cats infected with *C. parvum* are a potential human health risk. Techniques for the detection of *C. parvum* should be included in the diagnostic evaluation of all cats with diarrhea and all cats in the homes of immunosuppressed people. Infected cats generally do not shed large numbers of cryptosporidial oocysts, but acid-fast staining or immunofluorescent antibody staining of feces helps to identify the parasite (approximately 5 microns). Alternatively, fecal antigen ELISAs are available. Drugs for the treatment of cryptosporidiosis are discussed in Chapter 19. Because oocysts are immediately infectious, care should be taken in handling feces of infected cats.

15. Define toxoplasmosis.

Toxoplasma gondii is one of the most common small animal zoonoses; approximately 30–40% of adult humans in the world are seropositive, suggesting previous or current infection.

People are most commonly infected by *T. gondii* after ingestion of sporulated oocysts or tissue cysts. Thus, prevention of toxoplasmosis in people can be achieved by avoiding these two life stages. Clinical disease is generally mild after primary infection of immunocompetent people. Self-limiting fever, malaise, and lymphadenopathy are the most common clinical abnormalities, and most people do not know when their first *T. gondii* infection occurred. The disease is potentially confused with infectious mononucleosis. Clinical disease can be much more severe in immunosuppressed people, including fetuses, people with AIDS, and people treated with immunosuppressive agents for cancer and prevention of organ transplant rejection. *T. gondii* is a common opportunistic infection of the central nervous system (CNS) in people with AIDS; as T-helper cell counts decline, toxoplasmic encephalitis may result from activation of bradyzoites in tissue cysts. If a mother has her first *T. gondii* infection during gestation, stillbirth, CNS disease, and ocular disease are common clinical manifestations in the fetus.

16. What role do cats play in human toxoplasmosis?

Cats are the only known definitive host for *T. gondii* and thus are responsible for passage of oocysts into the environment. Once passed into the environment, sporulated oocysts survive for months to years. It is likely that some people acquire toxoplasmosis when working with soil or drinking contaminated water. Clinical toxoplasmosis developed in a group of people after a common exposure in a riding stable and in a group of soldiers drinking contaminated water in Panama. Although it cannot be stated definitively that a person will not acquire toxoplasmosis from a household cat, it is probably unlikely.

Cats shed oocysts for days to several weeks after primary inoculation. Thus, an individual cat passes oocysts into the human environment for only a small fraction of its entire life span. *T. gondii* oocysts are not infectious when passed by cats; sporulation requires 1–5 days in the environment. Most cats are fastidious and do not leave feces on their fur for this time period. Bioassay failed to detect oocysts on the fur of cats 7 days after they were shedding millions of oocysts in feces.

In general, veterinary health care providers are no more likely than the general population to be seropositive for *T. gondii* infection. Because oocysts are passed in an unsporulated and non-infectious form, working with fresh feline feces (< 1 day old) is not a risk for veterinary health care personnel. People with HIV infection that owned cats were not more likely to acquire toxoplasmosis during their illness than people with HIV infection that did not have contact with cats.

17. Does oocyst shedding recur in previously infected cats?

After primary inoculation of cats, it is difficult to induce repeat oocyst shedding. Prednisolone (10–80 mg/kg orally) or methylprednisolone (10–80 mg/kg intramuscularly) induces repeat oocyst shedding in some cats with toxoplasmosis. However, these doses are not routinely used in clinical practice. Administration of methylprednisolone acetate at 5 mg/kg weekly for 4–6 weeks to cats infected with *T. gondii* for 14 weeks or 14 months failed to induce oocyst shedding.

In one unpublished study, cats infected with *T. gondii* were given feline immunodeficeincy virus (FIV) followed by feline leukemia virus (FeLV). Although they developed immunodeficiency-associated syndromes, repeat *T. gondii* oocyst shedding could not be demonstrated. Cats with FIV or FeLV infections have been inoculated with *T. gondii*; oocyst shedding periods and number of oocysts shed were similar to those for cats without FIV or FeLV infections.

Gut immunity to *T. gondii* in cats is not permanent; 4 of 9 cats inoculated 6 years after primary inoculation shed oocysts, although each had high serum antibody titers. However, *T. gondii*-infected cats with and without FIV infection failed to repeat oocyst shedding when reinfected with *T. gondii* 16 months after primary inoculation. Thus, cats that are exposed to *T. gondii* frequently probably do not shed large numbers of oocysts after the first infection.

18. What are other means of transmission of *T. gondii* to people?

Ingestion of *T. gondii* in tissues can result in human toxoplasmosis. Meats (particularly pork in the United States) should be cooked to medium or well-done to inactivate tissue cysts. Gloves should be worn for handling raw meats (including field dressing) for cooking, or hands should be cleansed thoroughly afterwards. Freezing meat at −12°C for several days kills most tissue cysts. Ingestion of raw goat's milk also can result in human toxoplasmosis.

19. Should healthy cats be evaluated serologically for toxoplasmosis?

No serologic assay accurately predicts when a cat shed *T. gondii* oocysts in the past, and most cats that are currently shedding oocysts are seronegative. Most seropositive cats have completed the oocyst shedding period and are unlikely to repeat shedding; most seronegative cats will shed the organism if infected. But since humans are probably not commonly infected with *T. gondii* from contact with cats and since serologic test results cannot accurately predict the oocyst shedding status of seropositive cats, testing healthy cats for toxoplasmosis is of little clinical use. Fecal examination is an adequate procedure to determine when cats are actively shedding oocysts but cannot predict when a cat has shed oocysts in the past. Owners who are concerned that they may have toxoplasmosis should see their doctor for testing.

20. How can people avoid developing toxoplasmosis?

- All water collected from the environment should be boiled or filtered before drinking.
- Care should be taken to wash hands carefully after working with soil; alternatively, gloves should be worn.
- Produce from the garden should be washed carefully before ingestion. The children's sandbox should be covered when not in use.
- A litterbox liner should be used, and the litterbox should be cleaned daily. Oocysts require 1–5 days to sporulate.
- Immunosuppressed or pregnant cat owners should not clean the litterbox.
- Sporulated oocysts are extremely resistant to most disinfectants. Thus, cleaning with scalding water or steam is most practical.
- Oocysts measuring 10 × 12 μ in a cat fecal sample may be *T. gondii*. *Hammondia hammondi* and *Besnoitia darlingi* are morphologically similar coccidians passed by cats but are not human pathogens. The feces should be collected daily until the oocyst shedding period is complete; administration of clindamycin (25–50 mg/kg/day orally), sulfonamides (100 mg/kg/day orally), or pyrimethamine (2.0 mg/kg/day orally) can reduce levels of oocyst shedding.
- Cats should not be allowed to hunt and should be fed only processed or cooked foods.
- Potential transport hosts such as flies and cockroaches should be controlled.
- Meat should be cooked to medium well-done.
- Gloves should be worn or hands washed after handling meat.

21. What are the common bacterial zoonotic agents?

Salmonella spp., *Campylobacter jejuni*, *E. coli*, and *Yersinia enterocolitica* infect cats and can cause disease in humans. Gastroenteritis may occur in both species after infection. *Y. enterocolitica* is probably a commensal agent in cats but induces fever, abdominal pain, and bacteremia in humans. *Helicobacter pylori* causes ulcers in people and has been isolated from a colony of cats; the zoonotic risks are currently undetermined but appear to be minimal. Infected cats and people in the same family have been found to be infected with *Helicobacter* spp. Three other studies, including one of veterinarians, found no epidemiologic association of cat contact with human helicobacteriosis. *Salmonella* spp. infection in cats is often subclinical, but in one study the incidence was only 1% in client-owned and shelter cats with and without diarrhea. Approximately 50% of clinically affected cats have gastroenteritis; many are presented with abortion, stillbirth, neonatal death, or signs of bacteremia. Some cats with salmonellosis have a history of ingesting a songbird (songbird fever). If neutrophils are noted on rectal cytology, culture for *Salmonella* and *Campylobacter* spp. is indicated. Human infection with *Campylobacter* spp. has been associated with cat contact. Infection occurs after fecal-oral or fomite exposure, and prevention is based on sanitation and control of exposure to feces. See Chapter 20 for a discussion of the clinical management of these infections.

22. What is the recommended diagnostic evaluation for enteric zoonotic agents?

If enteric zoonotic agents are of concern, procedures that should be performed include fecal flotation for giardial cysts and helminth eggs, fecal wet mount for protozoal trophozoite identification, acid-fast monoclonal antibody staining of fecal smears or fecal antigen testing for *C. parvum*, and fecal culture for enteric bacteria.

BIBLIOGRAPHY

1. Angulo FJ, Glaser CA, Juranek DD, et al: Caring for pets of immunocompromised persons. J Am Vet Med Assoc 205:1711–1718, 1994.
2. Blagburn BL, Conboy G, Jutras P, et al: Strategic control of intestinal parasites: Diminishing the risk of zoonotic disease. Comp Cont Educ Pract Vet 19S:4–20, 1997.
3. Deming MS, Tauxe RV, Blake PA, et al: *Campylobacter* enteritis at a university: Transmission from eating chickens and from cats. Am J Epidemiol 126:526–534, 1987.
4. Dubey JP, Lappin MR: Toxoplasmosis and neosporosis. In Greene CE (ed): Infectious Diseases of the Dog and Cat, 2nd ed. Philadelphia, W.B .Saunders, 1998, pp 493–503.
5. Eberhard ML, Alfano E: Adult *Toxocara cati* infections in U.S. children: Report of four cases. Am J Med Hyg 59:404–406, 1998.
6. Glaser CA, Angulo FJ, Rooney JA: Animal associated opportunistic infections among persons infected with the human immunodeficiency virus. Clin Infect Dis 18:14–24, 1994.
7. Glaser CA, Safrin S, Reingold A, et al: Association between *Cryptosporidium* infection and animal exposure in HIV-infected individuals. J AIDS 17:79–82, 1998.
8. Hill S, Lappin MR, Cheney J, et al: Prevalence of enteric zoonotic agents in cats. J Am Vet Med Assoc 216:687–692, 2000.
9. Homan WL, Gilsing M, Bentala H, et al: Characterization of *Giardia* duodenalis by polymerase-chain-reaction fingerprinting. Parasitol Res 84:707–714, 1998.
10. Hopkins RM, Meoni BP, Groth DM, et al: Ribosomal RNA sequencing reveals differences between the genotypes of *Giardia* isolates recovered from humans and dogs living in the same locality. J Parasitol 83:44–51, 1997.
11. Juranek DD: Cryptosporidiosis: Sources of infection and guidelines for prevention. Clin Infect Dis 21:S57–S61, 1995.
12. Jutras P: Important zoonotic helminth infections. Comp Cont Educ Pract Vet 10S:4–9, 1997.
13. Kirkpatrick CE and Green GA: Susceptibility of domestic cats to infections with *Giardia lamblia* cysts and trophozoites from human sources. J Clin Microbiol 21:678–680, 1985.
14. Lu SQ, Baruch AC, Adam RD: Molecular comparison of *Giardia lamblia* isolates. Int J Parasitol 28:1341–1345, 1998.
15. Meloni BP, Lymbery AJ, Thompson RCA: Isoenzyme electrophoresis of 30 isolates of *Giardia* from humans and felines. Am J Trop Med Hyg 38:65–73, 1988.
16. McReynolds C, Lappin MR, McReynolds L, et al: Regional seroprevalence of *Cryptosporidium parvum* IgG specific antibodies of cats in the United States. Vet Parasitol 80:187-195, 1998.
17. Neiger R, Simpson KW: *Helicobacter* infection in dogs and cats: Facts and fiction. J Vet Intern Med 14:125–133, 2000.
18. Sargent KD, Morgan UM, Elliot A, et al: Morphological and genetic characterisation of *Cryptosporidium* oocysts from domestic cats. Vet Parasitol 77:221–227, 1998.
19. Tan JS: Human zoonotic infections transmitted by dogs and cats. Arch Intern Med 157:1933–1943, 1997.
20. Thompson RCA, Hopkins RM, Homan WL: Nomenclature and genetic groupings of *Giardia* infecting mammals. Parsitol Today 16:210–213, 2000.
21. Wallace MR, Rossetti RJ, Olson PE: Cats and toxoplasmosis risk in HIV-infected adults. J Am Med Assoc 269:76–77, 1993.

85. BITE- OR SCRATCH-ASSOCIATED ZOONOSES

Alice J. Johns, D.V.M.

1. What infectious agents are transmitted by scratches or bites?

Multiple bacteria can induce infection of people after bites and scratches. *Bartonella hense-lae* (cat scratch disease [CSD]) and oral flora such as *Pasteurella* spp. are most common. Rabies is the only significant viral disease transmitted by this means. Although *Blastomyces dermatitidis* has been transmitted by dog bites, systemic fungal diseases usually are not transmitted directly from animals to humans.

Common Feline Bite- and Scratch-associated Zoonoses

ORGANISM	CLINICAL SYNDROME	RELATIVE RISK FROM CATS TO HUMANS
Bacteria		
Bartonella spp.	Cats: subclinical; rarely uveitis, fever	Common
	Humans: lymphadenopathy, fever, malaise, bacillary angiomatosis, bacillary peliosis	
Capnocytophaga canimorsus	Cats: subclinical	Rare
	Humans: bacteremia	
Francisella tularensis	Cats: septicemia, pneumonia	Extremely rare
	Humans: ulceroglandular, glandular, oculo-glandular, pneumonic, or typhoidal (depending on route of infection)	
Yersinia pestis	Cats: bubonic, bacteremic, or pneumonic	Rare; regional
	Humans: bubonic, bacteremic, or pneumonic	
Fungus		
Sporothrix schenkii	Cats: chronic draining cutaneous tracts	Extremely rare
	Humans: chronic draining cutaneous tracts	
Virus		
Rabies	Cats: progressive CNS disease	Rare
	Humans: progressive CNS disease	

CNS = central nervous system.

2. Are bites and scratches common?

Animal bites result in approximately 300,000 emergency department visits per year in the United States. The majority of the aerobic and anaerobic bacteria associated with bite or scratch wounds lead only to local infection in immunocompetent people. However, 28–80% of cat bites become infected, and uncommon severe sequelae, including meningitis, endocarditis, septic arthritis, and septic shock, can occur. Most bite wounds are located on the hands, arms, or face. Bite wounds are contaminated with aerobic and anaerobic flora from the cat's mouth and aerobic bacteria from the skin. Cat bites may be at higher risk of infection than dog bites because they create small, deep puncture wounds that are difficult to irrigate and debride.

3. What bacteria are usually involved with bites or scratches?

Bite wounds typically have multiple bacterial isolates. *Pasteurella multocida* is responsible for 90% of infections resulting from cat bite wounds. Also commonly isolated are alpha-hemolytic *Streptococcus* spp., *Staphylococcus* spp., *Bacteriodes* spp., and *Fusobacterium* spp. Immuno-compromised people or those exposed to *Pasteurella* spp. or *Capnocytophaga canimorsus* (DF-2) more consistently develop systemic clinical illness after bites or scratches. Local cellulitis is noted initially, followed by evidence of deeper tissue infection. Bacteremia and the associated clinical signs of fever, malaise, and weakness are common. Death can occur from either genus, particularly in splenectomized individuals. At least two cases of mycoplasmal infection associated with cat bites have been reported in humans.

4. How should cat bites and scratches be treated?

Wounds should be irrigated voluminously with sterile saline and scrubbed. Refer to a physician any client or staff member who is bitten. Delay in seeking treatment may result in a more serious infection, requiring hospitalization for intravenous antibiotics. Diagnosis of bacterial infections is confirmed by culture. Treatment includes local wound drainage and systemic antibiotic therapy. Penicillin derivatives are highly effective against most *Pasteurella* infections. Penicillins and cephalosporins are effective against *Capnocytophaga* spp. in vitro.

5. How can cat bites and scratches be prevented?

Cats should not be teased, and appropriate restraint techniques should be used at all times to attempt to avoid being bitten or scratched.

6. What causes CSD?

CSD is most commonly associated with infection by *Bartonella henselae* (formerly *Rochalimaea henselae*). The organism is a small (0.3–3 μm), highly pleomorphic, gram-negative bacillus. It is facultatively intracellular and hemotropic and stains with Warthin-Starry silver stain. *B. henselae* also causes bacillary angiomatosis and bacillary peliosis in immunocompromised people. Cats also carry *B. clarridgeiae* and *B. koehlerae*.

7. Describe the epidemiology of *B. henselae* infection in cats.

Subclinical bacteremia is common in the feline population; as many as 54.6–81% of cats in some geographical areas of the United States are seropositive for *Bartonella* spp. and presumably were infected at one time. *B. henselae* has been cultured from the blood of many naturally exposed cats; cats infected with the organism by inoculation intradermally, subcutaneously, intravenously, or intramuscularly; and cats infected by *Ctenocephalidies felis*. Bacteremia occurs in cats within 2 weeks of exposure to infected fleas. Once infected, cats are intermittently bacteremic for months. *B. henselae* can be cultivated from 9-day-old flea feces, and it is likely that contact with fleas or their feces can transmit the organism to humans. The organism is present in feline red blood cells and may reside in or be excreted into the oral cavity. The organism probably is transferred to the claws during grooming or by bite wounds or licking open sores.

8. Do infected cats develop clinical illness?

Most cats have subclinical *B. henselae* infections. However, intravenous, intramuscular, and intradermal inoculation has resulted in fever, lymphadenopathy, and neurologic diseases in some cats. Uveal tract inflammation and other clinical signs of disease, including gingivitis and lymphadenopathy, have been reported in some naturally infected cats..

9. Describe the clinical signs of CSD.

CSD is the most common cause of chronic, benign lymphadenopathy in children and young adults. Typically, a nonpruritic, erythematous papule or pustule develops at the inoculation site 3–10 days after exposure. Regional lymphadenitis without lymphangitis follows within several weeks and may persist for weeks or months. Affected lymph nodes may abscess and drain spontaneously. Systemic signs may include fever, malaise, headache, anorexia, and myalgia. Weight loss, sore throat, splenomegaly, nausea, and vomiting occur in some patients. The syndrome is usually self-limiting. Immunocompromised or immunosuppressed people can develop hypotension, septic shock, metabolic acidosis, pulmonary infiltrates, and persistent fever. In unusual cases, ocular disease (Parinaud's oculoglandular disease), neurologic signs (convulsions or delirium), osteolytic lesions, or cutaneous eruptions may develop. In rare cases, splenic abscesses, hemolytic anemia, granulomatous hepatitis, pulmonary granuloma or atypical pneumonia may develop.

10. How is CSD diagnosed?

In people, a diagnosis is made if three of the four following criteria are met:
1. History of traumatic cat contact (scratch or bite)
2. Regional lymphadenopathy with characteristic nodal lesions
3. Negative laboratory investigation for unexplained lymphadenopathy
4. Detection of antibodies to *B. henselae* or detection of *B. henselae* DNA using polymerase chain reaction (PCR) analysis of tissue samples or lymph node aspirates.

11. How is *B. henselae infection* diagnosed in cats?

Several tests available can be used to assess the *B. henselae* infection status of individual cats. Cats should be screened for antibodies as well as by an organism demonstration technique (culture or PCR).
- Antibodies against *B. henselae* can be detected in serum. Positive test results suggest current or previous infection. Negative test results suggest peracute exposure (< 3 weeks) or absence of infection.
- Detection of local production of antibodies in aqueous humor was used to document ocular bartonellosis in 1 cat.
- The organism can be grown from the blood (EDTA anticoagulant). Positive test results prove current infection. Negative results suggest peracute exposure (< 2 weeks) or absence of infection. However, intermittent bacteremia commonly occurs and may lead to false-negative results on a single test.
- *B. henselae* DNA can be detected in blood or aqueous humor by PCR. Positive test results suggest current infection. Negative test results suggest peracute exposure (< 2 weeks) or absence of infection. However, intermittent bacteremia commonly occurs and may lead to false-negative results on a single test.
- An antibody-negative, PCR/culture-negative cat is probably not infected.

12. Should infected cats be treated?

Whether to treat bacteremic cats is controversial. To date, administration of antimicrobials has led to rapid resolution of bacteremia, but some treated cats become bacteremic again after treatment is discontinued. The following drugs, used singly, have been reported:
- Doxycycline (25–50 mg/cat orally every 12 hr for 30 days)
- Enrofloxacin (22.7 mg/cat orally every 12 hr for 4 weeks)
- Amoxicillin (100–200 mg/cat orally every 12 hr for 1–4 weeks)

13. Describe the clinical course of CSD.

Most cases resolve spontaneously in a few weeks or months. Antibiotics (rifampin, ciprofloxacin, trimethoprim-sulfa, or gentamycin) are used by some clinicians. Treatment is continued for 2 weeks in severe cases in immunocompetent patients and for 6 weeks in immunocompromised patients.

14. What is the prognosis of CSD?

The prognosis is excellent for immunocompetent people. Primary infection is likely to result in life-long protection. Life-threatening or relapsing infections can occur in immunocompromised people.

15. How can CSD be prevented?

1. Avoid traumatic contact with cats or avoid behaviors that may lead to a bite or scratch.
2. Do not kiss cats or allow them to lick open wounds.
3. Wash hands thoroughly after handling cats.

4. Wash bites, scratches, and cuts promptly with antiseptic soap.
5. Contact a physician for any bite wound.
6. Maintain good flea and tick control and prevention programs.

16. Can *Yersinia pestis* be transmitted by the bite of an infected cat?

Plague is considered endemic in the southwestern United States (see Chapter 86). Because many cats are infected by ingesting bacteremic rodents and have *Y. pestis* replication in the oropharynx, infection of humans may occur after bites or scratches. The organism also can be transmitted to humans by respiratory secretions and is a shared vector zoonosis.

17. What causes tularemia?

Tularemia is a syndrome caused by *Francisella tularensis*, a gram-negative bacillus found throughout the continental United States.

18. How is tularemia acquired?

The disease is vector-borne by *Dermacenter variabilis, D. andersoni,* and *Amblyomma americanum.* Human tularemia results most commonly from tick exposure and less commonly from contact with infected animals, including cats. Cats are infected most frequently by tick bites or by ingesting infected rabbits or rodents. Cat-associated tularemia in humans has occurred most frequently via bites.

19. How is *F. tularensis* managed clinically?

Ulceroglandular, oculoglandular, glandular, oropharyngeal, pneumonic, and typhoidal forms have been described in humans. The specific form depends on the route of exposure. Infected cats exhibit generalized lymphadenopathy and abscess formation in organs such as the liver and spleen, which leads to fever, anorexia, icterus, and death. Cultures and documentation of increasing antibody titers can be used to confirm the diagnosis in cats and humans. Ectoparasite control should be maintained, and cats should not be allowed to hunt to lessen risk of exposure.

20. What causes rabies?

Rabies is caused by a single-stranded RNA virus in the genus *Lyssavirus*, family Rhabdoviridae. There are 10 genetically distinct rabies variants in the United States.

21. Describe the pathogenesis of rabies.

The rabies virus enters the body through a wound, usually a bite, or the mucous membranes. After replicating in monocytes, it spreads to neuromuscular junctions and neurotendinal spindles. The virus travels to the central nervous system (CNS) via intraaxonal fluid within peripheral nerves, then spreads throughout the CNS. From the CNS it spreads to the peripheral sensory and motor neurons. Large quantities of virus are present in saliva.

22. What are the clinical signs of rabies?

Atypical presentations of rabies are common. Rabies must be included on the differential list for any cat showing unusual mood or behavior changes or exhibiting any unaccountable neurologic signs. Handle cases with extreme caution to prevent exposure of personnel. The three stages of rabies are prodromal, furious, and paralytic. Rabies should be suspected in animals with the following symptoms:
- Change in attitude (apprehension, nervousness, anxiety, unusual aggressiveness or shyness)
- Anxious, staring, wild, spooky, or blank look in the eyes
- Erratic behavior (biting, snapping, licking, or chewing at a wound site, biting at cage, wandering or roaming)
- Excitability, irritability, or viciousness
- Muscular incoordination, abnormal gait (especially involving the rear limbs), disorientation, seizures, or paralysis

- Change in sound or pitch of voice or increased frequency of vocalization
- Excessive salivation or frothing
- Physical examination may reveal mandibular and laryngeal paralysis with dropped jaw, inability to swallow, and hypersalivation. Fever may be present.

23. What are the differential diagnoses for rabies?
- Other neurologic disease (brain tumor, viral encephalitis)
- Head wound or trauma
- Laryngeal paralysis
- Choking
- Pseudorabies

24. How is rabies diagnosed?
Complete blood count and serum biochemical panel reveal no characteristic abnormalities. Cerebrospinal fluid may show a slight increase in protein or leukocyte counts. Direct immunofluroescent antibody testing must be done on nervous tissue (brain) or dermal tissue (skin biopsy of sensory vibrissae of maxillary area, including deeper subcutaneous hair follicles).

25. How is rabies treated?
Nearly 100% of cats die within 7–10 days of the onset of symptoms. There is no treatment. Once the diagnosis is certain, the cat should be humanely euthanized.

26. How can rabies be prevented?
Cats should be vaccinated according to local ordinances with an inactivated vaccine (see Chapter 81). Previously vaccinated cats should be given a booster vaccine if treated for wounds that may be bite-related. Quarantine procedures should be used for any rabies suspect, and the case should be reported to the authorities. The virus can be inactivated by disinfection with a 1:32 dilution of bleach. Personnel at risk should be immunized.

27. Can people be infected by feline retroviruses?
Feline leukemia virus (FeLV) and feline foamy virus (syncycia-forming virus) grow in human cell cultures; feline immunodeficiency virus (FIV) does not. Studies of people with chronic fatigue syndrome (FeLV), leukemia (FeLV and FIV), and veterinarians (FeLV, FIV, feline foamy virus) have failed to find evidence that these viruses infect people in vivo.

BIBLIOGRAPHY

1. Bonilla HF, Chenoworth CE, Tully JG, et al: *Mycoplasma felis* septic arthritis in a patient with hypogammaglobulinemia. Clin Infect Dis 24: 222–225, 1997.
2. Butera ST, Brown J, Callahan ME, et al: Survey of veterinary conference attendees for evidence of zoonotic infection by feline retroviruses. J Am Vet Med Assoc 217:1475–1479, 2000.
3. Carpenter PD, Heppner BT, Gnann JW: DF-2 bacteremia following cat bites: Report of two cases. Am J Med 82:621, 1987.
4. Chomel BB, Kasten RW, Floyd-Hawkins K, et al: Experimental transmission of *Bartonella henselae* by the cat flea. J Clin Microbiol 34:1952–1956, 1996.
5. Clark KA: Rabies. J Am Vet Med Assoc 192:1404–1406, 1998.
6. Fogelman V, Fischman HR, Horman JT, et al: Epidemiologic and clinical characteristics of rabies in cats. J Am Vet Med Assoc 202:1829–1833, 1993.
7. Gasper PW: Plague. In August JR (ed): Consultations in Feline Internal Medicine, vol. 3. Philadelphia, W.B.Saunders, 1997, pp 12–22.
8. Guptill L, Slater L, Ching-Ching W, et al: Experimental infection of young specific pathogen-free cats with *Bartonella henselae*. J Inf Dis 176:206–216, 1997.
9. Kordick DL, Breitschwerdt EB: *Bartonella* infections in domestic cats. In Bonagura JD (ed): Current Veterinary Therapy XIII—Small Animal Practice. Philadelphia, W.B. Saunders, 2000, pp 302–307.
10. Lappin MR, Black JC: *Bartonella* spp. associated uveitis in a cat. J Am Vet Med Assoc 214;1205–1207, 1999.

11. Lappin MR, Jensen W, Kordick DL, et al: *Bartonella* spp. antibodies and DNA in aqueous humor of cats. Feline Med Surg 2:61–68, 2000.
12. Rohrbach BW: Tularemia. J Am Vet Med Assoc 193:428–432, 1988.
13. Talan DA, Citron DM, Abrahamian FM, et al: Bacteriologic analysis of infected dog and cat bites. N Engl J Med 340:85–92, 1999.
14. Trevejo RT: Rabies preexposure vaccination among veterinarians and at risk staff. J Am Vet Med Assoc 217:1647–1650, 2000.
15. Valtonen M, Lauhio A, Carlson P, et al: *Capnocytophaga canimorsus* septicemia: Fifth report of a cat-associated infection and five other cases. Eur J Clin Microbiol Infect Dis 14:520–523, 1995.

86. RESPIRATORY ZOONOSES

Michael R. Lappin, D.V.M., Ph.D., and Alice J. Johns, D.V.M.

1. How often do cats and people share respiratory tract infections?

Although infectious causes of respiratory disease are extremely common in cats (see Section I), most causes are not transmissible to humans (feline herpesvirus 1, calicivirus). Humans are potentially exposed to *Bordetella bronchiseptica* and *Chlamydia psitacci* but rarely develop clinical infection. *Yersinia pestis* is a notable exception; both cats and people can develop pneumonic plague, which is a life-threatening disease. Group A streptococcal infections are a reverse zoonosis: humans are the primary reservoir, and cats are infected by contact with humans. *Pasteurella multocida* from a cat was cultured from the lungs of a man with AIDS who had had only passive contact with the cat.

Common Zoonoses Associated with Direct Contact with Respiratory or Ocular Secretions of Cats

ORGANISM	CLINICAL SIGNS	RELATIVE RISK FROM CATS TO HUMANS
Bordetella bronchiseptica	Cats: upper respiratory, rarely, pneumonia Humans: pneumonia in immunosuppressed patients	Extremely rare
Chlamydia psittacii	Cats: conjunctivitis, mild upper respiratory disease Humans: conjunctivitis, bacteremia	Extremely rare
Coxiella burnetii	Cats: subclinical, abortion, or stillbirth Humans: fever, pneumonitis, lymphadenopathy, myalgia, arthritis	Unknown; probably rare
Francisella tularensis	Cats: septicemia, pneumonia Humans: ulceroglandular, oculoglandular, glandular, pneumonic, or typhoidal (depending on route of inoculation)	Extremely rare
Pasteurella multocida	Cats: normal flora Humans: one case of pneumonia from passive contact with a cat has been reported	Extremely rare
Streptococcus group A	Cats: subclinical, transient carrier Humans: strep throat, septicemia	Extremely rare
Yersinia pestis	Cats: bubonic, bacteremic, or pneumonic Humans: bubonic, bacteremic, or pneumonic	Extremely rare and regional

2. How common is bordetellosis in cats?

B. bronchiseptica commonly causes infectious tracheobronchitis in dogs. Many cats from crowded environments have serologic evidence of exposure or are culture-positive, but most infected cats are clinically normal (see Chapters 2 and 12).

3. Do people develop bordetellosis from contact with cats?

Bordetella pertussis commonly infects and causes disease in people but is not a disease of cats. By 1998, 39 cases of *B. bronchiseptica* infection in people had been reported; most patients were immunodeficient. One person who was coinfected with *B. bronchiseptica* and HIV owned a cat. Because cats are commonly exposed but people are rarely infected, *B. bronchiseptica* infection of people from contact with cats appears to be unlikely. However, a diagnostic work-up and antimicrobial therapy should be considered for cats with suspected bacterial respiratory disease if the household has an immunosuppressed member. Definitive diagnosis is based on culture. Tetracycline derivatives, axomicillin-clavulanate, and quinolones are effective in controlling clinical signs of disease, but treated cats can be culture-positive for months.

4. Describe the clinical findings of chlamydiosis in cats.

Chlamydia psittaci infection of cats commonly causes conjunctivitis (see Chapter 2). If respiratory disease occurs, it is a mild rhinitis; lower respiratory tract disease is uncommon.

5. Are cats and people commonly exposed to *C. psittaci*?

In a recent study from Japan, antibodies against a feline strain of *C. psittaci* were detected in 45.5% of stray cats, 17.3% of pet cats, 1.7% of the general human population, and 8.8% of small animal veterinarians, suggesting that exposure is common.

6. Do feline strains of *C. psittaci* cause disease in people?

Although exposure to *C. psittaci* seems common, it has been associated with disease only in rare cases. Conjunctivitis in humans after direct contact with ocular discharges has been suspected. A chlamydial species isolated from an infected person was inoculated into cats, resulting in conjunctivitis and persistent infection. This experiment suggests that the isolate was from a cat. Feline *Chlamydia* spp. were indirectly associated with atypical pneumonia in an apparently immunocompetent 48-year-old man; with malaise and cough in an immunosuppressed woman; and with endocarditis and glomerulonephritis in a 40-year-old woman. Care should be taken to avoid direct conjunctival contact with discharges from the respiratory or ocular secretions of cats, especially by immunosuppressed persons. Topical or oral tetracycline derivatives are effective for the treatment of infected cats.

7. Do cats harbor group A streptococci?

It has been proposed that cats can be infected with group A streptococci and transmit the infection to children, ultimately causing strep thoat. Humans are the principal natural hosts for group A streptococci, but cats may develop a transient (about 2 weeks), subclinical infection from contact with an infected human. Because cats are occasionally infected, it is plausible that cat contact can lead to infection of people. However, this scenario is poorly documented and believed to be unlikely. Culture of a group A streptococcal organism from the tonsillar crypts can document a feline infection. Administration of penicillin derivatives is generally effective. However, if the cats are treated in an attempt to stop a strep throat problem in humans, all family members should be treated because humans can have a prolonged subclinical carrier phase.

8. What is feline plague?

Yersenia pestis is a gram-negative, bipolar staining coccobacillus in the family Enterobacteriaceae. It is endemic in rodent populations worldwide, including the western United States, where prairie dogs, rock squirrels, and ground squirrels are the commonly involved rodents.

9. Describe the pathogenesis of plague.

Fleas ingest a blood meal from an infected animal. The blood clots and blocks the gut of the flea. When the flea bites the next victim, it regurgitates *Y. pestis* onto or into the skin. Cats also are infected by ingestion of infected rodents when the organism enters via the mouth or esophagus. The bacteria migrate from the skin lymphatics to the regional lymph nodes. The organism is transmitted to humans by the bite of infected rodent fleas, aerosalization, bites and scratches from infected animals (including cats), or direct contact with infected people. The organism has a capsular glycoprotein with antiphagocytic properties and potent endotoxins. It proliferates rapidly and massively in susceptible hosts.

10. What are the three forms of plague in cats and people?
1. Bubonic (from a flea bite or ingestion of an infected transport host)
2. Pneumonic (via droplets or hematogenous spread)
3. Septicemic (via direct blood injection or extension of the bubonic or pneumonic form)

11. Describe the clinical signs of plague in cats and people.

In **cats**, the symptoms include lethargy, anorexia, fever (103–105°F), and lymphadenopathy (typically the submandibular, anterior cervical and medial retropharyngeal lymph nodes). Dyspnea and cough also can occur. The incubation period is 2–7 days after a flea bite or ingestion of an infected rodent.

In **people**, the symptoms are fever, lymphadenopathy, intense local inflammation, depression, vomiting and diarrhea, dehydration, enlarged tonsils, ocular discharge, weight loss, ataxia, coma, and oral ulcers. The lymph nodes become hemorrhagic, necrotic, and edematous. The lymph nodes may abscess, rupture, and drain through fistulous tracts to the skin. Septicemia may occur.

12. How is plague diagnosed?

History and physical examination findings can be used to place the disease high on the differential list. Most cases of feline plague are diagnosed between April and October when rodent fleas are most active. Any outdoor cat from an endemic area with fever and submandibular lymphadenopathy or fever and signs of pneumonia should be considered a plague suspect and immediately placed in isolation. The following steps should be taken:
1. Sedate the cat to avoid bites and scratches while collecting tissue aspirates.
2. Place a small amount of material on a swab for bacterial culture and label as plague suspect.
3. Make more than 1 thin smear of material so that routine cytology as well as fluorescent antibody staining can be performed.
4. The diagnosis is confirmed by culture of exudates, tonsillar area, and saliva, fluorescent antibody staining of exudates, and documentation of increasing antibody titers.
5. Contact county and state public health officials as well as the Centers for Disease Control if plague is suspected.

13. How is feline plague treated?

Infected cats should be treated with enrofloxacin (5 mg/kg/day intramuscularly) or aminoglycosides for the first 4 days of treatment. Doxycycline (5–10 mg/kg/day orally) then is prescribed for at least 14 days. Oral antibiotics should not be used while the cat is hospitalized to avoid placing your hands in the cat's mouth, where large numbers of the organism are present. Most treated cats survive. Cats are not considered infectious after 3–4 days of antibiotic therapy and can be discharged.

14. How is plague prevented?

Hospitalized cats are maintained in isolation and handled by as few people as possible. Handlers should wear a barrier gown, safety goggles, and surgical mask. Some recommend that cats with pneumonic plague be humanely euthanized because of the high zoonotic potential.

People in contact with the infected cat should seek medical advice about prophylactic antibiotic treatment. Untreated pneumonic plague is 100% fatal in people. The mortality rate is 5–20% with appropriate antibiotic treatment but much higher if antibiotics are started later than 24 hours after the onset of pneumonic or septicemic forms of the disease. Flea control should be initiated immediately for the affected cat and other client pets. Cats should be housed indoors and not be allowed to hunt.

15. How can respiratory zoonoses be prevented?
* House cats indoors to avoid contracting respiratory diseases.
* Have a veterinarian evaluate cats with clinical evidence of respiratory disease.
* Have someone other than an immunosuppressed person treat cats with suspected infectious respiratory diseases.

BIBLIOGRAPHY

1. Bart M, Guscetti F, Zurbriggen A, et al: Feline infectious pneumonia: A short literature review and a retrospective immunohistological study on the involvement of *Chlamydia* spp. and distemper virus. Vet J 159:220–230, 2000.
2. Binns SH, Dawson S, Speakman AJ, et al: Prevalence and risk factors for feline *Bordetella bronchiseptica* infection. Vet Rec 144:575–580, 1999.
3. Cotton MM, Partridge MR: Infection with feline *Chlamydia psittaci*. Thorax 53:75–76, 1998.
4. Eidson M, Thilsted JP, Rollag OJ: Clinical, clinicopathologic and pathologic features of plague in cats: 119 cases (1977–1988). J Am Vet Med Assoc 199:1191–1197, 1991.
5. Dworkin MS, Sullivan PS, Buskin SE, et al: *Bordetella bronchiseptica* infection in human immunodeficiency virus-infected patients. Clin Infect Dis 28:1095–1099, 1999.
6. Drabick JJ, Gasser RA, Saunders NB, et al: *Pasteurella multocida* pneumonia in a man with AIDS and nontraumatic feline exposure. Chest 103:7–11, 1993.
7. Greene CE, Prescott JF: Streptococcal and other gram-positive bacterial infections. In Greene CE (ed): Infectious Diseases of the Dog and Cat, 2nd ed. Philadelphia, W.B.Saunders, 1998, pp 205–214.
8. Griffins PD, Lechler RI, Treharne JD: Unusual chlamydial infection in a human renal allograft recipient. BMJ 277:1264–1265. 1978.
9. Hoskins JD, Williams J, Roy AF, et al: Isolation and characterization of *Bordetella bronchiseptica* from cats in southern Louisiana. Vet Immunol Immunopathol 65:173–176, 1998.
10. Macy DW: Plague. In Greene CE (ed): Infectious Diseases of the Dog and Cat, 2nd ed. Philadelphia, W.B. Saunders , 1998, pp 295–300.
11. Ostler HB, Schacter J, Dawson R: Acute follicular conjunctivitis of epizootic origin. Arch Ophthalmol 82:587–591, 1969.
12. Regan RJ, Dathan JRE, Treharne JD: Infective endocarditis with glomerulonephritis assocated with cat chlamydia *(C. psittaci)* infection. Br Heart J 42:349–352, 1979.
13. Stefanelli P, Mastrantonio P, Hausman SZ, et al: Molecular characterization of two *Bordetella bronchiseptica* strains isolated from children with coughs. J Clin Microbiol 35:1550–1555, 1997.
14. Yan C, Fukushi H, Matsudate H, et al: Seroepidemiological investigation of feline chlamydiosis in cats and humans in Japan. Microbiol Immunol 44:155–160, 2000.

87. EXUDATE AND CUTANEOUS ZOONOSES

Michael R. Lappin, D.V.M., Ph.D., and Tammy P. Sadek, D.V.M.

1. What infectious agents can be transmitted to people directly from contact with the skin or exudates of cats?

Several bacterial agents, fungal agents, and ectoparasites that cause skin or exudative diseases of cats are transmittable to people. Dermatophytes and fleas are most common.

Common Feline Cutaneous and Exudate-associated Zoonoses

ORGANISM	CLINICAL SYNDROME	RELATIVE RISK* TO HUMANS
Bacteria		
Francisella tularensis	Cats: septicemia, pneumonia Humans: ulceroglandular, glandular oculoglandular, pneumonic, or typhoidal (depending on route of infection)	Extremely rare
L-form bacteria	Cats: chronic draining tracts, polyarthritis Humans: chronic draining tracts, polyarthritis	Extremely rare
Yersinia pestis	Cats: bubonic, bacteremic, or pneumonic Humans: bubonic, bacteremic, or pneumonic	Rare; regional
Ectoparasites		
Cheyletiella spp.	Cats: superficial dermatologic disease Humans: superficial dermatologic disease	Common
Ctenocephalides felis	Cats: superficial dermatologic disease; anemia; transmission of vector-borne diseases Humans: superficial dermatologic disease; transmission of vector-borne diseases	Common
Noteodres cati	Cats: superficial dermatologic disease Humans: superficial dermatologic disease	Rare
Sarcoptes scabei	Cats: superficial dermatologic disease Humans: superficial dermatologic disease	Rare
Ticks	Cats: superficial dermatologic disease; anemia; transmission of vector-borne diseases Humans: superficial dermatologic disease; transmission of vector-borne diseases	Common
Fungi		
Dermatophytes	Cats: superficial dermatologic disease Humans: superficial dermatologic disease	Common
Sporothrix schenkii	Cats: chronic draining cutaneous tracts Humans: chronic draining cutaneous tracts	Extremely rare

* Frequency of infection from direct contact with infected cats.

2. What is the most common dermatophyte of cats?

Microsporum canis is the most common dermatophyte of cats; it is also the organism most commonly associated with zoonotic transfer to people.

3. How common is human infection with feline dermatophytes?

Approximately 50% of people exposed to dermatophytes become infected; most people that live in a household with infected cats become infected.

4. Describe the range of clinical symptoms in cats and humans.

Cats can be subclinical carriers or develop superficial dermatologic disease characterized by broken haired alopecia, crusts, and scale.

Humans develop characteristic red, raised, circular, pruritic lesions at infection sites; invasive infection may occur in immunocompromised people.

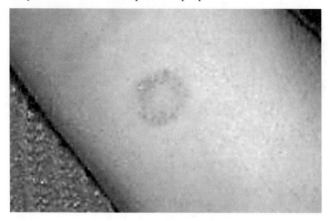

Ringworm lesion on a human. (Courtesy of Rodney Rosychuk, M.D., Colorado State University.)

5. What are the most common risk factors for dermatophytosis?
- Kittens from shelters with known history of infection
- Exposure to pet cats housed with large numbers of other animals
- Age of both human and cat (children and kittens are most likely to be infected)

6. How is dermatophytosis diagnosed?

Microconidia are noted within hair shafts on cytologic examination after KOH clearance; definitive diagnosis is made by culture of hair.

7. How can zoonotic transfer be prevented?

To lessen potential for zoonotic transfer of infection from infected cats, the body should be shaved, and both topical and systemic treatment should be instituted.

The vaccine is not recommended by most authorities as a preventive measure. Some believe that the vaccine can be used beneficially in cats that are difficult to handle or treat, but vaccination may increase the rate of subclinical carriers.

8. Do fungi associated with systemic infections cause human disease from direct contact with infected cats?

Cats are rarely infected by *Blastomyces dermatitidis, Coccidioides immitis, Histoplasma capsulatum, Cryptococcus neoformans*, and *Sporothrix schenkii*. Each of these fungi can cause exudative skin disease, but only *S. schenkii* has a high rate of transmission from infected cats to people. The others are acquired from environmental exposure.

9. How does *S. schenkii* infect the host?

S. schenkii is a soil saprophyte that usually infects the host through wound contamination or penetrating foreign objects; there is no known geographical distribution. Infection of cats and humans usually occurs after the organism contaminates broken skin. Cats are thought to be infected by scratches from contaminated claws of other cats. Multiple cases have been reported in cats; infection is most common in outdoor males. Exudates from infected lesions of cats usually contain numerous organisms and are another source of human infection.

10. What are the clinical manifestations of *S. schenkii* infection in cats and humans?

Cats usually develop a lymphocutaneous form of disease. Dermal and subcutaneous nodules spread from the inoculation site along lymphatics. This process causes tissue cording and ulceration and eventual pyrexia and depression. The cat may inoculate itself at sites distal to the primary lesion via grooming. If the immune response is strong, the lesion usually remains localized and appears ulcerated or acne-like. In rare cases, the organism disseminates throughout the body and infects multiple organs.

In **humans**, infections are commonly associated with rosebushes, sphagnum moss, and armadillo hunting. Most human infections are localized cutaneous lesions, although disseminated disease in immunocompromised people has been reported.

11. How is *S. schenkii* infection diagnosed?

Presumptive diagnosis is based on cytology of exudates or histopathology; the organism is round, oval, or cigar-shaped and may be extracellular or intracellular after being engulfed by macrophages. Definitive diagnosis is based on culture.

12. Describe the treatment for *S. schenkii* infection.

Potassium iodide is used to treat cats and people. The usual regimen in cats consists of 20 mg/kg orally every 12–24 hours for at least 3 weeks after resolution of signs. Alternative therapy includes itraconazole (5 mg/kg orally every 24 hr) or ketoconazole (5–15 mg/kg orally every 12–24 hr).

13. What bacterial diseases of cats can be transmitted to people by contact with exudates?

Theoretically, any bacterial disease of cats can infect a person if the organism is inoculated by biting or into an open wound. *Yersinia pestis* (see Chapter 86) and *Fransicella tularensis* (see Chapter 85) are of most concern because they are associated with life-threatening bacteremia in people.

14. Do ectoparasites of cats infest people?

In addition to being the vector or reservoir of some zoonotic agents (see Chapter 90), ectoparasites also can induce cutaneous disease in people. *Ctenocephalides felis, Cheyletiella* spp., *Sarcoptes scabei, Notoedres cati*, and various ticks parasitize both cats and people. Multiple species of *Cheyletiella* exist, and cross-infection to dogs and rabbits may occur.

15. Describe the clinical manifestations of *Cheyletiella blakei* mite infestations in cats and humans.

Cats with *C. blakei* may be subclinically infected or have scales of variable severity, primarily over the dorsum. Pruritus is also variable. Long-haired cats such as Persians are common subclinical carriers.

In **humans**, infestation causes a self-limited but intensely pruritic dermatitis with papules progressing to pustules and then to erythemic areas with areas of central necrosis.

16. How is *C. blakei* infestation diagnosed?

Diagnosis is made by demonstrating the mites after taking skin scrapings or acetate tape preparations of affected areas. Occasionally, a presumptive diagnosis is made by response to treatment in difficult-to-diagnose cats.

17. How is *C. blakei* infestation treated and controlled?

Once a diagnosis is made, all pets in the household must be treated. Lime sulfur 2% dips have been successful if applied weekly for 6–8 weeks. Two or three treatments with ivermectin (0.2–0.3 mg/kg subcutaneously every 2–3 weeks) is generally effective but not approved for use in cats.

Environmental control with an effective flea spray of the premises, disinfection of grooming brushes, and thorough vacuuming is essential to eradicate *C. blakei*, which can live off the body for a number of days.

18. How common are *Notoedres cati* infections of cats and humans?

Notoedric mange has a worldwide distribution but is relatively uncommon in the U.S.

19. Describe the presentation of *N. cati* infections in cats and humans.

Cats present with intense pruritus of the head and neck, with marked crusting, scaling, erythema, and hair loss in affected areas. Kittens may show a severe moist dermatitis of the ventrum, perineum, and legs, which may be fatal if left untreated.

Humans occasionally develop transient notoedric infestation and may experience intensely pruritic urticarial lesions on the arms, legs, and chest.

20. How is *N. cati* infection diagnosed and treated?

The mites usually are found easily on microscopic examination of skin scrapings.

Treatment with ivermectin (0.25 mg/kg subcuatneously every 2 weeks for 3 treatments) is usually successful. Lime sulfur dips and pyrethrin dips also have been used successfully; lime sulfur may be preferred in debilitated cats.

21. How is *N. cati* infection controlled?

As for cheyletielliosis, all animals in the household must be treated, and the premises must be disinfected with an effective flea spray.

22. What are the clinical manifestations of *Sarcoptes scabei* infections in cats and humans?

Cats are rarely infested by *S. scabei* but occasionally present with a miliary type of dermatitis similar to flea allergy dermatitis. More severe cases may show allergic sensitization with intense pruritus, crusting, alopecia, and lichenification spreading from the head and ears to encompass the entire body. Hyperkeratosis of the ears has been reported in cats that test positive for feline immunodeficiency virus.

Human infestations from contact with cats are transient and result in intensely pruritic, small, linear grooves, papules, and vesicles with possibly purulent secondary infections.

23. How is *S. scabei* infection treated?

Treatment is the same as for notoedric mange.

24. How can cutaneous and exudate-associated zoonoses be avoided?

All cats with exudative or cutaneous diseases should be taken to the veterinarian for appropriate diagnostic tests and appropriate treatment. Tick, flea, and mite control should be maintained. Kittens from crowded environments are most likely to carry cutaneous zoonoses.

BIBLIOGRAPHY

1. Chakrabarti A: Human notoedric scabies from contact with cats infested with *Notoedres cati*. Int J Dermatol 25:646–648, 1986.
2. Davies C, Troy GC: Deep mycotic infections in cats. J Am Anim Hosp Assoc 32:380–391, 1996.
3. Dunston RW, Langham RF, Reimann DA, et al: Feline sporotrichosis: A report of five cases with transmission to humans. J Am Acad Dermatol 15:37, 1986.
4. Foil CS: Dermatophytosis. In Greene CE (ed): Infectious Diseases of the Dog and Cat, 2nd ed. Philadelphia, W.B. Saunders, 1998, pp 362–370.
5. King D, Cheever LW, Hood A, et al: Primary invasive cutaneous *Microsporum canis* infections in immunocompromised patients. J Clin Microbiol 34:460–462, 1996.
6. Merchant SR: Zoonotic diseases with cutaneous manifestations. Part I. Compend Cont Educ Pract Vet 12:371–377, 1990.
7. Merchant SR: Zoonotic diseases with cutaneous manifestations. Part II. Compend Cont Educ Pract Vet 12:515–521, 1990.
8. Morriello KA, DeBoer DJ: Feline dermatophytosis: Recent advances and recommendations for therapy. Vet Clin North Am Small Animal Pract 25:901–921, 1995.
9. Romano R, Valenti L, Barbara R: Dermatophytes isolated from asymptomatic stray cats. Mycoses 40:471–472, 1997.
10. Rosser EJ, Dunstan RW: Sporotrichosis. In Greene CE (ed): Infectious Diseases of the Dog and Cat, 2nd ed. Philadelphia, W.B. Saunders, 1998, pp 399–402.

88. UROGENITAL TRACT ZOONOSES

Michael R. Lappin, D.V.M., Ph.D.

1. What infectious agents of the urogenital system of cats are capable of infecting people?
Coxiella burnetii and *Leptospira* spp. potentially infect both people and cats and are considered zoonotic.

Feline Urinary and Genital Tract Zoonoses

ORGANISM	CLINICAL DISEASE	RELATIVE RISK FROM CATS TO HUMANS
Bacteria		
Leptospira spp.	Cats: usually subclinical infection	Extremely rare
	Humans: fever, malaise, inflammatory urinary tract or hepatic disease, uveitis, central nervous system disease	
Rickettsia		
Coxiella burnetii	Cats: subclinical disease, abortion, or stillbirth	Unknown;
	Humans: fever, pneumonitis, lymphadenopathy, myalgia, arthritis	probably rare

2. Define Q fever.
Q fever in people is a clinical syndrome caused by *C. burnetii*, a rickettsial agent found throughout the world, including North America. Ticks and other arthropods are natural hosts for the organism, which is maintained in a sylvan cycle with reservoir hosts. Cats, cattle, sheep, and goats are commonly infected subclinically and pass the organism into the environment in urine, feces, milk, and parturient discharges. Acute clinical signs in people include fever, malaise, headache, interstitial pneumonitis, myalgia, and arthralgia. In cat-associated infections, clinical signs develop 4–30 days after contact. In approximately 1%, chronic Q fever can develop years after primary infection and may manifest as hepatic inflammation or valvular endocarditis.

3. How are cats and humans infected?
Infection of **cats** most commonly results from tick exposure, ingestion of contaminated carcasses, or aerosolization from a contaminated environment.

Humans usually are infected by ingesting the organism in raw milk or meat from infected food animals or by inhaling the organism in parturient secretions. Thus, people associated with livestock are particularly susceptible to infection. Human infection has been associated with aborting cats and normal parturient cats. Tick-borne infection also may occur. Because the organism is present in body secretions, person-to-person infection may occur in rare cases.

4. How common is *C. burnetti* infection of cats?
The true incidence of disease in cats has not been determined. In two studies, 20% of cats from a humane society in southern California and 20% of cats in maritime Canada were seropositive, suggesting that exposure is common. The organism was grown from the vagina of normal cats in Japan. Although the organism has been associated with aborting cats, infection is considered subclinical in most cases.

5. How is Q fever managed clinically?
Diagnosis in people can be based on organism isolation, polymerase chain reaction, or serologic test results. Tetracyclines, chloramphenicol, and quinolones are usually effective therapeutic agents in people.

6. How can infection with *C. burnetii* be prevented?

Gloves and masks should be worn while attending to parturient or aborting cats. Arthropod control should be maintained. The organism is extremely resistant to environmental extremes and disinfectants once it has sporulated.

7. Define leptospirosis.

Various bacteria are included in the *Leptospira interrogans sensu lato* group. Leptospires are maintained in nature in subclinically infected reservoir hosts; infection of incidental hosts results in clinical disease. People are incidental hosts to multiple serovars and develop fever as well as manifestations of liver, and kidney disease. Leptospires are passed by reservoir host in large numbers in infected urine and can enter the body through abraded skin and mucous membranes.

8. What are the clinical manifestations of leptospirosis in cats?

In one study, cats were experimentally inoculated with a *L. interrogans* serovars *icterohaemorrhagiae* and *canicola*. Although most cats seroconverted and *L. canicola* was shed in the urine, clinical abnormalities were not detected. Several other serovars have been isolated from cats, but reports of naturally occurring disease are rare. Ascites due to infection may have occurred in one cat; pleuritis, pericarditis, hepatitis, and uveitis occurred in another. Seropositive cats are common; exposure may be from contact with dogs or rodents.

9. Are cats a likely reservoir host for leptospires that infect humans?

Cats appear to be an unlikely source for human leptospirosis. In fact, two studies found that cat owners were less likely to be seropositive than people who did not own cats.

BIBLIOGRAPHY

1. Agunloye CA, Nash AS: Investigation of possible leptospiral infection in cats in Scotland. J Small Anim Pract 37:126–129, 1996.
2. Bryson DG, Ellis WA: Leptospirosis in a British domestic cat. J Small Anim Pract 17:459–465, 1976.
3. Childs JE, Schwartz BS, Ksiazek TG, et al: Risk factors associated with antibodies to leptospires in inner-city residents of Baltimore: A protective role for cats. Am J Public Health 82:597–599, 1992.
4. Greene CE, Miller MA, Brown CA: Leptospirosis. In Greene CE (ed): Infectious Diseases of the Dog and Cat, 2nd ed. Philadelphia, W.B. Saunders, 1998, pp 272–281.
5. Higgins D, Marrie TJ: Seroepidemiology of Q fever among cats in New Brunswick and Prince Edward Island. Ann NY Acad Sci 590:271–274, 1990.
6. Larsson CE, Santa Rosa CA, Larsson MH, et al: Laboratory and clinical features of experimental feline leptospirosis. Int J Zoonoses 12:2 111–119, 1985.
7. Levesque B, Serres de G, Higgins R, et al: Seroepidemiologic study of three zoonoses (leptospirosis, Q fever, and tularemia) among trappers in Quebec, Canada. Clin Diagnos Lab Immunol 2:496–498, 1995.
8. Nagaoka H, Sugieda M, Akiyama M, et al: Isolation of *Coxiella burnetii* from the vagina of feline clients at veterinary clinics. J Vet Med Sci 60:251–252, 1998.
9. Marrie TJ: *Coxiella burnetii* (Q Fever) pneumonia. Clin Infect Dis 21:S253–S264, 1995.
10. Marrie TJ, Durant H, Williams JC, et al: Exposure to parturient cats: A risk factor for acquisition of Q fever in maritime Canada. J Infect Dis 158:101–108, 1988.
11. Marrie TJ, Langille D, Papukna V, et al: Truckin' pneumonia: An outbreak of Q fever in a truck repair plant probably due to aerosols from clothing contaminated by contact with newborn kittens. Epidemiol Infect 102:119–127, 1989.
12. Marrie TJ, MacDonald A, Durant H, et al: An outbreak of Q fever probably due to contact with a parturient cat. Chest 93:98–103, 1988.
13. Pinsky RL, Fishbein DB, Greene CR, et al: An outbreak of cat-associated Q fever in the United States. J Infect Dis 164:202–204, 1991.
14. Randhawa AS, Dieterich WH, Jolley WB, et al: Coxiellosis in pound cats. Feline Pract 4:37–38, 1974.

89. ENVIRONMENTAL ZOONOSES

Tammy P. Sadek, D.V.M.

1. What environmental agents commonly infect both cats and humans?

Various infectious agents are acquired by cats and people from environmental sources. For some agents, soil and other environmental materials are the primary reservoir:

Blastomyces dermatitidis	*Mucor* spp.
Coccidioides immitis	*Sporothrix schenkii*
Histoplasma capsulatum	*Mycobacterium* spp.
Cryptococcus neoformans	*Rhodococcus equi*
Aspergillus spp.	

For other infectious agents, people or other animals are the primary host and reservoir. They contaminate the environment with infected secretions or excrement, allowing infection of others. Common examples include the enteric zoonoses, such as *Toxoplasma gondii, Cryptosporidium parvum, Toxacara cati, Ancylostoma tubaeforme,* and *Giardia* spp. (see Chapter 84). However, any infectious agent that survives outside the host may be acquired from contact with infected fomites in the environment.

2. Are systemic fungal infections acquired from direct contact with infected cats?

With the exception of *Sporothrix schenkii,* human infection by any of the systemic fungal agents is unlikely from contact with an infected cat. If both a cat and human in the same household are infected with a fungal agent, the likely source is a shared environmental exposure.

3. How does infection with *Blastomyces dermatitidis* occur?

B. dermatitidis survives in soil in a mycelial stage. Spores are released from the mycelium and result in infection by inhalation. The mycelial phase develops in culture and on bandages and is contagious to people.

The yeast form of the organism that occurs in the body does not spread by aerosal transmission between infected animals or from animals to people. It is possible to induce infection by contamination of wounds with the yeast phase.

4. How common is blastomycosis?

B. dermatitidis has highest concentrations in the regions of the Ohio, Missouri, and Mississippi Rivers and mid-Atlantic states. It seems to be confined to small areas within endemic regions; exposure is generally uncommon. Blastomycosis is uncommon in cats but has been associated with dyspnea, panopthalmitis, anorexia, weight loss, and granulomatous skin lesions (see Chapter 12).

5. How does infection with *Coccidiomyces immitis* occur?

The organism grows as a mycelium in the environment. Multinucleate arthroconidia are formed, dispersed by the wind, and inhaled by susceptible hosts to induce infection. The spherules and endospores found in tissues of infected individuals are not considered contagious. As for *H. capsulatum* and *B. dermatitidis,* the mycelial phase that develops in cultures or bandages used on draining tracts is infectious to people.

6. How common is *C. immitis* infection?

C. immitis is limited geographically to the desert Southwest. In endemic areas, most people and dogs have serologic evidence of exposure. The same is probably true for cats. Clinical illness occurs in approximately 40% of exposed humans; most develop transient respiratory disease.

Increased incidence of infection occurs in dry periods following periods of rain because more arthroconidia are produced and dispersed.

7. Describe the mechanisms by which *Cryptococcus neoformans* is transmitted.

  C. neoformans lives in the soil as a saphrocytic yeast-like stage. Cats and people are thought to be infected by inhalation. There are no reports of animal-to-animal or animal-to-human infections. Risk of infection increases with the presence of pigeon droppings (*C. neoformans* var *neoformans*) and eucalyptus trees (*C. neoformans* var *gatti*).

8. Where is *C. neoformans* infection most common?

  C. neoformans is considered to have worldwide distribution, but larger numbers of infections are reported in Australia and southern California.

9. How does infection with *C. neoformans* manifest in cats?

  In cats, infection usually localizes in the upper respiratory tract, but disseminated infections can occur (see Chapter 4).

10. Describe the mechanisms by which *Histoplasma capsulatum* infection is spread.

  The organism is a dimorphic fungus; macroconidia and microcondia of the myelial environmental stage probably are inhaled or ingested by cats and people to initiate infection. The yeast form that occurs in the body of infected mammals is not contagious from cat to cat or from cats to people. The mycelial phase that develops in cultures or bandages used on draining tracts is infectious to people.

11. How common is infection with *H. capsulatum*?

  H. capsulatum is a common systemic mycosis in cats of some regions (see Chapter 22). The agent is ubiquitous in the soil, particularly soil contaminated with bird or bat droppings. The regions of the Ohio, Missouri, and Mississippi Rivers have the highest numbers of cases.

12. How does infection with *Sporothrix schenkii* occur?

  S. schenkii is a dimorphic soil saprophyte. The organism exists as a mycelium in soil and as a yeast in infected people or animals. Infection usually occurs through wound contamination or penetrating foreign objects. Human infections are commonly associated with rosebushes, sphagnum moss, and armadillo hunting. Exudates from infected lesions of cats may contain numerous organisms and are another source of human infection (see Chapter 87). There is no known geographical distribution.

13. By what mechanisms does infection with *Rhodococcus equi* occur?

  R. equi is a gram-positive soil bacillus. The primary route of infection appears to be aerosolized soil, but local wound contamination also occurs.

14. Describe the clinical manifestations of *R. equi* infection.

  R. equi most frequently causes suppurative bronchopneumonia in foals. In cats, local infections may appear as caseating pyogranulomatous abcesses that ulcerate and drain. Occasionally, spread via the lymphatic system leads to pyothorax and visceral organ infection. HIV-positive people are most at risk and may develop cavitary pneumonia and pleural effusion.

15. How are *Mycobacterium tuberculosis* and *M. bovis* transmitted?

  M. tuberulosis and *M. bovis* do not survive well outside the host and are not environmental zoonoses. Although cats can be infected, they are not considered a primary host. When infection occurs, it is the result of reverse zoonosis: the cat was infected by the owner. Cats can be infected with an *M. tuberculosis–M. bovis* variant by ingestion of infected prey species. However, this variant is not known to infect people.

16. Describe the mechanisms by which the *Mycobacterium avium* complex is transmitted.

The *M. avium* complex is a group of organisms, passed by birds, that survive well in soil. Infection probably occurs by ingestion of the organism from a contaminated environment—not from direct contact with cats.

17. What are clinical manifestations of *M. avium* infection?

Infection results in skin granulomas in immunocompetent cats and disseminated infections in immunosuppressed cats. Infection with *M. avium* is common in immunocompromised people.

18. What causes feline leprosy? Can it be transmitted to humans?

M. leprae and *M. lepraemurium*, which cause multiple cutaneous nodules that are often ulcerated and draining. There are no known cases of transfer of infection from cats to people.

19. Summarize the significance of atypical mycobacterial infections in cats and humans.

Agents associated with atypical mycobacterial infections include *M. fortuitum, M. chelonae, M. phlei,* and *M. smegmatis*. These free-living, saprophytic organisms usually do not cause disease in immunocompetent animals. Cats seem to be more susceptible than other species and develop cutaneous nodules and draining tracts. Humans are rarely infected, and the agents are not considered direct zoonoses from infected cats.

20. How can infection by zoonotic agents in the environment be avoided?

• Housing cats indoors is the best way to reduce the potential for infection by organisms that colonize the environment.
• Control of transport hosts, such as flies, cockroaches, and rodents, may decrease environmental contamination by enteric zoonoses.

BIBLIOGRAPHY

1. Evans RH: Public health and important zoonoses in feline populations. In August JH (ed): Consultations in Feline Internal Medicine. Philadelphia, W.B. Saunders, 1997, pp 611–629.
2. Greene CE, Gunn-Moore DA: Tuberculous mycobacterial infections. In Greene CE (ed): Infectious Diseases of the Dog and Cat, 2nd ed. Philadelphia, W.B. Saunders, 1998, pp 313–321.
3. Hill SL, Cheney JM, Taton-Allen GF et al: Prevalence of enteric zoonotic organisms in cats. J Am Vet Med Assoc 216:687–692, 2000.
4. Lappin MR: Feline zoonotic diseases. Vet Clin North Am Small An Pract 23:57–78, 1993.
5. Legendre AM: Systemic mycotic infections. In Sherding RG (ed): The Cat: Diseases and Clinical Management. New York, Churchill Livingstone, 1994, pp 553–564.
6. Lewis DT, Kunkle GA: Feline Leprosy. In Greene CE (ed): Infectious Diseases of the Dog and Cat, 2nd ed. Philadelphia, W.B. Saunders, 1998, pp 321–322.
7. Lewis DT, Kunkle GA: Opportunistic rapid-growing mycobacterial infections. In, Greene CE (ed): Infectious Diseases of the Dog and Cat, 2nd ed. Philadelphia, W.B. Saunders, 1998, pp 322–325.
8. Malik R, Wigney DI, Dawson D et al: Infection of the subcutis and skin of cats with rapidly growing mycobacteria: A review of microbiological and clinical findings. J Feline Med Surg 2:35–48, 2000.
9. Stevenson K, Howie FE, Cameron ME et al: Feline skin granuloma associated with *Mycobacterium avium*. Vet Rec 143:109-110, 1998.
10. Werner AH, Werner BE: Feline sporotrichosis. Compend Cont Educ Small Anim Prac 15:1189–1197, 1993.

90. VECTOR-ASSOCIATED ZOONOSES

Tammy P. Sadek, D.V.M.

1. Define vector-borne diseases.

A vector is a carrier that transfers an infective agent from one host to another. Fleas, ticks, reduviid bugs (*Trypanosoma cruzi*), mosquitoes (*Dirofilaria repens*), and sandflies (*Leishmania* spp.) may transmit agents that infect cats and people. For some agents, cats serve only to bring infected vectors into the human environment (e.g., *Borrelia burgdorferi* and *Rickettsia rickettsii*). For others, the cat is also an effective reservoir and maintains the infectious agent (e.g., *Bartonella henselae* and *Rickettsia felis*). Disease in people can be induced by the parasitism itself or by the organism transmitted by the vector.

Vector-associated Zoonoses in Cats

ORGANISM	VECTOR	CLINICAL SYNDROMES	ROLE OF CAT IN HUMAN SYNDROME
Bartonella spp.	*Ctenocephalides felis*	Cats: subclinical, fever, uveitis Humans: lymphadenopathy, fever, malaise, bacillary angiomatosis, bacillary peliosis	Reservoir; transmitted by bites and scratches
Borrelia burgdorferi	*Ixodes* ticks	Cats: subclinical Humans: polyarthritis, cardiac disease, neurologic disease	Transport host for ticks
Coxiella burnetti	Many ticks	Cats: subclincal, abortion, stillbirth Humans: fever, pneumonitis, lymphadenopathy, myalgia, arthritis	Direct transmission to humans by aerosol; transport host for ticks
Diplyidium caninum	*Ctenocephalides felis*	Cats: subclinical, failure to thrive Humans: pruritus ani	Transport host for fleas
Dirofilaria immitis	Mosquitoes	Cats: cough, dyspnea, vomiting, death Humans: asymptomatic	None
Erlichia spp. (granulocytic)	(Ticks; undetermined)	Cats: fever, polyarthritis Humans: fever, polyarthritis, death	Unknown reservoir potential; transport host for ticks
Fransicella tularensis	Ticks	Cats: septicemia, pneumonia Humans: ulceroglandular, glandular, oculoglandular, pneumonic, or typhoidal (depending on route of transmission)	Direct transmission to humans by bites; transport host for ticks
Leishmania spp.	Sand flies	Cats: both visceral and cutaneous forms are rare; extremely rare in North America Humans: visceral and cutaneous	Minimal reservoir potential
Rickettsia felis	*C. felis*	Cats: subclinical Humans: fever, malaise	Reservoir likely: transhost for fleas
Rickettsia rickettsii	*Dermacenter* spp. *Ambylomma americanum* *Rhipicephalus sanguineus*	Cats: subclinical Humans: fever, malaise, petechiae, death	Reservoir unlikely; transport host for ticks

Table continued on following page

Vector-associated Zoonoses in Cats (Continued)

ORGANISM	VECTOR	CLINICAL SYNDROMES	ROLE OF CAT IN HUMAN SYNDROME
Rickettsia typhus	*C. felis*	Cats: subclincal Humans: fever, malaise	Reservoir likely; transport host for fleas
Trypanosoma cruzi	Reduviid bugs	Cats: subclinical Humans: cardiac disease, megaesophagus	None; reservoir unlikely
Yersinia pestis	Rodent fleas	Cats: bubonic, bacteremic, or pneumonic Humans: bubonic, bacteremic, or pneumonic	Direct transmission by exudates or aerosol; transport host for fleas

2. Which infectious agents are carried by fleas?

The significant infectious agents that are transmitted by fleas and involve cats include:
Bartonella spp. (cat scratch disease, bacillary angiomatosus, bacillary peliosis)
Yersinia pestis (plague)
Rickettsia typhus (murine typhus)
Rickettsia felis
Dipylidium caninum

3. Are *Bartonella* spp. infections important vector-borne diseases in humans?

Cats and people can be infected with *B. henselae* and *B. clarridgeiae*; cats are infected by *B. koehlerae* (see Chapter 85). *Ctencephalidies felis* can transmit *B. henselae* between cats. Cats are a chronic reservoir host for *B. henselae* and *B. clarridgeiae*, both of which cause cat scratch disease. Epidemiologically, cat scratch disease has been linked most often with cat contact, but flea transmission also may be important. Bacillary angiomatosis and bacillary peliosis in immunosuppressed people are also caused by *B. henselae*.

4. Are cats important in the vector-borne pathogenesis of plague?

Both cats and people have the potential to develop bubonic, pneumonic, or septicemic plague when infected by *Y. pestis* (see Chapter 86). Approximately 35% of reported human cases of plague in the United States have occurred in veterinarians or their assistants. The organism is maintained in a cycle between rodent fleas and infected rodents. *Y. pestis* infects over 230 species of rodents and over 1500 species of fleas, but *C. felis* is thought to be a poor vector. It is plausible that cats preying on rodents may be infested by rodent fleas and bring the *Y. pestis*-infected fleas into the human environment. However, it appears more likely that feline-associated plague in humans results most commonly from contact with exudates or respiratory secretions of infected cats.

5. Which rickettsial agents are transmitted by fleas?

Murine typhus (endemic typhus) is caused by *Rickettsia typhi*. Infection is usually through a flea bite or by contaminating flea bite wounds with flea feces. Opossums are the reservoir host in Texas and California. In a study in Los Angeles County, most cats tested were seropositive, suggesting that they may play a role infection of people. However, it is unknown whether the cats were infected with *R. typhi* or the related organism, *R. felis*. At the very least, cats serve to bring the infected flea vector into contact with the susceptible human host.

Using polymerase chain reaction and restriction fragment length polymorphism, *R. felis* was discovered in a person with clinical signs similar to typhus. Subsequently, it was shown that *C. felis* could be infected by *R. felis*; infected fleas have been found in many states. Cats infected experimentally seroconvert, but the infection appears to be subclinical. Whether cats are a reservoir, whether infection can result from direct contact, and the prevalence of naturally occurring disease are as yet unknown. Both *R. felis* and *R. typhi* can exist in the same flea.

6. Describe the clinical signs of murine typhus in humans.

Clinical signs in humans are similar to those of Rocky Mountain spotted fever: fever, headache, generalized pain, weakness, and rash.

7. What problems do *D. caninum* infections cause in people?

D. caninum is spread to people through ingestion of infected fleas. Young children are most likely to be affected. Clinical signs include mild abdominal discomfort, diarrhea, and anal pruritus. The infection is usually self-limiting.

8. Do ticks infest cats?

In many areas of the country, tick infestation is rarely noted by owners or veterinarians. Cats may be infested with the nymphal stages of ticks, which are so tiny that they are easily missed on physical examination. In addition, the meticulous grooming habits of cats may remove attached ticks after spread of disease but before examination. Because ticks that infect cats can transmit some tick-borne diseases to humans, tick control should always be maintained.

9. What are the common tick-borne infections in humans and cats?

- *B. burgdorferi* is transmitted by *Ixodes* spp. ticks and causes Lyme disease in people. Most cats exposed to *B. burgdorferi* are subclinically infected (see Chapter 65). People are unlikely to develop Lyme disease from direct contact with cats or their secretions, but cats can transport *B. burgdorferi*-infected ticks into human households.
- *Francisella tularensis* can infect both cats and humans (see Chapter 85). Contact with infected cats has resulted in human infection most commonly via bites and scratches, but it is also possible that cats could transport *F. tularensis*-infected ticks into human households.
- *Coxiella burnetti*, the cause of Q fever, infects over 40 species of ticks. Both cats and people can become infected via tick bite, and cats may bring ticks into the human environment. People, however, are more likely to be infected through inhalation of aerosolized material from parturient cats than via tick exposure (see Chapter 86).
- Cats seem to be very resistant to infection by *R. rickettsii*, the cause of Rocky Mountain spotted fever in people. People are unlikely to develop Rocky Mountain spotted fever from direct contact with cats or their secretions, but cats may transport *R. rickettsia*-infected ticks into human households.
- Several *Ehrlichia* spp. have been documented in cats (see Chapter 78). An isolate from a cat in Sweden was shown to be genetically identical to the agent causing human granulocytic ehrlichiosis. To date, no information suggests that direct contact with cats results in human ehrlichiosis, but cats may bring infected vectors into the human environment.

10. Do cats play a role in human dirofilariasis?

Although cats can be infected with *Dirofilaria immitis*, first-stage larvae (microfilaria) are rarely produced because of an intense immune response against the organism (see Chapter 10). Thus, it is unlikely that infected cats function as a reservoir for heartworm disease in humans. In the tropics, however, *D. repens* is a subcutaneous parasite in dogs and cats that uses mosquitos as a vector and has been implicated as a cause of abscesses and tumors in humans.

11. Is Chagas disease important in cats?

American trypanosomiasis, or Chagas disease, is caused by *Trypanosoma cruzi*, which is carried by the reduviid bug, *Triatoma* spp. It is common in South America and also has been identified in the southern United States. Dogs are considered important hosts in South America. Although infection in cats is not well documented, clinical disease in dogs appears to be similar to that in humans. The acute symptoms of fever and palpebral edema are followed by hepatomegaly, cardiac disease, and central nervous involvement. The chronic form generally causes myocardial disease and megaesophagus. Transmission occurs when a reduviid bug infected with *Triatoma* spp. deposits metacyclic trypanosomes on the host's skin after its blood meal. Treatment is relatively unrewarding in both humans and animals. Environmental control to eliminate contact with the reduviid bug vector is required. In North America, cats are unimportant reservoirs.

12. Is leishmaniasis of cats an important zoonosis?

Leishmania spp. are protozoan parasites endemic in South and Central America and portions of Africa, Europe, and the south central United States. Transmission occurs through the bite of blood-sucking sandflies, especially those of the genera Phlebotomus and Lutzomyia. Although common in dogs of endemic areas, infection is rare in cats, particularly in North America. Cutaneous lesions of the ear pinna of cats appear nodular. Visceral forms of the disease are extremely rare in cats. Definitive diagnosis is based on demonstrating the organisms cytologically or histologically. Treatment with pentavalent antimony compounds, allopurinol, and amphotericin B have been used successfully in dogs but minimal information about cats is available. Leishmaniasis appears to be an emerging opportunistic infection in humans and is seen regularly in HIV-infected humans in endemic areas. Cats are unlikely reservoir hosts in North America. Contact with exudates or open wounds of affected animals should be avoided.

13. What are the recommendations for control of vector-associated zoonosis?

• Keep house cats indoors at all times.
• Control potential transport hosts, such as rodents.
• Use flea- and tick-control products.

BIBLIOGRAPHY

1. Bjoersdoerff A, Svendenius L, Owens JH, et al: Feline granulocytic ehrlichiosis: A report of a new clinical entity and characterization of the infectious agent. J Small Anim Pract 40:20–24, 1999.
2. Chomel BB, Kasten RW, Floyd-Hawkins K, et al: Experimental transmission of *Bartonella henselae* by the cat flea. J Clin Microbiol 34:1952–1956, 1996.
3. Couto CG: Rickettsial diseases. In Birchard SJ, Sherding RG (ed): Saunders' Manual of Small Animal Practice. Philadelphia, W.B.Saunders, 1994, pp 124–127.
4. Davenport DJ: Bacterial and rickettsial diseases. In Sherding RG (ed): The Cat: Diseases and Clinical Management. New York, Churchill Livingstone, 1994, pp 527–551.
5. Evans RH: Public health and important zoonoses in feline populations. In August JR (ed): Consultations in Feline Internal Medicine, vol. 3. Philadelphia, W.B. Saunders, 1997, pp 611–629.
6. Hart CA, Trees AJ, Duerden BI: Zoonoses. J Med Microbiol 46:4–33,1997.
7. Kordick DL, Breitschwerdt EB: *Bartonella* infections in domestic cats. In Bonagura JD (ed): Current Veterinary Therapy XIII–Small Animal Practice. Philadelphia, W.B. Saunders, 2000, pp 302–307.
8. Lappin MR: Feline zoonoses. In Kirk RW, Bonagura JD (eds): Current Veterinary Therapy XI. Philadelphia, W.B. Saunders, 1992, pp 284–291.
9. Macy DW: Plague. In Greene CE (ed): Infectious Diseases of the Dog and Cat, 2nd ed. Philadelphia, W.B. Saunders, 1998, pp 295–300.
10. Noden BH, Radulovic S, Higgins JA, et al: Molecular identification of *Rickettsia typhi* and *R. felis* in coinfected *Ctenocepahlides felis* (Siphonaptera: Pulicidae). J Med Entomol 34:410–414, 1998.
11. Schreifer ME and Azad AF: Arthropod-borne diseases. In August JR (ed): Consultations in Feline Internal Medicine, vol. 2. Philadelphia, W.B. Saunders, 1994, pp 47–51.
12. Stubbs CJ, Holland CJ, Reif JS, et al: Feline ehrlichiosis. Comp Cont Educ Prac Vet 22: 307–318, 2000.
13. Walker DH, Barbour AG, Oliver JH, et al: Emerging bacterial zoonotic and vector-borne diseases: Ecological and epidemiological factors. J Am Med Assoc 275:463–469, 1996.
14. Weber DJ, Rutala WA: Zoonotic infections. Occup Med State Art Rev 14:247–285, 1999.

APPENDIX

Drugs Commonly Used in Feline Internal Medicine Practice

DRUG	DOSE REGIMEN	INDICATIONS	CHAPTER(S)
Acarbose	12.5–25 mg/cat PO with meals	Diabetes mellitus	56, 23, 21
Acepromazine	Up to 0.1 mg/kg IV q 12–24 hr 1.1–2.2 mg/kg PO q 12–24 hr	Smooth muscle relaxant for functional urethral obstruction; sedative for restraint	49
N-Acetylcysteine (5% solution)	140 mg/kg IV or PO, followed by 5–7 additional treatments of 70 mg/kg IV or PO q 4 hr	Acetaminophen toxicity	34, 73
Acyclovir	10–50 mg/kg PO q 8–12 hr	Feline herpesvirus 1 keratitis, conjunctivitis, and possibly rhinitis	3
Alprazolam	0.125–0.25 mg/cat PO	Skeletal muscle relaxant for functional urethral obstruction	49
Aluminum carbonate	30-120 mg/kg/day divided, with meals	Phosphate binder	40
Aluminum hydroxide	30–100 mg/kg/day divided, with meals	Phosphate binder	40
Aminophylline	4–5 mg/kg PO, IM, IV q 8–12 hr	Acute small airway disease	9
Amitriptyline	2.5–12.5 mg/cat/day PO	Idiopathic lower urinary tract disease syndrome	47
Amlodipine	0.625–1.25 mg/cat/day PO	Antihypertensive	40
Amoxicillin	11–22 mg/kg PO q 12 hr	Susceptible bacteria; gram-positive, anaerobes including *Clostridium perfringens*	2
Amoxicillin-clavulanate	11–22 mg/kg PO q 12 hr	Susceptible bacteria; gram-positive, anaerobes, and select gram-negative; *B. bronchiseptica*	2
Amphotericin B (regular)	0.25 mg/kg IV 3 times/wk 0.5–0.8 mg/kg SQ 2 times/wk diluted in 400 ml of 2.5% dextrose and 2.5% saline	Systemic fungal infections	4, 12, 22
Amphotericin B (lipid or liposomal)	0.5 mg/kg IV as test dose, then 1.0 mg/kg IV 3–5 times/wk	Systemic fungal infections	4, 12, 22
Ampicillin	10–20 mg/kg PO q 8 hr 10–20 mg/kg IV or SQ q 8 hr	*Clostridium perfringens* Anaerobic or gram-positive sepsis	20 20
Amprolium	60–100 mg/day PO for 5 days	*Cystoisospora* spp.	19
Arginine	1 gm/cat/day PO	Supplement for cats with hepatic lipidosis	30
Ascorbic acid	30 mg/kg SQ or PO q 6 hr for 7 doses	Acetaminophen toxicity	34, 73
Aspirin	12–25 mg/cat PO q 48–72 hr	Platelet function inhibition to lessen risk of thrombosis; fever control; arthritis; uveitis	17, 64, 65, 67
Atenolol	6.25–12.5 mg/cat PO q 12–24 hr	Cardiomyopathy; systemic hypertension	17, 63

Table continued on following page

Drugs Commonly Used in Feline Internal Medicine Practice (Continued)

DRUG	DOSE REGIMEN	INDICATIONS	CHAPTER(S)
Atropine sulfate	0.5% and 1% solution and ointment, 1 drop or ⅛ inch q 8–24 hr	Uveitis	67
Aurothioglucose	1 mg/cat IM q 7 days, then 1 mg/kg IM q 7 days until remission, then monthly	Polyarthritis; lymphocytic-plasmacytic stomatitis	3, 65
Azathioprine	0.3 mg/kg PO q 48 hr indefinitely	Inflammatory bowel disease; polyarthritis; primary immune diseases	23, 65, 72
Azithromycin	5–10 mg/kg/day PO for 3 days, then q 72 hr	Susceptible bacteria; *B. bronchiseptica*, *Mycoplasma* spp., *C. psittaci*, gram-negative and anaerobes	2
	7–15 mg/kg PO q 12 hr for 5–7 days	*Cryptosporidium parvum*	19, 84
Benazepril	0.25–0.5 mg/kg/day PO	Cardiomyopathy	17
Betamethasone	0.75 mg/eye, subconjunctival	Uveitis	67
Bethanechol	1.25–7.5 mg/cat PO q 8–12 hr	Increase bladder contractility	49
Bisacodyl	5 mg/cat/day PO	Stimulant laxative for use with megacolon	27
Bovine lactoferrin	350 mg/cat/day	Lymphocytic-plasmacytic stomatitis	3
Bupivicaine	2 mg/kg maximal dose SQ or IM	Local anesthetic for chest tube placement and other simple procedures	14
	0.75 mg/kg in chest tube q 8 hr	Topical anesthetic for pleural space pain	
Buspirone	2.5–5.0 mg/cat PO q 12–24 hr	Inappropriate urination	51
Butorphanol	0.1–0.8 mg/kg q 4 hr IV, IM, SQ	Analgesic	36
	1 mg/cat PO q 12 hr	Polyarthritis	65
Calcitriol	2.5–3.5 ng/kg/day PO; pulse dose at 20 ng/kg PO 2 times/wk	Chronic renal failure	40
	0.03–0.06 µg/kg/24 hr PO	Hypocalcemia	57
Calcium acetate	20–30 mg/kg q 8–12 hr PO with meals	Phosphate binder	40
Calcium carbonate	30–50 mg/kg q 8–12 hr PO with meals	Phosphate binder	40
Calcium gluconate (10%)	0.5–1.0 mg/kg IV over 10–15 min	Hypocalcemia	40
Calcium phosphate	0.5–2.0 mmol/kg/day PO	Hypophosphatemia	40
Carbimazole	2.5–5 mg/cat PO q 8–12 hr for 7–10 days, then as needed q 12–24 hr	Control of hyperthyroidism	53
Carnitine	250–500 mg/cat/day	Used in cats with hepatic encephalopathy	30
Carprofen	4 mg/kg PO once	Analgesic, anti-inflammatory, polyarthritis	65
Cefadroxil	22 mg/kg PO q 12–24 hr	Susceptible bacteria; gram-positive and anaerobes	
Cefoxitin	22 mg/kg IV, IM, SQ q 8 hr	Susceptible bacteria; gram-positive and anaerobes	
Cephalexin	22–50 mg/kg PO every 8–12 hr	Susceptible bacteria; gram-positive and anaerobes	

Table continued on following page

Drugs Commonly Used in Feline Internal Medicine Practice (Continued)

DRUG	DOSE REGIMEN	INDICATIONS	CHAPTER(S)
Cephalothin	22-44 mg/kg IV or IM q 8 hr	Susceptible bacteria; anaerobic or gram-positive sepsis	20
Chloramphenicol	25–50 mg/cat PO q 12 hr	Susceptible bacteria; *B. bronchiseptica, Mycoplasma* spp., *C. psittaci,* anaerobes, gram-positive	2
	10–15 mg/kg PO or SQ q 12 hr	*Campylobacter* spp.	20
Chlorambucil	2 mg/cat PO q 48 hr	Inflammatory bowel disease; other primary immune-mediated diseases	23, 72
Chlorpheniramine	2–4 mg/cat PO q 12 hr	Decongestant and antihistamine	
Chlorpromazine	0.25–0.5 mg/kg q 8 hr IM, IV, SQ	Antiemetic	25, 36
Cimetidine	4–5 mg/kg q 6–8 hr PO, IM, IV	H_2 receptor blocker antacid	
Cisapride	0.1–0.5 mg/kg PO q 8 hr	Esophagitis, increase colonic motility in megacolon	26
Clarithromycin	7.5 mg/kg PO q 12–24 hr	*Helicobacter* spp.	20
Clindamycin	11-24 mg/kg PO q 24 hr	Susceptible bacteria; gram-positive and anaerobes, good tissue penetration	
	10–12 mg/kg PO q 12 hr for 4 wk	*Toxoplasma gondii*	11
Clomipramine	1–5 mg/cat PO every 12–24 hr	Behavioral abnormalities including inappropriate urination	51
Cobalamine	125–250 µg/wk SQ or IM for 6–8 wk	Supplement for inflammatory bowel disease	23
Cyclophosphamide	50 mg/m² PO 4 times/wk When in remission, use chlorambucil	Inflammatory bowel disease, other primary immune mediated diseases	23, 72
Cyclosporine	5–8.5 mg/kg PO q 12–24 hr indefinitely	Inflammatory bowel disease, other primary immune diseases	23, 72
Cyproheptadine	2 mg/cat PO q 12 hr	Small airway inflammatory disease; appetite stimulant	9, 62
Dantrolene	0.5–2.0 mg/kg PO q 8 hr 1.0 mg/kg IV	Skeletal muscle relaxant for functional urethral obstruction	49
Desoxycorticosterone pivalate	10–12.5 mg/cat/month IM	Hypoadrenocorticism	55
Dexamethasone sodium phosphate	0.1% solution or 0.5% ointment 1 drop or ⅛ inch/eye q 6–8 hr	Uveitis	67
Diazepam	0.2–0.3 mg/kg q 12 hr SQ, IV	Appetite stimulant	40
	0.2–0.5 mg/kg IV 2.5–5.0 mg/cat PO q 8 hr or as needed	Skeletal muscle relaxant for functional urethral obstruction	49
Diclofenac	0.1% solution, 1 drop/eye q 6–12 hr	Uveitis	67
Digoxin	Cats < 3.0 kg: 0.031 mg PO q 48–72 hr Cats 3.0–6.0 kg: 0.031 mg PO q 24 hr Cats > 6.0 kg, 0.031 mg PO q 12–24 hr	Dilated cardiomyopathy	17

Table continued on following page

Drugs Commonly Used in Feline Internal Medicine Practice (Continued)

DRUG	DOSE REGIMEN	INDICATIONS	CHAPTER(S)
Diltiazem (extended release)	30 mg/cat PO q 12 hr	Cardiomyopathy; systemic hypertension	17, 63
Dimethylglycine	50–250 mg/cat PO indefinitely	Supplement for inflammatory bowel disease	23
Dimenhydrinate	8.0 mg/kg PO q 8 hr	Antihistamine, antiemetic	36
Diminazine aceturate	2.0 mg/kg/wk IM for 2 doses	*Cytauxzoon felis*	75
Dioctyl calcium sulfosuccinate	50 mg/cat PO q 12–24 hr as needed	Emollient laxative for use with megacolon	27
Dioctyl sodium sulfosuccinate	50 mg/cat/day PO as needed	Emollient laxative for use with megacolon	27
Diphenhydramine	2.0–4.0 mg/kg PO q 8 hr 2.0 mg/kg IM q 8 hr	Antihistamine, antiemetic	36
Dopamine	3 µg/kg/min	Possibly improves pancreatic blood flow in cats with pancreatitis	36 36
Doxycycline	5–10 mg/kg PO q 12–24 hr	*B. bronchiseptica, Mycoplasma* spp., *C. psittaci, H. felis*; possibly anti-inflammatory	2, 74
Enalapril	0.25–5.0 mg/kg PO q 12–24 hr	Cardiomyopathy; systemic hypertension	17, 63
Enrofloxacin	5 mg/kg PO q 12–24 hr	Susceptible bacteria; gram-negative, select gram-positive, *Mycoplasma* spp. *Campylobacter spp, Salmonella* spp., *Clostridium difficile*	2, 20
Ephedrine	2–4 mg/cat PO q 8–12 hr	Increase smooth muscle urethral tone	52
Epsiprantel	2.75 mg/kg PO once	Cestodes	19
Erythromycin	10 mg/kg PO q 8 hr	Susceptible bacteria; gram-positive and *Campylobacter* spp.	20
Erythropoietin	50–100 U/kg SQ 3 times/wk	Anemia of chronic renal disease	40
Famotidine	0.5–1.0 mg/kg/day PO	*Helicobacter* spp.	20
Feline facial phermone	Spray area daily	Urine marking	51
Fenbendazole	25–50 mg/kg PO q 12 hr for 10–14 days	*Aelurostrongylus abstrusus, Capillaria aerophilia, Paragonimus kellicotti*	11
	50 mg/kg/day PO for 3–5 days	*Giardia* spp. *Taenia* spp., helminths	19
Fentanyl	1 µg/kg IV bolus	Sedation for short-term procedures (e.g., chest tube placement)	14
Ferrous sulfate	50–100 mg/cat/day PO	Iron deficiency anemia	40
Flurbiprofen	0.03% solution, 1 drop/eye, q 6–12 hr	Uveitis	67
Fluconazole	50 mg PO q 12–24 hr	Systemic fungal infections	4, 12, 22
Flucytosine	50 mg/kg PO q 8 hr	*Cryptococcus neoformans* CNS infections	4, 12
Fludrocortisone	0.1 mg/cat/day PO	Hypoadrenocorticism	55
Folate	0.5 mg/day PO for 1 month	Supplement for inflammatory bowel disease	23
Furazolidone	8–20 mg/kg PO q 12–24 hr for 5 days	*Cystoisospora* spp.	19
	4 mg/kg PO q 12 hr for 7 days	*Giardia* spp.	19
Furosemide	6.25 mg/cat PO q 24–48 hr up to 12.5 mg/cat PO q 8 hr	Diuretic for pulmonary congestion	17

Table continued on following page

Drugs Commonly Used in Feline Internal Medicine Practice (Continued)

DRUG	DOSE REGIMEN	INDICATIONS	CHAPTER(S)
Furosemide *(cont.)*	2–6 mg/kg IV q 6–8 hr; incrementally increase dose q 1 hr up to 6 mg/kg if urine output remains poor	Anuric or oliguric renal failure	40
Gentamicin	2.2 mg/k IV or SQ q 8 hr	Gram-negative sepsis (including *E. coli* and *Salmonella* spp.)	20
Glipizide	2.5–5.0 mg/cat/day PO	Diabetes mellitus	56
Glutamine	250–500 mg/cat PO indefinitely	Supplement for inflammatory bowel disease	23
Heparin	100–200 U/kg IV once, then 100–300 U/kg SQ q 8 hr	Factor inhibition to lessen risk of thrombosis	17
Hydromorphone	0.08–0.2 mg/kg IV, IM, SQ q 4 hr	Analgesic	36
Imidocarb	5.0 mg/kg/wk IM for 2 doses	*Cytauxzoon felis, Ehrlichia* spp.	75, 76
Insulin	Multiple types and regimens	Diabetes mellitus	56
Interferon alpha	30 U/day PO	Chronic viral infections, FeLV, FIV, feline herpesvirus 1, FIP	3, 76, 77
	10,000–20,000 U/kg/day SQ	Acute viral infections; FeLV, FIV, feline herpesvirus 1, calicivirus	
Itraconazole	5 mg/kg PO q 12 hr for 4 days and then 5 mg/kg/day PO	Systemic fungal infections	4, 12, 22
Ivermectin	24 µg/kg PO monthly	Heartworm preventative; control of hookworms	10, 19
	300–400 µg/kg/day PO for 1–3 days	*Aelurostrongylus abstrusus, Capillaria aerophila,* ear mites	11
Ketamine	0.05–0.1 mg/kg IV with diazepam	Sedation; short-term anesthesia	
Ketoconazole	5–10 mg/kg/day PO	Systemic fungal infections	4, 12, 22
Ketoprofen	1 mg/kg/day PO for 5 days	Polyarthritis	65
	2 mg/kg/day SQ for 3 days	Polyarthritis	65
Ketorolac	0.5% solution, 1 drop/eye, q 6–12 hr	Uveitis	67
Lactobacillus acidophilus	50–500 × 10^6 organisms/cat until stool returns to normal	Supplement for inflammatory bowel disease	23
Lactulose	0.25-0.5 ml/kg PO q 8–12 hr as needed	Osmotic laxative for use with megacolon	27
Levothyroxine	0.1 mg/cat/day PO	Hypothyroidism	53
Lidocaine (2%)	0.75 mg/kg SQ or IM	Local anesthetic for chest tube placement and other simple procedures	14
	0.25-0.75, IV or 5 min	Ventricular arrhythmias	
Lisinopril	0.25–0.5 mg/kg/day PO	Systemic hypertension	63
L-Lysine	250 mg PO q 12 hr	Feline herpesvirus 1 keratitis, conjunctivitis, and possibly rhinitis	3
Magnesium chloride	0.75–1.0 mEq/kg/day IV for 3–5 days, mixed with 5% dextrose in water	Hypomagnesemia	40
Mannitol (20%)	0.25–1.0 g/kg; give as slow IV bolus over 15–20 min; can repeat q 4–6 hr	Osmotic diuresis for anuric or oliguric renal failure	40
Meclizine	6.25–12.5 mg/cat PO q 12–24 hr	Antiemetic	25

Table continued on following page

Drugs Commonly Used in Feline Internal Medicine Practice (Continued)

DRUG	DOSE REGIMEN	INDICATIONS	CHAPTER(S)
Medroxyproges- terone acetate	25–50 mg/cat SQ q 3–6 months	Eosinophilic granuloma complex; miliary dermatitis; endocrine alopecia	
Megestrol acetate	0.5 mg/kg/day PO for 3–5 days, then once q 5 days	Appetite stimulation	62
	2.2–4.4 mg/kg/day PO for 1 wk and then 1.1–1.2 mg/kg q 1–2 wk	Aggression; urine marking; eosinophilic granuloma complex	
Meperidine	1–5 mg/kg IV, IM to effect	Analgesia	
Methimazole	2.5–5 mg/cat PO q 12 hr for 7–10 days, as needed q 12–24 hr	Control of hyperthyroidism	53
Methylprednisolone acetate	10–20 mg/cat IM q 2 wk until controlled, then as needed	Eosinophilic and lymphocytic-plasmacytic inflammatory diseases	9
	4 mg/eye, subconjunctival	Uveitis	67
Metoclopramide	0.25–0.5 mg/kg PO, SQ q 8–12 hr	GI motility disorders; esophagitis	62
	1–2 mg/kg/day IV CRI	GI motility disorders; esophagitis	
Metoprolol	2–15 mg/cat PO q 8 hr	Cardiomyopathy	17
Metronidizole	7.5-10 mg/kg PO q 8–12 hr	Tissue infections; anaerobes; possibly anti-inflammatory	2
Metronidazole	10–25 mg/kg PO q 12 hr for 8 days	*Giardia* spp, *Pentatrichomonas hominis, Clostridium perfringens, Helicobacter* spp., inflammatory bowel disease	19. 23
Milbemycin	0.5–0.99 mg/kg PO monthly	Heartworm preventative; control of hook-worms and roundworms	10, 19
Mineral oil	10–25 ml/cat/day PO	Lubricant laxative for use with megacolon	27
Morphine	0.05-0.4 mg/kg, IV, IM, SQ q 4 hr	Analgesic	36
	0.05–0.1 mg/kg, IM, SQ q 6–8 hr	Pulmonary edema	
Neomycin	10–20 mg/kg PO q 8–12 hr	Used with hepatic encephalopathy	35
N-acetyl glucosa- mine	250–1500 mg/cat PO indefinitely	Supplement for inflammatory bowel disease	23
Nitroglycerine (2%)	¼–½ inch cutaneously to pinna, q 6–8 hr for first 24–48 hr	Acute congestive heart failure	17
Nizatidine	2.5–5.0 mg/kg/day PO	Prokinetic agent for use with megacolon	27
Nystatin	100,000 U/cat PO q 6 hr	Candidiasis	22
Omeprazole	0.7–1.0 mg/kg/day PO	*Helicobacter* spp.; antacid	20
Ondansetron	0.1–0.15 mg/kg slow push IV q 6–12 hr as needed	Antiemetic	25, 36
Oxazepam	0.2–0.4 mg/kg PO q 12 hr	Appetite stimulant	40
Oxybutynin	0.5 mg/cat PO q 12 hr	Decrease bladder contractility	52
Oxymorphone	0.025–0.1 mg/kg q 4 hr IV, IM, SQ	Analgesic	36
Oxytocin	0.5–3 U IV infusion	Uterine inertia	
	0.5–3U IM q 20 min for 2 doses	Uterine inertia	
Paromomycin	150 mg/kg PO q 12–24 hr for 5 days	*Cryptosporidium parvum*	19, 84

Table continued on following page

Drugs Commonly Used in Feline Internal Medicine Practice (Continued)

DRUG	DOSE REGIMEN	INDICATIONS	CHAPTER(S)
Pentosan poly-sulfate	2–10 mg/kg PO q 12 hr	Idiopathic lower urinary tract disease	47
Petrolatum	1–5 ml/cat/day PO	Lubricant laxative for use with megacolon	27
Phenoxybenzamine	1.25–7.5 mg/cat PO q 8–12 hr	Smooth muscle relaxant for functional urethral obstruction	49
Phenylpropanola-mine	1.1–2.2 mg/kg PO q 8–12 hr	Increase urethral smooth muscle tone	52
Plasma	1 ml/kg SQ, IV, IP	Passive immunotherapy for feline pan-leukopenia	21
Piperazine	110 mg/kg PO once, repeat in 2 weeks	Hookworms and roundworms	19
Piroxicam	1 mg/cat PO q 24–48 hr	Nasal adenocarcinoma, transitional cell carcinoma, polyarthritis	7, 46, 65
Potassium gluco-conate	2–6 mEq/cat/day PO	Hypokalemia; chronic renal failure	40
Prazosin	0.25–0.5 mg/cat PO q 12–24 hr 0.03 mg/kg IV	Smooth muscle relaxant for functional urethral obstruction	49
Prednisolone	1 mg/kg PO q 12 hr for 10–14 days, then tapered to 2.5 mg/kg PO q 48 hr	Eosinophilic and lymphocytic-plasmacytic inflammatory diseases	9
Prednisolone acetate	1% suspension, 1 drop/eye q 6–12 hr	Uveitis	67
Praziquantel	5 mg/kg/day for 2–3 days PO	*Alaria marcianae*	19
	23 mg/cat PO or 56.8 mg/ml SQ or IM once	Cestodes	19
	25 mg/kg PO q 8 hr for 2 days	*Paragonimus kellicotti*	11
Proanthocyanidin	10–200 mg/cat PO indefi-nitely	Supplement for inflammatory bowel disease	23
Prochlorperazine	0.1 mg/kg q 6 hr IM	Antiemetic	25, 36
Prochlorperazine + isopropramide	0.5–0.8 mg/kg q 12 hr IM, SQ	Antiemetic	36
Propanolol	2.5–5 mg/cat PO q 8–12 hr	Systemic hypertension	63
Propantheline	5.0–7.5 mg/cat PO q 24–72 hr	Decrease bladder contractility	52
Propofol	2–4 mg/kg IV to effect	Sedation for short-term procedures (e.g., chest tube placement, TTW)	14
Pumpkin (canned)	1–4 tbsp/day mixed with food	Bulk laxative for use with megacolon	27
Pyrantel pamoate	20 mg/kg PO once; repeat in 2–3 wk	Hookworms and roundworms	19
Pyrantel + prazi-quantel	72.6 mg pyrantel and 18.2 mg praziquantel, 1 tab/cat PO	Hookworms, roundworms, and cestodes	19
Psyllium	1–4 tsp mixed with food q 12–24 hr	Bulk laxative for use with megacolon	27
Ranitidine	2.5 mg/kg IV q 12 hr	H_2 receptor blocker antacid	
	3.5 mg/kg PO q 12 hr	H_2 receptor blocker antacid	
	1.0–2.0 mg/kg PO q 8–12 hr	Prokinetic agent for use with megacolon	27
Rutin	250–500 mg/cat PO q 8 hr	Chylothorax	15
Selamectin	6 mg/kg topically once/month	Heartworm preventative; control of hook-worms, roundworms, fleas, and ear mites	10, 19

Table continued on following page

Drugs Commonly Used in Feline Internal Medicine Practice (Continued)

DRUG	DOSE REGIMEN	INDICATIONS	CHAPTER(S)
Selenium	15 μg/cat/day PO indefinitely	Supplement for inflammatory bowel disease	23
Sodium bicarbonate	0.5-2.0 mEq/kg IV over 20–30 min; 5–10 mg/kg PO q 8–12 hr	Extreme acidosis; extreme hyperkalemia	40
Spironolactone	1–2 mg/kg PO q 12 hr	Diuretic used for systemic hypertension	63
Stanozolol	1–2 mg/cat PO q 12 hr	Appetite stimulation	62
Sucralfate	¼ gm crushed and mixed with 6 ml of water PO q 8 hr or 1.0–2.5 ml of 100 mg/ml commercially available suspension PO q 12 hr	Esophagitis and gastrointestinal ulcers	26
Sulfadimethoxine	50–60 mg/kg/day PO for 5–20 days	*Cystoisospora* spp.	19
Sulfasalazine	10–20 mg/kg/day PO for 7–10 days	Inflammatory colitis	23
Suprofen	1% solution, 1 drop/eye q 6–12 hr	Uveitis	67
Taurine	250–500 mg/cat PO q 12 hr	Cardiomyopathy	17
Terbutaline	0.625 mg/cat PO q 12 hr	Small airway inflammatory disease	9
Theophylline	50–100 mg/cat/day PO	Small airway inflammatory disease	9
Thiamine	50–100 mg/cat/day	Used in cats with hepatic encephalopathy	30
Triamcinolone	4 mg/eye, subconjunctival	Uveitis	67
Trimethoprim-sulfonamide	15 mg/kg PO q 12 hr for 5 days	Susceptible bacteria, *Cystoisospora* spp., *T. gondii*	19
Tropicamide	0.5% and 1% solution q 6–12 hr	Uveitis	67
Tylosin	10–15 mg/kg PO q 8–12 hr for 21 days	*Cryptosporidium parvum, Clostridium perfringens*	19, 84
Ursodeoxycholic acid	10–15 mg/kg/day PO	Choleretic agent for biliary or gallbladder disease	29
Vitamin A	1000–5000 IU/day PO as beta carotine, indefinitely	Supplement for inflammatory bowel disease	23
Vitamin C	250–300 mg/cat PO, indefinitely	Supplement for inflammatory bowel disease	23
Vitamin E	200 IU/cat/day PO as alpha tocopherol, indefinitely	Supplement for inflammatory bowel disease; hepatic diseases	23
Vitamin K$_1$	0.5–1.0 mg/kg/day SQ for 3–4 days, then once weekly	Cholestatic liver disease	29
	0.3–0.8 mg/kg PO q 12 hr	Vitamin K antagonism	71
Warfarin	0.25–0.5 mg/cat/day PO	Factor inhibition to lessen risk of thrombosis	17
Wheat bran (coarse)	1–2 tbsp/day mixed with food	Bulk laxative for use with megacolon	27
Zafirlukast	5 mg/cat PO q 12 hr	Small airway inflammatory disease	9
Zidovudine	5 mg/kg PO, SQ q 12 hr	Clinical FIV infections	77
Zinc	7.5 mg/cat/day PO, indefinitely	Supplement for inflammatory bowel disease	23

Drugs for the treatment of lymphoma are described in chapter 68; drugs for use with reproductive disorders are described in chapters 29 and 60.

Most doses listed are starting doses. Duration of treatment varies with the use. Please see individual chapters for complete descriptions for the use of these drugs and a description of toxicities.

IV = intravenously, IM = intramuscularly, SQ = subcutaneously, PO = orally, CRI = constant-rate infusion.

INDEX

Page numbers in **boldface type** indicate complete chapters.

Toxoplasmosis (*cont.*)
  as alveolar lung disease cause, 34
  clinical features of, 328
  definition of, 422–423
  gastrointestinal, 419
  hepatic, 151
  in hunting cats, 135
  ocular, 330, 343
  pancreatic, 167, 170
  pneumonitis, 55
  polymyositis, 339
  polysystemic, 92
  pulmonic, 30, 31, 49–50
  treatment of, 328
  uveitis, 343
  as zoonotic disease, 417, 422–424
Trachea
  cancer/tumors of, 31, 69–70
  foreign body in, 32
  rupture of, as pneumothorax cause, 61
Tracheoscopy, 70
Tractotomy, olfactory, 250
Transitional cell carcinoma, 221, 222–223
Transudates, as ascites cause, 172, 174
Trauma
  as chylothorax cause, 65
  as pneumothorax cause, 61, 62
Trematode infections, gastrointestinal, 91
Tremors
  hyperthyroidism-related, 339
  myopathy-related, 337
Triaditis, 121, 137, 139, 168
Trichinella spiralis infections, 339
Trichobezoars, 114, 116
Trichomonas, 94
Trichuris, 85
Trichuris campanula, 88
Trichuroidea, 47
Triiodothyronine (T3), 259
Triiodothyronine (T3) suppression test, 260–261
Troglotrematids, 47
Trypanosomiasis, 445, 446–447
Trypsin-like immunoreactivity assay, 120–121, 168, 171
Tularemia, 327, 329, 426, 429, 431, 435, 444, 446
Tympanic membrane, nasopharyngeal polyp-related
    abnormalities of, 17
Typanum, bulging or discoloration of, 2
Typhus, murine, 445, 446

UCCR (urine cortisol:creatinine ratio), 267–268
Ulcers, oral, uremia-related, 196–197
Ultrasound
  abdominal
    in biliary tract disease, 155, 156
    in cholangitis/cholangiohepatitis complex, 138
    for fever evaluation, 330
    for urinary incontinence evaluation, 256
  in gastrointestinal tract disease, 84
  in intestinal obstruction, 116
  in lower urinary tract disease, 225
  in pancreatitis, 120, 168
  in polyuria/polydipsia, 183
  in portosystemic shunt, 164, 165
  in pyometra, 296
  in pyothorax, 57
  renal, 186–187
    for tissue biopsy, 211–212
Ultraviolet light exposure, as squamous cell carcinoma
    cause, 23

Uncinaria stenocephala infections, 85, 86, 419, 420, 421
Urea, excretion of, in chronic renal failure, 242–243
Urease, as helicobacteriosis marker, 84, 96
Uremia, 119, 196–197
Uremic syndrome, 185
Ureter, ectopic, 256
Ureteral obstruction, 221
Urethra, hypercontractile, 232–233
Urethral incompetence, 257–258
Urethral obstruction
  idiopathic feline lower urinary tract disease-related, 244
  lower urinary tract disease-related, 223, 224
  portosystemic shunt-related, 163
Urethral plugs, 223, 224, 227, 228
Urethral relaxant drugs, 234
Urethral resistance, assessment of, 256
Urethrospasm, 232
Urethrostomy, 230
  perineal, 214, 229
Urinalysis
  in biliary diseases, 154
  in cough or dyspnea, 33–34
  in icterus, 136
  in lower urinary tract disease, 225, 226
  in myopathy, 337
  in neutropenia, 361
  in pollakiuria, 215
  in polyuria/polydipsia, 182
  in portosystemic shunt evaluation, 164
  in pyelonephritis, 204
  in renal failure, 186
  in urinary calculi, 217
  in urinary incontinence, 256
  in urinary tract infections, 230–231
Urinary calculi, **216–219**
  ammonium urate, 244
  calcium oxalate, 215, 216, 219, 236, 244, 289
  cystine, 236, 244
  hypercalcemia-associated, 290
  as lower urinary tract disease cause, 223
  as pollakiuria cause, 215
  struvite, 215, 216, 219, 227, 236, 243–244
  urate, 236
  as urinary tract infection risk factor, 230
Urinary incontinence, **255–258**
  congenital, 256, 257
Urinary tract, obstruction of
  azotemia associated with, 184
  functional, **232–235**
  as secondary gastrointestinal disease cause, 119
Urinary tract disease
  idiopathic feline lower, 222, **223–230**, 236, 244
  as pollakiuria cause, 214
Urinary tract infections, **230–231**
  bacterial, 214, 222, 227, 230–231
    dietary modification prevention and treatment of, 243
  fungal, 243
  lower, differentiated from kidney infection, 204
  recurrent, 205–206
Urinary tract neoplasia, **220–223**
Urination
  inappropriate, **245–254**
    definition of, 245
    inflammatory bowel disease-related, 108
    lower urinary tract disease-related, 223, 312
    management of, 248–249, 250–254
    pollakiuria-related, 214
    polyuria/polydipsia-relaetd, 182
    pain during, 254

Weight gain. *See also* Obesity
 as diabetes mellitus treatment, 278
 hypercortisolism-related, 266
Weight loss, 315–317
 cholangitis/cholangiohepatitis complex-related, 138
 chylothorax-related, 66
 as diabetes mellitus treatment, 278
 exocrine pancreatic insufficiency-related, 121, 171
 hepatic lipidosis-related, 142
 hyperthyroidism-related, 259
 hypoadrenocorticism-related, 265, 266, 273
 as idiopathic feline lower urinary tract disease treatment, 244
 inflammatory bowel disease-related, 108
 intestinal obstruction-related, 114
 nasal tumor-related, 23
 as ostoearthritis treatment, 333
 pancreatitis-related, 135, 168
 Platynosomum concinnum infection-related, 152
 pneumonia-related, 50, 51
 primary lung tumor-related, 70
 urinary tract neoplasia-related, 220
Weight-loss programs, 312–313
Wheezing
 asthma-related, 37
 Capillaria aerophila infection-related, 48
 nasopharyngeal polyps-related, 16
Whipworm. *See Trichuris campanula*
"White coat effect," 322
White-haired cats, squamous cell carcinoma in, 23

Xanthine uroliths, 244
X-rays
 abdominal
  in biliary tract disease, 154–155
  in constipation and megacolon, 129, 130
  in gastrointestinal tract disease, 84
  in hyperadrenocorticism, 267
  in hyperbilirubinemia or icterus, 136
  in lower urinary tract disease, 225, 226
  in pancreatitis, 168
  in portosystemic shunt, 164, 165

X-rays (*cont.*)
 in bacterial rhinitis, 5
 chest
  in *Aelurostrongylus abstrusus* infections, 48
  in dirofilariasis, 44, 45
  in *Paragonius* infections, 47
  in pneumonia, 53
 in chylothorax, 66
 in fungal rhinitis, 14
 in hypoadrenocorticism, 274
 in intestinal obstruction, 115
 open-mouth, in nasal disease, 24
 in pneumothorax, 62
 in polyuria/polydipsia, 183
 thoracic
  in asthma, 39, 40
  in cardiomyopathy, 76
  dorsoventral, 34
  in dyspnea, 33
  lateral, 34
  in pyothorax, 56

Yersinia enterocolitica infections, 424
Yersinia pestis, 30, 52. *See also* Plague
 bite or scratch-related transmission of, 426, 429, 437
 as zoonotic respiratory disease cause, 431

Zafirlukast, as small airway disease treatment, 41
Zinc sulfate fecal flotation test, 48, 83, 86
Zinc supplementation
 in hepatic lipidosis, 147
 in inflammatory bowel disease, 111
Zoonoses, **417–419**
 bite- or scratch-associated, **426–431**
 definition of, 417
 ehrlichiosis as, 399
 enteric, **419–425**, 441
 environmental, **441–443**
 gastrointestinal, 95
 respiratory, **431–434**
 urogenital, **439–440**
 vector-associated, **444–447**